Principles and Practice of
SURGERY

Commissioning Editor: Laurence Hunter
Project Development Manager: Janice Urquhart
Project Manager: Frances Affleck
Design direction: Erik Bigland
Illustrated by: Gillian Lee, Ethan Danielson

www.harcourt-international.com

Bringing you products from all Harcourt Health Sciences companies including Baillière Tindall, Churchill Livingstone, Mosby and W.B. Saunders

- ▶ **Browse** for latest information on new books, journals and electronic products

- ▶ **Search** for information on over 20 000 published titles with full product information including tables of contents and sample chapters

- ▶ **Keep up to date** with our extensive publishing programme in your field by registering with eAlert or requesting postal updates

- ▶ **Secure online ordering** with prompt delivery, as well as full contact details to order by phone, fax or post

- ▶ **News** of special features and promotions

If you are based in the following countries, please visit the country-specific site to receive full details of product availability and local ordering information

USA: www.harcourthealth.com

Canada: www.harcourtcanada.com

Australia: www.harcourt.com.au

Baillière Tindall   CHURCHILL LIVINGSTONE   Mosby   W.B. SAUNDERS

Principles and Practice of
SURGERY

EDITED BY

O. James Garden BSc MB ChB MD FRCS(Glas & Ed)

Regius Professor of Clinical Surgery, University of Edinburgh, Honorary Consultant Surgeon,
The Royal Infirmary of Edinburgh, Edinburgh, UK

Andrew W. Bradbury BSc MD FRCSEd

Professor of Vascular Surgery and Consultant Vascular Surgeon,
University of Birmingham and Heartlands Hospital, Birmingham, UK

John Forsythe MD FRCS

Consultant Transplant Surgeon, The Royal Infirmary of Edinburgh; Honorary Senior Lecturer,
University of Edinburgh, Edinburgh, UK

PAEDIATRIC ADVISER

Graham Haddock MB ChB MD FRCS(Glas & Ed) FRCS(Paed)

Consultant Paediatric Surgeon and Clinical Director of Surgery, Royal Hospital for Sick Children, Glasgow

FOURTH EDITION

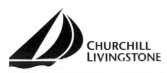
CHURCHILL
LIVINGSTONE

EDINBURGH LONDON NEW YORK PHILADELPHIA ST LOUIS SYDNEY TORONTO 2002

CHURCHILL LIVINGSTONE
An imprint of Harcourt Publishers Limited

© Longman Group Limited 1985
© Harcourt Brace and Company Limited 1998
© Harcourt Publishers Limited 2002

◿ is a registered trademark of Harcourt Publishers Limited

The right of O. James Garden, Andrew W. Bradbury and John
Forsythe to be identified as authors of this work has been asserted
by them in accordance with the Copyright, Designs and Patents
Act 1988.

First published 1985
Second edition 1991
Third edition 1995
Fourth edition 2002

ISBN 0 443 06493 8
International Student Edition ISBN 0 443 06492 X

British Library Cataloguing in Publication Data
A catalogue record for this book is available from the British
Library

Library of Congress Cataloging in Publication Data
A catalog record for this book is available from the Library of
Congress

Note
Medical knowledge is constantly changing. As new information
becomes available, changes in treatment, procedures, equipment
and the use of drugs become necessary. The editors, contributors
and the publishers have taken care to ensure that the information
given in this text is accurate and up to date. However, readers are
strongly advised to confirm that the information, especially with
regard to drug usage, complies with the latest legislation and standards of practice.

The
publisher's
policy is to use
**paper manufactured
from sustainable forests**

Printed in China

PREFACE

The continuing success of *Principles and Practice of Surgery* and its companion volume *Davidson's Principles and Practice of Medicine* suggests that there remains a need for an undergraduate medical textbook which provides a readable account of those facts which are important in surgery. It is also apparent that such texts should not specifically be focused on the preparation for final examinations but rather guide the student through key core surgical topics which will be encountered throughout an integrated undergraduate curriculum and in subsequent clinical practice.

The current editors have undertaken considerable restructuring and revision of the previous edition. In previous editions a substantial proportion of the book was written by the editors. Now we recognize that increasing specialization in surgery makes it vital that each chapter is assigned to clinicians who command both knowledge and experience in these areas. The editors have endeavoured to ensure that a consistent style has emerged and is in harmony, where appropriate, with the medical management which may be covered in greater detail in *Davidson's Principles and Practice of Medicine*.

A further innovation for this edition has been a review of the text to ensure that paediatric surgical issues have been dealt with adequately. An icon has been placed in the text to indicate paediatric matters. We are grateful to Mr. Graham Haddock for his input and constructive criticism.

We are indebted to the retiring editors Professors Sir Patrick Forrest, Sir David Carter and Mr Ian Macleod who have been responsible for establishing the reputation of the textbook with medical students and doctors around the world. We are also grateful to Laurence Hunter and Janice Urquhart of Churchill Livingstone for keeping the project on track. Anne McKellar, Bridget Kerr and Ann Murray provided invaluable secretarial support.

We very much hope that this edition continues the tradition and high standards set by our editorial predecessors and that the content and presentation of the fourth edition meets the needs of tomorrow's doctors.

OJG   2002
AWB
JF

CONTRIBUTORS

Andrew W. Bradbury BSc MB ChB(Hons) MD FRCSEd
Professor of Vascular Surgery and Consultant Vascular
Surgeon, University of Birmingham and Heartlands
Hospital, Birmingham, UK

Timothy M. Buckenham MD FRACR FRCR
Professor of of Radiology, Christchurch Clinical School of
Medicine, Christchurch, New Zealand

Roderick T. A. Chalmers MD FRCSEd
Consultant Vascular Surgeon, Vascular Surgery Unit, The
Royal Infirmary of Edinburgh, Edinburgh, UK

Trevor J. Crofts BSc FRCS FRACS FCSHK MS
Consultant Surgeon, Upper Gastrointestinal Unit, The
Royal Infirmary of Edinburgh, Edinburgh, UK

J. Michael Dixon BSc(Hons) MB ChB MD FRCS
FRCSEd
Senior Lecturer in Surgery, Edinburgh Breast Unit,
Western General Hospital, Edinburgh, UK

Malcolm G. Dunlop MB ChB FRCS MD
Professor of Coloproctology, University of Edinburgh;
Honorary Consultant Surgeon, Western General Hospital,
Edinburgh, UK

Andrew S. Evans MB ChB
Senior House Officer in Surgery, The Royal Infirmary of
Edinburgh, Edinburgh, UK

John R. Farndon BSc MD FRCS(Eng) FRCS(Ed)
Professor of Surgery, Bristol Royal Infirmary, Bristol,
UK

Kenneth C. H. Fearon MD FRCS(Gen)
Professor of Surgical Oncology, University of Edinburgh;
Honorary Consultant Surgeon, The Royal Infirmary of
Edinburgh, Edinburgh, UK

John Forsythe MD FRCS
Consultant Transplant Surgeon, The Royal Infirmary of
Edinburgh; Honorary Senior Lecturer, University of
Edinburgh, Edinburgh, UK

O. James Garden BSc MB ChB MD FRCS(Glas & Ed)
Regius Professor of Clinical Surgery, University of
Edinburgh; Honorary Consultant Surgeon, The Royal
Infirmary of Edinburgh, Edinburgh, UK

Rachel Green MB ChB BMedBiol FRCP FRCPath
Regional Director, Glasgow and West of Scotland Blood
Transfusion Service, Law Hospital, Carluke, UK

Ian F. Laurenson MA MB ChB MRCP MSc MRCPath MD
Consultant in Medical Microbiology and Infection Control,
Victoria Hospital, Fife, UK

David Brian Lorimer McClelland BSc(Hons) MB ChB
MRCP(UK) Dotoraat in de Geneeskunde – Leiden
(Cumlaude), FRCP(Edin) FRCPath
Director, Edinburgh and South East Scotland Blood
Transfusion Service and Department of Transfusion
Medicine, The Royal Infirmary of Edinburgh; Senior
Lecturer, Department of Medicine, University of
Edinburgh, Edinburgh, UK

Robert P. Mills MB BS MS MPhil FRCS(Eng) FRCS(Ed)
Consultant Otolaryngologist, The Royal Infirmary of
Edinburgh; Senior Lecturer, University of Edinburgh,
Edinburgh, UK

Kirsty Munro MB BS BSc(Hons)
Senior House Officer in General Surgery, The Royal
Infirmary of Edinburgh, Edinburgh, UK

Lynn M. Myles BSc(Hons) MD FRCS(SN)
Senior Lecturer and Consultant Neurosurgeon, Department
of Clinical Neurosciences, Western General Hospital,
Edinburgh, UK

Rowan W. Parks MD FRCSI FRCS(Ed) FRCS(Gen)
Senior Lecturer in Surgery, University of Edinburgh;
Honorary Consultant Surgeon, The Royal Infirmary of
Edinburgh, Edinburgh, UK

Simon Paterson-Brown MB BS MPhil MS FRCS(Ed)
FRCS(Engl)
Consultant General and Upper Gastrointestinal Surgeon,
The Royal Infirmary of Edinburgh; Honorary Senior
Lecturer, University of Edinburgh, Edinburgh, UK

William D. Plant BSc MB MRCPI FRCP(Edin)
Consultant Renal Physician, Department of Renal
Medicine, The Royal Infirmary of Edinburgh; Honorary
Senior Lecturer, Department of Clinical and Surgical
Sciences, The University of Edinburgh, Edinburgh, UK

Henry Pleass MB BS MD FRCS(Ed) FRCS(Gen)
Consultant Surgeon, The Royal Infirmary of Edinburgh, Edinburgh, UK

Anthony J. Pollock BSc MB ChB FRCA
Consultant Anaesthetist, Intensive Care Unit, The Royal Infirmary of Edinburgh, Edinburgh, UK

Mark Potter MB ChB MD FRCS
Specialist Registrar in Surgery, The Royal Infirmary of Edinburgh, Edinburgh, UK

Colin E. Robertson FRCSEd FRCPEd FFAEM FSAScot
Consultant, Department of Accident and Emergency Medicine, The Royal Infirmary of Edinburgh, Edinburgh, UK

Geoffrey C. S. Smith MB ChB
Senior House Officer in General Surgery, The Royal Infirmary of Edinburgh, Edinburgh, UK

Laurence H. Stewart MB ChB FRCS(Ed) MD FRCS(UrolEd)
Consultant Urological Surgeon, Department of Urological Surgery, Western General Hospital, Edinburgh, UK

Sonia J. Wakelin MB ChB BSc
Senior House Officer, Department of Surgery, The Royal Infirmary of Edinburgh, Edinburgh, UK

Timothy S. Walsh MB ChB(Hons) BSc(Hons) MRCP FRCA MD
Consultant in Anaesthetics and Intensive Care, The Royal Infirmary of Edinburgh, Edinburgh, UK

William S. Walker MA MB BChir FRCS FRCSEd
Consultant Cardiothoracic Surgeon, Department of Cardiothoracic Surgery, The Royal Infirmary of Edinburgh, Edinburgh, UK

James D. Watson MB ChB FRCSEd FRCSG(Plast)
Consultant Plastic Surgeon, St John's Hospital, Livingston; Honorary (Clinical) Senior Lecturer in Surgery, University of Edinburgh, Edinburgh, UK

Ian R. Whittle MD PhD FRACS FRCS(SN) FRCPE
Forbes Professor of Surgical Neurology, Department of Clinical Neurosciences, Western General Hospital, Edinburgh, UK

CONTENTS

CONTENTS

SECTION 1
PRINCIPLES OF SURGICAL CARE

1 The metabolic response to injury

T.S. Walsh

Following accidental or deliberate injury a characteristic series of changes occurs both locally at the site of injury, and within the body generally, which are intended to restore the body to its preinjury condition. These changes are mediated via many different systems, which interact in a complex manner and may be modified by external factors, such as drugs and other treatments administered to the patient. The metabolic response to injury is usually of benefit because it helps to return an individual to normality. However, if the balance or control of the changes that occur is abnormal, recovery may be delayed or incomplete. Occasionally the metabolic response to injury can actually be harmful, for example by damaging organs distant to the injured site itself.

Early descriptions of the metabolic response to injury were made in patients before the advent of medical treatments such as intravenous fluids. This unmodified response was divided into two phases: the 'ebb' and the 'flow'. During the ebb phase, which usually comprised the first few hours after injury, the individual was cold and hypotensive. In current medical practice this corresponds to the period of traumatic shock before or during resuscitation. The flow phase followed if the individual survived, and was described in two parts. The initial *catabolic* phase was characterized by a high metabolic rate, breakdown of proteins and fats, a net loss of body nitrogen (negative nitrogen balance) and weight loss. This phase usually lasted about a week and was followed by an *anabolic* phase, during which protein and fat stores were restored and weight gain

occurred (positive nitrogen balance). This recovery phase usually lasted 2–4 weeks.

This pattern of events probably occurs to some degree after any traumatic or surgical injury, but the extent and duration vary enormously. Modern surgical techniques which minimize tissue damage, such as laparoscopy, are usually associated with a mild, short-lived metabolic response and rapid patient recovery. In contrast, a critically ill patient in the intensive care unit may have an exaggerated metabolic response lasting for many months.

This chapter describes the principal physiological systems involved in the metabolic response to injury, how they function and are controlled, and at what stage they are important.

FACTORS MEDIATING THE METABOLIC RESPONSE TO INJURY

The acute inflammatory response

Inflammatory cells (neutrophils, macrophages and eosinophils) and cytokines (molecules with the capacity to act on a wide range of cell types, both at the site of injury and at distant sites in the body) are mediators of the acute inflammatory response. Physical damage to tissues results in local activation of cells such as tissue macrophages. These cells release a variety of cytokines (Table 1.1). Some of these, such as IL-8, attract large numbers of circulating macrophages and neutrophils to the site of injury. Other cytokines, such as TNF-α, IL-1 and IL-6, activate these

Table 1.1 Some cytokines involved in the acute inflammatory response	
Cytokine	Relevant actions
TNF-α	Proinflammatory, release of leukocytes by bone marrow, activation of leukocytes and endothelial cells
IL-1	Fever, T-cell and macrophage activation
IL-6	Growth and differentiation of lymphocytes, activation of the acute-phase protein response
IL-8	Chemotactic for neutrophils and T cells
IL-10	Inhibits immune function

inflammatory cells, enabling them to clear dead tissue and kill bacteria. Although these cytokines are produced locally, their release into the circulation probably initiates some of the systemic features of the metabolic response, such as fever (IL-1) and the acute-phase protein response (IL-6, see below). This cascade of events results in rapid amplification of the initial injurious stimulus, so that within a few hours large numbers of inflammatory cells are present at the injured site, controlling and mediating the inflammatory response via cytokines (Fig. 1.1).

Other proinflammatory substances are released in association with tissue injury, leukocyte activation and cytokine production. These include prostaglandins, kinins, complement, various proteases (such as elastase and cathepsin) and free radicals. Anti-inflammatory substances and mechanisms also exist, such as antioxidants (for example glutathione, vitamin A, vitamin C), protease enzyme inhibitors (for example α_2-macroglobulin) and IL-10. The balance between pro- and anti-inflammatory processes is extremely important but is not yet fully understood.

The endothelium

Endothelial cells lining the blood vessels within or adjacent to injured tissues are involved in a number of the changes that follow injury.

Leukocyte accumulation in injured tissues relies on a stepwise process whereby cells initially adhere to the endothelium 'lightly', subsequently adhere 'tightly', and then migrate between endothelial cells into tissues (Fig. 1.1). These processes are controlled via specific molecules released by endothelial cells and inflammatory cells following cell activation: 'light' adhesion is mediated via the *selectins*, and 'tight' adhesion via *integrins* and the *intercellular adhesion molecule family* (ICAM).

When tissues are injured the local blood flow increases because of vasodilatation. This increases the local delivery of inflammatory cells, oxygen and nutrient substrates which are important in the healing process. Vasodilatation is caused by substances such as kinins, prostaglandins and nitric oxide, which are generated in response to injury and inflammation. Nitric oxide, which is synthesized in endothelial cells, is particularly important in controlling blood flow to tissues both in health and following injury. In addition to vasodilation, capillaries in injured tissues become more permeable to plasma because endothelial activation increases the size of intercellular pores. As a result, fluid and colloid particles (principally albumin) leak into injured tissues, resulting in oedema formation. If tissue injury is severe and widespread, for example following severe burns, fluid loss into tissues can amount to many litres.

Afferent nerve impulses and the neuroendocrine response

Impulses generated in afferent nerve endings at the site of tissue injury have a role in mediating the metabolic response to injury. The most important nerves are probably pain fibres which comprise both unmyelinated C fibres and myelinated A fibres. These are stimulated via direct trauma or the release of nerve stimulants such as prostaglandins. Nerve impulses reach the thalamus via the dorsal horn of

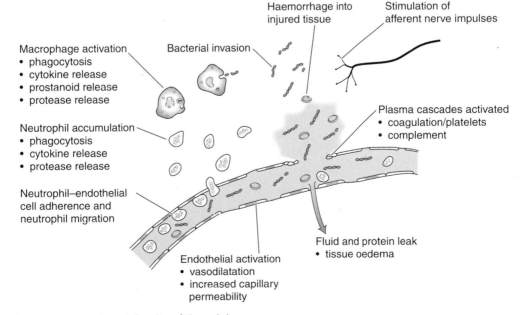

Fig. 1.1 Key events occurring at the site of tissue injury.

the spinal cord and the lateral spinothalamic tract. Afferent impulses reaching the thalamus mediate the metabolic response via several mechanisms:

1. *Stimulation of the sympathetic nervous system* Increased discharge of sympathetic nerves results in tachycardia and increased cardiac output. Noradrenaline (norepinephrine) release from sympatheic nerve endings and adrenaline (epinephrine) release from the adrenal gland increases circulating catecholamine concentrations. This contributes to the changes in carbohydrate, fat and protein metabolism that occur following injury (see below). Interventions that reduce sympathetic stimulation, such as epidural or spinal anaesthesia, may attenuate these changes.

2. *Stimulation of pituitary hormone release* Following injury, plasma concentrations of many pituitary hormones increase, notably antidiuretic hormone (ADH), growth hormone (GH) and adrenocorticotrophic hormone (ACTH) These changes are probably mediated partly via increased afferent nerve impulses.

In addition to pituitary hormones and catecholamines, changes in other hormones occur following injury, notably increased circulating concentrations of glucagon (in response to sympathetic stimulation) and of aldosterone.

Bacterial infection

Direct injury to tissues, whether from surgery or from unintentional trauma, can disrupt the normal physical barriers to infection by bacteria. Another mechanism of barrier breakdown occurs if tissues suffer impaired blood supply as a result of hypovolaemia, or because local blood flow is reduced by vasoconstriction. The resulting tissue ischaemia may cause cell dysfunction or death. The epithelial lining of the intestine is particularly sensitive to ischaemic injury because intestinal blood flow is reduced proportionally more by hypovolaemia than is blood flow to other organs. Even if blood supply is restored, for example by fluid resuscitation, further tissue injury may occur by a process termed the *ischaemia–reperfusion syndrome*, which activates an acute inflammatory response in the previously ischaemic tissues.

Bacteria that invade tissues can stimulate a local acute inflammatory response, which may spread to the systemic circulation. This is initiated by bacterial substances such as endotoxin. Endotoxin is a component of the cell walls of Gram-negative bacteria which has the capacity to directly initiate many of the features of the acute inflammatory response.

SUMMARY BOX

Factors mediating the metabolic response to injury

- The acute inflammatory response
  - inflammatory cells (macrophages, monocytes, neutrophils)
  - proinflammatory cytokines and other inflammatory mediators

- Endothelial cell activation
  - adhesion of inflammatory cells
  - vasodilatation
  - increased permeability

- Afferent nerve stimulation

- Release of stress hormones

- Bacterial infection and endotoxin

Table 1.2 Causes of fluid loss following surgery and trauma		
Nature of fluid	Mechanism	Contributing factors
Blood	Haemorrhage	Site and magnitude of tissue injury Poor surgical haemostasis Abnormal coagulation
Electrolyte-containing fluids	Vomiting	Anaesthesia/analgesia (e.g. opiates) Ileus
	Nasogastric drainage	Ileus Gastric surgery
	Diarrhoea	Antibiotic-related infection Enteral feeding
	Sweating	Pyrexia
Water Plasma-like fluid (third space losses)	Evaporation Capillary leak/ sequestration in tissues	Prolonged exposure of viscera during surgery Acute inflammatory response Infection Ischaemia–reperfusion syndrome

CONSEQUENCES OF THE METABOLIC RESPONSE TO INJURY

Hypovolaemia

A reduced circulating volume is characteristic following moderate to severe injury. It results from hypovolaemia due to fluid loss from the body, from fluid sequestration in tissues, and from reduced oral fluid intake (Table 1.2).

- *Fluid loss* may be in the form of blood (haemorrhage), as electrolyte-containing fluid (for example nasogastric suction, vomiting, sweating), or as water (evaporation from exposed organs during surgery).
- *Fluid sequestration* of plasma-like fluid in injured tissues (sometimes termed third-space losses) occurs in proportion to the severity and extent of injury. It results from the increased 'leakiness' of the endothelium described above, usually lasts 24–48 hours, and after major surgery can amount to several litres. The extent and duration of this leakiness may be prolonged if the acute inflammatory response is exaggerated, for example by infection or the ischaemia–reperfusion syndrome.

The neuroendocrine response to hypovolaemia and a reduced circulating volume attempts to restore normal fluid status and maintain perfusion to vital organs. These inter-related processes can be considered as *fluid-conserving measures* and *blood flow-conserving measures*.

Fluid-conserving measures

Oliguria, together with sodium and water retention is characteristic and is hormonally mediated.

Antidiuretic hormone (ADH) ADH synthesis in the hypothalamic supraoptic nuclei and secretion by the posterior pituitary is increased in response to the following stimuli:

- Direct afferent nerve impulses from the site of injury
- Increased plasma osmolality (principally sodium ions) detected by hypothalamic osmoreceptors
- Afferent nerve impulses from atrial stretch receptors (responding to reduced volume) and the aortic and carotid baroreceptors (responding to reduced pressure)
- Input from higher centres in the brain (pain, emotion, anxiety).

ADH promotes the retention of free water (without electrolytes) by cells of the distal renal tubule and collecting duct. If excess water is administered during the period of increased ADH secretion plasma hypotonicity and hyponatraemia may occur.

Aldosterone Aldosterone secretion from the adrenal cortex is increased by the following mechanisms (Fig. 1.2):

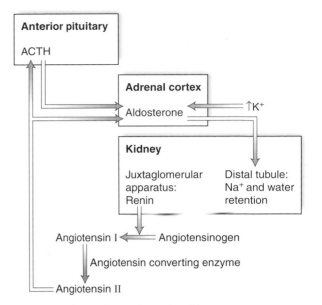

Fig. 1.2 The renin–angiotensin–aldosterone system.

- Via the renin–angiotensin system at the juxtaglomerular apparatus within nephrons. Renin is released from afferent arteriolar cells in response to stimuli activated during hypovolaemia and reduced renal blood flow. These include reduced afferent arteriolar pressure, tubuloglomerular feedback (signalling via the macula densa of the distal tubule according to electrolyte concentration), and activation of the renal sympathetic nerves. Renin, a proteolytic enzyme, converts circulating angiotensinogen to angiotensin I. Angiotensin I is converted to angiotensin II by angiotensin-converting enzyme (ACE), which is found in plasma and in various tissues, particularly the lung. Angiotensin II has several actions, which include potent vasoconstriction of arterioles and stimulation of aldosterone secretion by the adrenal cortex.
- ACTH secretion by the anterior pituitary is increased in response to hypovolaemia and hypotension via afferent nerve impulses from stretch receptors in the atria, aorta and carotid arteries.
- Hyponatraemia or hyperkalaemia directly stimulate adrenal cortex cells to increase secretion.

Aldosterone acts mainly via receptors on distal renal tubular cells. The net effect is reabsorption of sodium ions and simultaneous excretion of hydrogen and potassium ions into urine. Aldosterone also effects ion transfer across some other cell types, for example cardiac muscle.

The duration of increased ADH and aldosterone secretion is usually 48–72 hours. Urine volume is often reduced during this period (about 0.5 mL/kg/h), and is concentrated as a result of water retention. Urinary sodium excretion decreases, typically to 10–20 mmol/24 h (normal 50–80 mmol/24 h). Urinary potassium excretion increases, typically to >100 mmol/24 h (normal 50–80 mmol/24 h), but hypo-kalaemia is relatively rare in the 24–48 hours following injury because a net efflux of potassium from cells occurs. This typical pattern may be modified by fluid and electrolyte administration.

> **SUMMARY BOX**
>
> *Urinary changes during the metabolic response to injury*
>
> - Reduced urine volume in response to hypovolaemia and ADH release
> - Low urinary sodium and increased urinary potassium excretion due to aldosterone release
> - Increased urinary nitrogen excretion due to the catabolic response to injury

Blood flow-conserving measures

An important potential result of hypovolaemia is reduced cardiac output resulting in decreased blood flow to organs. Cardiac output is determined by the cardiac preload (the amount of blood returning to the heart), the heart rate, the contractility of cardiac muscle (the rate at which each con-traction occurs), and the afterload (a measure of the resist-ance against which the heart pumps). Blood pressure is determined by the cardiac output and the peripheral resis-tance of blood vessels (mainly arterioles). Following injury several mechanisms act to maintain or increase cardiac output and blood pressure despite hypovolaemia.

- The distribution of the available circulating volume is altered to reduce blood flow to the gut and to the skin and peripheries. These changes are mediated by increased sym-pathetic tone and circulating catecholamines. Veno-constriction within the skin and gut increases venous return to the heart.
- Increased circulating catecholamines and sympathetic activity to the heart increase heart rate and contractility.
- Increased sympathetic tone to arteries and arterioles, and the effect of vasoconstrictors such as angiotensin II, increase vascular resistance to maintain blood pressure.

Increased energy metabolism and substrate cycling

Metabolic rate (the energy expenditure of the body) can be considered in three parts: energy required for physical work, energy associated with heat production (thermogene-sis), and basal metabolic rate (BMR, comprising the energy

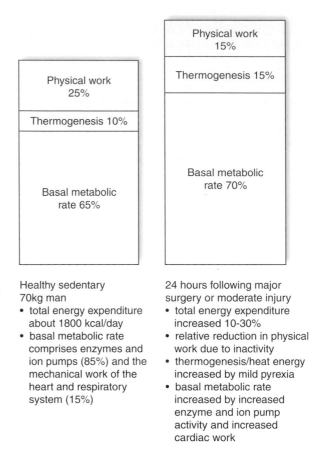

Fig. 1.3 Components of body energy expenditure in health and following injury.

Healthy sedentary 70kg man
- total energy expenditure about 1800 kcal/day
- basal metabolic rate comprises enzymes and ion pumps (85%) and the mechanical work of the heart and respiratory system (15%)

24 hours following major surgery or moderate injury
- total energy expenditure increased 10-30%
- relative reduction in physical work due to inactivity
- thermogenesis/heat energy increased by mild pyrexia
- basal metabolic rate increased by increased enzyme and ion pump activity and increased cardiac work

needed for enzyme reactions and ion pumps). Following injury physical work is usually decreased because of inac-tivity, although heart and respiratory muscle work may increase. Resting energy expenditure (the sum of BMR and thermogenesis) is increased by up to 50% following severe injury as a result of metabolic changes (Fig. 1.3).

Thermogenesis Patients are frequently mildly pyrexial for 24–48 hours following injury. This occurs because cyto-kines, principally IL-1, reset temperature-regulating centres in the hypothalamus. Pyrexia may also complicate infection occurring after injury. Metabolic rate increases by 6–10% for each 1°C change in body temperature.

BMR Following injury there is increased activity of protein, carbohydrate and fat-related metabolic pathways (see below) and increased activity of many ion pumps. The activity of some cycles is apparently 'futile', for example glucose–lactate cycling and triglyceride turnover involve simultaneous synthesis and degradation. This general increase in substrate cycling is energy dependent, but is thought to optimize metabolic control and the ability of the body to respond to altering demands.

Catabolism and starvation

Catabolism is the breakdown of complex substances, such as muscle proteins, to form simpler molecules (glucose, amino acids, fatty acids) which are basic substrates for metabolic pathways. Starvation is the inadequate intake of food to meet metabolic demand. Following severe injury or major surgery these two processes generally occur simultaneously. The metabolic changes associated with each process are different, and so the changes occurring in any individual patient depend on which process predominates. Generally, uncomplicated surgery or moderate trauma are followed by a period of starvation but little catabolism. Major trauma or surgery complicated by sepsis may result in marked catabolism, which outweighs any effect of simultaneous starvation.

Catabolism

Catabolism is probably mediated by catecholamines, cytokines and other substances generated in response to injury and released into the circulation. These bring about changes in carbohydrate, protein and fat metabolism (Table 1.3).

Carbohydrate metabolism Glycogenolysis in the liver results in rapid depletion of glycogen stores, which only lasts for 8–12 hours. Gluconeogenesis is increased, particularly in the liver, which converts substrates released from other tissues such as amino acids into glucose. Insulin resistance occurs, meaning that tissues become less sensitive to the effects of insulin. Together these factors result in hyperglycaemia. The increased circulating glucose is thought to provide a substrate for the inflammatory and repair processes that follow injury.

Catecholamines and pancreatic islet sympathetic nerve impulses increase glucagon secretion and inhibit insulin release. Glucagon and catecholamines stimulate gluconeogenesis. Insulin resistance may be mediated in part by the increased growth hormone concentrations that follow injury.

Fat metabolism Adipose tissue is a large triglyceride store and the principal source of energy following trauma. The stress hormones released as part of the metabolic response to injury (catecholamines, glucagon, cortisol and growth hormone) are all capable of activating the enzyme triglyceride lipase within fat cells. Triglycerides are broken down into glycerol and free fatty acids. Glycerol is a substrate for gluconeogenesis, and free fatty acids can be directly metabolized by most tissues to generate energy. The brain is unable to use free fatty acids for energy production, and in health relies on glucose supply. Animals are unable to convert free fatty acids into glucose, but the liver converts them into ketone bodies which are water soluble and can support cerebral energy metabolism. Following severe trauma 200–500 g of fat may be broken down daily.

Protein metabolism Skeletal muscle is the major labile protein store in the body. Following major injury skeletal muscle is broken down, releasing amino acids into the circulation. These are metabolized principally in the liver, which converts a major proportion into glucose for re-export to tissues for energy metabolism. Amino acids are also used in the liver as substrate for the 'acute-phase protein response'. This response involves the liver increasing the production of one group of proteins (positive acute-phase proteins) and decreasing the production of others (negative acute-phase proteins) (Table 1.4). The acute-phase response is mediated in the liver by cytokines, especially IL-1, IL-6 and TNF. Its function is not fully

---

Table 1.3 Physiological changes occurring during catabolism

Carbohydrate metabolism
↑ glycogenolysis (stores last about 10 hours)
↑ hepatic gluconeogenesis
Insulin resistance of tissues
Hyperglycaemia

Fat metabolism
↑ lipolysis
Free fatty acids used as energy substrate by tissues (except brain)
Some conversion of free fatty acids to ketones in liver (used by brain)
Glycerol converted to glucose in the liver

Protein metabolism
↑ skeletal muscle breakdown
Amino acids converted to glucose in liver and used as substrate for acute-phase protein production
Negative nitrogen balance

Total energy expenditure increased in proportion to injury severity and other modifying factors
Progressive reduction in fat and muscle mass until stimulus for catabolism ends

---

Table 1.4 Proteins synthesized by the liver which alter as part of the acute-phase protein response

Positive acute-phase proteins (↑ after injury)
C-reactive protein
Haptoglobins
Ferritin
Fibrinogen
α_1-Antitrypsin
α_2-Macroglobulin
Plasminogen

Negative acute-phase proteins (↓ after injury)
Albumin
Transferrin

understood, but is probably concerned with fighting infection and promoting healing.

The mechanism by which muscle catabolism occurs is incompletely understood. It is mediated by inflammatory mediators and hormones released as part of the metabolic response to injury. Trauma or surgery associated with a minimal metabolic response is usually accompanied by minimal muscle catabolism. In patients with major tissue injury marked catabolism and loss of skeletal muscle can occur, especially when factors that enhance the metabolic response, such as sepsis, are present.

In health 80–120 g/day dietary protein (12–20 g nitrogen) are ingested (1 g nitrogen = 6 g protein). Normally approximately 2 g/day nitrogen is lost in faeces and 10–18 g/day in urine (mainly in the form of urea). During catabolism nitrogen intake is often reduced but urinary losses can increase markedly, reaching 20–30 g/day in patients with severe trauma, sepsis or burns. Following uncomplicated surgery this negative nitrogen balance usually lasts only 5–8 days, but in patients with prolonged sepsis, burns or conditions associated with prolonged inflammation (for example acute pancreatitis) it may persist for many weeks. Severe catabolism and negative nitrogen balance cannot be reversed by feeding, but the provision of protein and calories can attenuate the processes. Even patients undergoing uncomplicated abdominal surgery can lose about 600 g muscle protein (1 g protein = 5 g wet muscle mass), amounting to 6% of total body protein. This is usually regained within 3 months.

Starvation

Starvation occurs in relation to trauma and surgery for several reasons:

- The illness requiring treatment, for example gastric carcinoma, may have reduced nutritional intake for weeks/months prior to surgery
- Fasting prior to surgery
- Fasting after surgery, especially to the gastrointestinal tract
- Loss of appetite associated with illness.

The response of the body to starvation can be described in two phases (Table 1.5).

1. *Acute starvation* is accompanied by metabolic changes that preserve the glucose supply to the brain. Glycogenolysis and gluconeogenesis occur in the liver, releasing glucose for cerebral energy metabolism. Lipolysis in fat stores releases free fatty acids for use by other tissues, and glycerol which is converted to glucose in the liver. These processes can sustain the normal energy requirements of the body (about 1800 kcal/day for a 70 kg adult) for approximately 10 hours.

2. *Chronic starvation* is initially accompanied by muscle breakdown to release amino acids, which are converted to glucose by hepatic gluconeogenesis. In addition, fatty acids released from adipose tissue are converted by the liver to ketones. Tissue energy supply is in the form of glucose, fatty acids and ketones. The brain is unable to utilize free fatty acids and uses about 70% of the glucose generated by hepatic gluconeogenesis. With prolonged starvation the brain adapts to utilize ketones as the primary energy substrate, rather than glucose. This adaptation reduces muscle protein loss and switches metabolism to increase fat consumption, so that net body nitrogen loss is reduced. Hepatic gluconeogenesis from amino acids decreases to about 25% of its previous rate, and overall metabolic rate and energy requirement falls from 1800 kcal/day to about 1500 kcal/day (Table 1.5). This state is termed *compensated starvation*, which continues until body fat stores are depleted. At this stage, when an individual is often close to death, muscle protein breakdown again increases to provide glucose for cerebral metabolism.

Changes in blood coagulation

Following tissue injury the blood may become hypercoagulable. This is usually a transient feature lasting 1–2 days, but increases the risk of thromboembolism after surgery or trauma. Contributing factors include:

- Endothelial injury and activation, which activates the coagulation pathways
- Increased activation of platelets in response to circulating mediators such as adrenaline and cytokines
- Dehydration and/or reduced venous blood flow due to immobility
- Increased circulating fibrinogen concentrations as part of the acute-phase protein response.

Table 1.5 A comparison of energy and nitrogen losses in a moderate to severe catabolic state and during the different phases of starvation			
	Catabolic state	Acute starvation	Compensated starvation
Nitrogen loss (g/day)	20–25	14	3
Energy expenditure (kcal/day)	2200–2500	1800	1500
Values are approximate and relate to a 70 kg man.			

Rarely, patients develop hypocoagulable states. These usually occur in association with shock, massive blood transfusion or sepsis. The most extreme form of coagulopathy is disseminated intravascular coagulation.

SUMMARY BOX

Consequences of the metabolic response to injury

- Sodium and water retention in response to hypovolaemia, and aldosterone and ADH release
- Pyrexia for 24–48 hours
- Increased energy expenditure
- Increased glucose and fat turnover
- Breakdown of adipose tissue as principal energy source
- Catabolism of skeletal muscle to provide amino acids for gluconeogenesis and hepatic synthesis of acute-phase proteins
- Altered blood coagulation

FACTORS MODIFYING THE METABOLIC RESPONSE TO INJURY

The magnitude and duration of the metabolic response to injury are influenced by many factors, including:

- *Severity of injury*. In general the greater the amount of tissue damaged, the greater is the response.
- *Nature of the injury*. Some forms of tissue injury cause a proportionately greater metabolic response. The classic example of this is severe widespread burn injury, which can cause more than 100% increases in total energy expenditure of an individual
- *Infection* potentiates the metabolic response because organisms contribute to the activation of inflammatory processes. Infection often results in prolongation of the response.
- *Genetic factors* probably contribute to the variation in response seen between different individuals to similar degrees of injury or infection. This may be due to interindividual differences in genes for central inflammatory mediators such as TNF-α.
- *Nutritional status*. Malnutrition may modify the metabolic response to injury owing to factors such as depletion of antioxidants and other cofactors essential to normal metabolic and immune function. Malnourished patients are at greatly increased risk of complications such as infection following surgery or injury.
- *Coexisting disease*. The presence of cancer and chronic disease, such as renal failure, haematological disorders and chronic liver disease, may alter the metabolic response.
- *Ambient temperature*. The body uses energy to maintain body temperature. Excessive cold or heat are both associated with increased energy expenditure, and metabolic rate is lowest within a range of ambient temperature of about 27–29°C (the 'zone of thermal neutrality'). Burn injury results in a shift of this range to higher temperatures, so that elevating room temperature to >30°C can markedly decrease body energy expenditure.
- *Anaesthesia and drugs*. Some drugs, such as synthetic opioids, can inhibit many of the neuroendocrine responses to injury, particularly if given in high doses. Non-steroidal anti-inflammatory drugs used for analgesia may reduce prostaglandin production. Regional anaesthesia can block afferent nerve pathways, which may modulate parts of the metabolic response.

ANABOLISM

Anabolism is the process of regaining weight, restoring skeletal muscle mass and strength, and the replenishment of fat stores. Anabolism is unlikely to occur until the processes associated with catabolism, such as the release of inflammatory mediators, have subsided. This point is often associated with an obvious clinical improvement in the patient, who feels better and regains his or her appetite. Hormones contributing to the process of anabolism include insulin, growth hormone, insulin-like growth factors, androgens and the 17-ketosteroids. The factors controlling the rate of anabolism are complex, but nutritional support and the activity level of the patient are important contributing factors.

2 Principles of fluid and electrolyte balance in surgical patients

T.S. Walsh, A.J. Pollok

Many patients undergoing surgery do not ingest oral fluids, either in preparation for surgery or as a result of the surgery itself. If fluid ingestion is restricted for a prolonged period, fluid requirements need to be met by intravenous administration. In addition to reduced intake from fasting, surgery can alter fluid and electrolyte status by:

- Stimulating the secretion of stress hormones (ADH, aldosterone, cortisol) that alter the body's handling of water and electrolytes (see Chapter 1);
- Causing fluid and electrolyte loss from the gastrointestinal tract, including the preoperative use of laxatives for bowel preparation;
- Increasing insensible fluid losses, for example sweating secondary to fever;
- Sequestration of fluids and electrolytes at the site of surgery ('third-space' losses);
- Fluid loss from surgical drains or fistulae.

Fluid and electrolyte status may also be altered during the perioperative period by the patient's normal medical treatments, such as diuretic and antihypertensive drugs. Careful monitoring of fluid balance (input and output) is therefore important in the perioperative period. An adequate volume of water, together with an appropriate amount of sodium and potassium, needs to be given. In surgical conditions associated with excessive and prolonged fluid loss (such as prolonged gastrointestinal loss or fistulae), consideration should be given to other electrolytes, such as calcium, magnesium and phosphate.

This chapter describes the important aspects of fluid and electrolyte balance relevant to the surgical patient. A broader account of disturbances in fluid, electrolyte and acid–base balance is given in Chapter 5 of Davidson's *Principles and Practice of Medicine*.

NORMAL WATER AND ELECTROLYTE BALANCE

The body of a healthy 70-kg male contains about 42 L of water, which is distributed into compartments as shown in Figure 2.1A. Electrolytes are dissolved in body water, but distributed differently between the various compartments (Fig. 2.1B). This distribution is maintained by membrane ion pumps, is essential for normal cellular function, and is an energy-dependent process that uses a significant proportion of basal energy requirements. The osmolality of extracellular fluid is determined primarily by sodium and chloride concentrations, whereas the major intracellular ions are potassium, magnesium, phosphate and sulphate. The distribution of fluid between the intra- and extravascular compartments is dependent on the *oncotic* pressure of plasma and the permeability of the endothelium. The plasma oncotic pressure is determined by the presence of *colloid* particles, of which albumin is the most important. Both the colloid oncotic pressure and the endothelial permeability may alter following surgery (see Chapter 1). The control of total body electrolytes and water is primarily a function of the kidneys in conjunction with hormonal regulation by factors such as aldosterone, antidiuretic hormone (ADH) and atrial natriuretic peptide. It follows that patients with abnormal renal function are more likely to develop fluid and electrolyte abnormalities in the perioperative period.

A healthy individual loses fluid and electrolytes by three routes: the kidneys, the gastrointestinal tract, and by evaporation from the skin and respiratory tract. Over 24 hours, a 70-kg adult in normal fluid balance will lose 1500–2000 mL of urine, 300 mL of fluid via the faeces, and 700–1000 mL as water vapour from the skin and respiratory tract (insensible water loss). An increase in core temperature (pyrexia) and/or sweating increases insensible fluid and electrolyte losses significantly. In health, water is taken in as fluids and in solid foods, and an additional

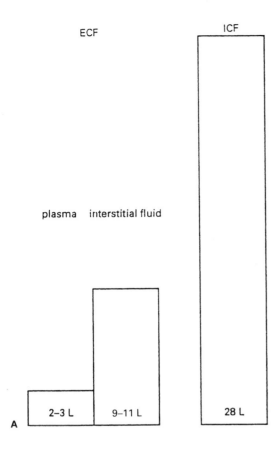

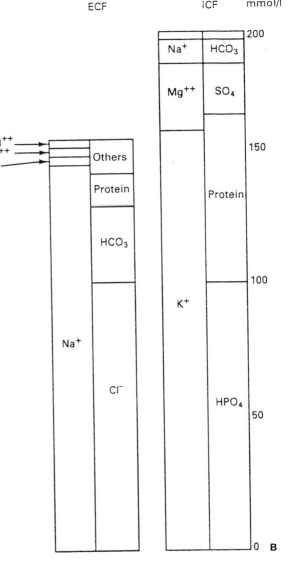

Fig. 2.1 **A** Distribution of water between the intracellular and extracellular compartments. Values shown are approximate values in a 70 kg man. **B** Distribution of cations and anions in the extracellular and intracellular fluid compartments.

200–300 mL per 24 hours are provided endogenously by oxidation of carbohydrate and fat (i.e. metabolic water).

In the absence of sweating almost all sodium loss is via the urine. Under the influence of aldosterone the kidney can reduce sodium loss to a minimum of approximately 10–20 mmol/24 h. Potassium is also excreted mainly via the kidney (60–100 mmol/24 h) and about 10 mmol/day are lost via the gastrointestinal tract. In severe potassium deficiency losses can be reduced to about 20 mmol/day, but increased aldosterone secretion, high urine flow rates and metabolic alkalosis all limit the ability of the kidneys to conserve potassium. The normal daily losses and the requirements to maintain fluid and electrolyte balance are summarized in Table 2.1.

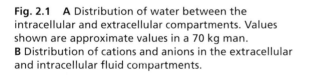

The percentage water content of newborn babies and children is higher than in adults. As a consequence, the maintenance fluid requirements of the paediatric surgical patient are higher than the adult counterpart. In the first few days of life, the newborn is relatively waterlogged and the kidneys relatively immature. The maintenance fluid requirement at birth is about 75 mL/kg body weight (BW)/day. This increases during the first week of life to 150 mL/kg BW/day. Premature infants can require

Table 2.1   Normal daily losses and requirements for fluids and electrolytes

	Volume (mL)	Na$^+$ (mmol)	K$^+$ (mmol)
Urine	2000	80	60
Insensible losses	700	–	–
Faeces	300	–	10
Minus endogenous water	300	–	–
Total	2700	80	70

as much as 200 mL/kg BW/day of maintenance fluids. After the first month of life fluid requirements decrease. The '4/2/1 formula' is widely used to calculate the fluid requirements of the average paediatric patient after the neonatal period. The first 10 kg BW requires approximately 4 mL/kg BW/hour (equates to 100 mL/kg/day); the next 10 kg BW requires approximately 2 mL/kg BW/hour (equates to 50 mL/kg BW/day); every kg BW thereafter requires approximately 1 mL/kg BW/hour (equates to 25 mL/kg BW/day). Using this formula a 35 kg child would require $(10 \times 4 \text{ mL}) + (10 \times 2 \text{ mL}) + (15 \times 1 \text{ mL}) = 40 + 20 + 15 = 75$ mL/hour of maintenance fluids.

Electrolyte and mineral requirements are also calculated by body weight e.g. the daily requirement for sodium and potassium in children is approximately 2–3 mmol/kg BW/day. It will be clear that the sodium content of normal saline (150 mmol/L) would result in serious sodium overload if this was used as the maintenance fluid for neonates and children. A 3 kg neonate whose daily fluid requirement is 450 mL/day (150 mL/kg BW/day) needs approximately 9 mols of sodium per day. 450 mL of normal saline contains 67.5 mmol of sodium; 450 mL of fifth strength (0.18%) contains 13.5 mmol of sodium. It is for this reason that the normal maintenance intravenous fluid used in children is not normal saline.

ASSESSING LOSSES IN THE SURGICAL PATIENT

Insensible fluid losses

Hyperventilation increases insensible water loss via the respiratory tract, but this increase is not usually very large unless the normal mechanisms for humidifying inhaled air (the nasal and upper airways) are compromised. Such a state can occur in patients receiving high-flow non-humidified oxygen in the postoperative period, or in patients undergoing mechanical ventilation without humidification of gases. In these situations gas humidifiers should be used.

Pyrexia increases water loss from the skin by approximately 200 mL/day for each 1°C rise in temperature. Sweating increases fluid loss considerably, by up to 1 L per hour, but is difficult to quantify. Sweat contains significant amounts of sodium (20–70 mmol/L) and potassium (10 mmol/L), which should be considered when assessing losses. After re-equilibration in the body, these forms of fluid and electrolyte loss result in depletion of all body compartments.

Effect of surgery

The stress response

This was considered in Chapter 1. ADH release conserves water and typically reduces urine volume to 1000–1500 mL for 2–3 days following major surgery. Excess water administration during this period is therefore likely to result in excess total body water, which may cause hyponatraemia (see later). Aldosterone secretion conserves sodium and further contributes to oliguria. In the first 2 days after operation, urinary excretion of sodium typically falls to approximately 30 mmol/24 h. Potassium excretion is increased during this period to approximately 120 mmol/day, as a result of aldosterone and the release of intracellular potassium from damaged tissues. Hypokalaemia is the commonest electrolyte disorder in the perioperative period, typically occurring 2–3 days after major surgery.

'Third-space' losses

Sequestration of extracellular fluid (ECF) at the site of operation produces local oedema. This fluid contains water, electrolytes and colloid particles because it results from local tissue injury, inflammation and capillary leak. As a result, third-space losses can significantly decrease the circulating fluid volume in the immediate postoperative period. Sequestration persists for approximately 48 hours and may involve up to 4 L of fluid, depending on the severity of the operation or injury. For example, it is estimated that about 500 mL/day are sequestered after partial gastrectomy. Third-space losses are an important consideration in the postoperative period because they significantly reduce extracellular fluid status and circulating volume.

Loss from the gastrointestinal tract

The magnitude and content of gastrointestinal fluid losses depend mainly on the site of loss. The approximate electrolyte content and volumes of various gastrointestinal fluids are shown in Table 2.2. Gastrointestinal losses may result from various factors:

• **Intestinal obstruction**. In general, the higher an obstruction occurs in the intestine the greater the fluid loss. This

Table 2.2 The approximate daily volumes and electrolyte concentrations of various gastrointestinal fluids. If gastrointestinal loss continues for more than 2–3 days, samples of fluid and urine should be collected regularly and sent to the laboratory for measurement of electrolyte content

	Volume	Na^+	K^+	Cl^-	HCO_3
Plasma		140	5	100	25
Gastric juice	2500	50	10	80	40
Intestinal fluid (upper)	3000	140	10	100	25
Bile and pancreatic juice	1500	140	5	80	60
Mature ileostomy	500	50	5	20	25
Diarrhoea (inflammatory)		110	40	100	40

Table 2.3 Conditions associated with increased risk of adynamic ileus

Trauma to the GI tract (including operative handling)

Infection

Electrolyte imbalance (particularly potassium, calcium and magnesium deficiency)

Hypoproteinaemia

Retroperitoneal trauma or haemorrhage

Hypoxaemia

Head injury or neurosurgical operations

Shock

is because fluids secreted by the upper gastrointestinal tract fail to reach the absorptive areas of the distal jejunum and ileum. Thus a patient with a high small bowel obstruction loses fluid more rapidly than one with a low small bowel obstruction.

- **Adynamic ileus**. This condition, in which propulsion in the small intestine ceases, has various possible causes (Table 2.3). The most common is probably handling and

surgical trauma to the bowel during surgery, which usually resolves within 1–2 days of the operation. Occasionally adynamic ileus persists for longer, when the less common causes should be sought and corrected if possible. During adynamic ileus the stomach should be decompressed using nasogastric tube drainage, and fluid losses monitored by measuring nasogastric aspirates. Adynamic ileus can sometimes be distinguished from obstruction by the presence or absence of bowel sounds.

- **Intestinal fistula**. Losses of fluid and electrolytes from an intestinal fistula can be considerable. As with obstruction, fistulae occurring high in the gut are usually associated with the greatest fluid losses. The electrolyte content of fistula losses can be large and the composition can vary depending on the site of the fistula. It can be useful

Table 2.4 Composition of commonly administered intravenous fluids

	Na^+ (mmol/L)	K^+ (mmol/L)	Cl^- (mmol/L)	HCO_3^- (mmol/L)	Misc. (mmol/L)	Oncotic pressure (mmH$_2$O)	Typical plasma half-life	pH
5% dextrose	–	–	–	–	–	0	–	4.0
0.9% NaCl	154	0	154	0	0	0	–	5.0
Ringer's lactate (Hartmann's solution)	131	5	112	29*	Ca^{2+} 1 Mg^{2+} 1	0	–	6.5
Haemaccel (succinylated gelatin)	145	5.1	145	0	Ca^{2+} 6.25	370	5 hours	7.4
Gelofusine (polygeline gelatin)	154	0.4	125	0	Ca^{2+} 0.4 Mg^{2+} 0.4	465	4 hours	7.4
Hetastarch	154	0	154	0	0	310	17 days	5.5
Human albumin solution 4.5% (HAS; PPF)	150	0	120	0	0	275	–	7.4

*The lactate present in Ringer's lactate solution is rapidly metabolized in the liver. This generates bicarbonate ions. Bicarbonate cannot be directly added to the solutions because it is unstable (tends to precipitate).

to measure the electrolyte content of fistula fluid in order to determine the type of fluid replacement required to maintain balance.

- **Diarrhoea**. Patients may present with diarrhoea or develop it during the perioperative period, for example as a result of antibiotic use. Fluid and electrolyte loss from diarrhoea may be considerable.

SUMMARY BOX

Causes of fluid and electrolyte loss from the gastrointestinal tract

- Vomiting
- Intestinal obstruction (greater loss from high obstructions)
- Paralytic ileus (increased intestinal secretion with reduced absorption)
- Intestinal fistula (high fistulae cause the greatest loss)
- Diarrhoea (may involve losses of up to 10 L/day)

INTRAVENOUS FLUID ADMINISTRATION

The composition of commonly administered intravenous fluids is shown in Table 2.4. When choosing and administering intravenous fluids it is important to decide:

1. From what deficiencies the patient suffers;
2. The compartments that require replacement;
3. Which fluid is most appropriate.

Dextrose solution 5% (5 g of dextrose/100 mL water) does not contain any electrolytes. The dextrose is rapidly metabolized in the body, such that dextrose solution is equivalent to administering water, which rapidly distributes evenly throughout the entire body fluid compartments. It follows that 1 L of intravenous dextrose solution expands the extracellular fluid compartment by 330 mL and the intravascular compartment by only about 70 mL (Fig. 2.2); 5% dextrose is therefore of value for replacing water losses but has no use as a resuscitation fluid to expand the intravascular volume.

Sodium chloride 0.9% ('normal saline') and *Ringer's lactate* are isotonic to extracellular fluid and have a similar composition. After intravenous administration these fluids distribute rapidly into the extracellular fluid compartment, and are appropriate when the main fluid deficiency derives from this source, for example gastrointestinal losses or intraoperative losses other than bleeding. It follows that 1 L of these fluids administered intravenously will increase the intravascular volume by about 220 mL after equilibration

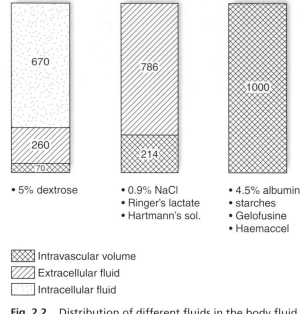

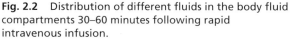

- 5% dextrose
- 0.9% NaCl
- Ringer's lactate
- Hartmann's sol.
- 4.5% albumin
- starches
- Gelofusine
- Haemaccel

▨ Intravascular volume
▨ Extracellular fluid
▢ Intracellular fluid

Fig. 2.2　Distribution of different fluids in the body fluid compartments 30–60 minutes following rapid intravenous infusion.

(Fig. 2.2). These fluids are therefore useful for resuscitation of the circulating volume, but it must be remembered that only about one-quarter remains in the circulating volume after redistribution. Under normal conditions redistribution is complete within 30–60 minutes, but this time may be considerably shorter in conditions such as sepsis and burns that cause capillary leakiness.

Colloid solutions are those containing particles that exert an oncotic pressure. These particles may occur naturally or be synthetic (Table 2.4). When a colloid solution is administered the solution remains in the circulation until the colloid particles are removed (predominantly by the reticuloendothelial system), after which it distributes into the extracellular fluid volume because it also contains electrolytes. Most solutions remain in the circulation for between 6 and 24 hours, but this time can be shorter in conditions associated with leaky capillaries. Colloid solutions are good resuscitation fluids because all the volume administered stays in the circulation. Some starch solutions have a greater oncotic pressure than normal plasma, so fluid is drawn into blood vessels and the circulating volume is increased by more than the volume administered. This is also the case for hypertonic saline, which is not a true colloid but is useful for resuscitation.

Maintenance fluid requirements

When prescribing the normal daily fluid and electrolyte requirements (Table 2.5) sodium and chloride are usually

Table 2.5 Provision of normal 24-hour fluid and electrolyte requirements by intravenous infusion

Intravenous fluid	Additive	Duration (h)
500 ml 0.9% NaCL	20 mmol KCl	4
500 ml 5% dextrose	–	4
500 ml 5% dextrose	20 mmol KCL	4
500 ml 0.9% NaCl	–	4
500 ml 5% dextrose	20 mmol KCl	4
500 ml 5% dextrose	–	4

provided as a 0.9% sodium chloride solution. Under normal conditions daily sodium and chloride requirements are contained in 1 L of 0.9% saline. Potassium requirements are usually met by adding potassium chloride according to plasma potassium concentrations (typically 60 mmol in 24 hours). Potassium should not be administered at a rate greater than 10–20 mmol/h except in severe potassium deficiency (continuous electrocardiogram (ECG) monitoring is then essential). It must never be given as an intravenous bolus, as cardiac arrest can occur. The remaining water requirement to maintain hydration is typically provided as 5% dextrose solution. In the postoperative period, when intravascular and extracellular fluid losses are increased by the factors described earlier, the additional fluid is best provided as crystalloid and colloid. The amount of extra fluid needed can be judged by the patient's blood pressure, pulse rate, urine output and peripheral skin temperature (a good indicator of peripheral blood flow). If a central venous

Table 2.6 How to estimate fluid and electrolyte requirements in a patient with ileus. Assuming that the patient is in electrolyte balance and is losing 2 L/day as nasogastric aspirate and 1.5 L/day as urine, 24-hour losses can be calculated as follows

	Volume	Na$^+$	K$^+$
Urine	1500	80	60
Nasogastric aspirate	2000	240	20
Insensible loss	800	–	–
Minus endogenous water	–300	–	–
Net losses/requirements	4000	320	80

2 L of normal saline would supply 300 mmol of Na$^+$
2 L of 5% dextrose would supply water
The required 60–80 mmol of K$^+$ can be added as 20 mmol to alternate 500 mL bags.

catheter is in place central venous pressure is very useful. An example of how short-term requirements may be provided for a patient with ileus is shown in Table 2.6.

In patients requiring replacement for more than 3–4 days correction of 'trace' ions may be needed, particularly if intestinal fluid loss is significant. Magnesium, calcium and phosphate are most commonly required (see later), and are best guided by direct measurement of plasma concentrations. In this situation the provision of parenteral nutrition also requires consideration (Chapter 5).

SPECIFIC WATER AND ELECTROLYTE ABNORMALITIES

Water and sodium imbalance

Water depletion

A decrease in total body water of 1–2% (350–700 mL) causes an increase in blood osmolarity sufficient to stimulate brain osmoreceptors and produce the sensation of thirst. Clinically obvious dehydration, with thirst, a dry tongue and loss of skin turgor, indicates at least 4–5% deficiency of total body water (1.5–2 L). Pure water depletion is rare in surgical practice, and is usually combined with sodium loss. The most frequent causes are inadequate intake or the excessive loss of gastrointestinal secretions.

Water excess

Water excess is common in surgical patients, particularly in postoperative patients who receive large volumes of intravenous 5% dextrose during the period of increased ADH secretion (see Chapter 1). In this situation the patient is commonly hyponatraemic (see below). Patients with water excess usually remain well, but may develop dependent oedema. In patients with poor cardiac function or renal failure, water accumulation can result in pulmonary oedema.

Sodium balance

Sodium is the principal extracellular cation. Changes in the concentration of sodium in extracellular fluid therefore result in changes in the tonicity of this fluid compartment. Sodium concentration is closely related to the relative amount of water in the extracellular fluid space. The presence of hypo- or hypernatraemia therefore reflects the balance between sodium and water content.

- *Hypernatraemia* is most commonly a result of water depletion or pure dehydration. The causes of water depletion resulting in hypernatraemia are listed in Table 2.7. In the surgical patient the common causes are

Table 2.7 The aetiology of hyper- and hyponatraemia. Causes commonly encountered in the surgical patient are denoted with an asterisk

Hypernatraemia
Reduced intake
  Fasting*
  Nausea and vomiting*
  Ileus*
  Reduced conscious level
Increased loss
  Sweating (pyrexia, hot environment)*
  Respiratory tract loss (increased ventilation, administration of dry gases)
  Burns*
Inappropriate urinary water loss
  Diabetes insipidus (pituitary or nephrogenic)
  Diabetes mellitus
Excessive sodium load (hypertonic fluids, parenteral nutrition)

Hyponatraemia
Low extracellular fluid volume
  Volume depletion (vomiting, diarrhoea, burns, decreased fluid intake)*
  Salt-losing renal disease
  Hypoadrenalism
  Diuretic use*
Normal extracellular fluid volume
  Hypothyroidism
  Syndromes of inappropriate ADH secretion (SIADH)
Increased extracellular fluid volume
  Excessive water administration*
  Excessive mannitol use
  Cardiac failure
  Cirrhosis
  Nephrotic syndrome
  Renal failure

Table 2.8 Causes of SIADH

Neoplasias
  Bronchial carcinoma
Non-malignant pulmonary disease
  Tuberculosis
  Pneumonia
  Legionnaire's disease
CNS disease
  Meningitis
  Encephalitis
  Brain abscess
  Head injury
  Cerebral tumours
  CVA
  Guillain–Barré syndrome
Drugs
  Narcotics/opiates
  Phenothiazines
  Carbamazepine
  Antidepressants
  Chlorpropamide

reduced water intake due to anorexia, nausea or fasting in relation to the surgical procedure. Increased water loss can result from fever, sweating and hyperventilation. The treatment is usually to increase the patient's water intake. This can be via the oral route by encouraging the patient to drink or adding additional water to nasogastric feeds, or by administering additional intravenous water as 5% dextrose solution.

- *Hyponatraemia* is a more complex disorder because it can occur in the presence of decreased, normal or increased extracellular volume. The common causes of hyponatraemia are listed in Table 2.7, and are discussed more fully in Chapter 5 of Davidson's *Principles and Practice of Medicine*. In the surgical patient the common causes of hyponatraemia are volume depletion, excessive administration of water as 5% dextrose (particularly

during the period of increased ADH secretion postoperatively), and diuretic use. Comorbidity, such as cirrhosis, cardiac failure and renal impairment, is a frequent contributing factor. The treatment of hyponatraemia depends on identifying its cause correctly. The most important assessment is to judge whether plasma and/or extracellular volume is increased, normal or decreased. In the surgical patient who does not have comorbidity such as cardiac failure or liver disease the most likely cause of hyponatraemia if ECF volume is normal or increased, is excessive intravenous water administration. This will correct spontaneously by decreasing water intake. In patients with decreased ECF volume the hyponatraemia usually indicates combined water and sodium deficiency, which will correct if adequate 0.9% sodium chloride is administered. *Severe* hyponatraemia (plasma sodium < 120 mmol/L) is usually a result of coexisting cardiac, liver or renal disease or, if these are not present, the syndromes of inappropriate ADH secretion (Table 2.8). Severe hyponatraemia requires careful management with water restriction, 0.9% sodium chloride therapy, and occasionally diuretic use. Hypertonic saline solutions are rarely indicated and can be dangerous. The condition can be complicated by confusion, cerebral oedema, seizures and coma. Plasma sodium requires slow correction (at about 1 mmol/h) with regular monitoring, because rapid increases in sodium concentration can cause permanent neurological damage.

Potassium imbalance

Potassium is the principal intracellular cation. Only 60 mmol of the normal total body potassium (typically

Table 2.9 Consequences of hyper- and hypokalaemia

Hyperkalaemia
Arrythmias (broad-complex rhythms, bradycardia, heart block, ventricular fibrillation)
Muscle weakness
Ileus

Hypokalaemia
ECG changes (flattened T-waves, U-waves)
Ectopic beats
Muscle weakness

Table 2.11 Management of severe acute hyperkalaemia (K$^+$ >7 mmol/L)

1. Identify and treat cause
2. 10–20 mL intravenous 10% calcium chloride over 10 min in patients with ECG abnormalities (reduces risk of ventricular fibrillation)
3. 50 mL 50% dextrose plus 10 units short-acting insulin over 2–3 min
   Monitor plasma glucose and K$^+$ over next 30–60 min)
4. Regular salbutamol nebulizers
5. Consider oral or rectal calcium resonium (ion exchange resin), although this is more effective for non-acute hyperkalaemia
6. Haemodialysis for persistent hyperkalaemia

about 3500 mmol) is extracellular. Plasma potassium concentration (typically 4 mmol/L) is therefore a poor indicator of the total body potassium. Changes in the distribution of potassium between plasma and intracellular fluid can have a dramatic effect on the plasma K$^+$ concentration. Potassium distribution is tightly controlled by Na$^+$/K$^+$ ATPase and other ion pumps present in cell membranes. The Na$^+$/K$^+$ ATPase is pH sensitive, and during acidosis reduced activity results in a net efflux of potassium from cells and hyperkalaemia. Conversely, during alkalosis increased activity results in hypokalaemia. These abnormalities are exacerbated by renal compensatory mechanisms that correct acid–base balance at the expense of potassium homeostasis. The consequences of hyper- and hypokalaemia are listed in Table 2.9.

Hyperkalaemia has several causes (Table 2.10). Most are characterized by an increased efflux of potassium from cells as a result of tissue damage or altered membrane pump function. Hyperkalaemia is often asymptomatic until dangerous arrythmias develop, or is diagnosed incidentally as a result of ECG changes or measurement of plasma con-

centration. Severe hyperkalaemia (K$^+$ > 7 mmol/L) requires immediate treatment and identification of the likely cause (Table 2.11). *Hypokalaemia* is a common disorder in surgical patients. Dietary intake of potassium is normally 60–80 mmol/day, and > 85% is excreted via the kidneys. Maintenance of potassium balance depends on normal renal tubular regulation. Potassium excretion is increased by alkalosis, increased urine flow rates and increased aldosterone release, which all occur frequently in the surgical patient. The causes of hypokalaemia are listed in Table 2.12. Hypokalaemia is treated by administering additional potassium orally as a potassium salt, or intravenously. The oral or nasogastric route is preferable and safer whenever possible.

Table 2.10 Causes of hyperkalaemia. Frequent causes in surgical patients are denoted with an asterisk

Excess intravenous or oral intake
Efflux of potassium from cells
   Haemolysis
   Rhabdomyolysis (e.g. crush syndromes, compartment syndromes)*
   Massive tissue damage (e.g. ischaemic bowel or liver)*
Acidosis
Impaired excretion
   Acute renal failure*
   Chronic renal failure
   Drugs (ACE inhibitors, spironolactone)
Abnormalities of the renin–angiotensin system (e.g. Addison's disease)

Table 2.12 Causes of hypokalaemia. Common causes in the surgical patient are denoted by an asterisk

Reduced/inadequate intake*
Gastrointestinal tract losses
   Vomiting*
   Gastric aspiration/drainage*
   Fistulae*
   Diarrhoea*
   Ileus*
   Intestinal obstruction*
   Potassium-secreting villous adenomas*
Urinary losses
   Metabolic alkalosis*
   Hyperaldosteronism*
   Diuretic use*
   Renal tubular disorders (e.g. Bartter's syndrome, renal tubular acidosis, amphoteracin-induced tubular damage)

Other electrolyte disturbances

Abnormalities in calcium and magnesium balance are rarely of major significance in the surgical patient except in specific conditions such as acute pancreatitis (hypocalcaemia) or in relation to endocrine surgery (such as parathyroid surgery). These are described in the relevant chapters of this book. Hypophosphataemia is a frequent and important disorder in the surgical patient that merits specific consideration. About 80% of total body phosphate is in the skeleton, and the remaining 20% is a major intracellular anion. Phosphate molecules are critical in many biochemical processes, notably in storing energy as ATP, in signalling messengers, and in synthesizing nucleic acids during cell division and healing. Severe hypophosphataemia (< 0.4 mmol/L; normal range 0.8–1.4 mmol/L) causes widespread cellular dysfunction and, notably, muscle weakness. Hypophosphataemia commonly occurs in patients recovering from major illness and surgery, particularly after nutrition is reintroduced, either naturally or artificially. Like hypokalaemia, hypophosphataemia is also precipitated by alkalosis. Plasma phosphate concentration should therefore be measured regularly following major surgery and in patients receiving artificial nutrition. Phosphate can be replaced via oral supplements or by slow intravenous infusion.

ACID–BASE BALANCE

There are four main types of acid–base disturbance: *acidosis* or *alkalosis* can occur, and each may be *respiratory* or *metabolic* in origin. These disturbances can occur in isolation or as mixed disorders. The diagnosis of acid–base disturbance relies on the measurement of arterial blood gases, and occasionally on blood lactate concentration (see Chapter 10). A full description of acid–base abnormalities can be found in Chapter 5 of Davidson's *Principles and Practice of Medicine*. The common conditions encountered in the surgical patient are discussed below.

Metabolic acidosis

Metabolic acidosis is characterized by an increase in plasma hydrogen ions in conjunction with a decrease in bicarbonate concentration. Respiratory compensation decreases the $P\text{a}CO_2$ to levels lower than normal secondary to hyperventilation. Metabolic acidosis can occur as a result of increased production of lactic acid, the accumulation of acids other than lactic acid, or increased loss of bicarbonate. The causes of metabolic acidosis frequently encountered in surgical patients are listed in Table 2.13.

The most common cause in surgical practice is lactic acidosis as a result of impaired tissue perfusion due to shock

Table 2.13   Common causes of metabolic acidosis in the surgical patient. For a full list of the aetiology of metabolic acidosis refer to Chapter 5 of Davidson's *Principles and Practice of Medicine*

Lactic acidosis
Shock (any cause)
Severe hypoxaemia
Severe haemorrhage/anaemia
Accumulation of other acids
Diabetic ketoacidosis
Acute renal failure
Increased bicarbonate loss
Diarrhoea
Intestinal fistulae
Ureterosigmoidostomy (an old fashioned bladder bypass operation)

(see Chapter 3). A low total CO_2 estimation on routine blood urea and electrolytes should alert the physician to the possibility of the presence of a metabolic acidosis, particularly if there are clinical signs of tissue hypoperfusion, such as oliguria, hypotension or cold peripheries. Therapy is directed towards restoring the circulating blood volume and tissue perfusion. With normal cardiorespiratory and renal function the metabolic acidosis will correct spontaneously after adequate resuscitation.

Metabolic alkalosis

Metabolic alkalosis is characterized by a decrease in plasma hydrogen ion concentration and an increase in bicarbonate concentration. A compensatory respiratory acidosis may occur, resulting in an increase in $P\text{a}CO_2$. Metabolic alkalosis is commonly associated with hypokalaemia and hypochloraemia. The body has an enormous capacity to generate bicarbonate ions, and this is stimulated particularly by chloride losses that can only be reversed by exogenous administration. This is a major factor causing metabolic alkalosis following chloride losses from the gastrointestinal tract, especially when combined with loss of acid from conditions such as gastric outlet obstruction.

Table 2.14   Common causes of metabolic alkalosis in the surgical patient

Loss of sodium, chloride and water
Vomiting
Aspiration of gastric secretions (e.g. nasogastric suction)
Diuretic administration
Hypokalaemia

Hypokalaemia is often associated with metabolic alkalosis because hydrogen ions shift into cells, and because distal renal tubular cells retain potassium in preference to hydrogen ions. The major causes of metabolic alkalosis in the surgical patient are listed in Table 2.14. Treatment of most forms of metabolic alkalosis involves the administration of adequate 0.9% NaCl together with sufficient potassium to correct hypokalaemia.

Respiratory acidosis

Respiratory acidosis is characterized by increased Pa_{CO_2}, hydrogen ions and plasma bicarbonate concentration, and is a common postoperative problem. It usually results from excessive opiate administration because of a shift in the response of chemoreceptors to CO_2. This form of respiratory acidosis is harmless in most patients, requires no specific treatment, and will resolve as opiate requirements for pain decrease. Occasionally respiratory acidosis occurs because of pulmonary complications such as pneumonia, but usually only in very sick patients or those with pre-existing respiratory disease. Patients with this cause of respiratory acidosis may require respiratory support with artificial ventilation, because the problem is inadequate respiratory muscle strength, often in association with respiratory complications that increase the work of breathing.

Respiratory alkalosis

Respiratory alkalosis is caused by excessive loss of CO_2 owing to hyperventilation of the lungs. Pa_{CO_2} and hydrogen ion concentration decrease. The common causes of respiratory alkalosis are shown in Table 2.15. Respiratory alkalosis rarely needs specific treatment and usually corrects spontaneously when the precipitating condition resolves.

Mixed patterns of acid–base imbalance

Mixed patterns of acid–base disturbance are common, particularly in very sick patients. In this situation acid–base nomograms can be very useful in clarifying the contributing factors (Fig. 2.3)

Table 2.15 Causes of respiratory alkalosis encountered in surgical practice
Hyperventilation during mechanical ventilation
Pain
Apprehension/hysterical hyperventilation
Pneumonia
Central nervous system disorders (meningitis, encephalopathy)
Septicaemia

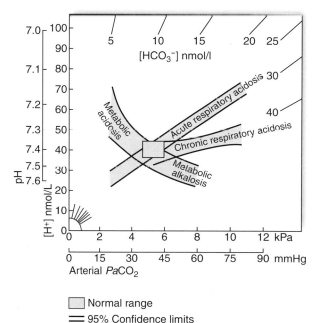

Fig. 2.3 Diagram showing changes in blood [H+]. The rectangle indicates limits of normal reference ranges for [H+] and Pa_{CO_2}. The bands represent 95% confidence limits of single disturbances in human blood in vivo. When the point obtained by plotting [H+] against P does not fall within one of the labelled bands, compensation is incomplete or a mixed disorder is present.

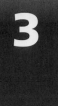

3 Shock

A.J. Pollok

DEFINITION OF SHOCK

The early stages of shock are characterized by an imbalance between oxygen supply and demand. This will result in cellular hypoxia and a switch from aerobic metabolism to an anaerobic state which, if not corrected, will lead to cellular dysfunction, organ failure and, ultimately, irreversible damage.

All patients with shock can be considered to have an inadequate oxygen delivery for their pathological or physiological state. Cardiac output can be low as a result of either the inability of the heart to pump on a background of adequate circulating blood volume, i.e. cardiogenic shock,

> **SUMMARY BOX**
>
> *Definition of shock*
>
> Shock is an imbalance between oxygen delivery and demand which results in cellular dysfunction and death, which is reflected in organ failure.

or an inadequate circulating blood volume (hypovolaemia) (Fig. 3.1). In sepsis there may be excessive systemic vasodilatation, which may be associated with a normal or high cardiac output. Despite this there is reduced perfusion of some vital vascular beds.

CAUSES OF SHOCK

Hypovolaemia

The loss of blood or any of its components will result in a reduction of circulating blood volume. With no compensation it will lead to a fall in the venous return to the right side of the heart and a decrease in cardiac output. The common causes are:

1. *Haemorrhage* This is frequently encountered in major trauma but can also be seen in the postoperative period. Clinical presentation and features will be influenced by the severity and duration of the bleeding and the patient's ability to compensate. This in turn depends on age, cardiac function and the adequacy of ongoing resuscitation. It is the young patient with a prolonged period of slow blood loss with efficient mechanisms of compensation (subclinical shock) in whom hypovolaemia may be difficult to identify early.

2. *Crystalloid/water loss* Increased GIT losses may occur as a result of prolonged vomiting or diarrhoea, fistulae, intestinal ileus, or may be iatrogenic due to aggressive preoperative bowel preparation without adequate fluid replacement.

3. *Plasma loss* Burns covering more than 20% of the body are associated with significant losses of plasma both from the burnt surface and from a generalized increase in capillary permeability, with extravascular sequestration of fluid. Severe sepsis can also lead to increased capillary permeability.

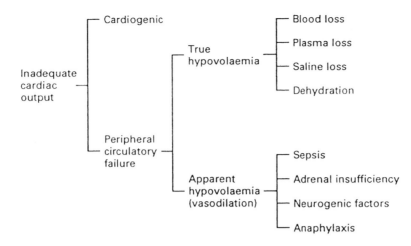

Fig. 3.1 Classification of the mechanisms underlying the shock process.

Pump failure

The inability of the heart to function as a pump will lead to a reduction in cardiac output on a background of an adequate circulating blood volume (normovolaemia) This condition is known as cardiogenic shock. Commonly this occurs following acute myocardial infarction, but may also be a sequelae of acute dysrrythmias, cardiomyopathy, or sudden and severe valvular incompetence.

Other causes include cardiac tamponade and massive pulmonary embolism, where the outflow to the right ventricle is obstructed, preventing blood from reaching the left side of the heart. In all shock states there is a fall in the perfusion of the myocardium via the coronary arteries. Myocardial oxygen delivery can be estimated from the coronary perfusion pressure, which can be calculated by subtracting the pressure in the left ventricle at the end of diastole (LVEDP) from the diastolic pressure. In addition, the compensatory increase in heart rate results in increased myocardial oxygen demand and reduced time for coronary blood flow (coronary blood flow only occurs during diastole, which is the component of the cardiac cycle that shortens as heart rate increases) and myocardial oxygen delivery. The result may be myocardial hypoxia, which adversely affects contractility and contributes to pump failure in shock.

Sepsis

Gram-negative organisms are most frequently implicated when shock is associated with severe sepsis. It is thought that the release of endotoxin by these organisms triggers a systemic inflammatory cascade within the vascular compartment which results in characteristic pathophysiological changes. The host's immune system plays a vital role in initiating this exaggerated inflammatory response, with the early activation of inflammatory cells such as polymorphs and macrophages. These cells in turn release a wide variety of inflammatory products and mediators, such as proteolytic enzymes (elastase), toxic oxygen radicals, vasoactive substances (platelet-activating factor, leukotrienes, prostaglandin E_2) and wound hormones (macrophage colony-stimulating factor). In addition, levels of circulating cytokines, such as tumour necrosis factor-α and interleukins IL-1 and IL-6, are increased. These are all essential components which act together with white blood cells, platelets, endothelial cells, the complement cascade and coagulation pathways to form the basis of the normal protective inflammatory response to infection and injury. In a minority of patients this local inflammatory response becomes greatly amplified and fails to remain limited to the site of the sepsis. This group of patients may go on to demonstrate systemic manifestations of the inflammatory

---

SUMMARY BOX

Determinants of myocardial oxygenation

Oxygen supply to the myocardium

Supply	Demand
Coronary perfusion pressure (CPP) (CPP = Diastolic pressure − LVEDP) Heart rate: coronary blood flow occurs during diastole Haemoglobin concentration Arterial oxygen saturation	Heart rate Afterload: systemic vascular resistance

response (SIRS). Increased capillary permeability and oedema can result in significant organ dysfunction, which may progress to failure. Other infective organisms (Gram-positive bacteria, fungi) and non-infective stimuli may act as triggers for the inflammatory cascades that underly SIRS.

Shock from any cause, if severe enough, will lead to splanchnic vasoconstriction and ischaemia. If prolonged this can lead to a breakdown of the gut mucosal barrier and a translocation of bacteria and/or their products (endotoxin) into the portal circulation. A failure by the liver to clear these would result in their reaching the systemic circulation and possibly triggering a systemic inflammatory response.

SUMMARY BOX

Definition of systemic inflammatory response syndrome (SIRS)

Systemic inflammatory response to infective or non-infective aetiologies (trauma, pancreatitis, vasculitis etc.) characterized by:

- Temperature > 38°C or < 36°C
- Heart rate > 90/min
- Respiratory rate > 20/min
- $Paco_2$ < 32 mmHg or ventilated
- White cell count > 12 000 or < 4000 mm³

SUMMARY BOX

Septic shock

- Commonly due to infections with Gram-negative bacteria, but can be due to Gram-positive bacteria or fungi.

- Endotoxin from bacterial cell wall triggers a localized inflammatory cascade within the vascular compartment, which in susceptible individuals becomes systemic.

- The haemodynamic response is vasodilatation due to a reduction in the systemic vascular resistance.

- A reflex increase in cardiac output may maintain the blood pressure, and the hyperdynamic circulation results in a patient who appears deceptively well, with pink warm peripheries.

- Significant organ hypoperfusion (splanchnic circulation) may be occurring, with arteriovenous shunting within the capillary beds of many organs, resulting in cellular hypoxia and organ dysfunction.

Whereas the pathophysiology responsible for the systemic inflammatory response remains complex and is yet not fully understood, the cardiovascular alterations are well documented. The final common pathway for a number of these processes is the local release of nitric oxide (NO), which is a potent vasodilator. This results in a marked reduction in the systemic vascular resistance and a fall in blood pressure. A reflex increase in the cardiac output occurs in response to this reduction in afterload. However, the presence of circulating myocardial depressant factors may limit this increase in cardiac output, and an increase in shunting from the arterial to the venous side of the vascular bed may contribute to paradoxical ischaemia and tissue hypoxia even with this increased cardiac output.

Anaphylaxis

Anaphylactic reactions can occur following the administration of any drug, colloid (predominantly synthetic) or blood. The underlying mechanism can be either the classic type 1 hypersensitivity reaction mediated by IgE antibodies, or anaphylactoid, where the clinical picture is identical but the underlying mechanism is unclear. Both stimulate the degranulation of basophils and mast cells, resulting in the systemic release of a number of vasoactive mediators such as histamine, bradykinin, prostaglandins, platelet-activating factor and leukotrienes. The immediate systemic vascular effects of these mediators is to produce smooth muscle contraction, vasodilatation and increased capillary permeability, the clinical manifestations of which are flush-

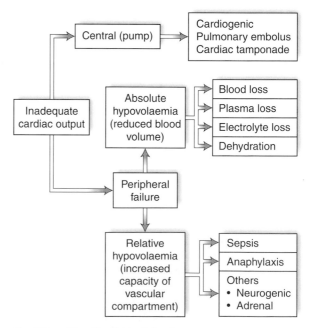

Fig. 3.2 Classification of shock.

ing and oedema. The hypovolaemia that occurs is responsible for the acute fall in cardiac output and the development of a shocked state (Fig. 3.2).

PATHOPHYSIOLOGY OF SHOCK

Irrespective of the aetiology underlying a low-output state (either hypovolaemia or 'pump' failure) the sympathetic stimulation and catecholamine release that occurs results in a similar clinical picture. Whereas slight differences can be detected at the level of the macrocirculation, alterations in the microcirculation are indistinguishable. Prolonged sympathetic overactivity and catecholamine release, due either to unrecognized shock or to an inability to correct the precipitating cause, will lead to organ and tissue hypoperfusion, with regional or generalized hypoxia reflected in a progressive deterioration in acid–base status. If this is allowed to continue, cell dysfunction and death will occur, leading to multiorgan failure. In septic shock elevated levels of circulating vasoactive substances are responsible for the physiological abnormalities observed. At the level of the macrocirculation there is a reduction in whole-body systemic vascular resistance. This picture masks serious inequalities in blood flow between various organs at tissue and capillary level, which can result in cellular hypoxia.

Macrocirculation

The classic signs associated with a low-output state are cold, pale, clammy skin along with collapsed peripheral veins reflecting increased activity of the sympathetic nervous system. This occurs because hypotension, reduced pulse pressure (with or without decreased venous return) and chemoreceptor stimulation from acidosis act to increase sympathetic activity and catecholamine release from the adrenal medulla. The resultant increase in heart rate, myocardial contractility and systemic vascular resistance helps to maintain venous return to the heart, cardiac output and mean arterial pressure. This mechanism to preserve blood flow and perfusion to vital organs will result not only in clinically obvious peripheral vasoconstriction but also less obvious splanchnic hypoperfusion. This reduced blood supply to the gut is now implicated in many of the complications associated with prolonged or untreated shock. A reduction in renal blood flow diverts blood from the cortex, stimulating the release of renin and activating the renin–angiotensin system. The resultant elevated levels of circulating angiotensin II further contribute to systemic vasoconstriction.

In a patient with sepsis the physiological changes are quite different and distinct. Elevated levels of circulating vasoactive substances such as cytokines result in pre-

capillary vasodilatation and a significant fall in systemic vascular resistance. This reduction in the afterload of the heart, along with possible hypovolaemia due to increased capillary permeability, results in a reduction in venous return (preload), mimicking a true hypovolaemic state. An increase in sympathetic activity results in tachycardia and increased cardiac output, with patients demonstrating a hyperdynamic circulation with warm pink peripheries and venodilatation. Patients with well preserved myocardial function may be able to compensate fully for this reduction in afterload by increasing their cardiac output sufficiently to maintain a satisfactory systolic pressure. Paradoxically whole-body oxygen delivery is increased, oxygen delivery

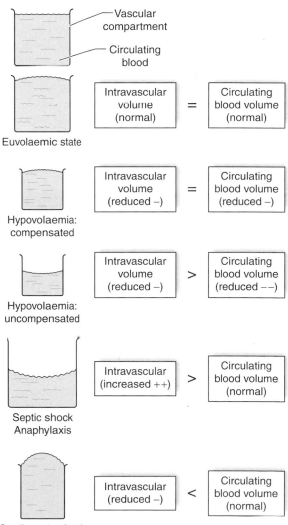

Fig. 3.3 Alterations in circulating blood volume and vascular compartment volume in various shocked states.

and utilization at capillary and cellular level is compromised. This leads to the apparently contradictory findings of a raised venous blood oxygen saturation together with a metabolic acidosis. It is the young, previously fit patient with subtle clinical signs, a blood pressure and heart rate within normal limits, but with an unexplained metabolic acidosis who should alert the physician to the possibility of serious sepsis. Myocardial contractility is affected in both the above forms of shock, as explained above. These effects may become clinically apparent earlier in older people with underlying ischaemic heart disease, as their ability for physiological compensation can be significantly reduced.

As cardiogenic shock is also a low-output state the physiological changes to the cardiovascular system are similar to those seen with severe hypovolaemia, but on a background of normovolaemia. As the precipitating cause is commonly severe myocardial damage resulting from infarction, dysrhythmias are very common. If there is associated left ventricular failure there will be an increased pressure in the pulmonary veins (measured by pulmonary artery catheter), resulting in pulmonary oedema which may manifest itself clinically as tachypnoea and shortness of breath. With right ventricular infarction the right side of the heart may begin to fail, either in isolation or as a consequence of left-sided failure, leading to an elevation in central venous pressure (CVP) (Fig. 3.3).

Microcirculation

Irrespective of the aetiology the microcirculatory abnormality is an imbalance between the supply and demand of oxygen at cellular level. Sympathetically mediated vasoconstriction, seen in early hypovolaemic and cardiogenic shock, results in the constriction of both precapillary arterioles and, to a lesser degree, postcapillary venules.

This helps to maintain a satisfactory mean arterial pressure by increasing the systemic vascular resistance, together with transferring the remaining circulating blood volume from the periphery to the centre, helping to maintain an adequate preload by maintaining the central venous pressure (CVP). This mechanism also results in a fall in the capillary hydrostatic pressure, encouraging (by Starling's law) a net transfer of fluid from the interstitial space into the vascular compartment in an attempt to augment the decreased circulating blood volume. In the early stages the changes in total body systemic vascular resistance reflect major increases in the vascular resistance in non-vital organs, specifically skin, muscle and splanchnic vascular beds. Whereas the reduced skin blood flow can be identified by an increase in the difference between core and peripheral temperatures, falls in muscle and splanchnic blood flow are not detected by routine cardiovascular measurements. A 10% reduction in circulating blood volume produces no alteration to heart rate or systolic blood pressure, but masks a significant reduction in splanchnic blood flow and oxygen delivery. In the case of septic shock the characteristic fall in systemic vascular resistance reflects a pathological increase in arteriovenous shunts in tissue capillary beds. This diversion of oxygenated blood away from capillary beds, together with an increase in capillary permeability, contributes to the hypoxia reflected by a metabolic acidosis. These microcirculatory responses to shock will be modified by underlying cardiovascular disease, such as hypertension or atherosclerosis, and explains why elderly patients frequently do not demonstrate the classic signs mentioned above and may decompensate at an earlier stage in the process. If shock remains uncorrected, the local accumulation of the products of anaerobic metabolism, such as lactic acid and carbon dioxide, together with the release of vasoactive substances

Table 3.1   Clinical signs associated with alteration to the macrocirculation in various shock states

	Normal	Hypovolaemia	Cardiogenic	Sepsis
Skin: Colour	Pink	Pale	Pale	Pink
Temp.	Warm	Cool	Cool	Warm
Feel	Dry	Damp	Damp	Dry
Cap. return	Prompt	Sluggish	Sluggish	Prompt
Pulse rate	Normal	Tachycardia	Tachycardia	Tachycardia
Pulse volume	Normal	Reduced	Reduced	Increased
Blood pressure	Normal	Low	Low	Low
JVP	Normal	Low	High	Low
Temp. gradient	Minimal	Increased	Increased	Minimal
Urine output	Normal	Reduced	Reduced	Reduced
Mental status	Normal	Obtunded	Obtunded	Obtunded

from the endothelium, reverses the sympathetic effects and leads to precapillary vasodilatation. However, if there is persistent postcapillary venoconstriction then the result is pooling of blood within the capillary bed and endothelial cell damage secondary to the presence of stimulants, such as microemboli, vasoactive substances, activated leukocytes and complement. Vessel permeability increases with the loss of fluid from the capillary into the interstitium, resulting in oedema. Haemoconcentration means increased viscosity, and this adds to the already increased viscosity associated with low-flow states. These conditions predispose to reduced red blood cell (RBC) deformability and a tendency for RBC and platelet aggregation. A combination of microemboli, increased local levels of noradrenaline, prostaglandins and thrombin, together with capillary endothelial damage on a background of low flow and increased viscosity, sets the scene for platelet aggregation and clot formation within the capillary beds. This will further exacerbate existing tissue ischaemia and oedema, contributing to ongoing damage to organs.

At the capillary level the activation of coagulation that is occurring in many tissue beds results in a consumption of both platelets and coagulation factors, leading to abnormal clotting with thrombocytopenia and prolonged prothombin and activated partial thromboplastin times. A parallel activation of the fibrinolytic pathway via plasminogen results in a breakdown of these intracapillary clots and an elevation in the circulating levels of fibrin and fibrinogen (D-dimers). These somewhat paradoxical findings of increased capillary coagulation and systemic antiocoagulation on a background of thrombocytopenia and elevated levels of D-dimers is referred to as disseminated intravascular coagulation (DIC). This serious abnormality of coagulation is uncommon and tends to be associated with more severe cases of shock, especially if there is underlying sepsis.

Cellular function

Aerobic metabolism requires a continuous supply of oxygen for the efficient extraction of energy from carbohydrate substrates such as glucose. This occurs within the mitochondria and results in the production of high-energy adenosine triphosphate (ATP). ATP is the energy source for the majority of active processes within the cell. The free hydrogen associated with ATP generation is temporarily scavenged by NAD^+ prior to its ultimate combination with oxygen and disposal as water. Early in shock the oxygen debt results in a saturation of NAD^+ and other scavengers and an accumulation of the intermediate metabolite pyruvic acid, which is prevented from entering the citric acid cycle. In the absence of oxygen, pyruvic acid itself can facilitate the oxidation of NADH to NAD^+ by converting to lactic acid. This allows limited ATP production to continue. Lactic acid accumulates in the systemic circulation and can

be monitored biochemically. In the absence of significant renal or liver disease it is a useful marker of cellular hypoxia and systemic oxygen debt. Sodium is a predominantly extracellular ion and the cell membrane 'sodium pump' is central to the maintenance of cellular homeostasis. The movement of the sodium ion against a concentration gradient is an active process requiring ATP. Any reduction in the ATP supply will lead to the intracellular accumulation of sodium. This in turn results in an osmotic gradient across the cell membrane, encouraging cell oedema. When this is combined with the failure of other vital cell functions and the breakdown of lysosomal membranes leading to the release of enzymes, cell death becomes the inevitable consequence. If the pathophysiological changes responsible for these cellular alterations are widespread and remain uncorrected, multiple organ failure supervenes and recovery is unlikely.

Acid–base balance

Tissue hypoperfusion leads to cellular hypoxia, anaerobic metabolism and the accumulation of lactic acid, which is a major component of the metabolic acidosis associated with shock. Blood gas estimations of both hydrogen ion and lactate concentrations are simple and useful measures of the severity of tissue hypoperfusion. Regular estimations can be helpful in monitoring the effectiveness of the resuscitation measures being undertaken, where a gradual fall in the value of both parameters over time would be expected. If renal function is not compromised the kidneys are able to increase their production of bicarbonate and are an important component of the physiological compensatory mechanisms which attempt to maintain a normal blood hydrogen ion concentration in the face of a metabolic acidosis. However, reduced renal blood flow and vasoconstriction significantly impair bicarbonate production. In cases of severe shock, established renal failure will actively contribute to the acidosis. Chemoreceptor stimulation results in an increase in rate and depth of breathing (minute ventilation), which causes a reduction in arterial carbon dioxide tension ($Pa\text{CO}_2$). In the early stages of shock, when both pain and anxiety may be present, centrally mediated hyperventilation may overcompensate for any metabolic acidosis present, resulting in a blood hydrogen ion below the normal range (respiratory alkalosis). Arterial blood gas assessment

> **SUMMARY BOX**
>
> *Metabolic monitoring in shock*
>
> Regular arterial blood gas sampling with measurement of acid–base status will assist the physician in assessing the effectiveness of the resuscitation.

SUMMARY BOX

The underlying acid–base abnormality in shock is a 'metabolic acidosis' resulting from cellular hypoxia and anaerobic metabolism. An arterial blood gas sample will reveal an elevated H^+, a reduced HCO_3^- level and, if available, an increased lactate concentration.

of $Paco_2$, H^+ and bicarbonate concentrations should be made in order to accurately identify the primary abnormality, its severity and the magnitude of any compensatory mechanisms.

EFFECTS ON VARIOUS ORGAN SYSTEMS

Intrinsic organ autoregulation, combined with an increase in sympathetic activity and circulating catecholamines, is the major compensatory mechanism responsible for the maintenance of an adequate perfusion and oxygen supply to vital organs. This occurs at the expense of both the periphery and non-essential organs. However, these 'sparing' mechanisms have limits, and in the cases of severe, prolonged and uncorrected shock the clinical effects of vital organ hypoperfusion become apparent.

Nervous system

In early shock the effects of pain and increased sympathetic activity may predominate, with the patient appearing inappropriately anxious. As compensatory mechanisms reach their limit and cerebral hypoperfusion and hypoxia supervene there is increasing restlessness, progressing to confusion, stupor and coma. Unless hypoxia has been prolonged effective resuscitation will quickly correct the depressed conscious level. In septic shock the clinical picture may be complicated by the presence of an underlying encephalopathy caused by other factors. This should be considered if, after the shocked state has been reversed, the patient remains confused with altered cognitive function. Unlike the effects of hypoperfusion the encephalopathy may take significantly longer to recover.

Kidneys

The clinical effects of shock on the kidneys reflects the combined effects of the increased sympathetic activity, circulating catecholamines, antidiuretic hormone and aldosterone. Reduced renal blood flow, with diversion of blood from the cortex to the medulla, together with sodium and water conservation results in a low urine output, or oliguria (< 0.5 mL/kg/h). This prerenal abnormality is characterized

by urine which has a normal to high specific gravity and low sodium concentration. If the shocked state is not reversed prolonged hypoxia of the tubular cells will result in damage and ultimately cell death. Acute tubular necrosis (ATN) results in renal failure and is associated with a very low volume of urine, which has a low specific gravity, high sodium concentration and osmolality close to that of plasma. Over the subsequent days a rising blood urea and creatinine in the presence of normovolaemia and an adequate blood pressure will confirm the clinical impression of ATN. Temporary renal replacement therapy may be required while the return of renal function is awaited. Recovery of the tubular function may be signalled by the development of a marked diuresis on a background of high urea and creatinine (diuretic phase of acute renal failure).

Patients in septic shock may present with an inappropriately high urine output in the presence of hypotension. However, an increasing blood urea and creatinine will confirm the presence of acute renal failure (high-output renal failure).

Respiratory system

In the initial phase of shock the patient is frequently tachypnoeic. The reasons for this include the central effects of pain, anxiety and increased sympathetic drive, together with peripheral chemoreceptor stimulation. Early arterial blood gas estimation may reveal a predominantly uncompensated respiratory alkalosis. With the onset of a metabolic acidosis respiratory compensation involves an increase in depth (tidal volume) and rate of breathing in order to raise the minute ventilation and increase CO_2 excretion. In hypovolaemic states the reduction in systemic blood flow is mirrored by an identical reduction in pulmonary blood flow. This decrease in pulmonary perfusion pressure increases the mismatching between lung ventilation and perfusion, so that increased areas of the lung are ventilated but not perfused.

In contrast, during cardiogenic shock left ventricular failure and pulmonary oedema are frequently present. Here there are areas of lung where the presence of pulmonary oedema fluid compromises alveolar ventilation and gas transfer across the alveolar–capillary membrane. This results in alveoli being perfused but not adequately ventilated (increasing the shunt fraction Qs/Qt). This pathological process will contribute to a low arterial oxygen saturation, which may not be reversed by simply increasing the inspired oxygen concentration.

Direct thoracic trauma may lead to pulmonary contusion, fractured ribs, pneumothorax or haemothorax, which can all result in a deterioration in pulmonary gas exchange. Additional insults, such as aspiration of gastric contents, fluid overload following resuscitation, smoke inhalation or central respiratory depression, may contribute to pulmonary insufficiency or precipitate acute respiratory failure. Any severe insult, such as multiple trauma, shock or sepsis, can trigger a systemic cascade of inflammatory mediators mentioned earlier, resulting in increased capillary permeability. The pulmonary manifestation of this systemic process is pulmonary oedema. This pathophysiological process is thought to be responsible for the delayed (24–48 hours) failure of ventilation and oxygenation that is often seen. This is the non-specific but well defined syndrome of adult respiratory distress (ARDS). The diagnosis of ARDS can only be considered after other causes of pulmonary oedema such as pneumonia, left ventricular failure and pulmonary contusion have been excluded. Irrespective of the cause, hypoxia will have profound consequences in patients in whom oxygen delivery to tissues is already compromised by haemodynamic factors.

Heart

In cardiogenic shock the primary abnormality is one of sudden pump failure, commonly due to extensive muscle damage from myocardial infarction. Myocardial function may also be compromised indirectly by a variety of factors associated with other causes of shock. Despite the presence of coronary autoregulation, severe hypotension will eventually result in an imbalance between myocardial oxygen supply and demand. This global decrease in oxygen supply causes ischaemia in the watershed area of the endocardial layer and will impair myocardial contractility. Hypoxia and acidosis depletes myocardial stores of noradrenaline and diminishes the cardiac response to endogenous and exogenous catecholamines. Acid–base and electrolyte abnormalities, when combined with local hypoxia, create conditions which are ideal for increasing myocardial excitability and generating dysrhythmias. Myocardial contractility and ventricular function may be further depressed by the direct action of a variety of circulating humoral factors and activated inflammatory mediators implicated in sepsis and the systemic inflammatory response (see above).

GIT

The gut is considered a non-vital organ and a marked reduction in splanchnic blood flow occurs early in the genesis of shock. Although prolonged mucosal hypoperfusion and hypoxia predispose the gastric mucosa to acid damage, stress ulceration and haemorrhage, subtle mucosal barrier damage to the remainder of the gastrointestinal tract is now considered more important. This process has been implicated in the movement (translocation) of toxic substances, gut bacterial endotoxin as well as the bacteria themselves from the intestinal lumen to the portal bloodstream. Their presence in the systemic circulation has been closely linked to the mechanisms underlying both the sys-

temic inflammatory response syndrome (SIRS) and multiorgan failure (MOF).

Liver

The liver is somewhat protected from ischaemic damage by its dual blood supply from the portal vein and hepatic artery. A significant elevation in serum transaminase levels indicates a major hepatocellular ischaemic–hypoxic injury, and is more commonly observed in severe cardiogenic shock and hepatic venous congestion. Irrespective of the aetiology of the shock state, the presence of biochemical and haematological markers of severe liver damage carries a very poor prognosis.

Neurohumoral response

Many of the clinical signs of shock reflect the central nervous system's attempt to preserve oxygen delivery to

> **SUMMARY BOX**
>
> *Effects of shock on various organs*
>
> **CNS** Progressive hypopertusion – anxiety, restlessness, confusion, stupor, coma
> Sepsis: encephalopathy – prolonged alteration in conscious level
>
> **Renal** Oliguria: < 0.5 mL/kg/h
> Acute renal failure – increasing blood urea and creatinine
> Anuria – acute tubular necrosis (ATN)
> High-output renal failure
>
> **Lungs** Hypovolaemia: alveolar ventilation/perfusion mismatch (V/Q), leading to hypoxia. Reversed by increasing FiO_2
> Cardiogenic: pulmonary oedema – increased proportion of cardiac output through alveoli that are not ventilated, leading to an increase in shunt (Qs/Qt), increasing hypoxia which may not respond to increasing the FiO_2
>
> **Heart** Decrease in diastolic pressure → fall in coronary perfusion pressure
> Increase in heart rate → decrease in period of diastole → decreased coronary blood flow
> Reduced oxygen delivery → ischaemia → increased excitability.
> Depressed contractility
> Acidosis, electrolyte disturbances, hypoxia → dysrhythmias
>
> **GIT** Hypoperfusion → breakdown of gut mucosal barrier
> Translocation of bacteria/bacterial wall contents into bloodstream

vital tissues by maintaining an adequate circulating blood volume, cardiac output and perfusion pressure. Multiple afferent inputs (arterial and venous pressures, vascular volume, osmolality, acidosis, pain, anxiety and tissue damage) trigger an increase in sympathetic outflow activity, leading to peripheral sympathetic stimulation and increased circulating catecholamines from the adrenal glands. This increase in sympathetic activity results in a diversion of blood from the renal cortex to the medulla and stimulates the juxtaglomerular cells to release renin. This in turn activates the renin–angiotensin cascade, leading to elevated circulating levels of the potent vasoconstrictor angiotensin II. In the attempt to maintain the circulating blood volume angiotensin II stimulates the adrenocortical release of aldosterone, resulting in increased sodium and water retention. This early endocrine response is followed by elevations in the concentrations of a number of other stress hormones. Antidiuretic hormone (ADH) acts on the distal tubules of the kidney to conserve water. Adrenocorticotrophic hormone (ACTH) stimulates the adrenal cortex to release cortisol, which plays a major role in the initial protection from the effects of hypovolaemia. Elevated levels of growth hormone and glucagon can also be detected. The combined effects of this complex neurohumoral response is to activate mechanisms that will help to maintain an adequate circulating blood volume and, by mobilizing energy reserves in the form of increased blood glucose, prepare the body for stress.

Inflammatory response

A large number of vasoactive substances have now been identified which are thought to be significant in conditions such as prolonged resistant shock, sepsis, and major trauma. Some of these have a predominantly local action at the level of the microcirculation, whereas others have systemic effects. Lysosomal enzymes can be released in conditions commonly encountered in shocked states such as hypoxia, sepsis, acidosis and ischaemia. In addition to being directly cytotoxic, they act with other substances such as activated factor XII (Hageman Factor) to convert kininogens to active kinins such as bradykinin. Along with locally released histamine and serotonin, these substances are potent vasodilators which increase capillary permeability and tissue oedema. They also have systemic actions, predominantly on the pulmonary vasculature, causing vasoconstriction. The arachidonic acid metabolites are also implicated. PGI_2 acts as a vasodilator and inhibits platelet aggregation, and thromboxane causes vasoconstriction and platelet activation. $PGF_{2\alpha}$ is implicated in the early pulmonary hypertension seen in septic shock. Within the capillaries the activated leukocytes and macrophages release a variety of substances, such as proteolytic enzymes (elastase), oxygen free radicals, vasoactive compounds

(leukotrienes, prostaglandins, platelet-activating factor) and cytokines (tumour necrosis factor-α IL-1, IL-6). The inflammatory response should be viewed as a dynamic process, with the above only a selection of the many substances that are acting either together in a complementary fashion or in opposing ways to produce the metabolic and microcirculatory derangements associated with sepsis and shock.

> **SUMMARY BOX**
>
> *Principles of management*
>
> Irrespective of the cause, the first concern of the physician is the restoration of an adequate oxygen delivery to all organs, tissues and cells.

PRINCIPLES OF MANAGEMENT

Irrespective of the cause of shock, the primary concern of the physician should be the restoration of an adequate oxygen delivery to all organs, tissues and cells. This requires restoring the circulating blood volume and a sufficient functioning red blood cell mass in order to deliver sufficient oxygen to satisfy the body's aerobic demands. An adequate cardiac output and mean arterial pressure to produce a satisfactory perfusion pressure is also necessary. These aims will be addressed with attention to ABC (airway, breathing and circulation). Any early resuscitation measures can be undertaken in parallel with investigation of the underlying cause. Resuscitatation should not be delayed because of a lack of diagnosis; however, its ultimate success will depend largely on the detection and treatment of the cause (e.g. stopping haemorrhage, draining the source of sepsis).

Hypovolaemic shock
Clinical assessment

Although obtaining a history from either the patient or witnesses can be helpful it may often prove impossible when the patient's consciousness is impaired from head injury, alcohol or drugs, or as a direct result of cerebral hypoperfusion.

In many cases, such as major trauma or burns, the presence of volume loss is obvious. In other situations (diabetic ketoacidosis, diarrhoea and vomiting, dehydration), both assessment and diagnosis become more problematical.

Cardiovascular assessment begins with observing the patient's colour, a pale skin suggesting a reduction of oxygenated blood through the skin capillaries. Palpation of a peripheral pulse will give valuable information on rate and volume and whether the skin feels warm and dry or cold and clammy. Capillary refill following nailbed pressure can be assessed. With this information alone the physician can make a quick and often accurate assessment as to the patient's volume status. Clearly, if the patient is pale, with a rapid low-volume pulse, skin which is cold and moist, delayed capillary refill and collapsed veins, the clinical picture is one of reduced cardiac output on a background of hypovolaemia and excess sympathetic activity. In contrast, a lucid patient with warm, dry pink skin with rapid capillary refill is unlikely to have significant hypovolaemia. The volume status may be further assessed by observing the height of the JVP as an estimate of central venous pressure.

The successful management of shock depends on early and frequent clinical monitoring of the patient's volume status and perfusion, as described above. In addition, there are a number of simple measurements of cardiovascular function and organ perfusion that can be made to help in the clinical assessment.

SUMMARY BOX

Clinical features of hypovolaemic shock

- Patient often anxious, restless and confused
- Skin pale, cool and clammy, with collapsed veins
- Pulse fast and thready; may be difficult to palpate limb pulses
- JVP not seen
- The successful management of shock depends upon the early and frequent clinical assessment of the patient's peripheral perfusion and volume status.

Blood pressure

Blood pressure will depend on the patient's volume status (relative in the case of septic shock and absolute in hypovolaemic shock), myocardial function and efficiency of compensatory mechanisms initiated by the sympathetic nervous system. These in turn will be influenced by the patient's premorbid cardiovascular state, age (which influences 'normal' blood pressure), ongoing resuscitation measures and additional comorbidities present. Taken in isolation, a satisfactory blood pressure does not exclude the presence of a shocked state and is only of use when placed in the context of a full clinical assessment.

This is particularly true of children.

Electrocardiogram (ECG) monitoring

The ECG is a measure of myocardial electrical activity and not of the heart's ability to act as a mechanical pump. It will detect dysrhythmias and severe myocardial ischaemia. It is more useful in cardiogenic shock, myocardial dysfunction secondary to ischaemia, or contusion as a result of severe thoracic injury. Severe hypoxia, electrolyte abnormality or acid–base disturbance can aggravate or precipitate abnormalities in electrical activity and myocardial contractility.

Pulse oximetry

When attached peripherally to a finger or earlobe the pulse oximeter will give information on the pulse volume as an estimate of peripheral perfusion and measure the oxygen saturation of the haemoglobin on the arterial side of the capillary. The screen will display a pulse waveform and a value of the percentage oxygen saturation of haemoglobin. As a simple non-invasive monitor it gives valuable information on the adequacy of arterial oxygenation and peripheral tissue perfusion. In the poorly perfused state it will provide a visual and audible warning of a poor signal and confirm the clinical impression.

Core to periphery temperature gradient

Peripheral and core (axillary, nasopharyngeal) temperature measurement can be made and the gradient calculated Δt (Fig 3.4). This is a useful measure of peripheral perfusion, as the gradient can be significant in the presence of severe vasoconstriction (>10°C). With volume replacement, improved cardiac output and reduced sympathetic activity,

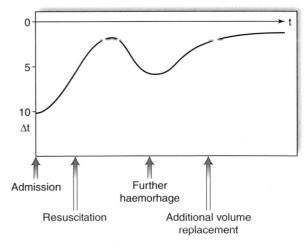

Fig. 3.4 Response of temperature gradient to resuscitation.

there will be an increase in the flow of warm blood through the skin, a rise in peripheral temperature and a decrease in the gradient. It can be used as a simple but accurate index of adequacy of resuscitation and an early indicator of ongoing blood loss. A lower than normal core temperature (hypothermia) is frequently found in trauma patients who have lain in a cold environment, but may also be seen in those who have received large volumes of unwarmed intravenous fluids.

The measurement of the core-peripheral temperature gradient is a particularly useful measurement in small children and neonates.

Urine output

Unless there is a contraindication (such as the possibility of urethral injury from severe pelvic fractures) the transurethral insertion of a bladder catheter connected to a graduated collecting device will allow an hourly measurement of urine output. This can be used as an indirect measurement of vital organ perfusion, namely the kidney. An adequate urine output (> 0.5 mL/kg/h) would suggest satisfactory renal perfusion. An increase in the urine output is frequently used as indicator of successful resuscitation.

Central venous catheterization

With the increasing availability of large-bore multilumen catheter packs, a catheter can be inserted percutaneously over a wire into a large central vein and the tip positioned in the superior vena cava. These catheters give the clinician secure vascular access to administer large volumes of fluid quickly at the same time as continuously monitoring the filling pressures on the right side of the heart (CVP). They are not essential in the early stages of the resuscitation process as fluid can administered by the insertion of one or two peripheral large-bore intravenous cannulae, and the volume status can be assessed by clinical examination. However, following the initial resuscitation CVP estimation can help in deciding the requirements for further measures. It can also aid the identification of patients who may appear to be clinically normovolaemic but remain volume deplete (subclinical hypovolaemia).

At the extremes of measurement the CVP gives an accurate indication of volume status (Fig. 3.5), with negative values being associated with significant hypovolaemia and high values (> 20 mmHg) indicating volume overload, seen in cardiac failure or cardiogenic shock. However, between these extremes isolated measurements become unreliable as an indicator of volume status. With minor to moderate hypovolaemia patients may not exhibit any classic signs of

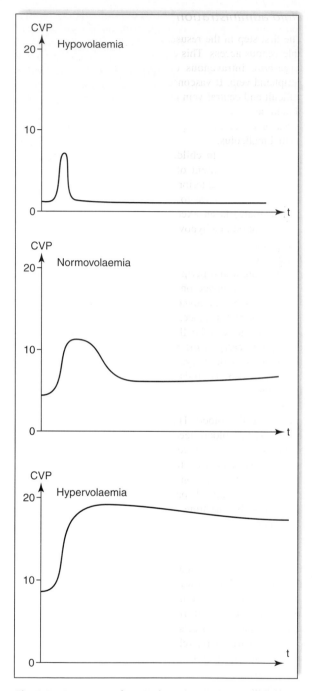

Fig. 3.5 Response of central venous pressure to fluid challenge.

shock and have a CVP value within the normal range. These patients can be identified by observing the response of their CVP to a fluid challenge (i.e. 200 mL colloid over 10 minutes).

Fluid administration

The first step in the resuscitation process is to obtain reliable venous access. This can be done by siting one or two large-bore intravenous cannulae (16 G or larger) in a peripheral vein. If vasoconstriction is intense access may be difficult and central vein cannulation or a formal cut-down should be considered. This is performed in the antecubital fossa or on to the long saphenous vein in front of the medial malleolus.

In children under the age of six, placement of an intraosseus needle into the anterior aspect of the upper tibia, (taking care to avoid damaging the epiphyseal growth plate) is an excellent alternative route for fluid administration in a hypovolaemic child.

Successful resuscitation depends on quick and adequate volume replacement in order to restore a satisfactory cardiac output and peripheral perfusion. The type of fluid lost has no influence on the initial choice of intravenous fluid replacement, both colloid and/or crystalloid being utilized in the first instance. In the case of continued haemorrhage and shock, red cell concentrates or whole blood will be required early in the resuscitation in order to maintain tissue oxygen delivery. Ideally, suitably cross-matched blood should be administered but in the emergency situation most accident and emergency departments hold a 'shock pack', which will include a quantity of group O rhesus-negative blood. This can be used until such time as cross-matched blood becomes available. Infusion of large volumes of crystalloid, colloid or stored blood will result in the dilution of clotting factors and platelets which, when combined with their consumption in major bleeding, may result in a generalized coagulopathy, contributing to further blood loss. By the time the volume transfused equates to the patient's calculated blood volume (approximately 5 L), consideration should be given to requesting a coagulation screen and administering replacement in the form of fresh-frozen plasma and platelet concentrate. Unless active measures are taken to warm all fluids to 37°C, the administration of large volumes of stored blood at 4°C or colloid/crystalloid at room temperature will result in hypothermia, with effects on coagulation and oxygen delivery being particularly relevant. The use of blood-warming equipment such as the 'Level 1' (Fig. 3.6) will allow the administration of up to 1000 mL/min of intravenous fluids warmed to body temperature.

Metabolic monitoring

In addition to venous blood being sent for full blood count and cross-matching, urea and electrolyte estimation should be undertaken. The results will provide a baseline and identify any pre-existing renal dysfunction. More importantly,

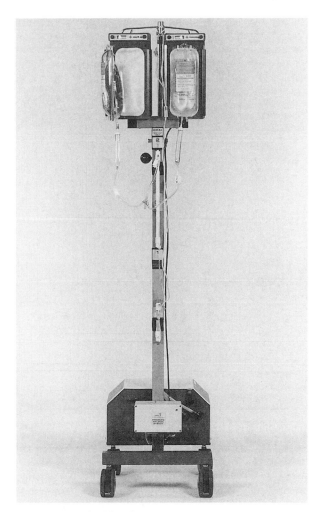

Fig. 3.6   Level 1 blood warmer.

arterial blood gas samples taken both early and frequently will aid in the early identification of respiratory failure, as indicated by the presence of hypoxia and/or hypercarbia. A low Pao_2 may simply require an increase in inspired oxygen concentration (40–60% via face mask), but should this prove to be inadequate, thought should be given to potential causes and assisted ventilation considered. An elevated arterial $Paco_2$ indicates respiratory insufficiency which, if confirmed on clinical examination, requires assisted ventilation together with identifying the underlying cause. Metabolic acidosis with increased base deficit, reduced level of bicarbonate (HCO_3^-) and an elevated blood lactate are the most frequently encountered abnormalities. They will correct rapidly when the circulating blood volume and cardiac output are restored. In severe cases (pH < 7.2 and base excess > 10) not responding to volume replacement a small volume of intravenous 8.4% sodium bicarbonate (50–100 mL) may help to improve myocardial contractility and correct any associated hyperkalaemia. As with the clinical examination, it is the frequent estimation of acid–base status, arterial blood gases and lactate concentrations over time that will give the most information on the effectiveness of the resuscitation process.

> **SUMMARY BOX**
>
> *Aids to the clinical assessment of shock*
>
> - Blood pressure measurement
> - Electrocardiogram (ECG) monitoring
> - Pulse oximetry
> - Core to periphery temperature gradient
> - Urine output
> - CVP measurement
> - In isolation, single measurements are not helpful. They become useful when used in combination with the findings of the clinical examination to confirm the clinical impression. Repeated measurements over time, trends and patterns, together with the changes associated with therapeutic interventions, increase their usefulness.

Analgesia

In the conscious patient with severe trauma there is no indication for withholding effective analgesia. In addition to the primary purpose of relieving pain, it also reduces the associated sequelae of anxiety and sympathetic overactivity that may be contributing to the pathophysiological derangements underlying the shocked state. Short-acting analgesics are inappropriate and in hypovolaemic shock there is no place for subcutaneous or intramuscular administration, as the reduced peripheral blood flow results in unreliable and unpredictable absorption. A long-acting agent such as morphine, given in 1–2 mg increments and titrated against effect, is appropriate. With constant monitoring of conscious level and respiratory function it should be possible to obtain satisfactory pain control without any significant sequelae of parenteral opiate administration. With a reduced circulating blood volume and decreased hepatic and renal blood flows, the pharmocokinetics of drugs such as morphine will be altered, making analgesic requirements difficult to predict. In general, patients appear to be more sensitive to the effects of opiates, with a subsequent reduction in dose requirements. Their duration of action will also be unpredictable, making recommendations difficult, but additional doses may be required every 30–60 minutes. Although the use of local anaesthetic techniques such as local infiltration and regional nerve blockade should be considered, they are frequently impractical in the presence of multiple injuries and are contraindicated in coagulopathy. With unilateral rib fractures multiple intercostal nerve blocks will produce superior analgesia while reducing the requirements for parenteral opiates.

Summary

The most important principle in the acute management of hypovolaemic shock is the rapid restoration and maintenance of an appropriate circulating blood volume, necessary to maintain a cardiac output adequate for peripheral perfusion and oxygen delivery to all capillary beds. Continued pharmacological support of the cardiovascular system (inotropes) should not be required in uncomplicated hypovolaemic shock, and should alert the clinician to possible myocardial impairment, severe acid–base/electrolyte abnormalities, hypoxia or, in the case of the older patient, the presence of underlying ischaemic heart disease. The need for continued inotropic support will require a higher level of invasive monitoring, necessitating transfer to either a high-dependency or intensive care unit.

If hypovolaemic shock does not respond to simple measures of fluid replacement and oxygen administration consideration should be given to additional complicating factors, such as:

- Underestimation of the magnitude of blood/fluid loss
- Ongoing concealed haemorrhage
- Impaired myocardial contractility due to cardiac tamponade, tension pneumothorax or direct injury, leading to myocardial contusion
- Underlying sepsis
- Secondary cardiovascular effects due to delay in instituting treatment, resulting in severe acid–base and electrolyte disturbances.

Septic shock

The principles of resuscitation remain the same as those for hypovolaemic shock, that is, to maintain an adequate oxygen delivery to all capillary beds. This requires a sufficient amount of haemoglobin, together with an adequate circulating blood volume and a satisfactory cardiac output to produce perfusion in all capillary beds. Significant hypovolaemia confirmed by a low or static CVP in the face of a fluid challenge may initially be present. This will either be true hypovolaemia due to excessive fluid loss from increased capillary permeability, or a relative hypovolaemia as a result of systemic vasodilatation characteristic of this condition. This pathological reduction in systemic vascular resistance results in hypotension, a reduction in cardiac afterload and a compensatory increase in cardiac output.

This reduction in total body vascular resistance conceals marked differences between and within organs. The pathological development of arteriolar–venous shunts results in the effective bypassing of capillary beds, hypoperfusion and cellular hypoxia. When this occurs in vital organs their function becomes compromised. These abnormalities in capillary bed perfusion are characterized by a reduction in the arteriovenous oxygen difference and a decreased oxygen extraction ratio, both of which contribute, along with the elevated cardiac output, to an abnormally high oxygen saturation of the blood returning to the heart (SvO_2). The associated lactic acidosis is further confirmation of tissue hypoperfusion, cellular hypoxia and anaerobic metabolism. Despite the pathological increase in cardiac output myocardial function is frequently impaired, partly as a result of the above alterations in the myocardial microcirculation but also from the presence of a variety of circulating inflammatory mediators, which have myocardial depressant properties. Therefore, the principles of resuscitation in septic shock are:

1. Volume replacement in order to maintain the cardiac preload or CVP
2. The administration of oxygen to optimize total body oxygen delivery
3. Maintaining a blood pressure that would be considered appropriate for the individual patient, in the hope that it might ensure adequate organ perfusion
4. Investigate the cause of sepsis.

On a background of a high cardiac output an intravenous infusion of a vasoconstrictor, such as noradrenaline, may be considered. In the severest cases, where there is evidence of organ dysfunction despite aggressive resuscitation and cardiovascular monitoring, admission to an intensive care unit for additional monitoring and/or organ support may be indicated. Although an infective agent is frequently implicated, this is not always the case and the systemic inflammatory response syndrome (SIRS) can be associated with noninfective conditions such as severe pancreatitis, trauma or vasculitis. Where an infective organism is being considered common sites are the chest, abdomen and urinary tract. Blood cultures, together with appropriate samples (urine, sputum, discharges), should be sent for urgent Gram staining, culture and sensitivities. Where the source is not obvious repeated blood cultures should be obtained, and consideration should also be given to atypical organisms and, in certain groups of patients (immunocompromised), infections with fungi. Multiresistant organisms may be responsible in patients who have received broad-spectrum antibiotics or those who have had a long hospital stay. In the case of many intra-abdominal conditions, antibiotic therapy should only be considered as a supplement to surgical intervention. Initial therapy is usually empirical with a broad-spectrum antibiotic in order to cover the most likely organisms. Following bacteriological culture and sensitivity the antibiotic may have to be changed or the spectrum narrowed.

SUMMARY BOX

Clinical features of sepsis

- Restlessness and confusion: cerebral hypoperfusion
- Tachypnoea: metabolic acidosis
- Tachycardia: reflex in response to reduced systemic vascular resistance
- Warm, dry, pink extremities: systemic vasodilatation
- Large-volume pulse: elevated cardiac output
- Systolic pressure:
  (1) Normal: preserved myoardial function
  (2) Low: depressed myocardial function
- Oliguria

Cardiogenic shock

The stress and cardiovascular instability observed with many acute surgical emergencies and major elective surgery predispose an increasingly elderly population to the risk of myocardial ischaemia and infarction. The pathogenesis is more frequently due to an imbalance between myocardial oxygen supply and demand, rather than a discrete occlusion of a coronary vessel. This often results in a subendocardial distribution of myocardial damage, rather than the more classic transmural lesion. The clinical diagnosis of pump failure is made on the basis of a low-output state similar to that seen with hypovolaemia on a background of an adequate circulating blood volume (high JVP). Following the diagnosis the patient should be transferred to a high-dependency area for continuous monitoring of blood pressure, ECG, SaO_2, CVP and urine output. Immediate therapy may include the administration of high-flow oxygen (minimum of 40%), together with intravenous opiates (morphine in 1–2 mg increments) to control pain, reduce anxiety and produce vasodilatation. The presence of a severe metabolic acidosis will contribute to poor myocardial function, which will not improve until there is an increase in cardiac output. The administration of small volumes of 8.4% sodium bicarbonate (50–100 ml), together with the regular monitoring of acid–base status and serum sodium, will allow for temporary pharmacological correction in the hope that this will result in an improvement in myocardial contractility, reflected in an increase in cardiac output. High-dose intravenous diuretics may be required to manage oliguria.

Should these simple measures fail to improve the patient's clinical condition, consideration should be made to transfer them to a coronary care or intensive care area, as additional invasive monitoring in the form of a pulmonary artery flotation catheter, together with the intravenous administration of vasodilators and/or inotropes, may be required in order to optimize myocardial function. Along with cardiovascular monitoring and support, the clinical diagnosis should be confirmed. This will require serial 12-lead ECGs and cardiac enzyme estimations to confirm myocardial damage. A transthoracic echocardiogram will give useful information on the state of left ventricular contractility, as well as excluding other cardiac causes of cardiogenic shock, such as pericardial tamponade, acute valve rupture and massive pulmonary embolus.

Anaphylactic shock

The cardiovascular collapse and shocked state associated with acute anaphylaxis is due to a sudden generalized vasodilatation, resulting in an imbalance between the capacity of the vascular compartment and the circulating blood volume. This relative hypovolaemia is quickly followed by increased capillary permeability and intravascular fluid loss, adding a hypovolaemic component to the shocked state. The common precipitating antigens, such as antibiotics, synthetic colloids, blood and blood components, are frequently encountered in a surgical ward. The principles in the early management are similar to those of other causes of shock, namely the maintenance of a satisfactory circulating blood volume and cardiac output in order to maintain a supply of oxygen to meet requirements. Apart from the discontinuation of the precipitating agent, this will involve the administration of high-flow oxygen, either via a face mask or following endotracheal intubation and artificial ventilation in more severe cases. There may be apnoea, cardiac arrest, severe bronchospasm, or the upper airway can be compromised with laryngeal oedema.

Incremental doses of 1–2 mL 1:100 000 adrenaline will act to stimulate myocardial contraction and, through peripheral vasoconstriction, decrease the volume of the vascular compartment. In addition, it will relieve any bronchoconstriction present and reduce peripheral oedema. The loss of intravascular fluid from the increased capillary permeability should be corrected by the rapid administration of intravenous fluids. Patients should be transferred to a high-dependency area for intensive clinical, cardiovascular and respiratory monitoring. Continuous ECG monitoring will allow for the early detection of dysrrhythmias resulting from hypoxia, hypotension or inotropes administration. CVP monitoring will help to guide intravenous fluid requirements, which can be considerable. As with other causes of shock, regular monitoring of arterial blood gases and acid–base status must be undertaken along with urea

and electrolytes, full blood count and clotting screens. Prolonged organ support with infusions of inotropes, bronchodilators or artificial ventilation will require transfer to an intensive care unit.

ADVANCED MONITORING AND ORGAN SUPPORT

Whereas uncomplicated hypovolaemic shock can be managed adequately in the setting of a general ward or high-dependency unit, patients with additional complications, septic or cardiogenic shock, and those with evidence of significant organ dysfunction will require invasive monitoring and continuous nursing and medical care that can only be delivered in an intensive care unit.

In such a unit medical staff will not only diagnose and manage the underlying pathology responsible for the shocked state, but are able to monitor individual organ function and intervene with either support or replacement threrapy until the underlying pathophysiological process is corrected.

Cardiovascular monitoring

Intra-arterial measurement of blood pressure

Using the Seldinger technique, a 20 G cannula can be inserted percutaneously into the radial artery. If the patient is vasoconstricted the femoral artery is often used. Via a saline-filled line, the mechanical pressure wave can be electrically transduced at a point distal to the artery and a continuous pressure wave displayed on a monitor. These lines allow access for the multiple arterial blood gas sampling which is an integral part of patient monitoring.

Pulmonary artery flotation catheter (PAFC)

In those patients who do not respond to the normal resuscitation measures of fluid replacement and remain shocked despite CVP evidence of normovolaemia, the PAFC gives the physician the opportunity to measure and monitor additional variables of cardiac function. The PAFC is a 100 cm long catheter with multiple lumina, one of which opens at the tip. An additional channel is connected to a small balloon at the tip which can be inflated by means of a 2 mL syringe. The catheter is inserted percutaneously through a large-bore cannula sited in a central vein. Once the catheter is within the blood vessel the balloon is inflated. The catheter will then float with the blood flow through the right side of the heart, lodging itself in a branch of the pulmonary artery. By transducing the pressure within the catheter lumen that is in continuity with the tip, the passage of the catheter can be monitored by observing the characteristic changes in the pressure waveform as it passes down the SVC, through the right atrium and ventricle, before coming to rest in the pulmonary artery. The balloon is deflated and the pulmonary artery pressure monitored continuously. If the balloon is inflated in the pulmonary artery it will move forward and become wedged in a more distal arterial branch. A pressure measurement taken at this point is called a pulmonary capillary wedge pressure (PCWP). Because there is now a solid uninterrupted column of blood between the end of the catheter and the left atrium, the measurement taken will in most instances provide an accurate estimate of left atrial filling pressure. Modern catheters now have the additional facility of continuously and automatically measuring cardiac output. Thus a PAFC can directly measure CVP, right atrial pressure, right ventricular pressure, pulmonary artery pressure, PCWP (estimation of left atrial filling pressure) and cardiac output. By sampling blood from the distal lumen of the catheter oxygen saturation and content of the mixed venous blood from the pulmonary artery can be measured. From these values, together with heart rate and arterial blood pressure, it is possible to calculate a large number of derived values, such as systemic vascular resistance, oxygen delivery (DO_2) and oxygen consumption (VO_2), which help in the monitoring of shocked patients and the effectiveness of any therapeutic manoeuvres undertaken.

Gastric tonometry

It is now recognized that the splanchnic circulation is one of the earliest vascular beds to be compromised in shock. By monitoring the CO_2 gap between an air filled intragastric tonometry balloon in the stomach and an arterial blood sample one can identify splanchnic hypoperfusion and cellular hypoxia resulting in anaerobic metabolism and increasing acidosis.

Pharmacological agents used to treat shock

The pharmacological agents used in the treatment of shock come under the broad heading of inotropes.

Noradrenaline

This causes predominantly α stimulation, resulting in an increase in systemic vascular resistance, leading to peripheral vasoconstriction and an elevation in mean arterial blood pressure. It is commonly used in septic shock, where the underlying pathophysiological process results in an inability to maintain a satisfactory mean arterial pressure due to a greatly reduced systemic vascular resistance.

Adrenaline

This is used for its combined inotropic ($β_1$) and vasoconstrictor (α effects). It would not be considered as a first-line

drug but may be used for intractable shock which is not responsive to other inotropes.

Dobutamine

This is a synthetic inotrope with predominantly $β_1$ and $β_2$ action, causing increased myocardial contraction with vasodilatation of some vascular beds and a reduction in systemic vascular resistance, thereby offloading the heart. It is a first-line drug in cardiogenic shock.

Dopexamine

Dopexamine is a newer synthetic inotrope with actions similar to those of dobutamine. It has been demonstrated that it also has a more specific vasodilatory action on the splanchnic vascular bed, and may have an advantage in certain shocked states where splanchnic hypoperfusion is a significant component, such as septic shock.

These are very powerful drugs which are administered via a large central vein, with continuous monitoring of the patient's cardiovascular parameters in the setting of an HDU or ICU.

Respiratory support

As a result of the pathophysiological derangements in shock there is frequently an increase in the mismatch between perfusion and ventilation in the lungs. This abnormality results in an increase in venous blood mixing with the fully oxygenated blood entering the left atrium (increasing shunt), reducing the overall oxygen content of the blood entering the arterial circulation. This is reflected in a fall in the oxygen saturation as measured with the pulse oximeter. This defect can usually be corrected by increasing the fraction of inspired oxygen from room air (21%) by administering supplemental oxygen (40–60%).

In a small number of patients where the process is so severe that increasing the inspired oxygen concentration is not sufficient to correct the hypoxia, exhaustion will set in owing to the increased effort of breathing (identified on clinical examination and arterial blood gas evidence of an inability of excrete CO_2). In these patients additional measures must be taken to protect the airway and assist ventilation. This is also the case in patients where cerebral hypoperfusion or septic encephalopathy has resulted in a reduced level of consciousness, putting their airway at risk from obstruction or aspiration. Induction of anaesthesia is necessary to aid endotracheal intubation and artificial ventilation until the underlying cause is reversed.

Renal support

In the most severe cases of shock there is renal vasoconstriction and hypoperfusion. Acute tubular necrosis

(ATN) may occur if resuscitation is not adequate. ATN is irreversible in the short term, but if the premorbid renal function was normal and the underlying precipitating insult is treated, renal function will usually return within 3–6 weeks. In the interim renal replacement is required.

The indications for replacement therapy reflect the lost functions of the kidney, and include:

1. Control of fluid balance to prevent fluid overload and pulmonary oedema
2. Reduction of blood urea to avoid the systemic effects of severe uraemia.
3. Control of hyperkalaemia
4. Normalization of acid–base status.

Continuous veno-veno haemofiltration (CVVH)

This is the replacement therapy of choice in the early stage of the patient's ICU stay, when there may be ongoing CVS instability. Via a double-lumen large-bore catheter introduced into a large central vein, blood can be mechanically withdrawn and pumped through a haemofiltration circuit at 200–300 mL/min. This is sufficient to produce a filtrate volume in excess of 1000 mL/h, which can be replaced with an equal volume of an appropriate electrolyte solution. This technique is continuous and requires a minimal amount of anticoagulation to prevent clotting within the filter. As only a relatively small volume of blood passes through the extracorporeal circuit it confers a degree of cardiovascular stability not obtainable with other methods.

Intermittent haemodialysis

Although this technique is more effective than CVVH in solute removal it is rarely the initial choice for replacement therapy. It results in a greater degree of cardiovascular instability and disequilibrium (acute changes in osmolality), which would not be tolerated by the unstable patient. Haemodialysis is frequently started in the convalescent phase, when the patient is recovering and waiting for the return of native renal function. It can be undertaken over short periods (4 h), often on alternate days, and should not delay the patient's mobilization or further recovery.

NUTRITION

Consideration should always be given to the patient's nutritional state. The shocked state is an intensively catabolic condition in which there is rapid protein breakdown. This can have significant effects on both wound healing and immune status. In an attempt to attenuate these effects artificial nutrition should be considered early on in the disease process. If the GIT is intact and there is no contraindication, then enteral nutrition is the method of choice.

Failure to institute enteral nutrition will require a dedicated line inserted into a central vein and the administration of total parenteral nutrition in an attempt to attenuate the stress response to shock, thereby reducing complications and speeding up recovery.

4 Transfusion of blood and blood products

R. Green, D.B.L. McClelland

Blood transfusion can be life-saving and many areas of surgery could not be undertaken without reliable transfusion support. However, as with any treatment, transfusion of blood and its components carries potential risks, which must be outweighed by the patient's need. The magnitude of risk depends on factors such as the prevalence of infectious disease in the donor population, the resources and dedication of the organization collecting, processing and issuing the blood and blood products, and the care with which the clinical team administers these products.

BLOOD DONATION

In the UK whole blood is donated by healthy adult volunteers aged 17–65 years with normal haemoglobin levels. The standard 480 mL donation contains approximately 200 mg of iron, the loss of which can be withstood readily every 4 months by healthy donors. Blood components (platelets and plasma) can be separated from the donated blood or obtained from the donor as separate products by the use of a cell separator, a process called apheresis.

Strict donor selection and the testing of all donations is essential to exclude blood that may be hazardous to the recipient, as well as ensuring the welfare of the donor. All donations are ABO grouped, Rhesus D typed, antibody screened, and tested for hepatitis B antigen and antibody to hepatitis C, human immunodeficiency virus (HIV) I and II and syphilis. Antibody to cytomegalovirus (CMV) is also tested to provide CMV-negative blood for patients such as transplant recipients and premature infants. Where available, nucleic acid testing (NAT) for viral DNA/RNA is additionally performed, thereby reducing the risk of window-period transmission when antibody has not yet been formed or is lower than the detection limits of the current tests.

BLOOD COMPONENTS

The components that can be prepared from donated blood are shown in Figure 4.1 and their descriptions follow. Since 1999 all blood donated in the UK has been filtered to remove white blood cells (called leukodepletion), and UK

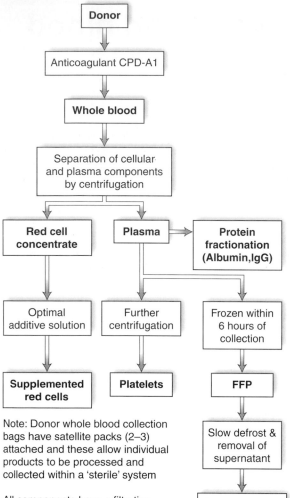

Note: Donor whole blood collection bags have satellite packs (2–3) attached and these allow individual products to be processed and collected within a 'sterile' system

All components have a filtration step at some stage in production

Fig. 4.1 Products which can be obtained from one unit of donated whole blood.

plasma has been excluded from fractionation as a precautionary measure to prevent the theoretical risk of transmission of variant Creutzfeldt–Jakob (vCJD) disease by transfusion.

FRESH BLOOD COMPONENTS

Whole blood

Donated whole blood is drawn into 63 mL of an anticoagulant (citrate) nutrient (phosphate, dextrose and adenine) solution in which it can be stored for up to 35 days at $4 \pm 2°C$. Despite the provision of nutrients, changes in the

red cells do occur during storage and the haemostatic properties of the blood decline. Platelets are non-functional after exposure to 4°C, and there are no functional granulocytes following leukodepletion. Concentrations of the labile factors V and VIII decrease quickly in the first week of storage, and are at only 30% of their original value at the end of their shelf-life. The blood is not sterilized, so that whole blood transfusion can transmit organisms not detected by donor screening.

There are few situations where plasma, proteins and red cells are all needed. Whole blood is therefore an inefficient means of giving red cells or haemostatic factors and can cause cardiac failure when used in patients with chronic anaemia. It may be indicated when rapid large-volume transfusion is needed, as in patients who have suffered major trauma. Transfused blood must be ABO and Rh(D) compatible with the recipient and transfused through a sterile blood administration set designed for the procedure. The filter in the administration set is intended to remove aggregates of cells, small clots etc. formed during storage. It may be less necessary with leukodepleted blood components, but no-one has proposed dropping the requirement. The set should be primed with saline and no other solutions transfused simultaneously.

Red blood cells in additive solution

This is prepared from a unit of donated whole blood by removing all of the associated plasma by centrifugation, and then adding a saline, adenine and glucose solution. The final product has a haematocrit of 55–65% and a volume of 300 mL. This product has a shelf-life of up to 42 days and is the most commonly available form of red cells for transfusion in the UK. The risk of infection, storage considerations and administration safeguards are those that apply to whole blood.

This product is indicated in most forms of anaemia, but should be used with caution in patients with renal failure because of the risk of the adenine in the additive solution crystallizing in the renal tubules.

Platelets

Some 50–60 mL of platelet concentrate can be produced from a unit of whole blood by centrifugation. The resulting unit contains more than 55×10^9 platelets and a small amount of red cells, and can be stored on an agitator for 5 days at 20–24°C. An adult dose is manufactured from four of these pooled together. Platelet concentrates therefore carry a greater infection risk than whole blood, as each transfusion exposes the recipient to the blood of four donors. Bacterial contamination is also more likely, as platelets cannot be refrigerated. Platelets are infused through a standard blood-giving set over less than 30 minutes. As the concentrate contains some red cells and plasma, it should ideally be ABO and Rh(D) compatible with the recipient. Females of childbearing age must receive Rh(D)-compatible platelets, or prophylactic Rh(D) immunoglobulin should be given. An adult dose (pool of four individual donations) should raise an adult platelet count by $20–40\,000 \times 10^9$/L.

Platelet concentrates are indicated in thrombocytopenia, when platelet function is defective, and when there is microvascular bleeding (oozing from mucous membranes, needle puncture sites and wounds) in patients receiving massive blood transfusions.

Fresh frozen plasma (FFP)

Some 200–300 mL of plasma can be removed within 6 hours of donation from a unit of whole blood and stored frozen at $-30°C$. FFP contains albumin, immunoglobulins and, most importantly, all of the coagulation factors. FFP can be stored at $-30°C$ for a year and is thawed to $37°C$ before issue. FFP must be ABO compatible with the recipient and should be given within 4 hours of thawing. The average adult dose is three to four units. Virally inactivated plasma is now available for use in recipients who will require repeated exposures to FFP, and for neonates.

FFP is used when there are multiple coagulation defects (e.g. disseminated intravascular coagulation (DIC)) and when there has been an overdose of the anticoagulant warfarin (bleeding with an INR of > 8.0); however, there are now heat-treated products which should be used in preference.

Cryoprecipitate

A single unit of cryoprecipitate can be removed from one unit of FFP after controlled thawing. After resuspension in 10–20 mL plasma the cryoprecipitate is frozen once more to $-30°C$. It contains fibrinogen, factor VIII and fibronectin, and can be stored for up to a year. Cryoprecipitate carries the same basic risk of transmitting infection as does whole blood, but as an adult dose is normally 10 units the recipient is exposed to material from 10 donors. ABO compatibility is achieved whenever possible, and the product is infused as soon as possible after thawing. It is used when fibrinogen levels are low, as in DIC, as well as in bleeding associated with uraemia.

PLASMA FRACTIONS

Fractionated products are manufactured from large pools (several thousand donations) of donor plasma which undergo some form of viral inactivation stage through the manufacturing process. Virus inactivation processes now

mean that these products should not transmit HIV I and II or hepatitis B and C, but this may not apply to heat-resistant viruses that have no lipid envelope (e.g. hepatitis A).

Human albumin

Albumin is prepared by fractionation of large pools of plasma that at the end of processing is pasteurized at $60°C$ for 10 hours. Because of this heat treatment these products have an excellent safety record in terms of viral transmission. There are no compatibility requirements. Recently a systematic review of clinical trials on the use of albumin suggested that there may be no clear benefit from the use of albumin solutions in the treatment of hypovolaemia or hypoalbuminaemia, and that in fact there was a higher mortality in patients treated with albumin for these indications. Clearly, careful consideration should be given before prescribing this product to individual patients.

Solutions of 4.5 or 5% are used to maintain plasma albumin levels in conditions where there is increased vascular permeability, i.e. burns, and are sometimes used in acute blood volume replacement, although crystalloid or non-plasma colloid solution are as effective and would be the recommended first-line volume expander until >20% of the blood volume has been replaced. Resuscitation with crystalloid requires three times greater volumes of fluid than with colloid.

Twenty percent solutions can be used when hypoproteinaemia is associated with oedema and is resistant to diuretics (e.g. liver disease, nephrotic syndrome); 20% albumin is hyperoncotic, so that there is a risk of acutely expanding the intravascular space and precipitating pulmonary oedema.

Prothrombin complex concentrates

This product contains factors II, IX and X, and may also contain factor VII. Prothrombin complex concentrates, which include other vitamin K-dependent factors (II, VII and X), may be used in warfarin overdose where there is major bleeding. Care must be taken in patients with liver disease as this therapy may be thrombogenic.

Immunoglobulin preparations (90% IgG)

These are prepared from fractionation of large pools of plasma from unselected donors or from individuals known to have high levels of specific antibodies. The product may be given intramuscularly or intravenously. The indications for some of the more commonly used immunoglobulins are shown in Table 4.1. Intravenous IgG was originally developed as replacement therapy for inherited immunodeficiency states. It is also used to treat immune thrombo-

Table 4.1   Indications and doses for human immunoglobulins

Problem	Patients eligible for IgG	Preparation	Dose
Hepatitis B	Needle-stick or mucosal exposure victims. Should also be immunized	Hepatitis B IgG	1000 iu for adults and 500 iu for children <5 years
Varicella zoster	Immunosuppressed contacts Infants exposed to case Pregnant contacts	Human normal IgG	0.5 mL/kg 0.25 mL/kg 0.2 mL/kg
Tetanus-prone wounds	Non-immune patients with heavily contaminated wounds Toxoid should be administered with IgG	Tetanus IgG	250 iu routine prophylaxis 500 iu if >24 h since injury or heavily contaminated wound
Accidental transfusions of Rh(D)-positive blood	Women of childbearing age	Anti-D IgG	125 iu/mL of transfused blood

cytopenia and other rare diseases such as Guillain–Barré syndrome.

RED CELL SEROLOGY

The red cell membrane is a bilipid layer with which a variety of blood group antigen systems are associated. Over 400 red cell antigens have been described, and although their precise role is uncertain they play a part in the recognition of self from non-self. Of the major antigens, the ABO, Lewis (Le) and P antigens are carbohydrates, whereas the Rhesus (Rh), Duffy (Fy) and Kidd (Jk) antigens are proteins.

ABO antigens

Nearly all deaths from transfusion error are due to ABO incompatible transfusion. ABO antigens are present on many cells of the body, and their presence depends on the inheritance of allelic genes on chromosome 9 which code for enzymes that change the carbohydrate structures on the cell membrane to the substance known as A or B antigen. In individuals belonging to group O the gene is silent, so that the basic carbohydrate structure is left unchanged. Only individuals who lack A or B antigens produce anti-A and anti-B antibodies, respectively. These are usually IgM antibodies (naturally occurring) and are present from the age of 3–6 months. ABO antibodies can react at body temperature and activate complement, and are of major clinical significance as a cause of rapid intravascular haemolysis. For example, transfusion of group A blood to a group B patient results in haemolysis of the transfused red cells because of the anti-A antibodies present in the recipient. Similarly, group O individuals have both anti-A and anti-B

Table 4.2   The antigens and antibodies of the ABO blood group system

Blood group	Frequency (UK) %	Red cell antigen	Plasma antibody	Compatible donor blood
A	42	A	Anti-B	A or O
B	8	B	Anti-A	B or O
AB	3	AB	–	AB, A, B or O
O	47	–	Anti-A,B	O only

antibodies in their plasma that will react with any red cells apart from group O cells (Table 4.2). Group O blood can be used in all recipients because of the processing that removes the plasma and hence the antibodies contained within.

Rhesus antigen (Rh)

Allelic genes at three closely linked loci on chromosome 1 code this complex blood group system. Phenotypes termed Rhesus(D) or no D (termed d), Cc and Ee exist. Individuals with Rh(D) are termed Rhesus positive and those without Rh(D) are termed negative. Rh(D) is by far the most immunogenic of the Rhesus antigens and is the only one currently cross-matched to ensure compatibility in blood transfusion. Individuals who are Rh(D) negative do not normally have anti-Rh(D) in their plasma unless they have been immunized by previous transfusion or pregnancy. Antibodies to Rh(D) are IgG antibodies and do not activate complement, although they do cause extravascular haemolysis. The Fc receptor of the IgG antibody is recognized by the macrophages of the reticuloendothelial system, and antibody-coated cells are removed from the circulation via the liver and spleen. Rhesus antibodies can cause transfusion reactions and haemolytic disease of the newborn (HDN). It is essential that Rh(D)-negative women of childbearing age are not transfused with Rh(D)-positive blood to avoid the stimulation of antibodies to Rh(D), which could cross the placenta in pregnancy and cause haemolysis of Rh(D)-positive cells in the fetus (HDN).

Other red cell antigens

Many different types of blood group systems exist: listed below are some of the more clinically significant.

Kell antigens The Kell (K) antigen is present in less than 10% of the population but is very immunogenic, so that the incidence of anti-K antibodies is high in the transfused K-negative population. The antibodies of the K system are IgG antibodies and can cause transfusion reactions and HDN.

Duffy antigens These antibodies are IgG and can activate complement, causing intravascular haemolysis and resulting in transfusion reactions and HDN.

Kidd antigens Although weakly immunogenic these produce IgG antibodies which can cross the placental membrane, activate complement, and cause intravascular haemolysis and HDN. Kidd antibodies may be undetectable in pretransfusion compatibility testing, and yet cause a severe delayed haemolytic reaction.

TRANSFUSION TRIGGERS

The decision to transfuse is a complex one which should not be taken without considering the benefits for each individual patient. Clear indications for the transfusion should be written in the patient's case notes. Healthy adults can

---

> **SUMMARY BOX**
> - Transfusion is likely to be required at haemoglobin levels <70 g/L.
> - Transfusion is unjustified at levels >100 g/L.
> - Patients with cardiovascular disease, or those expected to have a high incidence of covert cardiovascular disease (elderly, or those with peripheral vascular disease), are likely to benefit from transfusion at haemoglobin levels of < 90 g/L.
>
> Each unit should prepare a set of simple transfusion guidelines for the haemoglobin values/trigger they have demonstrated to have benefited clinical outcome.

---

tolerate significant blood loss without adverse effects. Elderly patients or those with myocardial disease may not tolerate the same level of anaemia. In the intensive care setting some studies have shown that maintaining a lower haemoglobin threshold was in fact better for patient outcomes than tranfusing to a higher level.

Although the decision to transfuse should be considered individually, in general terms transfusion above 100 g/L cannot be justified in the absence of continuing blood loss. There is no evidence that cardiovascular function is improved at haemoglobin levels above this.

PRETRANSFUSION TESTING

Two major forms of pretransfusion testing are available.

Type and screen involves determining the patient's ABO and Rh(D) type and screening a sample of patient serum for the presence of clinically significant antibodies. The sample is then held for up to 7 days, and if blood is needed it can be provided within 10–15 minutes after rapidly excluding ABO incompatibility. Thus, operations known to require blood transfusion infrequently can be covered without having to keep blood aside for a patient when it is unlikely to be needed.

Cross-matching normally takes about an hour and involves not only typing and screening, but also direct testing of the patient's serum for compatibility with red cells taken from the units of blood to be transfused. If the patient has an antibody, its specificity for a particular antigen is determined using a panel of red cells of known phenotype. Once the antibody(ies) has been identified, donor blood is screened and only units negative for the offending antigen(s) can be issued. This process may take several hours, depending on the population incidence of the antigen(s) in question. Cross-matched units are then allocated to the individual patient and held in reserve for 48 hours.

Emergency requirements for blood make the use of compatibility tests redundant. The laboratory must be told of the urgency and quantity of blood needed immediately, and asked what they can provide in the time required. Group O Rh(D)-negative blood is available in all hospitals for such emergencies. Patient samples can be rapidly ABO and Rh(D) typed, and compatible blood released after a rapid test of ABO compatibility while the antibody screen is ongoing and group O Rh(D)-negative blood is being transfused.

Computer cross-matching/issue

Direct compatibility testing may be bypassed in situations where there is accurate patient identification, in patients with no serum antibodies and a secure blood bank computer system that can reliably select and issue blood of compatible type. These systems are currently being investigated in the UK and may allow blood to be selected from remote blood fridges when the patient requires it. Concerns still arise regarding patient identification, as the system is critically dependent on it.

Maximal Surgical Blood Ordering Schedule (MSBOS)

MSBOS is a table of elective surgical procedures which lists the number of units of blood routinely cross-matched. This surgical tariff is based on retrospective analysis of actual blood use associated with the individual surgical procedure. The aim is to correlate as closely as possible the number of units cross-matched to the numbers of units transfused. When carefully controlled and monitored, this system uses scarce blood stock most efficiently.

BLOOD ADMINISTRATION

Acute haemolytic transfusion reactions due to ABO incompatibility can be fatal and are most often caused by *errors in identification of the patient at the time of blood sampling or administration*. Prior to transfusion the indication must be recorded in the case notes, and it is the clinician's responsibility to prescribe the blood.

It is crucial that the patient's identity is established verbally (if this is possible) and by checking the patient identi-

fication band before blood is taken. *The sample must be labelled fully before leaving the bedside, and sample tubes must never be prelabelled.* The blood request form should be completed, clearly and accurately providing the patient's full name, date of birth and hospital number (each patient must have a unique identification number). This is absolutely essential for emergency admissions, who might otherwise be unidentified.

The transfusion laboratory issues blood with a compatibility report, stating the patient's full name, ABO and Rh(D) type, and the unique number of the blood pack being transfused. The group of each unit is stated with its pack number. Each unit has a compatibility label attached which states the patient's full name, date of birth, hospital number, blood group and Rhesus type. The unique donation number and expiry date are also given on each pack.

Before commencing transfusion the following details must be checked by two individuals, at least one of whom must be a State Registered Nurse (SRN) or medical officer.

- *Full patient identity* on the patient wristband, compatibility label on the unit of blood and the accompanying report form
- ABO and Rh(D) type on the pack, compatibility label and report form
- Donation number on the pack, label and report form
- Expiry date of the pack
- Examination of the pack to ensure that there are no leaks or haemolysis.

If there are any discrepancies, the blood must not be transfused and the laboratory must be informed immediately. If there are no discrepancies, the compatibility form is signed by the person administering the blood and the person checking the documentation. The form is then placed in the case notes and a copy returned to the blood transfusion laboratory.

Before blood is administered the pulse rate, blood pressure and temperature should be recorded. Transfusion must be commenced within 30 minutes of removing the blood from the refrigerator and the transfusion of each unit should be completed within 4 hours. The blood is given through a standard sterile administration set designed for the procedure. The set may be primed with 0.9% saline, but nothing should be added to the blood. The giving set is flushed with 0.9% saline after each unit has been given. The patient must be observed closely during the first 15 minutes as this is when transfusion reactions are most likely. The vital signs should be repeated if the patient feels unwell during the transfusion. It is advisable to maintain a fluid balance chart in patients having blood transfusions, and pulse rate, temperature and blood pressure should be recorded once transfusion has been completed.

SUMMARY BOX

Transfusion errors

- Almost all deaths from transfusion reaction are due to ABO incompatibility.

- Errors in patient identification at the time of blood sampling or administration are the major cause, (occurring in at least 1/1000–1/2000 transfusions.

- When taking the initial blood sample:
  - check the patient's identity verbally and on the wrist identification band
  - label the sample fully before leaving the bedside
  - make sure that the blood request form is clearly and accurately completed.

ADVERSE EFFECTS OF TRANSFUSION

A voluntary anonymized reporting scheme for serious hazards of transfusion (SHOT) has been in place in the UK for the past 3 years, and the incidence of reported hazards is shown in Figure 4.2. The greatest concern for most patients is the risk of transfusion-transmitted infection, but by far the most common risk is the transfusion of an incorrect blood component.

Transfusion reactions can be divided into those that occur early (usually during the transfusion) and those that occur late (usually once the patient has been discharged).

Acute haemolytic reactions

These potentially lethal reactions are most often due to ABO incompatibility, with activation of complement and intravascular haemolysis. Procedural failure, such as inadequate identification checks or clerical errors, are the major causes. The reaction commonly begins very shortly after starting the transfusion, and even a few millilitres of incompatible blood can be fatal. The patient experiences distress, pain at the infusion site, flushing, abdominal pain and breathlessness. Hypotension ensues, with haemoglobinuria, disseminated intravascular coagulation and oliguria leading to acute renal failure.

If an acute haemolytic reaction is suspected *the transfusion must be stopped immediately* and the blood replaced with saline until the situation is fully understood. The next steps in management are outlined in Table 4.3.

Delayed haemolytic reaction

Patients previously immunized to red cell antigens by transfusions or pregnancy can have antibody levels that are too

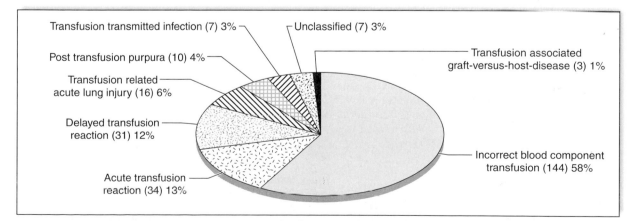

Fig. 4.2   SHOT report for 1999/2000 showing the rate (%) of serious hazards of transfusion reported in the UK out of 252 incidents

Table 4.3   Management of suspected haemolytic transfusion reaction

Investigation	Therapy
• Double-check the labelling of the blood unit with the patient's ID band and with any other identifiers • Take blood for investigation Haematology: FBC, platelet count, plasma Hb, coagulation screen Transfusion lab: repeat compatibility • Clinical chemistry: urea, creatinine & electrolytes	• Stop infusion and keep line open with 0.9% saline but avoid overhydration initially • Catheterize bladder and monitor urine flow • Maintain urine flow at >1.5 mL/kg/h: if falls below this give a fluid challenge ± frusemide 150 mg i.v.
	• If urine flow does not achieve >1.5 mL/kg/h 2 h post, assume acute renal failure and obtain specialist help • If urine flow >1.5 mL/kg/h adjust infusion rate to maintain this
• ECG–evidence of hyperkalaemia	• If hyperkalaemic, start glucose/insulin or calcium resonium therapy; seek specialist help
• Arrange repeat coagulation screens and biochemistry every 2–4 hours	• If DIC, give blood product support (platelets and cryoprecipitate)
	If patient needs transfusion use rematched blood. There is no increased risk of a second haemolytic reaction

low to be detected by pretransfusion screening. However, antibody concentrations may rise rapidly if the antigen is again transfused, and within a few days can attain levels that destroy the transfused cells. The patient presents some 5–10 days later with fever, haemoglobinuria and a falling haemoglobin level. Such delayed reactions occur once every 500 transfusions, and the Kidd, Duffy and Rhesus antibodies are commonly implicated. The reaction is seldom fatal but can cause significant morbidity in a patient who is already ill.

Febrile non-haemolytic reaction

Transfusion-associated fever and rigors are common, especially in patients who have had multiple transfusions or pregnancies. White cell antibodies in the recipient plasma reacting with the donor leukocytes are responsible, but since the use of leukodepletion of blood in the UK the incidence of this previously common reaction should be reduced. The reaction occurs late in the transfusion and is usually mild. Severe reactions may mimic the early stages of acute haemolytic transfusion reaction, and it is wise to stop the transfusion until a haemolytic reaction has been excluded. Febrile reactions normally respond to an antipyretic such as paracetamol (500–1000 mg).

Alloimmunization

Although blood is usually only cross-matched in respect of ABO and Rh(D) antigens, any antigen can give rise to antibodies. This is seldom significant in a surgical patient receiving a single episode of transfusion, but can be cata-

strophic in a woman of childbearing age as such antibodies can cause HDN. Platelets also have specific antigen systems, which can give rise to antibodies and cause the rare condition of post-transfusion purpura. The patient develops severe thrombocytopenia and haemorrhage some 10 days after transfusion. There is a significant risk of intracranial haemorrhage, and high-dose intravenous immunoglobulin or intensive plasma exchange should be considered.

Allergic reactions

Urticaria or itching within minutes of starting transfusion can result from plasma protein reactions and occur in 0.5–1% of all red cell transfusions. These reactions are occasionally severe and constitute anaphylaxis, particularly in patients with IgA deficiency who have developed antibodies against IgA. Mild reactions respond to an antihistamine alone (e.g. chlorpheniramine 10 mg given slowly i.v.), but anaphylactic reactions require urgent therapy. Transfusion is stopped immediately, although intravenous fluids are continued. Oxygen should be given and adrenaline and a salbutamol nebulizer may be required. If the patient does not respond promptly, specialist help must be summoned urgently.

Cardiac failure

Fluid overload is common in blood transfusion, particularly in patients with chronic anaemia (who have increased plasma volume) or cardiac dysfunction. It presents as acute left ventricular failure and is treated as such. The problem can be prevented by giving frusemide (20 mg orally or 40 mg i.v.) with alternate units of blood.

Graft-versus-host reaction

This rare complication follows the transfusion of viable lymphocytes into an immunocompromised host. It presents 1–4 weeks later with fever, a desquamating rash, abnormal liver function and neutropenia, and has a mortality rate of > 90%. Irradiating cellular blood components before transfusion can prevent it.

Transfusion-associated lung injury

Donor plasma very occasionally contains white cell antibodies that react with the recipient's leukocytes. The patient develops acute breathlessness, fever and chills; the chest X-ray shows nodular infiltration of the hilum and lower lung fields. This is a serious complication that requires intensive care support, and assisted ventilation may be needed.

Immune modulation

Allogeneic blood results in the down regulation of the recipient's immune response. This has led to concerns that blood transfusion, particularly in cancer patients, may have an adverse effect on long-term survival as well as postoperative infection risks. Many studies of postoperative infections have shown a reduction in those transfused with leukodepleted blood.

Transfusion-transmitted infections

Although plasma fractions are now treated to inactivate viruses, blood components such as red cells and platelets cannot yet be treated in this way. However, successive improvements in donor selection and virological screening of donated blood have greatly reduced the risks of transfusion-transmitted infection (Table 4.4). Any virus found in the blood, however, can be transmitted by blood transfusion, and agents such as prions have no suitable screening test as yet.

Table 4.4 Risks of a single red cell unit transmitting disease in the UK	
Infection	Estimated risk (per unit transfused) in the UK
Hepatitis B	1:50 000–1:200 000
Hepatitis C	1:200 000
HIV	1:2 500 000

Bacterial infection

Blood is occasionally contaminated during collection and storage, and is rarely collected from a bacteraemic donor. Sudden collapse during transfusion is mediated by endotoxin and can be misdiagnosed as an acute haemolytic reaction. Samples should be taken from the patient and the unit of blood for bacteriological culture, and broad-spectrum antibiotics commenced. Bacterial contamination is commoner in platelet transfusion, as these are stored at room temperature.

AUTOLOGOUS TRANSFUSION

As immunological and infective complications can result from donated blood, the use of the patient's own blood may be considered in certain situations.

Preoperative donation

Blood can be withdrawn from otherwise fit patients awaiting elective surgery and stored for up to 35–42 days. Assuming that the haemoglobin concentration is adequate before withdrawal of each unit and that iron therapy is used, up to five units of the patient's own blood can be made available. Sepsis and severe myocardial disease are absolute contraindications to autologous transfusion, and problems may arise if the operation has to be postponed. Autologous units undergo the same testing as allogeneic donations, including the pretransfusion compatibility test, and their use is restricted to the donor. Autologous blood should only be collected from patients who are likely to require blood during surgery.

Isovolaemic haemodilution

Up to 1.5 L of blood can be withdrawn into anticoagulant before the induction of anaesthesia and replaced by saline. The fall in haematocrit reduces the loss of red cells (and haemoglobin) during surgical bleeding while maintaining optimal tissue perfusion. The withdrawn blood can be reinfused either during surgery or postoperatively.

Cell salvage

Blood can be collected from the operation site either directly during surgery or by the use of collection devices attached to surgical drains. During surgery, blood can be collected by suction, processed by a cell salvage machine in which it is anticoagulated while the cells are washed, and then returned to the patient. The process is contraindicated in patients with malignancy or sepsis, and is only appropriate when there is substantial blood loss. Postoperative drainage can be returned to the patient, most commonly not washed. This process does require some positive suction pressure, and in some circumstances this may lead to increased blood loss. Cell salvage can significantly reduce the exposure of patients to allogeneic blood.

TRANSFUSION REQUIREMENTS IN SPECIAL SURGICAL SETTINGS

MASSIVE TRANSFUSION

Massive transfusion denotes the transfusion of the equivalent of the circulating blood volume within a 24-hour period (i.e. 10–12 units in an adult). It is needed most often in severe trauma and in bleeding from the gastrointestinal tract or various obstetric disorders. Although massive transfusion restores circulating blood volume and oxygen-carrying capacity, it is frequently complicated by coagulopathy, particularly in patients with an underlying disorder such as liver disease or DIC. The following problems may complicate massive blood transfusion.

Thrombocytopenia Stored blood contains no functional platelets, and consumption and dilution of the patient's own platelets is anticipated in conditions needing massive transfusion. Platelet counts should be kept above 50×10^9/L by platelet transfusion. Oozing from venepuncture sites and mucous membranes (microvascular bleeding) is a good indication of thrombocytopenia in these circumstances, and platelets should not be withheld while a platelet count is awaited.

Coagulation factor deficiency Stored blood contains little factor V and VIII, but has all other factors in amounts adequate for haemostasis. Red cell concentrates (supplemented) provide few coagulation factors. Dilutional deficiency occurs during blood transfusion, but coagulopathy is more often due to DIC caused by the underlying condition. When tests of the intrinsic and extrinsic coagulation pathways (prothrombin time or INR, and partial thromboplastin time (PTT), respectively) show values greater than 1.5 times control levels and/or a low fibrinogen count (< 0.8 g/L), FFP and cryoprecipitate (10–15 mL/kg) should be used as replacement therapy.

Hypocalcaemia Citrate used as an anticoagulant binds ionized calcium and can lower plasma calcium levels. The liver normally metabolizes citrate rapidly, so that this is only a problem in neonates, those with liver disease, and when blood is being infused more rapidly than 100 mL/min. If the electrocardiogram (ECG) shows changes of hypocalcaemia (prolonged QT interval), 5 mL of calcium gluconate should be infused over 5 minutes, the dose being repeated if the ECG remains abnormal.

Hyperkalaemia and hypokalaemia Red cell degeneration during storage increases the plasma potassium concentration, and rapid transfusion of large volumes of stored blood can cause hyperkalaemia. This may result in cardiotoxicity, particularly in patients with renal failure, hypothermia or extensive muscle damage. After transfusion, red cells normalize their Na/K equilibrium rapidly so that hypokalaemia then becomes the more common problem.

Hypothermia Rapid transfusion of blood at 4°C lowers core temperature, and in conjunction with other metabolic changes can cause cardiac arrest. A blood warmer must be used when the transfusion rate exceeds 50 mL/kg/h in adults and 15 mL/kg/h in children.

Adult respiratory distress syndrome (ARDS) The risk of developing ARDS is minimized if tissue perfusion is maintained, hypotension is corrected rapidly and overtransfusion avoided.

SUMMARY BOX

Massive blood transfusion

- This is defined as the transfusion of the equivalent of the circulating blood volume within a 24-hour period (in practice 10–12 units in an adult).

- Common indications for massive blood transfusion are major trauma, gastrointestinal bleeding and obstetric complications.

- Major problems associated with massive blood transfusion include:
  underlying coagulopathy
  thrombocytopenia (stored blood has no platelets)
  lack of coagulation factors V and VIII
  hyperkalaemia (although hypokalaemia may develop as transfused red cells normalize their Na/K equilibrium)
  hypothermia (risk reduced by use of blood warmers).

CARDIOPULMONARY BYPASS

Platelets and coagulation factors may be activated or lost in the extracorporeal circulation during cardiopulmonary bypass at open heart surgery (see Ch 28), so that FFP and platelet transfusion may be needed to deal with postoperative bleeding. The platelet count may be normal but the platelets are likely to be dysfunctional, having disaggregated during the extracorporeal circuit. Coagulation screens should be performed to assess therapy preinfusion of coagulation factors in all but life-threatening haemorrhage.

Heparin is used during bypass to prevent clotting in the extracorporeal circuit, and should be adequately neutralized with protamine when surgery is completed. There is no evidence that overneutralization with protamine causes coagulopathies. Late-onset bleeding (6 hours post-operatively) has been ascribed to heparin leaching out of the tissues and is dealt with by neutralization with protamine.

Both the antifibrinolytic drugs aprotinin and tranexamic acid have been shown to reduce the exposure to allogeneic blood as well as the reduction in resternotomy rate in coronary artery bypass grafting. Continuing doubts regarding the potential for aprotinin to influence graft patency have restricted its use to redo grafting, where surgical blood loss is significantly higher.

Aspirin is commonly administered to patients awaiting bypass surgery. This drug has a prolonged inhibitory effect on platelet function (5–7 days), and should therefore be stopped 7 days before surgery and commenced immediately postoperatively, when it significantly helps graft patency. It is prudent in the setting of unstable angina or in urgent coronary artery bypass grafting that aspirin is not stopped, and so the use of antifibrinolytics may have a role to play in these patients.

METHODS TO REDUCE THE NEED FOR BLOOD TRANSFUSION

Large variations in transfusion practice are currently seen in the European Union (Fig. 4.3). This is due to many factors, including the patient populations treated, differences in

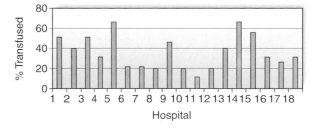

Fig. 4.3 Variation in transfusion practice (percentage of patients transfused with red cells for a primary hip replacement) between hospitals in the EU. Corrected for age, sex and preoperative Hb. Sanguis study.

surgical and anaesthetic techniques, attitudes to and availability of blood, as well as differences in pre- and post-operative care. Such differences in transfusion practice have not been shown to be associated with significant differences in mortality. These findings indicate that transfusion can be avoided or reduced by various interventions and that this does not appear to affect clinical outcomes.

Acute volume replacement

Non-plasma colloid volume expanders of large molecules, such as dextran (see Table 4.5), are a relatively inexpensive colloidal alternative to plasma in first-line management of volume-depleted patients. Anaphylactic reactions are rare and the products carry no risk of viral transmission. Hydroxyethyl starch (HES) increases red cell sedimentation rate and can cause difficulty in grouping and compatibility testing, whereas HES and dextrans can interact with factor VIII when given in large doses.

Table 4.5	Non-plasma colloid volume expanders				
Product	Source	Concentration of solution (%)	Average molecular weight (kDa)	Intravascular persistence	Frequency of acute reactions
Hydroxyethyl starch (HES)	Maize starch, chemically modified	6	450 000 or 265 000	Similar to or longer than Dextran 70	0.1/10 000
Dextran 70	Bacterial product	6	70 000	50% of infused volume persists 8 h	1.5/10 000
Dextran 40	Bacterial product	10	40 000	Shorter than Dextran 70	0.7/10 000
Urea-bridged gelatin (Haemaccel)	Heat-degraded cattle bone gelatin	3–4	35 000	50% of infused volume persists 4–5 h	14/10 000

Data from reviews and from Petz LD, Swisher SN 1987 Clinical practice of blood transfusion. Churchill Livingstone, Edinburgh.

In the initial resuscitation of patients with haemorrhagic shock, the adequacy of volume replacement is usually of much greater importance than the choice of fluid. A reasonable guide in adults is 1000 mL of crystalloid (0.9% saline or Ringer's lactate solution) followed by 1000 mL of colloid, and then replacement with red cells. In the elderly and those with cardiac impairment, red cell replacement is started earlier to maintain oxygen-carrying capacity without causing fluid overload.

Mechanisms for reduced blood use in surgery

Preoperative

When surgery is elective, significant reductions in blood use can be made by ensuring that the patient has a normal haemoglobin and by correcting any existing anaemia. Drugs that interfere with haemostasis should be stopped where appropriate, i.e. non-steroidal anti-inflammatory drugs, aspirin and warfarin. In suitable patients an autologous predeposit programme (see above) may be considered. Erythropoietin, the peptide hormone normally made in the kidney, is now available in recombinant form and can be used to raise the haemoglobin levels in patients thought likely to need blood, i.e. women with low haemoglobin levels who are undergoing a procedure with a high transfusion requirement. Erythropoietin should be used in conjunction with iron therapy.

Intraoperative

The training, experience and competence of the surgeon performing the procedure are the most crucial factors in reducing operative blood loss. The importance of meticulous surgical technique with attention to bleeding points cannot be underestimated. Other techniques, such as posture, the use of vasoconstrictors and tourniquets, should always be considered as these can have a significant impact on perioperative blood loss. Certain pharmacological agents, such as anti-fibrinolytics, can significantly reduce the requirements for blood and are indicated in certain operative procedures. Aprotinin is a serine proteinase inhibitor which exerts an antifibrinolytic effect. Its use is established in cardiac surgery, particularly in repeat surgery, although concerns still exist regarding graft patency in primary coronary artery bypass grafting (see section on cardiopulmonary bypass). Aprotinin is also proving to be effective in liver transplantation and orthopaedic surgery. Acute allergic effects have been described with repeated dosing. Tranexamic acid also has anti-fibrinolytic effects and has been shown to reduce allogeneic blood use in cardiac surgery.

Fibrin sealant mimics the final stage in the coagulation cascade, in which fibrinogen is converted to fibrin in the presence of thrombin, factor XIII, fibronectin and ionized calcium. Freeze-dried sterilized fibrinogen, fibronectin and factor XIII can be delivered from one barrel of a double-barrelled syringe while thrombin, calcium and aprotinin are delivered from the other. If the two mixtures meet at a surgical bleeding site the solution clots almost immediately, the clot resolving over a period of days. Fibrin sealant has been used in vascular, cardiac and liver surgery and in situations where even small amounts of bleeding can be problematic (e.g. middle ear surgery). The product is *not* for intravenous use.

Acute normovolaemic haemodilution and intraoperative blood salvage are two of the autologous methods of blood conservation that can be employed during surgery to reduce exposure to transfusion. They are described in more detail in the section above on autologous programmes.

Postoperative

Postoperatively blood can be salvaged from drains into collection devices that permit reinfusion. These procedures usually do not include a step to wash the red cells to remove cellular debris, and so may lead to activation of the coagulation cascade on reinfusion.

The decision to transfuse postoperatively should depend on several factors: the age of the patient and their ability to tolerate lower levels of anaemia (pre-existing myocardial disease), as well as the rate and amount of continuing blood loss.

FUTURE TRENDS

The demand for blood continues to rise yearly in the UK. Although local shortages occur from time to time, where high demand coincides with low rates of collection, the UK is still self-sufficient in red cells. With ever more stringent donor selection guidelines and an increasingly elderly population the number of available donors will continue to decrease. This means that blood should be considered a scarce and valuable commodity that should be responsibly prescribed.

Although red cell substitutes are in various stages of clinical trial, no cell free haemoglobin solution or fluorocarbon oxygen carrier is as yet licensed for clinical use. However, there is every expectation that transfusion therapy will be increasingly supplanted by the use of synthetic or biologically engineered substitutes. Until this occurs, the administration of human blood products will be required and must be practised responsibly.

Recombinant growth factors are making an increasing impact on blood requirements. For example, recombinant human erythropoietin raises haemoglobin levels in patients with chronic renal failure and has been used with some success to raise the haemoglobin level preoperatively with/without autologous prior deposit.

The objective in managing surgical patients should be to minimize anaemia and bleeding and hence the need for transfusion. Although it is clear that no patient should be transfused unnecessarily, it is equally certain that no patient should be allowed to exsanguinate because of concerns regarding blood safety.

5 Nutritional support in surgical patients

K.C.H. Fearon

INTRODUCTION

It goes without saying that without food there can be no life, that food is a basic human right, and that it behoves every doctor to pay attention to the nutritional needs of his or her patients. Nevertheless, approximately one-third of all patients admitted to an acute hospital will have evidence of protein–calorie malnutrition and two-thirds will leave hospital either malnourished or having lost weight.

Clearly, malnutrition has damaging effects on psychological status, activity levels and appearance. Paradoxically, in the surgical patient a low body fat content may sometimes be viewed as an advantage, making technical aspects of surgery easier. There is, however, clear evidence that patients with severe protein depletion have a significantly greater incidence of postoperative complications, such as pneumonia and wound infection, and a prolonged hospital stay.

Nutritional disorders in surgical practice have two principal components. First, starvation can be initiated by the effects of the disease, restriction of oral intake, or both. Simple starvation results in progressive loss of the body's energy and protein reserves (i.e. subcutaneous fat and skeletal muscle). Secondly, there are the metabolic effects of stress/inflammation, namely increased catabolism and reduced anabolism. These result in a variety of changes, including a low serum albumin concentration, accelerated muscle wasting and water retention. Although malnutrition may be the result of starvation, in most surgical patients it results from a combination of the two.

ASSESSMENT OF NUTRITIONAL STATUS

The main energy reserves in the body are found in subcutaneous and intra-abdominal fat. Fat reserves are generally in excess and their loss does not greatly impair function. In contrast, there are no true protein reserves in the body. Thus, in the face of starvation or stress, structural tissues such as skeletal muscle and the gut are autocannibalized, resulting in functional impairment which can eventually impede recovery.

The key elements of nutritional assessment include current food intake, levels of energy and protein reserves, and the patient's likely clinical course (Fig. 5.1). Patients who have not eaten for 5 days or more require nutritional

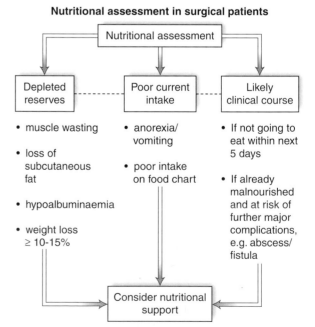

Fig. 5.1 Nutritional assessment in surgical patients.

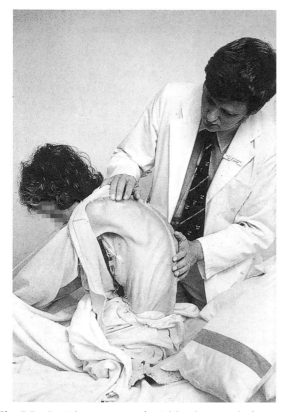

Fig. 5.2 Protein–energy malnutrition in a surgical patient, illustrating depleted muscle and subcutaneous fat stores.

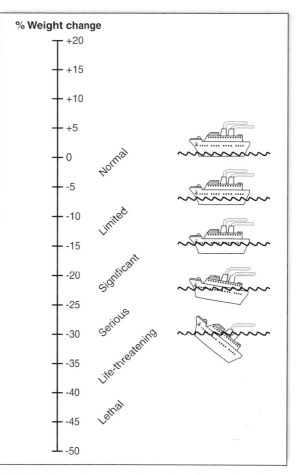

Fig. 5.3 Alterations in nutritional status associated with weight loss.

support, and those with symptoms such as anorexia, nausea, vomiting or early satiety are at risk of a reduced food intake and hence undernutrition. Levels of energy reserves are most easily assessed by examining for loss of subcutaneous fat (skinfolds), whereas protein depletion is most commonly manifest as skeletal muscle wasting (Fig. 5.2). A history of weight loss of more than 10–15% is highly significant. Patients can also be assessed according to their body mass index (BMI: weight (kg)/height (m^2)). The normal BMI is 20–25. A value less than 16 is suggestive of severe protein–calorie undernutrition. Finally, it is important to recognize that in assessing the nutritional status of a patient knowledge of their likely clinical course is vital (Fig. 5.3). For example, if a patient is well nourished they should be able to withstand the normal period of starvation associated with major surgery. However, if a patient is severely malnourished (e.g. weight loss of 20%, BMI 16) then even a short further period of starvation or catabolism may make them so critically undernourished that this becomes life-threatening in itself. Taken together, the elements of a patient's food intake, level of reserve and likely clinical course should alert the astute clinician to the

need for nutritional support and should be part of the routine daily appraisal of every patient during a surgical ward round.

SUMMARY BOX

Nutritional status

- Nutritional status in surgical patients may be adversely affected by starvation (effects of disease such as oesophageal cancer, restricted intake), the effects of inflammation (increased catabolism) and the effects of the operation itself (stress/inflammatory response).
- Nutritional status is assessed by current food intake, levels of reserves and likely clinical course.

ASSESSMENT OF NUTRITIONAL REQUIREMENTS

Energy and protein requirements vary, depending on weight, body composition, clinical status, mobility and dietary intake. Ideally, energy requirements should be measured using indirect calorimetry. However, for most patients an approximation based on weight and clinical status is sufficient. Relevant values are given in Table 5.1. Few patients require more than 2500 kcal/day. Additional calories are unlikely to be used effectively and may even constitute a metabolic stress. Particular caution must be exercised when refeeding the chronically starved patient because of the dangers of hypokalaemia and hypophosphataemia.

Table 5.1 Estimation of energy and protein requirements in adult surgical patients		
	Uncomplicated	Complicated/stressed
Energy (kcal/kg/day)	30	34–40
Protein (g/kg/day)*	1.0	1.3–2
*g of protein can be converted to the equivalent amount of nitrogen by dividing by 6.25.		

The most common method for assessing protein requirement is 24-hour urinary urea excretion. This is converted to an estimate of 24-hour urinary nitrogen loss. Most patients require 10–15 g nitrogen per day. (The equivalent amount of protein can be calculated by multiplying by a conversion factor of 6.25.) Even if losses are in excess of this, more than 18 g nitrogen/day (equivalent to 112 g protein) is seldom given because it is unlikely to be used effectively.

CAUSES OF INADEQUATE INTAKE

The ideal way for a surgical patient to take in enough nutrients is for them to eat or drink palatable food. Unfortunately, the catering budget is often far too low for the provision of appetising food, and wastage of unwanted food can account for up to 40% of that served. Other reasons for a poor food intake include the patient being too weak and anorexic, or having a mechanical problem such as obstruction of the gastrointestinal tract. Patients with increased metabolic demands may have some difficulty in taking sufficient food to meet such demands. Patients with a normal functional gut may also have a reduced food

intake due simply to the cumulative effects of repeated periods of fasting to undergo investigations such as endoscopy or contrast radiology.

Some patients suffer from what is best described as 'intestinal failure', i.e. a state in which the amount of functioning gut is reduced below a level where enough food can be digested and absorbed for nourishment. The four principal causes of intestinal failure are:

- *Short bowel syndrome*, which results from massive small bowel resection
- *Fistula formation*, in which bowel content is lost externally or short-circuited (internal fistula) before it can be adequately digested and absorbed
- *Motility disorders* such as paralytic ileus and chronic intestinal pseudo-obstruction
- Extensive *small bowel disease*, such as Crohn's disease.

In these difficult cases specialized nutritional treatment is required if the patient is to remain normally nourished. The situation of many of these patients, at least in the acute phase, is further complicated by the presence of ongoing inflammation or sepsis. As a general rule, nutritional treatment is not as effective as it might be in the presence of active sepsis. The priority in such patients is to eliminate sepsis at the same time as providing nutritional support.

METHODS OF PROVIDING NUTRITIONAL SUPPORT

Nutrients can be given via the gastrointestinal tract, i.e. enteral nutrition, or intravenously, i.e. parenteral nutrition. Parenteral nutritional is indicated only when enteral feeding is not feasible. Very few patients are not suitable for some form of enteral feeding, which is both safer and cheaper than parenteral nutrition. Certainly all those who have a normal length of functioning gastrointestinal tract, and most of those who have a reduced amount, can be fed by this route. Furthermore, the ingestion of even suboptimal amounts of food may help maintain the integrity of the intestinal mucosa, thereby reducing bacterial and endotoxin translocation, which may compound the metabolic upset in such patients.

ORAL ENTERAL NUTRITION

As stated previously, it is essential to provide warm, appetizing food on the wards, to make sure there are enough nursing and auxiliary staff available to help elderly/infirm patients take their food, and to encourage nursing staff to be aware of the nutritional needs of all patients. It is against this basic background of nutritional care that the need for artificial nutritional support should be considered.

Many patients suffer from early satiety (feeling full after a meal), and encouraging them to eat small amounts frequently or to sip an oral supplement between meals can help overcome this symptom. Oral supplements come in cartons of about 250 mL and each contains about 250 kcal and 10 g of protein. These should be available to all patients who require them. There is a range of flavours and the texture can be changed if chilled, for example. Most patients manage to take two or three cartons per day if required. However, fatigue with such supplements is commonplace and leads to reduced efficacy in the long run.

There are numerous reasons why surgical patients may suffer from anorexia (i.e. poor appetite) (Table 5.2). Before embarking on tube enteral feeding it is important to actively manage any symptoms that can be treated (e.g. oral thrush with nystatin, nausea with antiemetics) and thus boost spontaneous oral intake. For patients who are unable to swallow, or for those whose anorexia is resistant to other therapy, nasoenteral feeding via a fine-bore tube should be used.

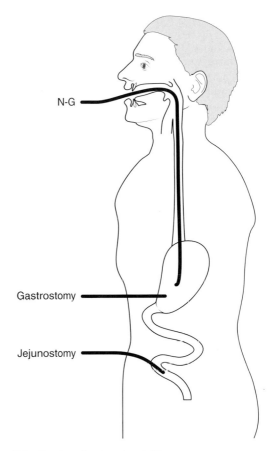

Fig. 5.4   Routes of enteral nutrition.

Table 5.2   Causes of anorexia in surgical patients
Intestinal obstruction
Ileus
Cancer anorexia
Depression, stress, anxiety
Drugs, e.g. opiates
Oral ulceration/infection
General debility/weakness

Methods of administration of enteral feeds

Nasogastric or nasojejunal tubes

If the patient cannot drink or sip a liquid feed for mechanical reasons, or if they are unconscious or on a ventilator, enteral nutrition can be given by a fine-bore nasogastric or nasoenteric tube. The position of the tube tip should be checked radiologically, or by injecting air while ausculating over the epigastrum, before nutrients are infused. Patients who need prolonged enteral feeding can learn to pass a fine-bore tube each evening and feed themselves overnight. When carried out at home this is known as home enteral nutrition.

Gastrostomy and jejunostomy

If nasogastric feeding is impossible because of disease or obstruction of the upper alimentary tract, nutrients may be given through a tube placed into the gastrointestinal tract below the lesion (Fig. 5.4). Thus a patient with pseudobulbar palsy or an oesophageal fistula can be fed through a gastrostomy, and a patient with a gastric or duodenal fistula can be fed through a jejunostomy.

Specially designed gastrostomy tubes can now be inserted by a combined percutaneous and endoscopic method, and are particularly valuable for prolonged feeding when there is no impairment of gastric emptying (e.g. stroke patients). Feeding jejunostomy tubes can be inserted at the time of laparotomy when the surgeon anticipates that prolonged nutritional support will be needed postoperatively (e.g. patients undergoing oesophagectomy and gastrectomy for cancer, or necrosectomy for severe pancreatitis).

Complications of enteral nutrition

Just because enteral feeds are administered directly into the gastrointestinal tract, it cannot be assumed that they are free from complications. Diarrhoea may be managed by reducing the rate of infusion and by ensuring the patient is not on broad-spectrum antibiotics. Vomiting can be managed by reducing the rate of feeding and by the use of prokinetic drugs such as cisapride. Monitoring of fluid and electrolyte balance is important, at least in the acute phase of a patient's illness (for metabolic complications see section on parenteral nutrition).

Complications also occur because of difficulty in placing the tubes. Examples include a fine-bore nasogastric tube inserted wrongly into the respiratory tract, or early accidental removal of a jejunostomy tube, with intraperitoneal leakage. As with other areas of nutrition supplementation, attention to detail is paramount.

SUMMARY BOX

Enteral nutrition

- If the patient cannot eat adequate amounts of food they should be reviewed by the ward dietitian. If oral supplements fail, a tube can be used for supplemental or total enteral nutrition.

- Most patients tolerate a whole protein feed (1 kcal/mL), which can be escalated to 100 mL/h and thus supply about 2400 kcal/day and 14 g N/day.

- If a tube cannot be passed down the oesophagus, gastrostomy and jejunostomy feeding should be considered.

- The main complications of enteral feeding relate to patient tolerance (nausea, vomiting and diarrhoea) and to the insertion site (gastrostomy or jejunostomy).

PARENTERAL NUTRITION

Intravenous feeding is indicated when patients cannot be fed adequately by mouth, nasogastric tube or gastrostomy/jejunostomy, or when they have complete or partial intestinal failure. The problem may be permanent, as in most cases of short bowel syndrome, or reversible, as in paralytic ileus or fistula formation. In some cases of short bowel syndrome the remaining intestine 'adapts' by undergoing mucosal hyperplasia over a period of weeks or months, and normal feeding can then resume.

Parenteral nutrition can provide the patient's total needs of protein, energy, electrolytes, trace metals and vitamins, i.e. total parenteral nutrition (TPN). The need to restrict volume means that concentrated solutions are used. As such solutions are irritant and thrombogenic, they have to be administered through a catheter positioned in a large high-flow vein, such as the superior vena cava.

Indications for TPN

The chief indications are those already mentioned. Although preoperative TPN has been advocated as a means of improving the condition of a patient prior to surgery, this is only relevant to those with severe protein–calorie undernutrition. In contrast, it is sensible to commence TPN in any patient with intestinal failure as soon as the condition is diagnosed. In general, operative removal or eradication of the lesion causing the nutritional disorder is followed by more rapid recovery if nutritional support continues without interruption.

In contrast to preoperative TPN, there is no doubt that postoperative TPN can be both effective and life-saving when complications develop, especially when these prevent enteral nutrition or are associated with infection. Situations in which TPN is invaluable include prolonged paralytic ileus, gross abdominal sepsis, and in dealing with the greatly increased metabolic demands that follow severe injury or burns.

TPN should continue until intestinal function has recovered sufficiently to allow nutrition to be maintained by the oral or enteral route. In cases of intestinal fistula, parenteral feeding is continued until the fistula has closed spontaneously or been closed surgically. When enteral nutrition cannot be resumed, the patient can be taught the necessary aseptic techniques to permit home TPN.

Composition of TPN solutions

Although TPN can be provided by sequential or simultaneous administration of individual glucose, fat or amino acid solutions, it is now standard practice to mix the day's requirements in a 3-L bag. This is made up in the pharmacy under sterile conditions, and its contents are infused over 12–24 hours using an infusion pump. Many pharmacies now use three or four standard regimens. The solutions contain fixed amounts of energy and nitrogen, and typically provide 1800–2500 kcal (50% glucose, 50% lipid) and 10–14 g nitrogen.

Fluid and electrolyte needs are also catered for. Many patients on TPN need additional water, sodium and potassium because of excess loss from, for example, a high-output fistula. Trace elements and vitamins can also be incorporated, and the demands created by infection and excessive loss can be met. An example of a standard TPN regimen is given in Table 5.3.

Administration of TPN

Hypertonic solutions have to be infused into a vein with a high flow. Vascular access to the superior vena cava is normally obtained through the internal or external jugular, subclavian or cephalic veins. Although veins of the lower limb can and occasionally have to be used, they are best avoided

Table 5.3 Standard parenteral nutrition regimen		
Non-protein energy	2200	kcal
Nitrogen	13.5	g
Volume	2500	mL
Sodium	115	mmol
Potassium	65	mmol
Calcium	10	mmol
Magnesium	9.5	mmol
Phosphate	20	mmol
Zinc	0.1	mmol
Chloride	113.3	mmol
Acetate	135	mmol
Adequate vitamins and trace elements		

because of the higher risk of thrombosis and infection. To allow patients greater mobility and to facilitate catheter care, the external portion of the catheter is usually run through a subcutaneous tunnel to emerge through the skin on the anterior chest wall.

Modern cannulae are made of silastic rubber or polyurethane and are of fine bore. For longer-term feeding a Hickman catheter is used; this type of silastic catheter has a Dacron cuff, which secures it in the tunnel without the need for suture fixation. Before use, the position of the catheter tip is checked radiologically. With good care, a correctly positioned catheter can remain in place for several months or years.

Complications of TPN

Catheter problems

Percutaneous insertion of a catheter may damage adjacent structures and can cause pneumothorax, air embolus and haematoma. Incorrect catheter positioning is excluded by taking a chest X-ray prior to commencing infusion.

Thrombophlebitis

Thrombosis is common when long lines are used, when the catheter tip is not in an area of high flow, and when very hypertonic solutions are infused. The telltale signs are redness and tenderness over the cannulated vein, together with swelling of the whole limb and engorgement of collateral veins if the thrombosis is more proximal. Occasionally, a superior mediastinal syndrome develops in patients with superior vena cava thrombosis. If major vessel occlusion is suspected, the diagnosis is confirmed by venography and anticoagulation is commenced with heparin. If vascular access has to be maintained, an attempt can be made to lyse the clot with urokinase or plasminogen activator. If the clot cannot be dissolved, the cannula must be removed and a

new one positioned in an unoccluded vein. The patient may need to remain on long-term anticoagulation.

Infection

Infection and septicaemia are the most frequent complications of TPN. The usual offending organisms are coagulase negative staphylococci, *Staphylococcus aureus* and coliforms, but the incidence of fungal infection is increasing, possibly because many of the patients requiring TPN are also taking broad-spectrum antibiotics. Most catheter infections are the result of poor care of the feeding line. The insertion site must be protected with an occlusive dressing and should be cleansed on alternate days with an antiseptic agent. The line must only be used for infusion of nutrients and never for taking or giving blood or administering drugs. Great care is taken to avoid contamination when changing bags. A nutrition support nurse is invaluable in avoiding catheter sepsis and supervising all aspects of catheter care. If the patient receiving TPN develops pyrexia the protocol outlined in Table 5.4 should be followed.

Metabolic complications

Metabolic complications include under- or overhydration. Patients with coexisting medical conditions (e.g. cardiac failure) should be carefully monitored. Hyperglycaemia may occur and requires either a reduction of the glucose load or

Table 5.4   Detection and treatment of catheter sepsis
If a pyrexia >38°C develops, or there is a further rise in temperature if already pyrexial • Stop parenteral nutrition and check for other sources of pyrexia (e.g. chest or urinary tract infection) • Take peripheral and central blood cultures • Administer intravenous fluids • Heparinize catheter • Consult senior medical staff
If blood culture is negative Restart parenteral nutrition
If blood culture is positive • Remove catheter and send tip for bacteriological analysis • Administer appropriate antibiotic therapy • If necessary, replace catheter and restart parenteral nutrition within 24–48 hours
Where central access must be preserved • Administer intravenous antibiotics for 5 days • Flush catheter with urokinase to remove infected fibrin clot at tip of catheter • Alcohol lock

the concomitant infusion of insulin via a separate pump. Hypokalaemia and hypophosphataemia are common when severely malnourished patients are re-fed after a long period of starvation because of the large flux of potassium and phosphate into the cells; correction is by further supplementation. Abnormal liver function tests may occur in severely stressed or septic patients. If the changes are marked and progressive, the overall substrate load should be reduced and discontinuation of parenteral nutrition considered.

Peripheral vein nutrition

Lipid emulsions and isotonic solutions of amino acids are available which are less irritant than conventional TPN solutions and which can be infused into peripheral veins. Such solutions can be used in the short term, but their prolonged use is associated with thrombophlebitis and conventional techniques should be employed if long-term support is needed. Peripheral catheters require the same level of care as central catheters, and the patient must still be monitored for signs of infection or metabolic complications.

MONITORING OF NUTRITIONAL SUPPORT

Patients receiving nutritional support are monitored to detect deficiency states, assess the adequacy of energy and protein provision, and anticipate complications. Patients receiving enteral feeding require less intense monitoring but are prone to the same metabolic complications as those who are fed intravenously.

Pulse rate, blood pressure and temperature are recorded regularly, an accurate fluid balance chart is maintained (remembering not to overlook insensible losses), and the

SUMMARY BOX

Parenteral nutrition

- Parenteral feeding is indicated if the patient cannot be fed orally or enterally. Intestinal failure is the commonest indication.

- The need to restrict volume when using total parenteral nutrition (TPN) means that concentrated solutions are used, which may be irritant and thrombogenic. TPN is therefore infused through a catheter in a high-flow vein (e.g. SVC).

- TPN is usually given in an 'all-in-one' 3-L bag with a mixture of glucose, fat and L-amino acids combined with fluid, electrolytes, vitamins, minerals and trace elements.

- The major complications with TPN can be classed as catheter related, septic or metabolic. A multidisciplinary approach to the management of TPN patients by a nutrition team will minimize such complications.

urine is checked daily for glycosuria. Body weight is measured twice weekly.

Serum urea and electrolytes are measured daily, as are blood glucose levels if there is glycosuria. Full blood count, liver function tests, and serum albumin, calcium, magnesium and phosphate are monitored once or twice weekly. Urine is collected over one or two 24-hour periods each week to measure sodium and nitrogen losses. To maintain a positive nitrogen balance, nitrogen intake should exceed daily losses by at least 2 g. For patients on long-term EN or TPN (i.e. longer than 2–3 weeks) less intense monitoring is appropriate once they are stable.

6 Infections and antibiotics

I.F. Laurenson

PATHOGENIC POTENTIAL OF MICROBES

Exaltation

When an organism is serially passaged in vivo its virulence may be exalted (increased) and its capacity to spread from one host to another increased.

The concept of increased pathogenic potential as a result of exaltation in vivo must be linked with the ability of some commensal or opportunist bacteria to acquire and pass on new, potentially dangerous genetic information. This may affect an organism's ability to colonize, to infect, to produce toxin or to develop multiple antibiotic resistance. The 'hospital staphylococcus' illustrates some of the alarming possibilities that can result when an organism acquires new genetic material in the course of its colonization. Gram-negative bacilli, especially klebsiellas, have also demonstrated a potential for dangerous genetic exchange. The extending range of β-lactamases in such widely different genera as *Haemophilus*, *Neisseria* and *Bacteroides* species is a matter for concern and may lead to treatment failure with commonly used β-lactams. The transmission of organisms from patient to patient, or between staff and patients, must be rigorously avoided. Handwashing on the ward is critical, as is the wearing and appropriate changing of disposable gloves in situations where transfer of flora from one patient to another may occur.

Pathogenic synergy

Two or more organisms may combine forces in a mixed infection and demonstrate enhanced virulence. Examples include acute ulceromembranous gingivitis (Vincent's infection), Meleney's synergistic gangrene, and various fusospirochaetal or mixed infections with anaerobic components, all of which may lead to progressive destruction of tissue or a fulminating invasive infection. Mixed infections are common in a wide range of conditions, e.g. cerebral, dental, lung and pelvic abscess, and peritonitis. When the anaerobic *Bacteroides* spp are present in such infections they may interfere with phagocyte function and produce detectable levels of β-lactamases in abscess fluid. These β-lactamases protect normally susceptible organisms of mixed infections from the actions of antimicrobials. These factors may explain the observed synergistic action of coexisting pathogens.

ASEPSIS

Surgical ritual

In surgical areas, clear and specific instructions must be given on preoperative skin cleansing of the patient and on adequate disinfection of the operation site. The relative advantages of masks, gowns and drapes at operation are debated, and the limitations of these precautions should be understood. Not only may they serve to protect the patient, they can also protect the operator from fluid splashes. Only suitable protective materials should be used.

There should be a clear disinfectant policy and an antibiotic policy to ensure that antimicrobial agents are used sensibly on the wards and in the operating theatres. Strict adherence to the principles of sterilization and disinfection is essential when cleansing and processing surgical instruments and anaesthetic equipment.

Sterilization

This is an absolute term denoting the complete removal or inactivation of viable microorganisms (protozoa, fungi, bacteria and viruses). It can only be achieved by strict attention to detail. Instruments or articles can be classified as sterile following thorough cleaning if they have been subjected to any of the following:

- Wet heat in an autoclave at 121°C for 20 minutes, or at a higher temperature for a shorter time (HTST) to provide an equivalent exposure (Fig. 6.1)
- Dry heat in a hot-air oven at 160°C for 1 hour (see Fig. 6.1)
- Irradiation under strictly controlled conditions (used predominantly in industry)
- Special sterilizing chemicals, liquids or gases, such as formaldehyde, glutaraldehyde or ethylene oxide, under strictly controlled conditions.

Some transmissible agents, known as prions, challenge these conventional assumptions; an example are those responsible for Creutzfeldt–Jakob disease (CJD). To prevent prion transmission instruments used in such patients should not be reused on any other patient. Prions of variant CJD have also been found in gut lymphoreticular tissue, raising the spectre of inadvertent transmission on instruments that have not been properly cleaned prior to standard sterilization methods, which are known to be ineffective.

Disinfection

This denotes a significant reduction in the numbers of organisms present, particularly those that might cause infection. With few exceptions, chemical disinfectants are not sterilizing agents. *Antiseptics* are relatively mild disinfectants that can be used on living tissues without causing undue harm.

Disinfection and preparation of the skin for surgery

Preoperative shaving at the site of incision is no longer recommended, as it leads to increased wound infection.

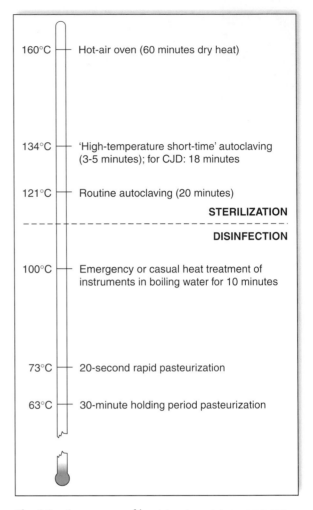

Fig. 6.1 A summary of heat-treatment temperatures. (After Collee J G. 1981, in Applied medical microbiology, p. 104. Blackwell, Oxford). Updated

---

SUMMARY BOX

- *Sterilization* = complete removal or inactivation of viable organisms. Accomplished by:
  - wet heat
  - dry heat
  - irradiation
  - chemicals.

- *Disinfection* = a significant reduction in the numbers of organisms present, particularly those that might cause infection.

However, if for convenience the site often has to be cleared of hairs immediately prior to the operation. This tends to be carried out in the anaesthetic room or in the operating theatre itself. Before a surgical incision is made in intact skin, the transient and resident flora at the operation site can be markedly reduced by thorough cleansing, and remaining flora largely inactivated by the application of a suitable antibacterial agent. This will inactivate vegetative forms of bacteria only: it cannot be expected to kill bacterial spores. Accessible vegetative bacteria on the skin can be quickly inactivated by applying 70% ethanol, or 70% isopropyl alcohol, in water. The addition of an antiseptic such as chlorhexidine or iodine 1–2% further enhances the bacterial kill. However, any surgery where diathermy is used has a risk of igniting any residual alcohol from the skin preparation. The aqueous solution of chlorhexidine or iodine is therefore used in most operating theatres. However, without the presence of alcohol the skin preparation is less effective, and this should be borne in mind by the surgeon. As its action is time dependent, the solution should be left in contact with the skin for as long as possible before being dried and the incision performed.

SURGICAL INFECTION

Infection, bacteraemia and septicaemia

The term *infection* means the presence of organisms in a normally sterile site, usually but not necessarily accompanied by an inflammatory host response. When bacteria are present in the blood as shown by blood culture the term *bacteraemia* is used. This phenomenon may be transient. *Septicaemia* is similar but a greater severity is implied.

Microbiological diagnosis of infection

In the appropriate clinical context symptoms and signs of infection should be sought. Before antibiotics are given appropriate specimens of pus (in a sterile container without additives), wound swabs, blood cultures, sputum and urine should be sent rapidly to the microbiology laboratory, accompanied by a clearly completed request form with full details of the patient, the clinical situation, antibiotic allergies and any treatment. Urgent Gram staining may guide initial therapy. It should be noted if mycobacterial infection is under consideration. In some cases serological or special techniques may be helpful. Microbiological advice should be sought.

Wound infection

Contamination usually denotes the passive presence of a relatively small number of various species of bacteria. An

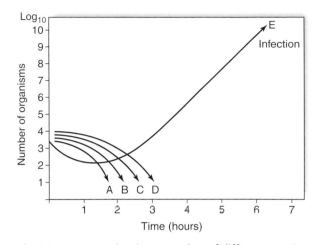

Fig. 6.2 In contamination a number of different species (A, B, C, D, E) may be present in small to moderate numbers. In infection one (or more) species expresses a survival advantage and multiplies to produce a significant challenge (E).

open wound is invariably contaminated with organisms, which may be derived endogenously from the patient's skin or exogenously from an external source such as the soil or air, or the hand of an attendant. The outcome of the microbial challenge depends on many factors, including the circumstances of contamination. When one or more contaminants has a survival advantage over the others and replicate in the wound, infection is initiated and microbial pathogenicity expressed (Fig. 6.2). There may be bacterial invasion, toxin production, or a combination of these. Occasionally there may be fungal or viral infection.

If contamination is minimal, as in an elective surgical incision performed under good conditions on a patient in good general health, the defences of the host cope completely. If contamination is severe, and particularly when other adverse factors operate, the challenge may rapidly result in a fulminating and overwhelming infection unless prompt and adequate action is taken to counter it. Such conditions arise, for example, with a lacerated wound following a road accident in an elderly person, or a perforated colon in a debilitated patient.

Thus a wound infection implies the implantation of a potentially infective inoculum under conditions that allow the organism to evade or overcome host defences; it is a function of the number of organisms in the inoculum, their quality or nature, and the efficacy of local and general host defences.

Factors predisposing to infection

In accidental wounds several infective organisms are likely to be present. Therefore, prompt and adequate surgical

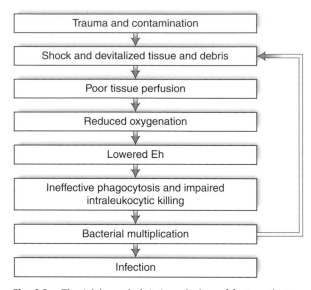

Fig. 6.3 The 'vicious circle'. Association of factors that may be involved in the change from contamination to infection in a wound. Eh = oxidation-reduction potential.

treatment should be given before the stage of bacterial contamination has led to proliferation and passed into that of active infection. Ideally this should be within 1–2 hours of injury, and must include thorough cleansing of the wound and the removal of all debris (surgical toilet), followed by the excision of all devitalized tissue (debridement). If primary surgical care is not given within 6 hours, infection must be presumed.

Factors concerned with healing, and the problems of wound management are considered in Chapter 13.

Tissue oxygenation

Primary host defences against wound infection include phagocytosis and intraleukocytic microbicidal systems. Effective phagocytosis, good tissue perfusion and oxygenation are requirements for the optimal function of these defences. All wounded tissue is less aerobic than normal tissue: impaired oxygenation persists for some days until healing is established. If the patient is initially shocked tissue perfusion is further constrained, and a vicious circle may result (Fig. 6.3): Postoperative hyperoxygenation of the patient lowers the incidence of infection following colorectal surgery.

Temperature

Both wound and patient hypothermia give rise to impaired tissue perfusion and oxygenation. This results in a number of adverse outcomes, such as delayed wound healing, increased infection rates, intra- and postoperative myocardial ischaemia, coagulation disturbances and prolonged hospital stay. Thus accidental hypothermia, particularly in the perioperative period, should be avoided.

Symptoms and signs of infection

It is important to detect infection in a wound early. Cardinal local symptoms and signs include pain, erythema, warmth, oedema, and possibly serous or seropurulent exudate. The patient's temperature may rise and local tenderness may increase, with muscle guarding in the affected part.

Pyogenic organisms provoke a polymorphonuclear leukocytosis. The erythrocyte sedimentation rate (ESR) and plasma viscosity increase and the level of C-reactive protein rises. In the immunocompromised or severely infected patient some of these features, such as temperature and white cell count, may be apparently 'normal' or depressed. If the infection is severe, with early progression to bacteraemia and septicaemia, the patient may quickly and insidiously develop bacteriogenic or 'septic' shock (see below).

When an operation involves an unavoidable and significant microbial challenge to the tissues, as in colonic surgery, it is standard practice to protect the patient by giving antimicrobial prophylaxis just before or at anaesthesia induction and to cover the period of challenge. It is important that this should be for a short time to prevent the selection of resistant organisms and side-effects. For example, a suitable antibiotic may be given just before surgery and continued for up to 24 hours postoperatively.

Postoperative wound infection

Bacterial infection of a surgical wound is still a common postoperative complication. It depends on a number of factors, including the type of operation and incision, the surgical team's skill, the patient's susceptibility to infection and the duration of operation. Regular surveillance and feedback of a surgical team's infection rates can result in a review of practice and lowering of such rates. The following generalizations reflect current experience.

Clean wounds in healthy tissue should heal promptly. With adequate facilities, an infection rate of less than 2% should be the aim of a good surgical team. Infections with *Staphylococcus aureus* occur from time to time. A series of such infections in a surgical unit suggests that a member of the team may be a carrier. Infections with coagulase-negative staphylococci are particularly associated with the implantation of heart valves, orthopaedic prostheses, vascular grafts, central venous catheters or other artificial materials.

'*Clean contaminated*' operations on the head and neck, oesophagus, stomach and proximal small bowel are at risk of infection with oropharyngeal flora such as cocci, oral anaerobes and coliforms. Peroperative antimicrobial prophylaxis has significantly reduced the incidence of infection in such operations. A 10% infection rate is not uncommon, especially if gastric achlorhydria allows bacterial multiplication in the stomach. This has special relevance to patients receiving drugs that raise gastric pH, such as H_2 antagonists or proton pump inhibitors. Antimicrobial prophylaxis is also important in surgery of the biliary tract, where potentially infective organisms include faecal streptococci (enterococci), coliforms, pseudomonads and *Clostridium perfringens*. Despite antimicrobial use, infection rates of 5–10% are still recorded in such patients.

Urological surgery, such as transurethral resection of the prostate, risks infection with coliforms and enterococci and similar postoperative infection rates.

'*Contaminated*' operations, such as colorectal surgery and those on patients with complicated appendicitis, are associated with higher postoperative infection rates, ranging from 5% to 20% or more. Coliforms and *Bacteroides* spp are common pathogens, often acting synergistically. Mixed infections with faecal streptococci and proteus or pseudomonads pose special problems in clinical management. 'Dirty' operations on abscesses or infected tissue may have an incidence of postoperative wound infection as high as 40%.

The hazard of infection can be reduced by careful choice of antimicrobial prophylactic agents, meticulous preoperative preparation of the patient and good anaesthetic and surgical techniques. Acute emergency cases are at special risk.

Peritonitis

Chemical ('abacterial') peritonitis arises when irritant substances such as pancreatic juice, gastroduodenal contents or blood gain access to the peritoneum. Staphylococcal peritonitis sometimes follows surgical intervention.

Various bacteria, e.g. streptococci, may be associated with a *primary* infection. Peritonitis occurring as a complication of continuous ambulatory peritoneal dialysis (CAPD) is a particular problem.

Infections most commonly associated with peritonitis are *secondary* to perforation of an abdominal or pelvic viscus. These infections are due to aggressive elements of the commensal flora and are mixed: coliforms, *Bacteroides* spp. and Gram-positive cocci are usually prominent. Clostridia are sometimes involved. Pure anaerobic infections may be encountered, especially in pelvic abscesses.

Pelvic inflammatory disease

This is a cause of much morbidity in female patients, who are especially prone to pelvic infection. It is most commonly acquired from the genital tract, with inflammation in the region of the uterus, fallopian tubes and ovaries giving rise to symptoms and signs of local peritoneal irritation. As in other forms of pelvic sepsis there may be mixed coliform organisms and anaerobes, usually *Bacteroides* spp and/or anaerobic cocci. Chlamydial infection, which frequently leads to infertility, is common and must not be missed. Expert advice should be sought and the appropriate swabs taken. Pelvic sepsis in male or female patients may follow peritoneal infection arising from a non-genital source, such as a perforated appendix.

Burns

Burned areas of skin are highly vulnerable to bacterial colonization with organisms such as *Streptococcus pyogenes* (group A β-haemolytic streptococcus), various staphylococci and Gram-negative aerobic bacteria (e.g. coliforms, proteus and pseudomonads) and faecal streptococci.

Pressure sores

Ulceration of the skin over pressure areas in immobilized patients results from ischaemia. There is direct pressure on small blood vessels which causes endothelial damage, leading to activation of the clotting system. Predisposing factors include vascular disease, anaemia, obesity, incontinence, malnutrition, loss of cutaneous sensation, chronic debilitating disease, and imposed restriction of movement associated with the control of fractures.

Prevention requires careful teamwork and vigilance. Quality nursing care, the identification of high-risk patients, regular (minimum 2-hourly) turning and special beds or mattresses (e.g. a water ripple mattress) may be necessary to avoid uneven distribution of the patient's weight. The skin should be kept dry and clean. Treatment of a pressure sore includes control of infection, debridement of necrotic tissue and eschar, cleansing, relief of pressure and nutritional support. Dietary supplements of vitamin C and oral zinc may help to promote good healing.

Sepsis, shock and SIRS

The non-microbiological term *sepsis* implies clinical evidence of infection, plus evidence of a systemic response to infection. This may be as two or more of:

- Hypo- or hyperthermia
- Heart rate > 90:bpm
- respiratory rate > 20 breaths/min or Pa_{CO_2} < 32 mmHg (<4 kPa)
- WBC > 12 000 cells/mm^3 or < 4000 cells/mm^3 or > 10% immature (band) forms.

These findings, with evidence of altered organ perfusion and hypoxemia, elevated lactate, oliguria or hypotension indicate the presence of the *sepsis syndrome*. The term 'septic shock' denotes sepsis with hypotension despite adequate fluid resuscitation, along with the presence of perfusion abnormalities. Dilated small vessels result in a reduction of systemic vascular resistance and leaky capillaries under the influence of inflammatory mediators such as kinins, complement components, histamine, cytokines and endogenous opiates.

Such shock syndromes are associated with a considerable spectrum of microbial challenges. These may occur postoperatively after abdominal or genitourinary operations, following invasive manipulations, or in patients in intensive care after serious injuries or major surgery. Blood cultures can be helpful in identifying the pathogens and guiding therapy, but it is necessary to start active antimicrobial treatment on a 'best-guess' emergency basis.

The shock syndromes are variously described as *bacteraemic*, *septicaemic* or *septic shock*. Other synonyms, such as *Gram-negative shock* and *endotoxic shock* reflect the fact that Gram-negative bacteria are often (but not invariably) responsible, and that bacterial lipopolysaccharide endotoxin is a significant mediator. Such endotoxin is a potent inducer of inflammatory mediators. Macrophage-derived mediators such as interleukin-1, tumour necrosis factor and interleukin-6 play important roles in the initiation and generation of the acute-phase inflammatory response to infection. The clinical use of the terminology is often rather loose, which may be confusing.

Although Gram-negative sepsis is more commonly associated with septic shock, Gram-positive sepsis may be too. Gram-positive shock is caused by other cell wall compo-

nents and lipoteichoic acid. It is clinically indistinguishable from Gram-negative sepsis. The possibility of septic shock should be considered whenever cardiovascular instability is evident in a patient with major infection, or in a postoperative or injured patient in whom a major infection may be developing. The condition may present suddenly, but some patients become progressively more shocked over a period of time. Clinical awareness and prompt action are essential.

Two phases are recognized, although in a fulminating case the patient's condition may deteriorate so rapidly that the dramatic features of the second phase may be all that are noted.

The *hyperdynamic* phase is characterized by tachycardia, hyperventilation, warm dry extremities, but an ominous degree of hypotension. The patient may be anxious and restless, and then confused, lethargic, drowsy and weak.

The patient's colour may progress to a curious facial flush with a slightly mauve cyanotic tinge, heralding the transition to the *hypodynamic* phase. Here there is cyanosis, marked hypotension, vasoconstriction, oliguria and mental confusion, followed by multiple organ failure, coma and then death.

The pulmonary component of multiple organ failure is the adult respiratory distress syndrome (ARDS), with acute dyspnoea and hypoxaemia, widespread infiltrates in the lungs with increased permeability and inflammatory changes, and pulmonary oedema. ARDS may be associated with a range of causes. In at least 50% of patients the cause is septicaemia and the mortality rate in this group is very high. ARDS as a complication of septicaemia is sometimes loosely called 'septic lung'. The term denotes acute respiratory failure in a patient with sepsis or septic shock, but the lung is not primarily involved in the bacterial infection and is reacting as one of the components of multiple organ failure.

In septic shock the organs that fail include the heart, the lungs, the brain, the kidneys and the liver.

The *systemic inflammatory response syndrome* (SIRS) is the response to a variety of clinical conditions where inflammation may be evident with fever and organ hypoperfusion. Non-infectious entities such as pancreatitis, trauma and severe burns, as well as infection, are potential causes.

Helicobacter pylori

Infection with *H. pylori* carries the risk of upper gastrointestinal inflammation and neoplastic disease. The prevalence varies with geography and increases with age. In developing countries infection is virtually universal by the age of 20 years, whereas in more developed countries acquisition is gradual and may reach 60% of the population by the age of 60. There are associations with peptic ulcer disease, gastric carcinoma and lymphoma. Pernicious anaemia is negatively associated, as is infection with certain (cag A⁺) strains and oesophageal reflux, Barrett's oesophagus and adenocarcinoma of the stomach. Diagnosis of *H. pylori* infection can be made endoscopically by biopsy and/or culture, or non-invasively by serology and urease breath tests. In the past management of peptic ulceration frequently included surgery, but now *H. pylori* eradication with triple therapy can be used in most cases of disease caused by this organism. A proton pump inhibitor or bismuth salt with two antibiotics, such as amoxicillin with clarithromycin or metronidazole, is used. Treatment failure is usually related to compliance difficulties or antibiotic resistance.

ANAEROBIC INFECTION

Tetanus

The key features of tetanus, which is caused by *Clostridium tetani*, are given in the summary box, below. When infection is established, *C. tetani* contributes little to local wound inflammation. However, it produces an exotoxin (*tetanospasmin* commonly called tetanus toxin). This enters the presynaptic terminals of the lower motor neurons, pro-

---

SUMMARY BOX

Tetanus

- *Clostridium tetani* is an anaerobic spore-forming bacillus found in soil and faeces.

- Tetanus may develop from small contaminated puncture wounds, which may be so small that they are ignored by the patient (one-third of cases).

- Survival in wounds is favoured by hypoxia and by haematoma formation, devitalized tissue, and the presence of soil and foreign bodies.

- Failure to cleanse, excise and debride wounds favours multiplication of the organism and the liberation of exotoxin.

- Tetanus contributes little to local inflammation but exotoxin increases muscle tone, leading to muscle spasms and exaggerated responses to trivial stimuli.

- The incubation period varies from a few days to 3 months (usually less than 2 weeks), and the longer the incubation period and delay to the onset of spasms, the better the prognosis.

- Antibiotics (penicillin or erythromycin) are an *adjunct* to correct surgical care of wounds.

---

ducing local failure of neuromuscular transmission. Retrograde axonal transport carries the toxin to the cell bodies of these neurons in the brain stem and spinal cord.

Clinical presentation

The clinical presentation of tetanus is often insidious. A tingling, ache or stiffness in the wound area is usually the first symptom. Jaw movements become restricted (hence the traditional name 'lockjaw'), facial muscle spasms produce a sardonic grin (risus sardonicus), and the muscles of the neck and back become stiff. Dysphagia, laryngeal spasm and spasm of the chest wall muscles and diaphragm can compromise ventilation and threaten life.

In severe cases, painful muscle spasms become more widespread and increase in frequency and duration. Arching of the back muscles can produce a state known as 'opisthotonos'. Sphincter spasm may cause micturition difficulties.

The patient remains conscious, although consciousness is frequently clouded. The muscle spasms are painful and exhausting and may be triggered by minor stimuli. The temperature is normal or only slightly elevated, despite profuse sweating and tachycardia, manifestations of autonomic dysfunction. These features are due to sympathetic overactivity, which may also cause worrying swings in blood pressure.

It is important to appreciate that these are the clinical features of a severe attack. Some cases are milder and do not progress to the full spectrum of generalized muscle spasms.

Diagnosis

The diagnosis is essentially clinical. It may be supported by the demonstration of typical slender bacilli with drumstick spores in material from the devitalized wound tissue, and confirmed by the demonstration of tetanus toxin in cultures by toxin–antitoxin neutralization tests in mice.

Prevention

Tetanus is a preventable disease – some call it an 'inexcusable disease'. Its low prevalence in countries with well-developed medical services depends on prompt and adequate attention to wounds (Fig 6.4) and programmes of active immunization.

Active immunization of all children in the UK is achieved by the use of a combined vaccine, the so-called triple vaccine (diphtheria, pertussis and tetanus), which includes adsorbed tetanus toxoid and is given in three doses within the first year of life, starting at 2 months of age. For primary immunization of children and adults the doses are

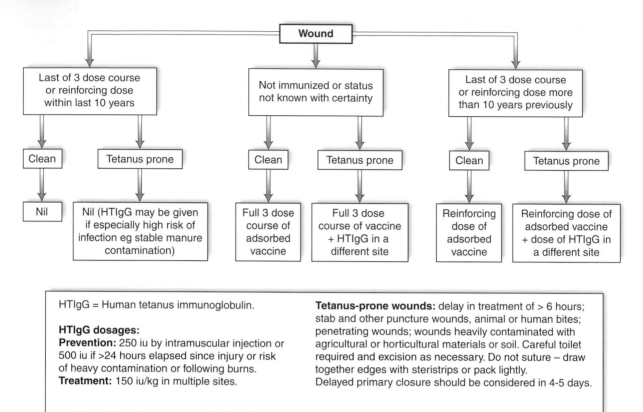

HTIgG = Human tetanus immunoglobulin.

HTIgG dosages:
Prevention: 250 iu by intramuscular injection or 500 iu if >24 hours elapsed since injury or risk of heavy contamination or following burns.
Treatment: 150 iu/kg in multiple sites.

Tetanus-prone wounds: delay in treatment of > 6 hours; stab and other puncture wounds, animal or human bites; penetrating wounds; wounds heavily contaminated with agricultural or horticultural materials or soil. Careful toilet required and excision as necessary. Do not suture – draw together edges with steristrips or pack lightly.
Delayed primary closure should be considered in 4-5 days.

Adapted from Department of Health, Welsh office, Scottish Department of Health, DHSS (Northern Ireland). Immunisation against Infectious Diseases HMSO 1996

Fig. 6.4   Antitetanus wound management.

given at 1-month intervals. Booster injections of adsorbed toxoid should be given at 5 and 15 years, and thereafter at 10-year intervals until a total of five doses have been administered. This probably gives lifelong immunity.

Human tetanus immunoglobulin (HTIgG) is available in many countries, rather than equine immunoglobulin (antitetanus serum, ATS), to give immediate transient protection to non-immune patients. Its use is reserved for those considered to be tetanus prone, and then as an adjunct to active immunization and antibiotic treatment (see below).

Antibiotic prophylaxis

Penicillin (or, if the patient is hypersensitive, erythromycin) should be started before the wound is cleaned and explored. A 5-day course is given, the first tablet being administered just before wound toilet. It must be stressed that antibiotic treatment does not replace the need for basic surgical care of the primary wound, but it may be a necessary adjunct.

Tetanus treatment

Treatment of tetanus is intensive and must begin as soon as the diagnosis is made. Surgical debridement of any wounds is indicated.

Life support   The airway and ventilation must be rapidly assessed and, if necessary, endotracheal intubation performed under benzodiazepine sedation and neuromuscular blockade. The effects of toxin that has been fixed to receptors in the nervous system must be countered if the patient is to survive. Muscle spasms are controlled by benzodiazepines such as diazepam, or a propofol infusion. Such sedation also helps to reduce the patient's awareness of a terrifying experience. Sometimes neuromuscular blockade is required.

Destruction of the infecting organism and neutralization of the toxin   Human tetanus immunoglobulin 150 iu/kg is given intramuscularly at multiple sites. The wound is excised, cleaned and left open. Penicillin 1 mega-unit 6-hourly by intramuscular injection, or intravenous infusion with metronidazole 500 mg intravenously or 1 g rectally 8-hourly by suppository, will kill surviving bacteria and prevent further production of toxin. In North America metronidazole is thought to be more efficacious than penicillin. Appropriate doses should be continued for 7–10 days. The first dose of antibiotic and the antitoxin should be given immediately, and before wound excision if possible. Active immunization with intramuscular tetanus toxoid should also be commenced early, and a further 2 doses given at monthly intervals.

Gas gangrene and other clostridial infections

Clostridium perfringens (previously called *C. welchii*) is the principal cause of clostridial myonecrosis or gas gangrene. Other clostridial species, alone or in combination, may also be associated with gas gangrene, often in concert with facultative organisms. The organisms form spores, which reside in soil and faeces and contaminate skin and clothing. They are strict anaerobes and their growth is favoured by failure to debride contaminated wounds.

The spectrum of infection extends from superficial contamination of an open wound, through the invasion of subcutaneous tissue, the production of crepitant cellulitis and localized painful myositis, to the full-blown picture of clostridial myonecrosis and gas gangrene. Localized forms of infection need not be associated with signs of systemic upset, or there may be relatively mild upset with fever and tachycardia. Diffuse myositis and gas gangrene produce profound systemic upset and quickly threaten the affected limb, as well as the life of the patient.

Infection typically takes 2–3 days to become manifest. The wound and surrounding tissues must be inspected, after the removal of plaster casts if need be. In the right clinical setting rapid onset of pain without local findings should alert the practitioner to gas gangrene. A brown seropurulent discharge with a characteristic odour, oedema, crepitus and pain on examination support the diagnosis, which is confirmed microscopically by the presence of Gram-positive rods. Subsequent culture and special tests determine the clostridial species involved. Blood culture sometimes helps to establish the diagnosis and to guide management.

Prevention

As with tetanus, prompt and adequate primary wound care by excision and debridement is essential. Contaminated wounds must not be closed by primary suture. Penicillin remains the prophylactic antibiotic of choice, with erythromycin as a good alternative. Polyvalent gas gangrene antitoxin was once available but its efficacy was in doubt and allergic reactions were common. It is no longer used.

Treatment

An established infection is treated radically. The wound is opened widely, fascial compartments are freely incised and dead tissue meticulously removed. Devitalized muscle must be excised widely until bleeding viable tissue is encountered. In some cases amputation is inevitable.

Wounds are loosely packed and left open, to be closed only when they appear healthy. Wide tissue defects may require subsequent tissue reconstruction and skin grafting. Amputation stumps are also left open in the first instance.

Intensive supportive therapy to correct and maintain fluid and electrolyte balance is necessary. Hypovolaemia is common and multiple transfusions may be required. Antibiotic therapy is essential. Penicillin is given in very high dosage, together with metronidazole to control anaerobes. Additional antibiotics may be needed to control the components of mixed infections that may be encountered. Intensive antibiotic therapy should be started before radical surgery, but not at the expense of losing valuable time.

Hyperbaric oxygenation in a pressure chamber has been used for over 30 years, but it remains controversial. It is not

SUMMARY BOX

Clostridial infection

- *Clostridium perfringens* is the principal cause of gas gangrene (clostridial myonecrosis), but other clostridial species may also be involved.

- The organism is a spore-forming strict anaerobe present in soil and faeces, and its growth in a wound is favoured by failure to debride.

- Toxins produced by clostridia (lecithinase, collagenase, proteinases, hyaluronidase, lipase and haemolysins) devitalize cells, destroy the microcirculation, and favour the spread of infection along tissue planes.

- The clinical manifestations of infection are first local (crepitus, brown seropurulent discharge and painful myositis) and then systemic (tachycardia, pallor and clouded consciousness).

- Infection may take 2–3 days to become manifest, but should be suspected if there is an unexplained deterioration in the general clinical condition.

- Clostridial myonecrosis is prevented by adequate *excision and debridement of contaminated wounds*, the prescription of antibiotics (penicillin or erythromycin), and avoidance of inappropriate primary closure.

- Established gas gangrene is managed urgently by opening the wound widely and excising all devitalized tissue, prescribing antibiotics in very high dosage, and (possibly) by hyperbaric oxygenation. Amputation may be unavoidable.

a replacement for adequate surgery and the other measures described above. An increased arterial PaO$_2$ cannot drive oxygen into dead tissues or eradicate established infection in devitalized tissues.

A particular mixed form of clostridial infection follows penetrating injury to the colon or rectum, the source of infecting organisms being the bowel. The mixed infection is likely to include clostridia and *Bacteroides* spp, anaerobic cocci, faecal streptococci, coliforms and pseudomonads. Wide debridement, free drainage, intensive broad-spectrum antibiotic therapy and a proximal colostomy are essential measures.

Progressive bacterial gangrene and necrotizing fasciitis

These form a spectrum of advancing bacterial gangrene which may occur after a seemingly trivial injury or an operation, typically in the lower abdomen or perineum.

Progressive bacterial gangrene (bacterial synergistic gangrene, dermal gangrene, Meleney's gangrene) involves only the skin and advances relatively slowly. A variety of organisms have been incriminated, and synergistic action between microaerophilic streptococci and associated organisms is considered important. Predisposing factors include general debility, diabetes and hypoxia.

The syndrome of *necrotizing fasciitis* can be divided into two entities. Type I involves at least one anaerobic species isolated in combination with one or more facultative anaerobic species such as streptococci (other than group A) and coliforms. Type II (haemolytic streptococcal gangrene) involves group A streptococci alone or in combination with other species, such as *Staphylococcus aureus*. Necrotizing fasciitis is an uncommon severe infection affecting primarily the subcutaneous fat and deep fascia. The skin dies as a result of thrombosis of its blood supply. It is a rapidly advancing, frequently fatal disease in which any part of the body may be involved, but most commonly the extremities. The rapidity and extent of tissue destruction are very alarming. The initial clinical feature of pain at the affected site in the setting of possible infection is key in alerting the clinician to the possible diagnosis. In 25% of patients there is no skin erythema. Initial cellulitis may be associated with the appearance of dusky purple patches in its centre, which progress to skin necrosis. There may be crepitus in 20% of cases. The patient becomes very ill and develops septic shock.

Fournier's gangrene is a term that refers to necrotizing fasciitis occurring around the male genitals. It may extend to involve the abdominal wall. Typically mixed bacterial cultures are grown.

Diagnosis and treatment

Prompt diagnosis should lead to the mainstay of treatment; immediate radical surgical excision of the affected area.

Haemoglobin, blood glucose, blood urea and electrolyte concentrations should be determined. Haemodynamic instability must be corrected with intravenous infusions. Swabs and excised tissue are sent for Gram filming and culture. Blood is also sampled and sent for culture. Intraoperative frozen section examination can confirm the diagnosis. Diabetes may coexist and predispose to this condition.

Intravenous antibiotics are started immediately: a combination of high-dose benzylpenicillin, metronidazole and gentamicin is recommended. Clindamycin should be included in group A streptococcal infection, as in-vitro animal data show this is more effective than penicillin. Where possible, cultures should be taken before antibiotics are given. Treatment is modified in the light of patient factors such as renal function and culture reports as they become available.

Urgent surgical review and radical excision of the affected area, including skin, subcutaneous tissue and deep fascia, is performed. Amputation may be necessary. The patient returns to theatre daily for inspection and further necessary excision until the infection is under control. The resulting defect in the skin and deep fascia, which frequently is very large, may require skin grafting.

Other anaerobic infections

The Gram-negative non-sporing anaerobic pathogens include *Bacteroides*-like spp (*Bacteroides fragilis*, *Prevotella* (*Bacteroides*) *melaninogenica*, *Porphyromonas asaccharolytica* etc.) and fusobacteria such as *Fusobacterium necrophorum*. These often occur in association with anaerobic cocci and other facultative organisms in a wide range of mixed putrefactive infections, including cerebral abscess, periodontal disease, ulceromembranous gingivitis and dental abscess, cancrum oris, Ludwig's angina, aspiration pneumonia, lung abscess, infected bite wounds, synergistic gangrene, necrotizing fasciitis, peritonitis, pelvic abscess, perianal and ischiorectal abscess, balanoposthitis, vaginitis/vaginosis and decubitus ulcers. The most important aspect of treatment of most abscesses, particularly those in the perianal and ischiorectal region, is surgical drainage to prevent damage and sequelae, such as anal sphincter dysfunction. Some abscesses are best drained under radiological guidance.

The common anaerobic component of many of these infections must be appreciated if the results of treatment are not to be disappointing. In some cases there is alarming pathogenic synergy, which overwhelms the patient if effective treatment is delayed.

HOSPITAL-ACQUIRED (NOSOCOMIAL) INFECTIONS

Nosocomial infection is the term used to describe infection that becomes manifest while the patient is in hospital, typically more than 48 hours after admission. Such infection may be endogenous, from the patient's own flora, or exogenous, from the hospital environment. Infection may spread from the environment, between patients, and between patients and staff. Patients who remain in hospital for some time acquire hospital organisms on the skin, in the nose and mouth and in the gut. Such hospital strains of bacteria may have evolved a special facility for colonization and infection. Examples include some strains of *Staphylococcus aureus*, particularly epidemic methicillin-resistant *Staph. aureus* (MRSA). A patient who is unwell and old has both reduced tissue and reduced general resistance, and is more susceptible to colonization and infection. An increased length of stay of such a patient in an acute hospital increases the risk of infection. After any prolonged series of inpatient investigations it is wise to allow patients to return home before surgical treatment, so that their normal flora can be restored away from the hospital environment.

Sites of colonization

Hospital practice often fails to recognize the significance of a patient's own endogenous flora in relation to both potential protective and pathogenic effects. For example, long-

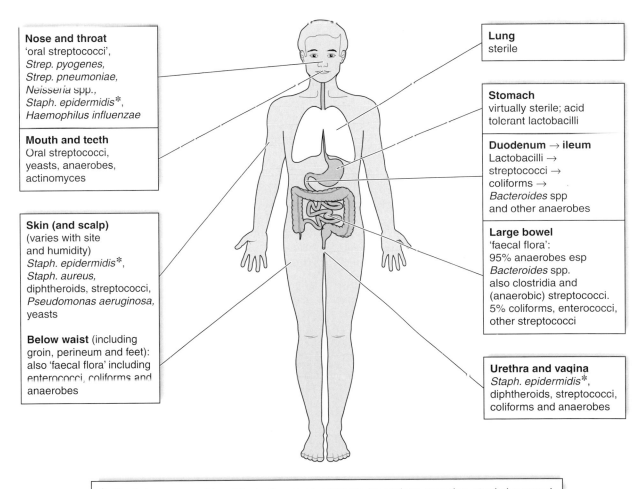

Nose and throat
'oral streptococci',
Strep. pyogenes,
Strep. pneumoniae,
Neisseria spp.,
Staph. epidermidis*,
Haemophilus influenzae

Mouth and teeth
Oral streptococci,
yeasts, anaerobes,
actinomyces

Skin (and scalp)
(varies with site
and humidity)
Staph. epidermidis*,
Staph. aureus,
diphtheroids, streptococci,
Pseudomonas aeruginosa,
yeasts

Below waist (including
groin, perineum and feet):
also 'faecal flora' including
enterococci, coliforms and
anaerobes

Lung
sterile

Stomach
virtually sterile; acid
tolerant lactobacilli

Duodenum → ileum
Lactobacilli →
streptococci →
coliforms →
Bacteroides spp
and other anaerobes

Large bowel
'faecal flora':
95% anaerobes esp
Bacteroides spp.
also clostridia and
(anaerobic) streptococci.
5% coliforms, enterococci,
other streptococci

Urethra and vagina
Staph. epidermidis*,
diphtheroids, streptococci,
coliforms and anaerobes

* *Staphylococcus epidermidis* is the most common 'coagulase negative staphylococcus' frequently found on skin. Density of colonization varies greatly with age and site.

Mucosal or skin breaches may allow normal flora to infect usually sterile sites. Overgrowth by potentially pathogenic members of the normal flora may occur with changes in normal composition (eg after antimicrobial treatment, local changes in pH (vagina and stomach) or defective immunity (eg AIDS or immunosuppressive treatment). The most common yeast is *Candida albicans.*

Fig. 6.5 Distribution of normal adult flora.

stay patients, particularly when old, should ideally not be treated in an acute surgical ward, as the dispersal of acquired skin flora, e.g. from an infected bedsore, into the ward environment and on to surfaces in toilet areas, poses a danger to other patients. The distribution of 'normal flora' in healthy adults is shown in Figure 6.5. The 'colonization resistance' of the gut is markedly reduced by some forms of antibiotic therapy. This allows the emergence of *Clostridium difficile*-associated diarrhoea, as well as opportunities for the exchange of antibiotic resistance between strains and species of gut bacteria.

Hospital microbial challenges

Hand-borne or surface-mediated challenges

The hands of patients and staff are of great importance in conveying microbes. Compliance with handwashing among healthcare workers is often poor, at about 40%. Medical staff are often the worst offenders, and until opinion formers (i.e. hospital consultants) lead by example in this area, rates of hospital-acquired infection are likely to remain higher than need be. Infection spread on the hands of staff may be considered iatrogenic and is increasingly the cause of litigation. Related hazards and possible control measures are summarized in Table 6.1. Some sophisticated measures, such as special containment facilities, are costly, but simple methods of control are not, and yet the latter are often neglected.

Airborne challenges

Potential microbial challenges from air and effective measures to control them are listed in Table 6.2. Some basic control measures are not unduly expensive and, if applied conscientiously, reduce the advantages of more costly measures, such as unidirectional filtered air systems.

Table 6.1 Hand-borne challenges and contact hazards, and possible control measures

Hazard	Control measures
Hand contact (direct and via surfaces)	Handwashing, antiseptics and disinfectants, gloves, no-touch techniques
Trolley surfaces etc., contaminated instruments, contaminated solutions	Disposable or 'dedicated' instruments, adequate staff adequately trained, adequate facilities
Shared facilities, e.g. shared toilets, basins, towels, cork mats	Separate facilities, special containment facilities

Table 6.2 Airborne hazards, associated problems and possible control measures

Hazard	Control measures
Contamination of ward and theatre air	Ventilation in theatre and ward. Adequate bed interspacing
Transmissible respiratory infections	Attention to anaesthetic equipment and ventilators
Wound dressing	Avoidance of contamination by restriction of this procedure in ward
Bedmaking	Avoidance of generation of airborne particles
Floor polishing, toilet flushing etc.	Avoidance of use of aerosols, treatment of fabrics, control of dangerous dispersers
Hot air blowers	Filtration and laminar flow systems, special containment facilities
Droplet *Legionella* spread	Expert engineering and maintenance of hospital water systems

Ingested challenges

Significant microbial challenges may be delivered to the gastrointestinal tract in hospital (Table 6.3). Food hygiene is of paramount importance and hospital catering systems must be of a high standard. The numbers of organisms

Table 6.3 Ingested challenges, associated problems and possible control measures

Hazard	Control measures
Contaminated hospital food	Strict food hygiene, isolation of patients with infective diarrhoea
Contaminated special diet formulations	Good, easily cleaned equipment, safe kitchen practices
Contaminated drug and TPN preparations	Microbiological monitoring, trained staff, sterile preparation facilities
Resistance factor transmission from animals	Control of antibiotics in animal husbandry, care in food preparation

delivered to patients in hospital food may be unacceptably high. Resistant organisms may reach the gut of patients as a result of the multiplication of animal strains that contaminate some foods.

Inoculated challenges

Inoculated challenges and controls are of increasing clinical significance (Table 6.4). 'Universal precautions' is the term

Table 6.4 Inoculated challenges, problems and possible control measures	
Hazard	Possible (current/?future) control measures
Bloodborne pathogen (e.g. protozoa–malaria, viruses, treponemes (syphilis))	'Universal precautions' Prevent inoculation of carrier's blood Immunization Exclude blood donations from high-risk donors Screen blood donations Emergency antiviral prophylaxis Routine antimalarial with blood infusion Removal of contaminated component (e.g. neutrophil filters – CMV, ?CJD) Heat treatment of blood donation Detergent treatment of blood donation?
Contaminated infusion (e.g. with staphylococci and aerobic Gram-negative bacilli)	Sterile infusion equipment and infusates Sterile pharmacy infusate preparation Once-only needle, connectors, infusion kits Careful management of connectors etc.
Percutaneous catheter infection	Handwashing, skin preparation with iodine, chlorhexidine or alcohol Sterile technique Multidisciplinary team for management Optimal management of the insertion site and limitations of entry into the system, administration set and catheter itself Tunnelling of catheter

used to convey the concept that appropriate barrier precautions should be routinely taken to prevent skin and mucous membrane contact with blood or other body fluids of any patient. Any patient may be 'high risk'. Infection with bloodborne viruses, such as hepatitis B (HBV), hepatitis C (HCV) and the human immunodeficiency virus (HIV), are important examples of the serious potential hazard of skin-penetrating injuries in patients and all clinical staff. This arises from cross-contamination with blood or other body fluids from someone with a recognized infection, or one who may be a known or unknown carrier. Following inoculation with infected blood the risk of infection to the naive injured party is approximately 30%, 3% and 0.3% for HBV, HCV and HIV, respectively. Such an injury should be encouraged to bleed and washed immediately with soap and water. If the eye is involved this should be copiously irrigated with water. Many other pathogenic agents, including bacteria, malaria and syphilis, can be transmitted by accidental inoculation of blood or blood products. In surgical staff, glove punctures occur in up to 30% of operations, and skin-penetrating injuries with needles and knives are common events, demanding constant caution for avoidance. The carrier rate for hepatitis B in the UK is around 0.1%; in some countries in Africa and Asia it is as high as 5–15%. In any country there are groups at higher and lower risk than these. Surgeons, obstetricians, dentists, haematologists, laboratory workers and workers in transfusion services are particularly at risk, and should take care to avoid skin-penetrating injuries and skin, eye and mucous membrane exposure in circumstances in which contamination with blood or blood products or other body fluids is likely.

The infective state of a patient or carrier in relation to HBV is demonstrated by the detection of hepatitis B surface antigen (HBsAg) in the serum. Detection of hepatitis B 'e' antigen (HBeAg) indicates an individual at particularly high risk of spreading infection.

At present in the UK medical, dental, nursing and midwifery students should be immunized against hepatitis B for their own protection, and their response checked. Non-responders should be shown to be non-infective.

If a non-immune person has a skin-penetrating injury or mucosal exposure to likely hepatitis B contamination, emergency (postexposure) passive protection can be given by intramuscular injection of hyperimmune hepatitis B immunoglobulin (HBIgG), preferably within 48 hours. Unless the non-immune person is a known non-responder, active immunization should also be commenced. In the case of penetrating HIV contamination urgent postexposure antiretroviral prophylaxis should be available. At present there are no such recommendations following HCV exposure. Knowledge is advancing rapidly and the detail of these recommendations may change. Should healthcare workers think that they may have been exposed to a bloodborne virus such as HBV, HCV and HIV, following counselling they should be tested and followed up. Advice on how to protect sexual partners may also be required. The sensitive and confidential handling of such individuals presents a significant challenge to Occupational Health Departments and Healthcare Organizations.

Hazards associated with intensive care

Special infective hazards may be posed by a variety of procedures performed in an intensive care unit, including the use of ventilators, nasogastric tubes, drugs reducing gastric acid secretion, suction apparatus, intravenous lines, percutaneous needles, and catheters. It is paradoxical that our most severely compromised patients should be exposed to such inadvertent challenges.

The remarks made above concerning the avoidance of hospital-acquired infection become vital in intensive care, where the patients are already critically ill. All units should have well developed policies to avoid the transfer of organisms from staff to patients, or from patients to patients.

Control of hospital-acquired (nosocomial) infection

An effective hospital infection control programme depends above all on teamwork, conscientiousness and communication. The specialized risks of bloodborne viruses are described above.

Prompt detection and treatment of hospital infection

Day-to-day monitoring in the wards and related areas is essential to ensure that infections are detected quickly and recorded. A wound infection record should be kept in each unit. Ward surveillance is particularly important in special areas such as intensive care units, neonatal units, renal units, and areas where neutropenic patients are nursed. There must be assured daily links, ideally including visits, with the laboratory, so that the nature of the infecting organisms is known, early notification of a particularly dangerous pathogen is ensured, and trends in antibiotic resistance are monitored. Close cooperation between the infection control team (doctors and nurses) and senior ward staff and laboratories is essential.

Prevention of transmission of infectious agents

Approaches to preventing the spread of infection in a hospital range from the provision of suitable isolation and containment facilities for those with special infections or at special risk of infection, to the prompt availability of an expert team to mount an immediate investigation and institute necessary control measures as required. Prompt diagnosis and treatment of an infection can contribute substantially to the prevention of transmission. Clear policies on the following matters are important to protect patients from cross-infection:

- Recording of infection
- The correct use of disinfectants
- Safe disposal of infected material
- Cleaning, disinfection and sterilization of instruments
- Management of patients who have infections associated with special risks
- Proper use of antibiotics
- Use of immunizing agents.

ANTIMICROBIAL MANAGEMENT OF WOUND INFECTIONS

It is important to know when a wound is being significantly colonized by a potential pathogen. Regular inspection of wounds is essential, and microbiological assistance should be sought when necessary. The decision to treat a wound infection should be based on clinical judgement and should not be an automatic response to a positive culture report. In some cases, removal of a suture at an inflamed point (minor stitch abscess) may be all that is needed to allow host defences to operate. Similarly, the isolation of coliforms from a mild superficial infection of an abdominal wound need not call for active antimicrobial therapy if the patient's general condition does not indicate a constitutional upset. On the other hand, a positive blood culture obtained from a patient with signs of impending shock, or the isolation of a significant pathogen (e.g. *Streptococcus pyogenes*) from a wound with signs of regional lymphadenitis, calls for immediate antimicrobial treatment.

Inconsistent or incompatible findings must be discussed with senior experts. For example, a report on a secondary plate culture obtained after a specimen of pus has been subjected to enrichment culture in cooked meat broth might yield a profuse, almost pure growth of *Clostridium perfringens* derived from spores contaminating skin adjacent to the wound. If the wound is giving no clinical cause for alarm and the patient's general condition is satisfactory, a diagnosis of gas gangrene is most unlikely to be justified. Heroic treatment must not be instituted on the basis of such evidence.

Suggestions for specific antibiotic therapy are given in Table 6.5, and initial ('best-guess') therapy is indicated in Table 6.6. The antibiotic sensitivities of common anaerobic pathogens are outlined in Table 6.7. Therapy should be guided by local epidemiology and antimicrobial sensitivity data.

Table 6.5	Antibiotics in surgery: suggestions for specific therapy 2001	
Organism	First choice	Alternative
Methicillin-sensitive *Staphylococcus aureus* (coagulase positive)	Flucloxacillin	Erythromycin, cefuroxime, clindamycin
Methicillin-resistant *Staphylococcus aureus*	Vancomycin	Teicoplanin, Linezolid
Coagulase-negative staphylococci	Vancomycin	Teicoplanin
Streptococcus pneumoniae (the pneumococci)	Benzylpenicillin	Erythromycin, cefuroxime, *ceftriaxone
Streptococcus pyogenes (group A β-haemolytic streptococcus)	Benzylpenicillin	Erythromycin, clindamycin
Streptococcus (*Enterococcus*) *faecalis*	Amoxicillin	Gentamicin with penicillin or amoxicillin, vancomycin
Bacteroides species	Metronidazole	Co-amoxiclav, clindamycin, erythromycin
Escherichia coli 1. Sepsis, including bacteraemia	Cefuroxime or gentamicin	*Ceftriaxone, ceftazidime, ciprofloxacin
2. Urinary tract infection	Trimethoprim or amoxicillin	Co-amoxiclav, cefuroxime, *cefotaxime, ceftazidime, norfloxacin
Haemophilus influenzae	Amoxicillin	Co-amoxiclav, cefuroxime, *ceftriaxone, trimethoprim, chloamphenicol (ocular)
Klebsiella species	Cefuroxime or gentamicin	*Cefotaxime, ceftazidime, ciprofloxacin, meropenem
Proteus species	Cefuroxime or gentamicin	*Ceftriaxone, ceftazidime, ciprofloxacin
Pseudomonas aeruginosa	Ceftazidime with gentamicin	Tazocin or ciprofloxacin
Clostridia	Benzylpenicillin, metronidazole	Clindamycin, erythromycin
Clostridium difficile	Stop predisposing antibiotic	Metronidazole or vancomycin (oral)

NB: These suggestions should be considered in the light of local epidemiology, sensitivities and drug availability.
*Ceftriaxone may be given once daily; same spectrum as cefotaxime, multiple daily dosing.

PRINCIPLES GOVERNING THE CHOICE AND USE OF ANTIBIOTICS

Antibiotics should be used with care. The clinician should attempt to recognize self-limiting infections while taking account of the potential toxicity and cost of any antibiotic. As antibiotic resistance is increasing, antibiotic abuse carries collective penalties for the individual patient and for the community.

In some situations, such as in the management of an infected ingrowing toenail (Fig. 6.6), antibiotics have a minimal role. Some consider that those managing these with antimicrobials should be strung up by the toenails! Careful removal of the nail is the appropriate management, with antimicrobial cover. In other situations, particularly in surgery, antibiotics are merely an adjunct to definitive drainage of an abscess or the removal of devitalized tissue.

If clinically indicated, the choice of therapy should be positively determined. Some organisms associated with certain illnesses are almost invariably sensitive to certain antibiotics. For example, the group A β-haemolytic streptococcus (*Streptococcus pyogenes*) is always sensitive to benzylpenicillin. On the other hand, hospital staphylococci are

Table 6.6 Initial ('best guess') therapy for acute infections

Type of infection	Antimicrobial
Chest infection	
uncomplicated	amoxicillin, erythromycin
community-acquired pneumonia	cefuroxime + erythromycin
hospital-acquired/postoperative	ceftazidime/ciprofloxacin + gentamicin
'aspiration' pneumonia	co-amoxiclav or amoxicillin + metronidazole
'atypical' or legionella likely	erythromycin or tetracyline
Urinary tract infection	
'lower' infection	trimethoprim/amoxicillin/cephalexin/nitrofurantoin
acute pyelonephritis or prostatitis*	cefuroxime/ceftriaxone/ciprofloxacin/gentamicin
Wound infection	
abdominal and pelvic	metronidazole, with (a) 2nd or 3rd generation cephalosporin or (b) benzyl penicillin and gentamicin
If *Staph. aureus* suspected	flucloxacillin or cefuroxime or erythromycin; vancomycin for MRSA or combination therapy as guided by sensitivities
amputations and ?gas gangrene	benzylpenicillin, metronidazole
Septicaemia and septic shock	benzylpenicillin with metronidazole and gentamicin/ciprofloxacin
Severe pseudomonas infections	ceftazidime or piperacillin with gentamicin for synergy; ciprofloxacin
Candida sepsis	amphotericin B; alternative fluconazole

Note: these suggestions are for occasions when immediate treatment is necessary. Amendments may be necessary in the light of local epidemiology and microbiological and clinical developments.
*4 weeks therapy with quinolone or trimethroprim for prostatitis, guided by sensitivities.
Note: 2nd generation cephalosporins such as cefuroxime have better Gram-positive action; 3rd generation cephalosporins such as ceftriaxone, cefotaxime and ceftazidime have better Gram-negative action. Ceftriaxone can be given once daily, which may be advantageous in some settings.

Table 6.7 In-vitro activity of antimicrobial drugs against anaerobic bacteria

Antibiotic	*B. fragilis*	Anaerobic cocci	Clostridia
Metronidazole	++++	++++	++++
Penicillin	+/– (often resistant)	++	++
Amoxicillin plus clavulanic acid (co-amoxiclav)	+++	+++	+++
Erythromycin	+	++	+++
Clindamycin	+++	++++	++
Chloramphenicol	++++	++++	++++
Tetracycline	+	+	+
Cephradrine	+	++	++
Cefuroxime	+	+++	++
Cefotaxime/ceftriaxone	+	++	+
Cefoxitin	+++	++	+++
Meropenem	+++	++++	++++
Gentamicin	R	R	R

Relative activity* against (column header spanning B. fragilis, Anaerobic cocci, Clostridia)

*+/–,+,++,+++, ++++ indicate increasing degrees of activity. R = resistant.

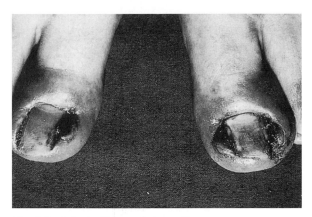

Fig. 6.6 Infected ingrown toenails.

resistance patterns of all pathogens isolated from sputum, urine, bile, pus and blood should be regularly recorded and periodically reviewed, e.g. at 6-monthly intervals. A policy may then be devised that restricts the use of those antibiotics to which resistance is developing. Knowledge of resistance permits more appropriate use of antibiotics in circumstances where it is necessary to give 'blind' treatment, for example in life-threatening infections where antibiotics must be prescribed before the results of culture and sensitivity tests are known. The guidelines below (see Box) should be observed when prescribing antibiotics.

virtually always resistant to penicillin. Antibiotic sensitivity tests are necessary to guide the clinician in many cases. It is reasonable to initiate therapy on clinical evidence, but the drugs selected must be reviewed once the microbiological report is available. When an antibiotic has been selected, an adequate dose must be given by the recommended route at the correct time intervals. In hospital practice there is often a disturbing difference between the practical interpretations of '8-hourly' and 'three times a day'.

When an organism acquires resistance to an antibiotic, it has an advantage over others of the same species in the presence of the relevant antibiotic. If the antibiotic is used extensively or carelessly in a ward, resistant organisms may become predominant.

The penicillinase-producing staphylococcal menace of the last two decades has been largely controlled, but staphylococci with multiple resistance are a threat. Many other bacteria exploit mechanisms of resistance to gain inroads into the patient they invade.

In general, an effort should be made to use a single effective antibacterial agent in the treatment of a particular infection. If a combination of antibiotics is used, the decision should be based on positive evidence that this is rational. In some cases, for example when a patient is seriously ill and a mixed infection is likely (as in acute peritonitis), it may be necessary to give more than one antibiotic to cover a likely combination of pathogens. This blunderbuss strategy should be reserved for such desperate situations and should be rationalized at the earliest opportunity in the light of the patient's progress and available microbiological guidance.

Antibiotic policy

A policy for the use of antibiotics is desirable and must be kept under regular review because of continuing changes in the patterns of bacterial resistance to antibiotics. Ideally the

---

SUMMARY BOX

Antibiotic policy

- Antibiotics should be avoided in self-limiting infections and due consideration should be given to expense, toxicity, and the need to avoid the emergence of resistant strains.

- Choice of therapy is determined positively by knowledge of the nature and sensitivities of the infecting organism(s). Therapy may be initiated on clinical evidence, but must be reviewed in the light of culture/sensitivity reports.

 Restrict the use of antibiotics to which resistance is developing (or has developed).

- Single agents are preferred to combination therapy, and narrow-spectrum agents are preferred to broad-spectrum agents whenever possible.

- Adequate doses must be given by the recommended route at correct time intervals.

- Antibiotics which are used systemically must not be used topically.

 The side-effects of antibiotics should be known and monitored.

 Expensive antibiotics are not used if equally effective and cheaper alternatives are suitable.

- With few exceptions (e.g. lung abscess), antibiotics should not be used to treat abscesses unless adequate surgical or radiological drainage has been achieved.

- Body fluids from patients receiving antibiotics must be disposed of carefully to avoid the emergence of antibiotic-resistant strains in staff, patients and the environment.

- Some policies may include automatic 'stop' orders.

Prophylactic use of antibiotics

The principle of antimicrobial prophlyaxis is to achieve high concentrations at the incision and site of operation at commencement, during and immediately after surgery. There is evidence that selective decontamination of the gut with non-absorbable antimicrobials may also help reduce some postoperative infection.

Skull fractures and meningitis

Patients with skull fractures may develop a cerebrospinal (CSF) leak or communication with a sinus or the middle ear. About 11–25% of individuals with CSF leaks become infected. The delay from the time of injury to the onset of meningitis is highly variable, from days to several years. Therefore, patients and their families should be taught how to recognize the symptoms and signs of meningitis and their doctors informed of the risks. Antibiotic prophylaxis is of uncertain benefit and is not advised.

The prophylactic use of antibiotics is established in the following situations.

Tetanus

Patients with tetanus-prone accidental wounds are given prophylaxis as described above, but the wounds must still be treated by meticulous debridement or, if treatment is delayed, by excision.

Gas gangrene

Patients with ischaemic limbs that require major surgery are at considerable risk of developing gas gangrene. Benzylpenicillin is given 1 hour preoperatively and continued 6-hourly for 3–5 days.

Prevention of endocarditis

Patients with a heart lesion, such as congenital, rheumatic or degenerative valve disease, septal defects, or prosthetic heart valves or past endocarditis are at risk of bacterial colonization if bacteraemia occurs. Before any operation that might expose them to such a risk they are given prophylactic antibiotics. The exact regimen depends on the predisposing risk factor, the nature of the operation, and whether there has been recent exposure to penicillin or a history of penicillin allergy.

Typical regimens include high-dose amoxicillin or clindamycin, amoxicillin with gentamicin and vancomycin, or teicoplanin with gentamicin. Prophylaxis may not be necessary for some (dermatological) procedures, but is indicated for dental, upper respiratory tract, genitourinary, obstetric, gynaecological and gastrointestinal procedures. A postoperative dose may also be required. It is advisable to consult expert guidelines such as those in the latest edition of the *British National Formulary* (BNF), or with an infection specialist for advice on a particular patient.

Clean surgery

Antibiotic prophylaxis is not routinely recommended for all cases, but may be beneficial in breast surgery and hernia repairs, especially where any artificial material is implanted.

Gastrointestinal and genitourinary surgery

Patients undergoing gastrointestinal and genitourinary surgery, whether elective or emergency, are at risk of wound infection, intra-abdominal infection and septicaemia. Many methods have been advocated in the past decade to reduce this risk. A single large dose of antibiotics appropriate for the predicted bacterial flora, administered intravenously on induction of anaesthesia, is probably the most convenient and effective method. Metronidazole in combination with a suitable cephalosporin has a good success record. Such regimens, particularly if prolonged, may lead to the selection of MRSA and *Clostridium difficile*-associated diarrhoea. In heavily contaminated surgery and in emergency surgery, additional doses at 8-hourly intervals postoperatively may confer further benefit. Lavage of the operative field with sterile saline is also often carried out.

Treatment of compound limb fractures

As a compound fracture is almost invariably associated with considerable contamination in an area of severely damaged tissue, it is reasonable to give antibiotic cover at once, and preferably before radical wound toilet and debridement if this does not delay essential surgical attention. Opinions differ on the choice of antibiotics. Staphylococci, coliform organisms and anaerobes are likely infecting organisms, often occurring together and with catastrophic potential. Some surgeons rely on penicillin and metronidazole to control at least two of the likely components. Others would use a second- or third-generation cephalosporin, or clindamycin or erythromycin.

Prosthetic implants

Prophylactic antibiotics are obligatory when any prosthetic material is inserted. Staphylococcal infection is the most serious problem, for example in heart valve replacement, cardiac pacemaker insertion, ventriculovenous shunts, vascular grafts, joint prostheses, mammary prostheses or polypropylene mesh repairs of massive abdominal wall defects. However, other bacteria may also be involved, and broad-spectrum cover is usually given immediately pre-operatively and 8-hourly postoperatively for 24 hours. It is important to have informed microbiological advice.

MANAGEMENT OF IMMUNOSUPPRESSED PATIENTS, INCLUDING THOSE WHO HAVE HAD SPLENECTOMY

Prophylaxis

Patients with suppressed immune mechanisms, as a result of either disease or therapy (e.g. transplant patients), should receive antibiotic prophylaxis when undergoing surgery. The choice of antibiotic is dictated by individual circumstances and expert microbiological help should be sought. Splenectomized patients are at increased risk of infection with encapsulated bacteria and protozoa. Those having elective splenectomy should be immunized with pneumo

coccal vaccine at least 2 weeks in advance of surgery. Amoxicillin should be commenced and continued for some years. In addition to routine vaccinations, *Haemophilus influenzae* type B, influenza and conjugate group C meningococcal vaccine are recommended. Travellers to areas endemic for meningococcus groups A, W135 or Y infection or malaria should take expert advice.

Treatment

Prompt *empirical antibiotic treatment* of suspected bacterial infections in immunosuppressed patients is advisable. A combination of an aminoglycoside with an anti-pseudomonal penicillin or cephalosporin is often relied upon to cover the range of likely organisms. In these patients it is also important to be on guard against fungal and protozoal infections, and to be aware of problems posed by viruses such as herpes simplex, varicella zoster and cytomegalovirus.

Ethical and legal principles in surgical practice

W.D. Plant

The practice of surgery requires a range of skills and a broad knowledge base. Prominent among these skills is the ability to identify, analyse and resolve ethical dilemmas. Medical ethics and the law as it applies to medicine have substantial overlap. In a pluralist society individuals hold different, but reasonable, views on how ethical issues should be resolved. Political, cultural and legal differences between societies and the complex new issues arising from advances in biotechnology mean that medical ethics and medical law are in an ongoing state of flux.

All patients are entitled to good standards of practice and care from their doctors. All societies recognize specific obligations, which are integral to the practice of medicine and which are expressed in various codes of practice, such as the Hippocratic Oath or the Declaration of Geneva. Regulatory authorities, such as the General Medical Council, issue guidelines specific to their jurisdictions. Statute and case law on issues such as euthanasia, abortion and medical negligence exist and are constantly modified.

Traditional medical ethics focuses largely upon the professional ethics of physicians and on the doctor–patient relationship. The term 'bioethics' has become popular in recent times. Traditional medical ethics is at its core, but it also acknowledges interplay with the more general ethics of biology, science, sociology and culture.

Fluency in the resolution of ethical dilemmas is not a part-time accomplishment for use only in theoretical debate: it is a full-time clinical and professional skill necessary for practical problem solving and decision making in the real world.

SYSTEMS AND PRINCIPLES IN MEDICAL ETHICS AND BIOETHICS

Western medicine is characterized by a number of ethical traditions that find expression in codes of practice and in the culture of healthcare workers. Among these are the deontological (duty based) and the utilitarian (consequence based) traditions.

The deontological tradition stresses the duties of practitioners and the rights of patients. This is often prescriptive and has much in common with the tenets of organized religion. Clinicians 'ought' to act in particular ways because this is 'right', often irrespective of the consequences. Statements such as 'Never kill', 'Never cause pain', or 'Always tell the truth' are classic expressions in this tradition.

The deontological tradition stresses the autonomy of the patient and the primacy of the doctor–patient relationship. Individuals should always be viewed as *ends* in themselves, never as *means* to an end. Generally speaking, ethical dilemmas should be resolved by the application of principles which are 'universal'.

Sometimes 'absolute' principles that are contradictory present as competing priorities in particular circumstances (e.g. 'Never cause pain', 'Always preserve life' – but what if a life-saving intervention causes pain?). Real-life situations often pose these difficulties.

Utilitarians, by contrast, suggest that doctors should always do that which leads to a 'good' or 'best' outcome. 'The greatest good of the greatest number' is commonly used as a summary of this approach. If the 'right' action does not lead to the 'best' outcome then it should be reviewed or abandoned. Rationing of healthcare resources brings utilitarian analyses into particular prominence. On occasion, the individual may be the 'loser' in the greater scheme of things, a common criticism of this approach.

Utilitarian analysis can be applied to an individual case – what is in the *patient's* best interest – as well as to a group of cases – what is in *patients'* best interests (or will lead to the best outcomes)? These are felt to be strands within the spectrum of utilitarianism.

For example, weighing up the consequences of acting according to a **general moral rule** (e.g. that patients over 80 years with type II diabetes should never have coronary artery bypass grafting, as the long-term survival of this group is likely to be less than that of a younger non-diabetic group) can be described as 'rule' utilitarianism. On the other hand, weighing up the consequences of **a particular act** (e.g. deciding not to proceed with an aggressive bowel resection in a relatively feeble man with mild dementia), could be described as 'act' utilitarianism.

These traditions are not opposite ways of viewing and acting upon ethical dilemmas. They tend to derive the same conclusions when 'working' moral issues are at stake. Both traditions have a strong flavour of universalisability. Ethical analyses, however, usually focus on particular cases. Because of this it is often argued that the importance of *context* may well have been understated in the past.

Some current intellectual traditions, notably Existentialism, Situation Ethics and Postmodernism are less convinced of the existence of general laws/principles that can be applied to particular cases. These focus more on how to solve specific problems as they arise, and are open to the insights of other religious, racial, philosophical and cultural traditions. Some doctors dislike this sense of moral relativism.

There is a spectrum between cases in which context and situation need to be the dominant consideration and those in which universally derived general principles can be applied. No one tradition or perspective is 'more correct': they offer different perspectives to problem solving, but often arrive at the same practical solution.

SUMMARY BOX

Systems

- Deontological   Duty based
- Utilitarian   Outcome based
- Existential/postmodern Context based

Principles

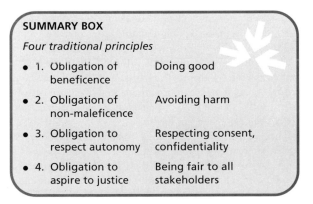

SUMMARY BOX

Four traditional principles

- 1. Obligation of beneficence   Doing good
- 2. Obligation of non-maleficence   Avoiding harm
- 3. Obligation to respect autonomy   Respecting consent, confidentiality
- 4. Obligation to aspire to justice   Being fair to all stakeholders

Beneficence: doing good

A number of principles (traditionally four) are accepted as the basis of medical ethics. In individual cases there is often conflict between simultaneous adherence to all of these. Depending on the context (and on whether a deontological or utilitarian approach is favoured), a 'least unsatisfactory' trade-off between principles must be negotiated or achieved. Skill is needed in identifying and achieving the best balance.

There is the obligation to do 'good' for the patient. Deontologists view this as a universal moral duty, utilitarians as achieving the universally desired best outcome. In the face of uncertainty, this may not be straightforward. It is worth reflecting as to whose view of 'good' should be taken as the outcome of importance. In the past, medical judgement as to 'best outcome' predominated, with relatively little input from the patient. This attitude may be less prevalent today.

Beneficence demands competence. In a multidisciplinary multispecialist environment doctors should not exceed their personal competence if a more appropriate practitioner or service is available. Accreditation and continuing medical education are central to this, as are elements such as professional development, research and audit. Communication skills are vital – weighing up possible outcomes is one thing; sharing them with the patient and negotiating choices quite another.

Non-maleficence: avoiding harm

The principle of *Primum non nocere* ('First, do no harm') has been a central tenet of medical ethics since the days of Hippocrates. All interventions, however well intentioned, may cause harm. Making sure that the balance between benefit and harm is appropriate and proportionate is an important clinical judgement. In the past, professional decisions (i.e. that the balance achieved by a particular course of action was acceptable) often paid scant attention to the patient's perspective of the balance. This is *paternalism* – according overwhelming weight to clinicians' judgement on the balance between beneficence and non-maleficence, with little weight given to respect for patient autonomy.

Sometimes the opposite may occur. A patient may demand a procedure which, in the considered opinion of the practitioner, may cause more harm than good. In this setting, after appropriate discussion with the patient, the proper course of action is to refer the patient for another opinion. There is no professional obligation to respond uncritically to *consumerism*.

Respect for autonomy

Individuals should be treated as ends not as means. Respect for the dignity, integrity and authenticity of the person is a basic human right. Deriving from this principle are the important issues of consent and confidentiality. As mentioned above, working through the first two principles seeks to arrive at a professional judgement as to what is in the patient's best interests. Moving from advice to action involves further consideration.

Informed consent is central to the doctor–patient relationship. Two issues arise here. The first relates to a patient's capacity to give or withhold consent. The second relates to the amount of information that needs to be shared with (or withheld from) the patient.

From both a legal and an ethical perspective, the patient retains the right to decide what is in his or her best interest. All conscious adults are held to have the capacity to make choices, unless evidence to the contrary can be advanced. Making a choice that seems irrational or is at variance with professional opinion does not alter that capacity.

Capacity to consent exists if a patient can:

1. Understand relevant information (explained in broad terms and with simple language)
2. Consider the implications of different options (in terms of his or her values)
3. Come to a communicable decision.

Jehovah's Witnesses illustrate this point well. Although the views of this church with regard to contact with blood products may not be in accordance with the majority view in western society, a decision to forego red-cell concentrate transfusion in a life-threatening situation must be respected if the above circumstances exist.

There are circumstances in which the capacity to consent may not exist:

- Minors
- Transient or irreversible cognitive impairment
- Mental illness
- Undue coercion.

These groups present different challenges. The law relating to children is complex, with differences between English and Scottish law in some important interpretations. Many children will be able to understand, reflect and decide on their wishes. The scenario becomes complex if a difference develops between the views of a child and those with parental responsibility. In some instances a competent child may refuse treatment, in contradiction to the wishes of the parents. An automatic right to overrule this by the parents may not exist. In these situations, legal advice is recommended.

Patients with mental illness may retain the capacity to consent to particular procedures. If not, treatment may be given in emergency or urgent situations with their compliance (subject to the remarks below). If the patient does not comply and is detained under the Mental Health Act, then treatment for the mental disorder may be administered compulsorily, subject to the safeguards included within the Act. Treatment for other physical disorders may not be enforced on the patient against their wishes, and legal advice is strongly recommended in these circumstances.

Patients with transient or irreversible cognitive impairment frequently require medical attention (including sur-

gical procedures). Acutely unwell patients often fall into this category. Some may have fluctuating capacity, owing to fever, drugs, anxiety etc. Regular assessment is mandatory, with clear record keeping. In emergencies, treatment may need to be administered in the patient's best interest. Certain guidelines are helpful (although seeking further advice from professional organizations or legal sources is always prudent). Clear communication with all relevant parties, careful documentation of the process, and broad consultation is appropriate.

SUMMARY BOX

1. Establish the various options available (including non-treatment).

2. Seek evidence of previously expressed views (e.g. advance directives).

3. Seek opinion of third parties to whom the patient may be known (e.g. parents, partner, GP, family) as to the patient's previously expressed views.

4. Administer the level of treatment that least restricts the patient's future choices (i.e. life-saving or stabilizing treatment, rather than physician-selected choice of 'definitive' treatment).

5. If substantial doubt or conflict exists, seek counsel from more experienced colleagues, from professional organizations, from legal sources.

6. If necessary, seek advice as to whether a court ruling is necessary.

Where non-therapeutic or controversial treatment is proposed (e.g. sterilization or withdrawal of feeding) for a patient who does not have the capacity to consent, then even greater care, communication and consultation is needed.

Informed consent presumes information sharing. If a patient does have the capacity to consent, then questions arise as to how much information should be provided, in what format should it be presented and recorded, and who should be responsible for this.

The legal basis of informed consent differs between states: in countries such as Australia and Canada there is a legal duty to provide patients with that information that a **prudent or reasonable patient**, in that patient's particular circumstances, would wish to know in order to arrive at a decision. In the UK, the amount of information that a **reasonable doctor** would provide, in that patient's particular circumstances, is required. (Although a court might decide that, in unusual circumstances, failure to disclose certain risks of procedures might be negligent, *even if this is accepted practice* as attested by a responsible body of medical opinion). As in the circumstances already discussed, further counsel should be sought if there is doubt.

Information about certain possible risks may be retained under so-called 'therapeutic privilege', if it is honestly felt that this would needlessly harm the patient psychologically (justified by an 'act' utilitarian attitude with heavy emphasis on non-maleficence). This privilege cannot be invoked when informed consent to participation in a research study is being obtained – for obvious reasons.

There should be no overt or covert pressure to consent. This may come from a variety of sources – employers, insurance companies, physicians or institutions deriving financial benefits from use of a specific therapy, or religious groups. Prisoners, other detainees and those detained under mental health legislation may be particular vulnerable.

The process of obtaining consent should be administered by a suitably trained and competent person, with sufficient knowledge of the treatment and its possible outcomes to engage in discussion with the patient. For many routine procedures a standardized information leaflet may be helpful. Providing sufficient time for discussion and reflection is important, particularly for complex procedures of uncertain outcome.

Ideally a written record of the patient's consent should be obtained, with sufficient detail to identify their express wishes (particularly if certain aspects of treatment have been declined). Assuming (implied) consent to a variety of procedures because of compliance with a perfunctory 'consent-form signed' interaction is not a prudent course of action.

The other major principle deriving from respect for autonomy is the right to confidentiality. This is of even greater moment in an age of electronic record holding, with multidisciplinary teams caring for patients. Information relating to patients must never be casually revealed to other persons. Within teams, only that information relevant to a team member fulfilling his or her part in the process of care should be shared. If individual cases are discussed to illustrate or inform teaching activities, then the identity of the patient must be concealed. There are some circumstances (e.g. notifiable diseases) in which there is a statutory obligation to reveal details about an individual patient. In general, confidentiality is an integral part of the doctor–patient relationship.

Justice: promoting fairness

In modern healthcare, demand outstrips supply. Consequently, access to healthcare interventions varies (by either explicit or implicit rationing). The principle of justice is important here. The allocation of resources requires a rank-ordering system with some philosophical justification for the method chosen. There are many theories of justice, some deriving from the deontological and utilitarian traditions. If scarce resources are to be allocated, how should this be done? Discrimination based on race, gender, age or 'social worth' obviously violates the principle of justice.

A 'rule' utilitarian might suggest that we seek to maximize the overall welfare of society and minimize the waste of resources. Many surgical services have allocation systems loosely built upon the premise that selecting and organizing allocation around a limited number of criteria predictive of best outcome best serves this purpose. This disadvantages some patients. Alternative models might prioritize on the basis of degree of pain or threat to life. Operating on 100 ingrown toenails will provide substantial relief to many patients; performing five cardiac transplants will save five lives that would otherwise be lost.

One approach that may improve equity is to apply the formal principle of justice of Aristotle (*Nicomachean Ethics*). This suggests that 'equals' should be treated 'equally', but where 'inequality' exists then 'unequal' treatment should occur to correct this imbalance. In the example, those with terminal cardiac failure clearly had a more immediate and life-threatening (unequal) need than those with ingrown toenails. Allocating resources to them acts, in part, to redress the 'inequality' in the situation.

There is usually broad societal consensus that some kind of system that seeks to balance welfare maximization with equity is acceptable, particularly if it is transparent and reactive to the identification of systematic imbalances. However, the individual patient may not share this view and may feel that his or her case is the 'most deserving'.

If there is an obligation to achieve the best outcome for each patient, how can a physician support an allocation system that does not place him or her 'top of the list?' A deontologist could argue that the patient's interests are best served by a transparent (respecting autonomy, communication, information-sharing) system with a commitment to justice (applying equally to this patient as to others). Abandoning this might lead to a free-for-all in which the patient's needs might have even less chance of being met.

The context in which these decisions need to be made is so wide-ranging that it is impossible to establish core rules. Doctors do need to be explicit when justifying why choices are made. The extreme of immediate clinical need (in which beneficence is likely to be the dominant relevant principle) is particularly challenging. Will the 'slightly less unwell' patients always get 'shoved back in the queue' when new emergencies present? Justice and fairness need to be applied broadly. These principles apply to the individual patient, but also to other patients whose circumstances may be influenced by events relating to that patient. Similarly, we need to be fair to other members of the healthcare team and to the broader needs of society.

It is probably fair to say that autonomy and justice are themes enjoying considerably more attention now than in the intermediate past, when medical paternalism may have been a more culturally dominant phenomenon than in the present.

SPECIFIC TOPICS

Euthanasia is a term used to describe the deliberate termination of life in circumstances where a patient suffers from an incurable, progressive and distressing (because of pain or disability) illness. Its motivation is usually compassionate, and frequently (but not always) the patient requests that it be done. It is both illegal and considered to be unethical in the UK.

It should be distinguished from other 'end-of-life' issues, such as withdrawal of or withholding 'extraordinary' measures in situations where these are deemed futile, or where a patient has expressed a wish that such measures not be implemented.

Similarly, the concept of the 'double effect' is felt to be a different issue. In this scenario, an action may lead to 'good' and 'bad' outcomes (e.g. treating cancer pain with opiates in a dose that might cause the patient to die more rapidly than if they were withheld). The primary intention is to relieve pain, not to cause death. It is the *intention* that is felt to distinguish this act from euthanasia.

Discussion on the distinction between 'killing' and 'letting die' merge into those distinguishing between active and passive therapeutic decisions. With an ageing population and ever more elaborate possibilities to prolong life, it is likely that this topic will continue to be both topical and controversial.

Abortion. Therapeutic abortion, whether legal or illegal, is the subject of extensive debate on philosophical, religious and political grounds. Currently in the UK, legal abortion is regulated by the Abortion Act 1967 (amended following the Human Fertilization and Embryology Act 1990). The broader debate on the ethics of abortion (particularly as it applies to abortion before 24 weeks' gestation, or if there is a substantial risk of severe physical or mental abnormalities in the unborn child) is beyond the scope of this chapter, but it is pertinent to note that abortion is legal in a number of circumstances that might be encountered in surgical practice.

Abortion may be performed in emergency circumstances after 24 weeks' gestation if there is a risk to the life of the pregnant woman, or if it is necessary to prevent grave permanent physical or mental injury to the woman. Furthermore, although conscientious objection to abortion normally excuses a healthcare worker from participation in the process of abortion, this does not extend to the emergency situations described above.

Negligence implies that a duty of care exists, that a breach of that duty of care has occurred, and that harm has occurred as a result of this. Fault is felt not to be as serious as when harm occurs as a result of either intention or recklessness (in either of these circumstances prosecution under the criminal law is likely).

The duty of care exists because of the nature of the professional relationship between the doctor and the patient. The standard against which performance is judged is derived from the outcome of the cases of *Bolam v Friern Hospital Management Committee (1957)* in England and Wales, and *Hunter v Hanley (1955)* in Scotland. A doctor is felt not to be negligent if his or her actions are '… in accordance with a practice accepted as proper by a responsible body of medical men skilled in that particular act' (*Bolam*), or if the actions cannot be described as those which '… no doctor of ordinary skill would be guilty of if acting with ordinary care.' (*Hunter*).

Support and advice is readily available from professional organizations such as the British Medical Association, defence organizations such as the Medical Defence Union, Medical Protection Society and Medical and Dental Defence Union of Scotland, or regulatory authorities such as the General Medical Council.

Some useful recent publications on the subject are: Boyd K. M., Higgs R., Pinching A. J. 1997 The new dictionary of medical ethics. BMJ Publishing, London; Davies M. 1998 Textbook on medical law, 2nd edn, Blackstone Press, London; General Medical Council 1998 Good medical practice, 2nd edn, GMC, London; General Medical Council 1999 Seeking patient's consent: the ethical considerations. GMC, London; Mason J. K., McCall Smith R. A. 1994 Law and medical ethics, Butterworth, London.

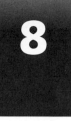

8

Principles of the surgical management of cancer

M.A. Potter, K.C.H. Fearon

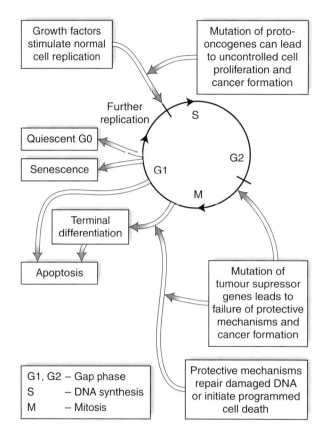

Fig. 8.1   Cell replication and cancer formation. Normal cell replication is under tight regulation by endogenous growth factors. Mutations that result in abnormal growth factor proteins can lead to cancer formation.

THE BIOLOGY OF CANCER

A neoplasm or new growth consists of a mass of transformed cells that does not respond in a normal way to growth regulatory systems. These transformed cells serve no useful function and proliferate in an atypical and uncontrolled way to form a benign or malignant neoplasm. The mechanisms by which this abnormal growth activity is induced (carcinogenesis) are complex and the subject of much research. In normal tissues cell replication and death are equally balanced and are under tight regulatory control (Fig. 8.1). However, when a cancer arises this is generally due to genomic abnormalities that either increase cell replication or inhibit cell death in an uncontrolled manner. Cellular insults (e.g. viral infection, exposure to ionizing radiation or chemical carcinogens) are thought to be the main factors giving rise to the relevant changes in nuclear DNA that lead to either activation or overexpression of proto-oncogenes (e.g. k-*ras*, c-*erbB*2) or the inactivation of tumour suppressor genes (e.g. *P53*), or a combination of the two.

Changes within the cellular genome occur frequently but do not necessarily result in a tumour. Natural protective mechanisms repair errors in DNA replication; similarly, immune surveillance, simple wastage (i.e. loss of cells from the surface) and programmed cell death (apoptosis) destroy

mutant cells before they proliferate. For persistence of growth and hence cancer formation these protective mechanisms must break down (e.g. mutations in the mismatch repair genes *MLHI* and *MSH2*, or failure of apoptosis). The host's internal environment may also have a role in the 'promotion' of tumour growth. Good examples are the 'hormone-dependent' cancers of the breast, prostate and endometrium, which require a 'correct' balance of hormonal secretion from the endocrine glands of the host for their continued growth. The natural history of a tumour is also related to its growth rate, which in turn is determined by the balance between cell division and cell death. Some tumours are slow growing and years may pass before deposits reach a size that threatens normal organ function. Others grow rapidly as a result of a high rate of cell proliferation, and some expand rapidly (despite a relatively normal rate of cell proliferation) if cell death is slow to occur.

SUMMARY BOX

Growth of a cancer is dependent on:

- increased cell proliferation
- decreased programmed cell death (apoptosis)
- a combination of the two

The adenoma–carcinoma progression

Neoplasms may be benign or malignant: the essential difference is the capacity to invade and metastasize. The cells of benign tumours do not invade surrounding tissues but remain as a local conglomerate. Malignant tumours are invasive and their cells enter blood and lymphatic channels, to be deposited at remote sites. This malignant genotype develops as a result of the progressive acquisition of cancer mutations (by point mutation, chromosomal loss or translocation). The acquisition of the malignant phenotype can be recognized histologically as a tumour develops from a benign adenoma through to a dysplastic lesion, and finally into an invasive carcinoma (Fig. 8.2). The progression from benign to malignant cancer is sometimes observed at one of the intermediate or preinvasive stages, known as carcinoma in situ. Although many cases of carcinoma in situ eventually progress to an invasive phase (over a period of months or years), there is evidence to suggest that this does not always happen. Nevertheless, the concept of tumour progression provides the rationale behind screening and early detection programmes, i.e. if benign or preinvasive lesions are removed, this will prevent invasive disease.

Invasion and metastasis

Malignant tumours are fatal because of their ability to grow into adjacent tissues (invasion) and spread to distant tissues (metastasize). Metastases are cancer deposits similar in cell type to the original cancer found at remote (secondary) sites in the body. The process of invasion and spread is complex (Fig. 8.3) and is clearly dependent on the biology

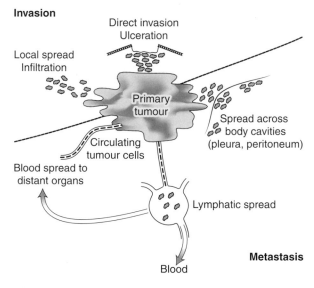

Fig. 8.3 Invasion and metastasis. Cancers invade adjacent tissues by direct infiltration. Spread to distant sites (metastasis) is via the bloodstream or lymphatics, or across body cavities (transcolemic spread).

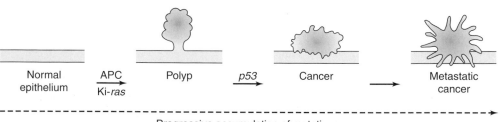

Mutations in mismatch repair genes e.g. *MSH2* and *MLH1* can accelerate the acquisition of malignant mutations

Fig. 8.2 Adenoma–carcinoma progression. By the progressive acquisition of genetic mutations normal colorectal epitheium forms a benign polyp, which can progress to an invasive cancer or metastatic cancer.

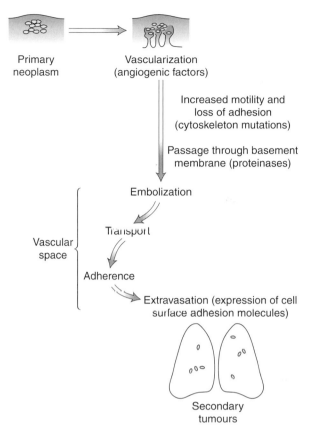

Fig. 8.4 Metastasis. Following initial growth, cancer cells lose local adherence and invade blood vessels. They are then transported via the bloodstream to adhere in distant organs and grow into secondary tumours.

sion and metastasis by degrading extracellular collagens, laminins and proteoglycans. Other proteases, such as urokinase, plasminogen-activating factor and the cathepsins, are also involved in metastasis formation. Clumps of cancer cells can then embolize to distant tissues and form metastases. The survival of metastatic deposits depends on angiogenesis, which is mediated by an imbalance between positive and negative regulatory molecules released by the tumour cells and surrounding normal cells. Negative factors such as angiostatin or endostatin will inhibit new vessel formation. Positive factors such as vascular endothelial growth factors or fibroblast growth factors will enhance metastasis. Cancer cells also secrete prostaglandins, which can induce osteolysis and may promote the development of skeletal deposits.

Natural history and estimate of cure

Benign tumours rarely threaten life but may cause a variety of cosmetic or functional abnormalities. In contrast, malignant tumours invade and relentlessly replace normal tissues, destroying supporting structures, disturbing function, and eventually causing death. Calculations based on an exponential model of tumour growth suggest that three-quarters of the lifespan of a tumour is spent in a 'preclinical' or occult stage, and that the clinical manifestations of the disease are limited to the final quarter.

For cure, every malignant cell must be eradicated. Not only should there be no recurrent tumour during the patient's lifetime, there should also be no evidence of residual tumour at death. This rigid definition of curability can rarely be applied. A normal duration of life without further clinical evidence of disease is generally accepted as evidence of cure even though microscopic deposits of tumour may still be present.

of the tumour. Some tumours metastasize earlier in their clinical course than others. This variation may depend on the tissue of origin of the primary tumour, but can also vary widely according to the phenotype of individual tumours. For example, cancer of the breast is thought to metastasize early and micrometastases are often present but not detectable when the patient first presents. Some patients with apparently localized colorectal cancer are cured by radical surgery, but others receiving the same treatment deteriorate rapidly with metastatic disease.

The mechanisms that control invasion and metastasis are obscure (Fig. 8.4). Local pressure effects from the expanding tumour and the increased motility of tumour cells may play a role in local invasion. Malignant cells secrete a number of factors that may determine their biological behaviour and promote growth at both primary and metastatic sites. The matrix metalloproteinases (MMPs) are a family of zinc-dependent endoproteinases with enzymatic activity directed against components of the extracellular matrix. Their enzymatic action facilitates tumour cell inva-

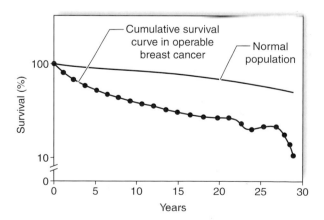

Fig. 8.5 Cumulative survival curve in operable breast cancer (dotted line).

'Cure' rates of individual cancers are assessed by survival rates at various times after treatment. Conventionally, 5- and 10-year intervals are used. Cumulative survival curves (life tables) can be constructed for individual cancers and compared with those of age-matched healthy subjects of the same population (Fig. 8.5). Divergence of these two curves indicates that patients with cancer are dying faster than their normal counterparts, whereas parallel curves indicate that patients with the disease are dying at no greater rate than their age-matched controls. The point at which these two curves become parallel is the time at which cure can be assumed.

Cure rates vary according to the aggressiveness of the disease and the success of treatment. In some patients with cancer (e.g. stomach and lung), metastases grow rapidly and cause death within a few years of clinical presentation. In others (e.g. cancer of the breast and melanoma), many years may elapse before metastatic spread becomes evident and, even when metastases have occurred, life may be long. It is for this reason that 5-year survival rates cannot provide a satisfactory estimate of cure for all tumours. Many regard the treatment of a malignant tumour as a matter of extreme urgency. When one considers the natural duration of a cancer, a week or two spent in careful investigation, counselling and planning of treatment is good practice. However, this period must not be unduly delayed, as patients with cancer are naturally worried and wish to have their initial treatment completed within a reasonable time.

THE MANAGEMENT OF PATIENTS WITH CANCER

Screening

If cancer can be detected before it causes symptoms, then it is generally smaller, has less chance of having metastasized and is therefore more amenable to cure. Detecting benign lesions with malignant potential, preinvasive cancer, and invasive malignancy before it becomes symptomatic is called screening. Screening is expensive and its effectiveness in relation to cost must be critically evaluated before routine use. Screening is most effective when targeted at specific risk groups and when the screening test has a high level of acceptability (i.e. the vast majority of the target population accept the invitation to undergo the screening procedure). For successful screening the test used must be able to detect the cancer at a stage when earlier treatment will lead to fewer deaths from the cancer. In any given population the likelihood of a cancer being present is generally low (<1%), and hence, the test must be sensitive in order to detect these relatively rare lesions. The test must also be specific (i.e. have a low false-positive rate), otherwise indi-

viduals will undergo unnecessary investigation or even inappropriate treatment. Finally, the proposed treatment of a cancer patient detected by a screening programme must be effective. In the UK cervical cytology is offered to women on a 3-yearly basis until the age of 60, and mammographic screening is offered to women between 50 and 64 years on a 2-yearly basis. Acceptance rates vary, but below 60–70% the viability of the programme is question-

> **SUMMARY BOX**
>
> *A test for use in cancer screening must:*
> - be sensitive
> - be specific
> - be acceptable
> - detect cancer at a stage when cure is possible
> - be a reasonable cost

Table 8.1 Examples of cancer types that are or could be the subject of screening programmes

Cancer	Screening test
Breast	Mammography
Cervix	Smear cytology
Colon	Faecal occult blood test+ colonoscopy
Prostate	Prostate-specific antigen (PSA)

able. Other tumour types that might be amenable to screening and their relevant screening tests are listed in Table 8.1.

Screening for inherited cancer

Some forms of cancer can be inherited: for example, about 5% of patients with colorectal cancer develop the disease because of an autosomal dominant inherited mutation either in the *APC* gene (polyposis coli) or in the mismatch repair genes *MSH* and *MLH1* (hereditary non-polyposis colorectal cancer). Alternatively, about 5% of women develop breast cancer as a result of an autosomal dominant inherited mutation on the *BRCA1* or *-2* genes. In these instances closely related family members should be offered the appropriate tests to detect these specific mutations. Carriers of the mutation can then be offered prophylactic surgery, e.g. bilateral mastectomy (for *BRCA1* and *-2* carriers) or restorative proctocolectomy (for *APC* carriers) in an attempt to eliminate subsequent cancer development.

The cancer patient's journey

The management of cancer frequently involves surgery, be it radical for cure or palliative to relieve distressing symptoms. Even in patients where the primary treatment is not surgical, the surgeon can play an important role, for example in obtaining diagnostic biopsies. The care of cancer patients is now commonly concentrated in specialist centres and the surgeon is an indispensable member of the multidisciplinary team (Table 8.2). Good communication with the patient and between team members forms the basis of optimal patient care. There are several key stages in the management of the patient with cancer, which can be regarded as a journey from the onset of symptoms to defini-

Table 8.2 Multidisciplinary team involved in cancer care	
Medical staff	Surgeon General physician Medical oncologist Radiotherapist Palliative care physician General practitioner
Nursing staff	Ward nurse Chemotherapy nurse Nurse counsellor Hospice nurse
Paramedical staff	Oncology dietitian Physiotherapist Occupational therapist Clergy

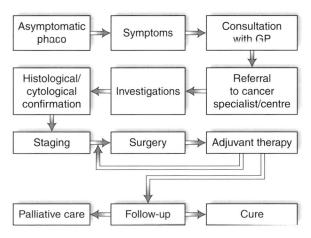

Fig. 8.6 Patient's cancer journey. During their management several key stages are encountered from symptoms to diagnosis and treatment.

tive treatment and subsequent follow-up (Fig. 8.6). The exact sequence of events may differ from one patient to the next. For example, it may be necessary to remove the tumour to obtain full information on staging before an adequate treatment plan can be evolved. Patients usually begin their 'cancer journey' by deciding that a symptom or symptoms they have developed are serious enough to merit consultation with their GP. These symptoms may be a result of local or systemic effects of the cancer.

Symptoms that may initiate a patient's 'cancer journey'

Local effects

A tumour that lies on the surface of the body may become visible, change in shape or pigmentation, bleed, or discharge mucus or pus. A hollow viscus or duct may be obstructed by a tumour, e.g. a bronchus, causing pulmonary collapse, a segment of bowel, causing intestinal obstruction, or the bile duct or pancreatic duct, causing jaundice. A tumour within a closed space may cause pressure symptoms. For example, increased intracranial pressure may complicate intracerebral tumours, and paraplegia from a spinal cord tumour. Invasion of an organ by a tumour may compromise its normal functions and cause organ failure. Invasion of tissues such as the pancreas, bone or nerves can cause severe pain. A cancer can also mimic the pain of benign disease, for example dyspeptic symptoms in stomach cancer.

> **SUMMARY BOX**
>
> *Symptoms that should initiate investigation*
>
> - Weight loss
> - Rectal bleeding/melaena
> - Haemoptysis/persistent cough
> - Haematuria
> - Breast lump
> - Dysphagia/dyspepsia
> - Persistent headache

Systemic effects

Weight loss is often the key symptom that alerts both the patients and his or her doctor to the possibility of malignant disease. A proportion of patients become so emaciated that they appear to die of starvation. This syndrome is known as cancer cachexia, and is clinically characterized by anorexia, severe weight loss, lethargy, anaemia and oedema.

The secretory products of some tumours can produce characteristic clinical syndromes. These products may be appropriate to the organ of origin. Thus, a tumour of the adrenal cortex may secrete excess corticosteroid and cause Cushing's syndrome; a parathyroid tumour may secrete excess parathormone and cause hypercalcaemia; and an islet cell tumour of the pancreas may secrete excess insulin and cause hypoglycaemia. On the other hand, secretory products may be inappropriate to the site of a tumour. Such 'ectopic' secretion occurs predominantly in tumours of neuroendocrine origin, and produces a variety of endocrine syndromes.

Consultation with the GP

Distressing or dramatic presenting symptoms, for example rectal bleeding, rightly produce a prompt referral from the GP to a hospital specialist. Frequently, however, the initial presenting complaint of a patient with cancer is non-specific, e.g. general malaise. Other symptoms, such as epigastric pain, are common complaints encountered by the GP and are usually associated with benign disease. These symptoms are more challenging to the GP and it can be difficult to decide which patient needs an urgent referral and which does not. Cancer patients presenting with such non-specific symptoms may consult their GP on more than one occasion before being referred to a hospital specialist.

Referral to a specialist/cancer centre

Because of the complexity of modern cancer management, cancer services in a hospital are currently organized around a multidisciplinary team approach. The team commonly includes surgeons, medical oncologists (chemotherapy), clinical oncologists (radiotherapy/chemotherapy), radiologists, pathologists and clinical nurse specialists. Individual aspects of patient care are undertaken by different members of the team, but the overall staging and treatment plan are discussed on a weekly basis at the multidisciplinary team meeting.

Patients who are referred with a suspected diagnosis of cancer are generally seen urgently in the surgical outpatient clinic appropriate to the probable site of origin of the tumour. In practice, the time taken to see the hospital specialist is a small proportion of that taken to diagnosis when other factors, such as delay to presentation, referral and investigation, are considered. At the initial consultation it is important to spend time taking a full and detailed history and examination. It is also important to spend time addressing any patient anxieties and provide the patient with a clear view of any investigations that are planned. Following the initial consultation the patient will be asked to attend for investigations either as an inpatient or an outpatient, to confirm or refute the diagnosis. Increasingly 'one-stop'

clinics are being provided, allowing the initial consultation and investigations to be performed at one clinic attendance. This approach is particularly suited to the diagnosis of breast cancer.

Investigation

Investigations serve two main purposes. First, they are aimed at histological or cytological confirmation of the diagnosis of cancer. Second, they are used to assess the extent of the primary disease (local invasion) and to look for the evidence of metastatic spread. This is known as 'staging' the disease.

Diagnostic investigation

Initial investigations to make the diagnosis should proceed in a logical order, starting with simple blood tests (e.g. tumour markers) and progressing through more complex imaging investigations, with the ultimate aim of obtaining histological or cytological confirmation of the diagnosis (Table 8.3). Plain radiology may demonstrate a soft tissue tumour, e.g. of the lung or bone, but for tumours of the stomach or intestine contrast studies are necessary. For some deep-seated tumours, e.g. of the pancreas or brain, other methods of imaging are needed. These may include

Table 8.3	Investigations for the diagnosis of cancer	
Blood tests	Haematology Biochemistry	FBC LFTs Tumour markers
Cytology	Sputum Urine Endoscopic brushings	
Radiology	Plain X-rays Contrast enhanced Ultrasound CT MRI	CXR Barium enema
Endoscopy	Upper GI endoscopy Colonoscopy ERCP	
Histology	Fine-needle aspiration, e.g. breast and thyroid cancer Radiologically guided FNA Endoscopic biopsy Excision biopsy, e.g. lymph node	
Operative	Examination under anaesthetic and biopsy Diagnostic laparoscopy and biopsy	

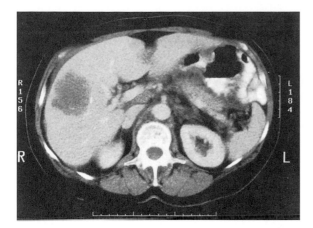

Fig. 8.7 Staging CT of the abdomen showing a large solitary liver metastasis in a patient with colorectal cancer.

angiography, radioactive scintigraphy and ultrasonography (US), but increasingly CT (Fig. 8.7) and MRI are the standard forms of investigation. Neoplastic disease can be confirmed cytologically, e.g. by the demonstration of malignant cells in secretions, in washings from hollow viscera, or in needle aspirates. Biopsies obtained at either upper or lower gastrointestinal endoscopy can provide material for histology, as can ultrasound or CT-guided Tru-cut needle biopsies. In some instances it may be necessary to perform an examination under anaesthetic or diagnostic laparoscopy to obtain suitable diagnostic material. In general, a treatment plan for the management of a patient cannot be formulated until a histological or cytological diagnosis has been made. However, there are circumstances when this is not possible (e.g. certain patients with pancreatic cancer), and then clear radiological evidence may be used instead.

Staging investigations

Staging investigations will depend on the site of the primary cancer and the relevant common sites of metastasis. Local invasion can be assessed, for example in oesophageal cancer, by endoscopic ultrasound. CT or MRI scans can also be usefully employed to assess local invasion. Metastatic spread can be determined by a variety of investigations, e.g. bone scans, CT scans and laparoscopy. Often staging investigations have been undertaken as part of the diagnostic process, e.g. CT scan.

The aim of staging is to define the extent of the disease, assess its likely prognosis, and permit the development of an appropriate treatment plan by the multidisciplinary team. The International Union Against Cancer (UICC) has described a system of staging (TNM) in which three components are assessed. These are the extent of the primary tumour (T), the presence and extent of metastases in regional lymph nodes (N), and the presence of distant metastases (M). The addition of numbers to each component indicates the extent of the disease within that category.

In the initial TNM system only clinical, radiological and endoscopic investigations were used (Table 8.3). Such clinical staging is still important in defining the extent of disease and may be used to plan the initial management of a patient. However, without histological confirmation such clinical staging can sometimes be highly inaccurate. For example, the palpability of regional lymph nodes is a poor indicator of their involvement by tumour. Impalpable nodes may still contain metastases, whereas palpable nodes may be the seat of reactive hyperplasia (sinus histiocytosis) rather than tumour. Small deposits of tumour in viscera and bones cannot be detected by routine radiology, and thus many patients who on clinical and radiological grounds appear to have localized disease have in fact unrecognized widespread microscopic tumour deposits. For this reason the TNM system has now been modified to include not only a pretreatment clinical classification, but also a postsurgical pathological classification, denoted as pTNM. Excision of regional lymph nodes is one way to provide such information. In some melanomas and skin tumours, and in cancer of the bladder and large bowel, histological assessment of the depth of tumour penetration provides important information about the extent and prognosis of the disease. It must be recognized that all staging has its limitations and that microscopic tumour deposits may not be detected, particular in terms of distant metastases. These staging systems are therefore used to provide a 'best-guess' scenario upon which to base the patient's treatment.

Prognosis is also affected by the biological characteristics of a tumour. For example, its degree of nuclear and cellular atypia and the extent of lymphocytic infiltration, inflammatory response and vascular invasion all influence outcome. These factors, as well as biochemical indices (e.g. oestrogen receptor status in breast cancer), can all be used in the planning of a patient's treatment.

> **SUMMARY BOX**
>
> *Purpose of staging*
> - Define the extent of disease
> - Assess likely prognosis
> - Allow the development of a treatment plan

Treatment

Following the initial diagnosis and staging, the patient may be discussed by the multidisciplinary team or may proceed to surgery, where the primary tumour and surrounding tissue and locoregional lymph nodes are excised and then sent for histopathology. Thus, the clinical staging is translated into histopathological staging; the multidisciplinary team can then discuss further aspects of management with the maximum amount of information available.

Benign tumours

Provided sufficient surrounding tissue is excised to ensure its complete removal, a benign tumour is cured by local excision. Some benign tumours, e.g. pleomorphic adenomas of the parotid, extend beyond their apparent macroscopic limits. Removal of the involved segment of the gland or organ is then the only sure way to cure.

Malignant tumours

A radical cancer operation implies complete or nearly complete removal of the organ or tissue bearing the tumour, together with a margin of unaffected surrounding tissue. In some tumours there is sequential spread, first locally, then to lymph nodes, and then to distant organs such as the liver and lungs. In this situation careful local removal, along with the locoregional lymph nodes (known as 'en bloc resection'), can be curative. Often, however, the spread of a tumour may be more unpredictable and in essence the removal of local lymph nodes is simply to provide information for the stage of the cancer, rather than being of true therapeutic benefit. The management of regional lymph nodes thus depends on the site and type of the tumour. With some tumours, e.g. those of the gastrointestinal tract, regional lymph nodes are routinely resected on the basis

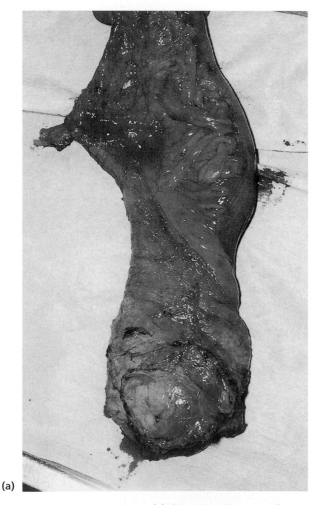

(a)

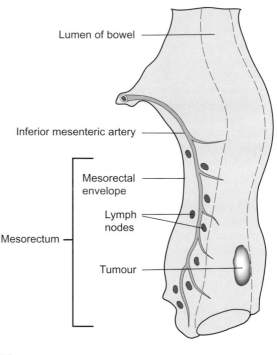

(b)

Fig. 8.8 Operative specimen **(a)** demonstrating a total mesorectal excision of a rectal cancer. The diagram **(b)** shows the structures that have been removed with this en bloc resection.

that sequential spread may have occurred. In other tumours lymph node sampling or sentinel node biopsy may be more appropriate (e.g. breast cancer), especially if en bloc lymph node resection may be associated with significant morbidity, for example limb lymphoedema.

Complete radical excision, which is confirmed by histological examination with no evidence of lymph node metastasis, carries a high chance of surgical cure. A good example is total mesorectal excision performed for rectal cancer (Fig. 8.8). During any operation for cancer, care is taken to try and avoid the spillage of malignant cells. In some sites (e.g. testis, large bowel) it is usual to ligate the main vessels draining the area before the tumour is mobilized, so that further malignant cells are not shed into the circulation. Care is taken to avoid handling a tumour of the bowel and to prevent spillage of cells into the lumen, which may cause cancer recurrence at the anastomosis. Many surgeons also irrigate the wound or body cavity with dilute cetrimide or betadine to destroy 'free-floating' cells and thus reduce the likelihood of local recurrence. Overall, a careful and meticulous approach to all aspects of the operation is vital. Attention to each detail improves the outcome of surgery.

There are data to suggest that surgery performed in specialist centres where surgeons are regularly performing radical operations produces better survival rates than surgery in non-specialists centres. Hence surgeons are increasingly subspecialized and concentrate on performing selected operations.

Adjuvant treatment

As mentioned previously, the most accurate staging of a patient with cancer is generally available after pathological evaluation of the resected specimen. Once this information is available the patient can be discussed by the multidisciplinary team with a view to the need for further therapy.

Clearly it is sometimes not possible to remove all the local disease. Moreover, early systemic dissemination may have occurred. Thus, an adjuvant to surgery is needed to provide both local and systemic control. For example, adjuvant chemotherapy may help prevent both local recurrence and distant metastasis, and this is commonly used in patients with colorectal or breast cancer who have lymph node involvement. However, surgical excision must be adequate, and adjuvant radiotherapy or chemotherapy must not be regarded as a safety net for careless surgical practice. Reduction of the tumour burden may also contribute to the success of systemic treatment, which is aimed at controlling the disease as a whole (e.g. ovarian cancer).

Achieving a balance between the relief of symptoms and the morbidity induced by radical cancer therapy is often difficult, and it is important to remember that the quality of life is as important as the duration of survival. Chemotherapy is potentially toxic: morbidity and quality of life must always be considered before undertaking this form of treatment.

The success of adjuvant chemotherapy varies from one histological type of cancer to another. In general, drugs are given in combination over a period of 6–12 months. Toxicity, such as mouth ulcers, diarrhoea, weakness and alopecia, is common but in general tolerable. Results in colorectal and breast cancer suggest that the likelihood of death from recurrent cancer is reduced by about 20–30% in patients with evidence of lymph node metastasis.

Because of the localized nature of radiotherapy, it is administered to reduce the chances of local recurrence rather than of distant metastasis. Radiotherapy may be given prior to surgery to try and 'downstage' or shrink a bulky and fixed tumour (e.g. rectal cancer) and thus make surgery easier to perform. Alternatively, it may be given to the postoperative patient in whom the chances of local recurrence are thought to be high (e.g. a patient in whom the margins at the edge of the resection specimen are involved with tumour). When tumours are relatively radiosensitive radiotherapy can reduce the need for radical surgery and a more cosmetically acceptable conservative operation is then possible (e.g. lumpectomy and radiotherapy, as opposed to mastectomy in breast cancer).

The impact of intensive chemo- and radiotherapy on growth in children with malignant disease can be significant. The potential for cure, which is possible in many childhood malignancies, has to be balanced against the long-term morbidity of growth failure as a side effect of such treatment.

Other modes of adjuvant therapy include less toxic therapies, such as administration of the antioestrogen tamoxifen in women with breast cancer. Experimental models have shown that monoclonal antibodies, synthetic peptides, antisense oligonucleotides and soluble adhesion molecules can inhibit tumour growth. Gene therapy carries the potential to restore the function of altered tumour suppressor molecules. MMP inhibitors and angiogenesis inhibitors offer other potential avenues for novel anticancer therapy.

Follow-up

In most patients with tumours amenable to surgical treatment it is important to check subsequently that there is no local recurrence of disease and that the patient is symptom free. In general, patients are seen more frequently in the early months after surgery, as this is the period when recurrence is most likely; it is also the period when it is necessary to detect and treat non-cancer related postoperative complications. The nature of the surgery will influence the follow-up strategy: patients undergoing palliative surgery will have different follow-up requirements from those undergoing curative surgery. However, it is often difficult to detect recurrence or metastasis in the asymptomatic postoperative patient, and some would question the value of routine sophisticated investigations to try to detect metastatic disease in such cases. Current evidence suggests that in some cases, once the primary therapy has been undertaken the patient could be discharged back to their GP for follow-up with re-referral to the multidisciplinary team as necessary.

SUMMARY BOX

Principles of surgery for cancer

- Multidisciplinary team approach
- Accurate pre- /postoperative staging
- En bloc radical surgery
- Appropriate pre-/postoperative adjuvant therapy
- Good communication with patient and relatives
- Audit of results

Palliation of advanced cancer

The management of patients with incurable disease involves the relief of distressing symptoms (palliative care). This is a specialist branch of medicine in its own right, and the palliative care physician and the associated team play an important part in the overall management of the cancer patient. The terminal stages of malignancy can be prolonged, and pain and other distressing symptoms are common. Effective palliation is achieved by a variety of means. Local and/or systemic adjuvant therapy can be used to induce tumour regression, for example to reduce the pressure effects of cerebral metastases. Surgery can be employed to resect symptomatic metastases or bypass a malignant obstruction. When a palliative operation is performed the patient and their relatives should understand that its object is to prevent additional suffering, and not to attempt cure. Medical treatments are used to relieve symptoms such as pain, nausea, depression, infections etc. A wide range of analgesic and narcotic drugs is available to relieve pain. The choice depends on the type of pain, its severity, and the stage of the illness. The aim is to achieve complete analgesia without impairing mental clarity or inducing side-effects. It is essential never to let the patient wait for the next dose of analgesic. Schedules of adminis-

tration are planned to prevent rather than treat pain. When pain is severe, narcotic drugs should be used; fear of addiction is irrelevant in this context. Treatment should start with simple analgesics for mild pain (e.g. paracetamol) and move to more potent agents if the pain is not readily controlled (e.g. dihydrocodeine, coproxamol). For severe pain, slow-release morphine sulphate tablets (MST) are usually administered 12-hourly, and can be combined with morphine elixir or dextromoramide for occasional breakthrough pain. For persistent pain, continuous subcutaneous infusions of analgesics can be administered. The psychological and social aspects of care for both the patient and the family should also be addressed.

Prognosis and counselling

Honesty is the basis of the doctor–patient relationship and it is almost always best to tell patients that they have cancer. However, in doing so one should reveal as much of the truth as the patient wishes to have or can understand. When therapy is undertaken with curative intent it is most important to emphasize that this is the goal in mind. Radical cancer surgery followed by radiotherapy or chemotherapy can be very arduous, and maintenance of morale is essential. When palliation is the objective it is important not to remove the patient's hope, as 'the end of hope is the beginning of death'. It is usually best to speak to patients in a quiet, private room with one of the nursing staff present.

Care of the dying

Death from malignant disease is usually a gradual process of withdrawal. A sympathetic doctor can greatly help the patient and their relatives. A dying patient must never feel abandoned in a surgical ward, and doctors and nursing staff must be prepared to spend time to help the patient to die with dignity. In general, however, most patients either die at home (with support from palliative care nurses etc.) or in a hospice, where the level of quiet and care is appropriate to the situation. Early involvement of the hospice/palliative care team helps allay patient fears and optimize the control of distressing symptoms.

Palliative care of children with terminal malignant disease is now becoming increasingly available in the UK. A number of Children's Hospices have now been established which offer this service and have proven to be of great support, not only to affected children, but also to their parents and families.

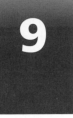

9 Trauma and multiple injury

C.E. Robertson

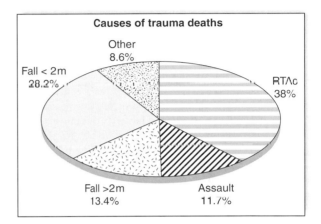

Fig. 9.1 Causes of trauma deaths. (Data kindly provided by the Scottish Trauma Audit Group 1992–1999).

TRAUMA EPIDEMIOLOGY

Despite the prominence given to ischaemic heart disease, cancer and AIDS, the commonest cause of death from birth to the fourth decade, and the fourth commonest cause overall, is trauma. It is not an overstatement to say that this situation is a pandemic, as for individuals between 15 and 24 years trauma leads to three times as many deaths as any other cause. On average, for individuals of working age, heart disease and cancer result in the loss of 10 years of potential life, but road traffic accidents (RTAs) alone cause the loss of 30–35 years. The economic cost is staggering. Patients with trauma occupy 10% of hospital beds in the UK, RTAs cost the Exchequer £4–5 billion annually; and globally trauma accounts for 1–2% of gross national product.

However, experience of trauma cannot be extrapolated from other countries to predict events or outcomes. For example, in the UK RTAs, falls and interpersonal violence account for the majority of major trauma (Fig. 9.1). Fewer than 1 in 10 patients with major trauma have penetrating injury, and this is usually caused by knives. In the USA approximately 20% of the population owns a gun, and RTA deaths are now exceeded by firearm injuries. Having a gun in the home increases the risk of homicide threefold, and of suicide fivefold. For 15–24-year-olds these figures increase by a factor of 10. Unsurprisingly, a recent UK study found the total number of homicides over a 2-year period for a population of 0.8 million was similar to that seen in a single day among the same-sized population of many American cities.

For so-called 'developed' countries, annually, one person in 50 will be involved in a road traffic accident. Of these, 1% will die, 10% will need hospital treatment and 25% will be temporarily disabled. But even within apparently similar nations RTA death rates vary enormously. For example, the death rate of 31/100 000 in Portugal is 400% greater than that for Norway or Sweden (the UK figure is 9).

The timing of death after injury illuminates the limitations of a trauma system. It is often said that trauma deaths have a trimodal distribution. The first 'peak', representing deaths occurring immediately or within a few seconds of injury, contributes up to 50% of the total. The second 'peak', up to 4 hours after injury, accounts for 30% of deaths, and the final 20% take place (usually in an intensive care unit) days or weeks after the event.

Much significance has been placed upon this alleged temporal relationship, particularly the second peak. On the basis that interventions for the second group of patients offered great potential for preventing unnecessary deaths, the provision and nature of prehospital and hospital trauma services in the USA and the UK were changed profoundly.

The concept of a second peak is attractive but is a myth, at least in the UK, where the vast majority of deaths occur immediately or within a very few minutes of injury. Furthermore, the subsequent deaths do not cluster into peaks. So, although attempts to improve care for those who initially survive must continue, the overwhelming message is that trauma prevention is far more important than any other aspect.

 Trauma is a common cause of death and morbidity in children. After the first year of life it is the commonest cause of death in the paediatric population. Injury prevention programmes have had little impact on this sad statistic to date. The commonest causes of serious injury seen in children are road traffic accidents and falls. Non-accidental injury accounts for a significant number of the remainder.

The pattern of injury seen in children differs from that seen in adults. The small mass of the child is less able to disperse the kinetic energy of impact; as a consequence multi-system injury is more common. The large paediatric head (in proportion to the rest of the body) means that head injuries are common. The larger body surface area to body mass results in increased heat loss after injury; this is particularly important to be recognized during the resuscitation phase of treatment – warmed fluids in a warm resuscitation room are essential.

There are often significant psychological sequelae to major trauma in children. It has been estimated that as many as 60% of such children are left with behavioural or learning difficulties after a serious accident.

INJURY BIOMECHANICS AND ACCIDENT PREVENTION

To anticipate the injuries from any given trauma event the clinician must understand the biomechanics involved. As with any surgical condition, an accurate history can identify or predict the great majority of an individual patient's injuries.

The magnitude of an injury is related to the energy transferred to the victim during the event, the volume/area of tissue involved, and the time taken for the interaction. Tissue characteristics such as elasticity, plasticity and fluid content are also important. These factors are summarized in the formula:

$$\text{Injury magnitude} \propto C \, \frac{E}{T \, V}$$

where E = energy transfer, T = time, V = volume of tissue, C = tissue factors (a constant).

Kinetic energy, the energy of motion, is proportional to the mass of the object but to the square of its velocity. This can have unexpected effects. For example, a pedestrian struck by a car, of mass 700 kg travelling at 100 kph, receives over three times the destructive energy than if hit by a heavy lorry mass 5000 kg travelling at 40 kph. If the car travels at 160 kph (100 mph), over 10 times the energy is involved. The longer the timeframe during which the kinetic energy is transferred to the body, the less the acceleration/deceleration forces sustained and the less the trauma that results.

These physical principles underpin various forms of accident prevention and protection. Obviously, reducing the chance of direct contact helps: separating pedestrians and traffic is the single most important factor in reducing pedestrian injury rates. This is illustrated by the fact that in the US < 2% of traffic fatalities are pedestrians, whereas in the UK they account for 36% of the total. In a similar fashion the central reservation barriers on motorways dramatically reduce the chances of high-speed head-on collisions.

If impact does occur then limitation of the velocities involved is the most important determinant in reducing injury. One in 10 drivers involved in RTAs travels inappropriately fast. Even a 1 mph (1.6 kph) reduction in average road speed reduces fatal accidents by 8%. When, in the late 1980s, a number of US states increased their speed limit to 65 mph, an immediate one-third increase in deaths followed. States maintaining the 55 mph limit had unchanged numbers. The 20 mph (32 kph) zones in residential areas, together with traffic calming measures, significantly reduce deaths and serious injuries, in particular to children and the elderly.

Contact factors can be minimized by vehicle design: crumple zones, energy-absorbing materials, preventing the ejection of passengers from the vehicle and reducing intrusion into the passenger compartment. For the occupants seatbelts, airbags, collapsible steering columns and soft fascia compartments enable contact deceleration to take place over a longer time period, reducing the potential for injury. Properly used, seatbelts reduce the risk of death/serious injury by 45%. Airbags further reduce the risk of death by 10% for belted drivers, and by 20% for unbelted front-seat passengers, but may not provide protection from side-impact events, or if the vehicle rolls over.

These devices can also modify the patterns of injury experienced, particularly if they are incorrectly positioned. Seatbelts and airbags do reduce deaths overall but certain injuries, e.g. sternal fractures and soft-tissue neck injuries, may be associated with their use. With lapbelts, pancreatic, renal, splenic and liver injuries are increased and hyperflexion of the trunk over the belt can produce anterior compression fractures of the vertebrae. Finally, seatbelts can only be protective if they are used. A recent study showed that 90% of rear-seat passengers were unrestrained. These passengers increase the severity of their own injuries, as well as causing injury to restrained individuals in the front seats.

ALCOHOL AND DRUGS

The message is often unwelcome, but few episodes of trauma are without direct human failing or causation (there is, for instance, a fourfold increase in the risk of being involved in a RTA while using a mobile telephone, a level similar to that seen when driving with a blood alcohol level at the legal limit).

The combination of youth, inexperienced motor skills, an innate belief in immortality and a powerful vehicle accounts for an extraordinarily high rate of events. Accident rates decline with increasing age and experience, but at the other end of the spectrum the elderly have a disproportionately high incidence of trauma because of coexisting medical conditions and visual/motor impairments that affect judgement.

At all ages alcohol is the major causal factor for all types of trauma: 60% of individuals sustaining trauma in assaults have consumed alcohol. For burns, homicides and drowning, alcohol is implicated in 30–50% of events. Its combination with young males and road vehicles is particularly lethal, where one-third of all fatalities, and 10% of all injuries, involve alcohol consumption. Drink–driving laws do reduce the proportion of fatal crashes involving intoxicated drivers, but high-risk behaviour remains common. Although death rates from alcohol-related events have fallen, the risk of being involved in an accident with a blood alcohol at the current UK driving limit is twice that for an individual with no alcohol in their blood. At higher levels the risk dramatically increases further. About 20% of RTA deaths are related to drug or substance misuse, but the difficulties of testing and the involvement of prescribed medications such as sedatives makes this area less completely evaluated.

WOUNDS

Classification and production

- *Abrasions or grazes* are caused by the tangential application of blunt force. Dirt is often ingrained in the surface layers of skin, with the risk of short-term infection and, if untreated, later permanent 'tattooing'. The abrasion's site and nature may give useful clues as to the direction and magnitude of injury forces.
- *Contusions, ecchymoses or bruises* result from blunt force disrupting superficial capillaries. The overlying skin is intact. When small blood vessels are involved a large collection of blood (haematoma) may develop. It is impossible accurately to 'age' a bruise by its colour, but if it is yellow the bruise is likely to be at least 18 hours old.

- *Lacerations* Blunt forces tear, shear or crush skin and soft tissues, producing lacerations. The wound edges are irregular and often abraded or contused, as are the surrounding tissues.
- *Incised wounds or 'cuts'* are produced by sharp edges such as knives or glass shards, and have characteristically clean edges with clear margins. The greatest dimension of an incised wound is its length (*cf.* puncture wound).
- *Puncture wounds* Sharp points or edges produce puncture wounds, in which the greatest dimension is the depth. When the wound pierces a body cavity it is 'penetrating'; if it passes through a viscus it is 'perforating'.

Gunshot wounds

Gunshot wounds highlight the gulf between UK and US practice. In the US, deaths from gunshot wounds are the fourth leading cause of years of potential life lost before the age of 65. Guns are used in over 60% of suicides and 70% of all homicides. Non-fatal gunshot wounds outnumber the fatal ones two- to threefold.

As with other injury, the exchange of energy is crucial. Low-velocity missiles cause local injury, involving tissue tearing and compression. When velocities exceed 500–600 m/s cavitation injury – a temporary space torn in tissues at right-angles to the direction of travel – is also produced. This process develops in microseconds and, depending upon the body tissues involved and their elasticity, can involve a volume many times the diameter of the bullet itself. The wounding potential can be further magnified by features specifically designed to increase the area of injury and the release of energy: examples include bullets that tumble in tissues and others designed to deform or fragment on impact (dum-dum or semijacketed bullets).

Shotgun events are relatively more common in the UK than handgun or rifle injuries. The muzzle velocity of these weapons is relatively high, but dissipation of the shot and air resistance on the pellets quickly decreases their velocity and limits the wounding potential. These weapons are lethal at close range but, unless 'choked', are relatively less wounding at greater distances, where they tend to cause superficial injury to skin and subcutaneous tissues.

FALLS

The major determinant of injury and the chance of death is directly proportional to the height fallen, as the accelerating force of gravity is constant. A body falling two storeys (10 m) has an impact velocity of ~50 kph. At impact the deceleration forces are determined by the individual's mass, the nature of the landing surface and the body's orientation on landing. Surfaces such as mud, snow, soft earth and, to a lesser extent, water can permit an increased duration of impact, reducing deceleration forces and hence injury. For an 'average' man, a 5 m fall on to a concrete surface produces a deceleration force of approximately $700g$, but if the landing is into a soft, yielding surface the stopping distance may be several centimetres, decreasing the force 10–20-fold.

The body's position during landing affects the contact area and the propagation of energy since, if the same force is dissipated over a larger area, there is less force per unit area and hence less damage. Feet-first falls involve a relatively small area of contact, but deceleration forces can be reduced by flexing the knees and hips. Regardless of the position on landing, however, for falls > 5 m there is a high incidence of deceleration injuries to intrathoracic and intra-abdominal structures, particularly where these are relatively immobile or tethered – for example the aortic root and the mesenteric arteries. Overall, a fall on to an unyielding surface from 15–20 m has a > 50% mortality.

INJURY SEVERITY ASSESSMENT

Audit of trauma patients, both individually and as a group, is essential. To allow objective comparison between systems or hospitals, injury classifications have become standardized.

Two types of classification are used. The first measures the severity of anatomical injury. The most commonly used is the Abbreviated Injury Scale (AIS). Once the patient's injuries have all been identified (this may only be possible at discharge or autopsy), each separate injury is assessed from a scoring 'dictionary' and awarded a numerical score from 1 to 6. It is important to recognize that these separate AIS values are not linear in terms of increasing severity.

The Injury Severity Score is then derived by adding the squares of the three highest AIS scores within six body areas (head and neck, abdomen and pelvic contents, bony pelvis and limbs, face, chest and body surface). The maximum ISS is 75 ($5^2 + 5^2 + 5^2$). Note that an AIS score of 6 (an injury which is, by definition, incompatible with survival) in any one body region automatically receives an ISS of 75.

Mortality increases predictably with increasing ISS, and patients with an ISS $\geq$ 16 have 'major trauma'. As with AIS scoring, ISS is non-linear and some values are numerically not possible. For these reasons, when comparing groups of patients mean values are inappropriate and non-parametric statistical analysis is required. The value of ISS, however, is that it provides an internationally recognized objective evaluation of anatomical injury.

The best-known physiological scoring system is the Glasgow Coma Scale, which is used to assess objectively the neurological state of injured patients, and which also has prognostic value. The GCS, in conjunction with two other physiological recordings, systolic blood pressure and respiratory rate, can be used to produce the 'Revised Trauma Score'.

Each of the three parameters is given a coded value between 0 and 4. This is then multiplied by a weighting factor reflecting the relative importance of each individual measurement. A Revised Trauma Score value can be between 0 and 7.8204.

Although widely used, the Revised Trauma Score has its own problems. Some patients with severe injury may not be identified initially, usually because the assessment has been performed before detectable physiological compromise has had time to occur. The RTS may also overestimate injury severity if physiological changes occur (due, for example, to alcohol) that are not reflected in the measured parameters, or which modify these factors.

When anatomical and physiological scoring systems are combined, using TRISS methodology (Fig. 9.2), comparisons can then be made between predicted and actual patient outcomes. The impact of age, and factors such as whether the injury was blunt or penetrating, can be incorporated. In general, for any given score mortality increases with increasing age, but TRISS analyses allow an objective and uniform assessment of patient outcome, so that comparisons between individual hospitals and trauma systems have validity.

TRISS methodology can also be used to highlight unexpected individual patient outcomes and prompt a review of the processes involved. For each patient, a probability of survival (P_s) can be derived. Thus, if a patient with a P_s of 90% dies, this outcome is unexpected in that it would normally be considered that nine of 10 patients with that particular P_s would survive. It must, however, be recognized that one out of those 10 patients with that combination of RTS and ISS would also die. So, whereas the identification of an individual patient for discussion at an audit meeting is useful, inappropriate extrapolations should be avoided.

PREHOSPITAL CARE AND TRANSPORT

The objective of prehospital care is to prevent further injury, initiate resuscitation and transport the patient safely and rapidly to the most appropriate hospital. The size and demographics of the population served, and geographical constraints, affect this directly.

In the USA basic trauma care is often provided by fire and police services. Emergency medical technicians and paramedics supply advanced care, with direct communication links to the receiving hospital. According to the nature of their injuries, patients may bypass the nearest hospital and be taken directly to a designated trauma centre.

TRAUMA SCORING:

Accident details: 72-yr-old female front-seat passenger (wearing seatbelt) in car involved in head-on collision with articulated lorry. Driver of car died at accident scene.

Recordings on arrival in hospital:

	Systolic BP	85 mmHg
	GCS	14 (E4, V4, M6)
	Respiratory rate	26/min

Revised Trauma Score Calculation:

	Weighting value
Resp. rate	
0	0
13–15	1
13–16	2
13–17	3
> 29	4
Systolic BP:	
0	0
13–15	1
13–16	2
13–17	3
> 89	4
GCS	
3	0
13–15	1
13–16	2
13–17	3
13–18	4

RTS = (Resp. rate weight × 0.2908) + (Syst. BP weight × 0.7326) + (GCS weight × 0.9368)

So: RTS = (3 × 0.2908) + (4× 0.7326) + (4 × 0.9368)

$\quad\quad$ = 0.8724 + 2.9304 + 3.7472

$\quad\quad$ = 7.56

Injury Severity Score Calculation:

	Score:
Flail chest (left side) with pulmonary contusion	4
Left pneumothorax	3
Myocardial contusion	3
Splenic tear (simple capsular tear)	2
6 cm scalp laceration	1
Right and left cerebral frontal lobe contusions	4
Undisplaced closed L tibial shaft fracture	2
8 cm laceration L knee (not involving joint)	1

The ISS is the sum of the numerical squares of the highest scoring injuries in the three highest scoring body regions. Here, there are two injuries in the thoracic domain, of which the 'Flail chest' scores higher at 4. In the head domain the cerebral contusions score higher at 4. Accordingly the three highest scores are 4, 4 and 2.

Hence: ISS = $4^2 + 4^2 + 2^2 = 36$

Probability of Survival (P_s) Calculation:

$P_s = 1/(1 + e^b)$ $\quad\quad$ e = 2.7182818 – the base for Naperian logarithms

For blunt trauma: b = 0.56 + (0.7281 × RTS) – (0.1132 × ISS) – 1.8339 (an age correction factor)

$P_s = 1/(1 + e^{-0.148055})$

$\quad$ = 0.53694

i.e. the probability of survival for this patient is ≈ 54%

NB: The coefficients used to calculate the P_s value are updated regularly to reflect changes in the standard of trauma care. The values here have been kindly supplied by the Scottish Trauma Audit Group (STAG), and for blunt trauma are those published by MTOS(UK).

Fig. 9.2 Trauma scoring.

In the UK and Europe ambulance services, augmented by physician-led teams, often transport the patient to the nearest hospital. In 1995, the Department of Health recommended the presence of a paramedic in each frontline ambulance. Paramedics can provide techniques such as tracheal intubation, peripheral i.v. access and the administration of i.v. fluids and drugs. Axiomatically, the use of such skills by ambulance paramedics at the scene of injury or en route to hospital should improve outcome for injured patients, but controlled studies have not demonstrated such benefits. There are two main reasons for this surprising result. First, paramedic treatment may increase prehospital time delaying definitive care. Such delay is closely related to increases in mortality. Secondly, the techniques used may themselves have intrinsically adverse effects. For example, i.v. fluids given to patients in whom bleeding cannot be controlled (e.g. intraperitoneal bleeding, or from pelvic or long bone fractures) can precipitate additional blood loss by increasing blood pressure.

Except for situations in which unavoidable delays will occur for a prehospital patient (usually entrapment or impalement; rural or inaccessible locations), advanced prehospital techniques are inappropriate.

Transport from accident locus to hospital must be safe and rapid, with constant communication. In the UK land-based ambulance service vehicles perform this, with additional support from helicopters and fixed-wing aircraft. Much experience has been obtained with helicopters in military medical environments, the USA and Australia: they dramatically increase costs and have additional risks for both patient and crew. Despite the potential to reduce journey times, the types of helicopters used in the UK have major operational difficulties with poor visibility, nighttime flying, high winds and urban environments. Recent audit in an urban environment in the UK failed to show an improvement in response times, with longer on-scene times and no increase in survival for trauma patients. There is a clear justification for helicopter use in offshore, mountain rescue and certain rural incident situations, but the majority of patients will continue to be transported by land ambulances.

TRAUMA CENTRES

A trauma patient should receive definitive surgical and intensive care facilities as soon as possible after injury. The problem is how to deliver this standard. In the 1970s and 1980s trauma centres were introduced in the USA and a few European cities, where they unequivocally reduced preventable, in-hospital trauma deaths. Some of the results were remarkable, with 'avoidable' deaths reduced 5–10-fold for patients taken directly to a Level 1 centre.

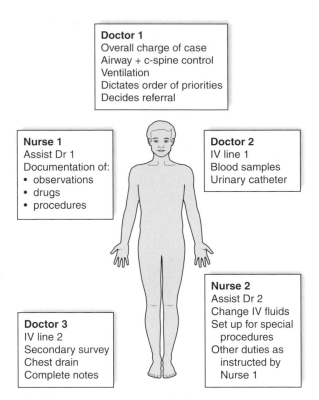

Doctor 1
Overall charge of case
Airway + c-spine control
Ventilation
Dictates order of priorities
Decides referral

Nurse 1
Assist Dr 1
Documentation of:
• observations
• drugs
• procedures

Doctor 2
IV line 1
Blood samples
Urinary catheter

Nurse 2
Assist Dr 2
Change IV fluids
Set up for special
   procedures
Other duties as
   instructed by
   Nurse 1

Doctor 3
IV line 2
Secondary survey
Chest drain
Complete notes

Fig. 9.3 Trauma team organization.

The key elements in these systems were: transfer of patients from the accident scene directly to the centre; reception by senior staff on a 24 hour basis; the availability of all appropriate specialties on the same site; and a high throughput of patients.

Independent evaluation of the pilot trauma centre in England, however, failed to show a reduction in death rates. Two facts may explain this disappointing result. The first is the difference in trauma epidemiology, in relation to both the nature of the trauma and the volume of patients presenting. Secondly, despite having run for several years, the centre was not fully integrated into a comprehensive regionalized system. For the foreseeable future in the UK, the provision of care will be by a trauma team approach (Fig. 9.3).

RESUSCITATION IN THE A&E DEPARTMENT

The first 10 minutes

The receiving department should have advance warning from Ambulance Control to permit an appropriate manpower and resource response.

Advance information required by the trauma team:

- Estimated time of arrival
- Numbers, ages and sex of patients
- Nature of incident and any special features e.g. associated chemical/radioactive contamination, helicopter transportation etc.
- Brief details of injuries, treatment given at scene/in transit and current condition.

The resuscitation room must have all equipment needed for at least the first 1–2 hours of resuscitation. A calm ordered approach is essential. Compliance with universal precautions for sharps/instruments disposal, the use of gloves, face/eye protection and protective clothing is mandatory. All personnel must be appropriately immunized for hepatitis B.

If the number and severity of injured patients involved exceeds the facilities immediately available, the hospital's major incident plan may need to be activated. In this event patients are triaged on arrival according to their priority for treatment.

During reception, a concise, relevant history is obtained from the ambulance crew and other emergency personnel, noting factors associated with an increased likelihood of severe injury.

A trauma team, of 4–5 experienced doctors and nurses, is used for the patient's initial assessment and treatment (Fig. 9.3). Each team member has a preassigned role and performs this, unless directed otherwise by the team leader, who must have sufficient seniority and competence to direct and control the entire resuscitation process. The team members must be entirely familiar with the tasks required of them and perform them with minimal delay or questioning.

SUMMARY BOX

Accident features associated with major trauma

- Death of another individual in the same accident
- High-velocity impact, e.g. pedestrian or cyclist (motor or pedal) struck at > 30 kph vehicle occupants in collisions with closing speeds >60 kph
- Entrapment or intrusion into the passenger compartment of the vehicle
- Ejection from a vehicle
- Falls from heights > 3 m
- Penetrating injury of the chest, abdomen or neck

The patient's clothing is removed completely (cut off, if necessary, to avoid patient movement), allowing adequate access for examination, and to avoid missing an occult external injury. Injured patients lose their normal themoregulatory ability, so they must then be kept warm and excessive exposure for examination or practical procedures avoided.

A traditional surgical approach, with history taking, clinical examination, investigation and treatment, is inappropriate in major trauma patients. An 'ABC' approach is logical and easy to remember, but although the steps are presented here sequentially, the trauma team performs and constantly reassesses all of these aspects *simultaneously*.

Airway

The patency of the airway is first assessed by direct inspection, identifying and removing obstructions. Loose-fitting dentures or dental plates are removed. Snoring or stridor implies airway obstruction. A rigid suction catheter, used carefully to avoid stimulation of the sensitive pharynx, will remove blood, vomit, secretions and other debris from the mouth and oropharynx. Larger items, e.g. lumps of food, are extracted with forceps under direct vision.

The commonest cause of airway obstruction is the tongue falling back and blocking the oropharynx. Airway clearance, together with the 'chin-lift' or 'jaw-thrust' manoeuvres, will correct this in the majority of cases. The airway is then constantly reassessed by **Looking** (to see the chest rise and fall), **Listening** (for abnormal airway sounds) and **Feeling** (for the patient's exhaled breath – using the side of the cheek).

Assessment of conscious level helps in airway assessment. A patient speaking in complete sentences does not have an immediate airway problem (although one may develop later). The Glasgow Coma Scale can identify patients with established or potential problems and, if < 8/15, usually mandates definitive airway intervention as the protective gag and swallow airway reflexes are likely to be absent or compromised. In the majority of cases the upper airway is secured with simple positioning, regular suction and the use of basic adjuncts such as oro- or nasopharyngeal airways.

Control of the cervical spine

Irrespective of the airway control technique used, the cervical cord is protected constantly by manual in-line cervical control with the neck in the neutral position or by using a carefully fitted rigid neck collar, sandbags and tape.

Tracheal intubation is the advanced technique of choice. It protects the airway from aspiration of vomit or blood, and allows ventilation with controlled levels of oxygen, and airway suctioning to remove debris. It does, however, require expertise in using anaesthetic and neuromuscular paralysing agents. Prior to intubation the patient is preoxygenated and must be carefully monitored throughout the process. A 'surgical' airway is extremely rarely needed and, if required, a percutaneous cricothyrotomy is the simplest, safest and quickest surgical approach.

Advanced airway techniques

- Absent protective airway reflexes (usually caused by altered consciousness)
- Basic techniques unable to cope with current or predicted airway compromise (e.g. major facial, burns/inhalation injury)
- Need for controlled ventilation (e.g. head &/or chest injury).

Breathing

Optimal ventilation requires a patent upper and lower airway and effective function of the thoracic wall, lungs and diaphragm. Clinical assessment is extremely helpful. Respiratory compromise is characterized by tachy- or bradypnoea, the use of accessory muscles of respiration, and paradoxical (seesaw movement) of the chest and abdomen, indicating failure of normal diaphragmatic function. Hypoxia may be manifest by restlessness, tachycardia, confusion, agitation, pallor or sweating, but cyanosis is uncommon, particularly if hypovolaemia is present.

Concern about oxygen toxicity in the initial phase of resuscitation is unnecessary, and until the patient is stable and adequate tissue oxygen delivery has been confirmed, the highest possible concentration of oxygen must be given. Pulse oximeters can detect arterial desaturation, but readings are unreliable in hypovolaemic or shocked patients, or if abnormal haemoglobins (including carboxyhaemoglobin) are present. Pulse oximetry does not replace arterial blood gas analysis, as hypercapnoea can occur with normal SaO_2 levels.

Clinical inspection, palpation and auscultation of the neck and chest (including the back) should detect immediately life-threatening injuries such as flail segment, penetrating wounds, tension or open pneumothoraces, major haemothorax and cardiac tamponade. These conditions need immediate treatment, e.g. needle thoracocentesis for tension pneumothorax, or the insertion of an intercostal drain for haemothorax. Open or sucking chest wounds are rare but, if present, allow equalization of atmospheric and intrathoracic pressures. With large defects, atmospheric air passes through the wound into the intrathoracic space with

each inspiration, and the lung collapses. To prevent this, the open wound is covered with a sterile occlusive dressing, taped on three sides. This acts as a flutter valve, and formal tube thoracostomy is then performed at a separate site from the open wound.

Repeated arterial blood gas analyses are needed to ensure that hypoxia is not present and that alveolar ventilation is sufficient to prevent hypercapnoea. For patients who are intubated and ventilated additional problems may develop. Positive-pressure ventilation may reduce cardiac output (manifest initially by tachycardia ± hypotension) because of decreased venous return to the heart resulting from increased intrathoracic pressure during the 'inspiratory' phase of ventilation. The risk of pneumothorax in patients with coexisting chest injuries is markedly increased by positive-pressure ventilation. If a pneumothorax is already present, tension may be induced. For these reasons tube thoracostomy is mandatory if a pneumothorax is present and positive-pressure ventilation, for whatever reason, is to be undertaken.

For patients in whom positive-pressure ventilation is instituted, the aim is to ensure adequate oxygenation (PaO_2 levels >12 kPa) and alveolar ventilation ($PaCO_2$ levels 3.5–4 kPa). Controlled ventilation is particularly important in patients with head injury, as hypercarbia causes dilation of the cerebral vessels and increased intracranial pressure, whereas hypocarbia produces cerebrovascular vasospasm, compromising cerebral perfusion.

The drugs necessary to permit intubation and controlled ventilation may themselves obscure important clinical features, particularly of neurological or abdominal injury. Before any drugs are used, the patient's neurological status must be recorded. Additional imaging, such as CT scanning, will be required if there is any suspicion of associated head injury. Abdominal injury is commonly missed in patients with altered consciousness of whatever cause. This is compounded in paralysed and sedated patients, and so additional investigations, such as ultrasound, CT or diagnostic peritoneal lavage are important (see below).

Gastric dilation is common in trauma patients. It results from a combination of factors including air-swallowing (in conscious patients), bag–mask ventilation (where the airway pressure exceeds the gastro-oesophageal closing pressure), and the effects of sympathetic nervous system overactivity and electrolyte disturbance on gastric peristalsis. A distended stomach full of air, fluid and food, in a patient with compromised airway protective reflexes, is a situation ripe for regurgitation and potentially fatal aspiration. In addition, the distended stomach will restrict diaphragmatic movement and impair respiration. To prevent these problems a nasogastric (if there is any suspicion of an anterior cranial fossa fracture, an orogastric) tube is routinely inserted and suction applied.

Circulation

The clinical detection of blood loss and the resulting haemo-dynamic effects is crude and non-specific. Pulse rate, cuff blood pressure and peripheral perfusion (assessed by capillary refill time) are routinely noted every 5–10 minutes in the initial stages, but these recordings have major limitations. Protective homeostatic mechanisms in previously fit healthy adults mean that, depending upon the rate and site of blood loss, 20% or more of total circulating blood volume can be lost without a measurable change in these recordings. Isolated readings are especially misleading. Trends in pulse rate and blood pressure are of much greater value. A rising pulse rate combined with a falling blood pressure strongly suggests uncontrolled, often occult, blood loss.

Absence of these features does not necessarily mean that all is well. The patient may not be able to respond to hypovolaemia by increasing the heart rate because of age, pre-existing cardiac disease or routine medications such as β-blockers. In addition, an individual's 'normal' values need to be considered. A blood pressure of 110/60 mmHg may represent severe hypotension if the patient's normal value is 190/120 mmHg, but may be normal for a healthy young adult. Unfortunately, this knowledge is rarely available in the early stages of resuscitation, and a high index of suspicion, bearing in mind the mechanism of injury, is therefore essential.

To reduce blood loss is essential. External haemorrhage can invariably be controlled by simple direct pressure. Haemostasis from the sometimes profuse bleeding of scalp wounds is best achieved with carefully applied sutures. Careful splinting of long-bone fractures reduces blood loss from fracture sites by up to 50%, makes the patient more comfortable, and reduces analgesic requirements. In contrast, blood loss into the peritoneal cavity, thorax or pelvis is usually concealed, can be life-threatening in magnitude, and cannot be controlled simply (see below).

The immediate priority is to insert and secure two large-bore (12–14 G) intravenous cannulae. The forearms or antecubital fossae are the most accessible peripheral sites, but the nature and location of the injuries may require alternative sites, such as the femoral or external jugular veins, to be used. Central venous cannulation is difficult and potentially hazardous in shocked hypovolaemic patients, so if percutaneous access cannot be obtained, a surgical cut-down at the saphenofemoral junction at the groin is preferable, although more time-consuming. At the time of cannulation initial venous blood samples should be taken, carefully labelled and sent for analysis, the laboratories having previously been alerted.

The effective resuscitation of the injured child requires an appreciation of the physiological differences that exist between children and adults. The normal cardiovascular and respiratory parameters that we measure vary with age e.g. the normal heart rate of a newborn infant is 160 beats/minute; the normal respiratory rate of a one-year-old is about 30 breaths per minute. A knowledge of what is normal is required to allow the confident identification of the abnormal.

Suitable equipment is essential to safely resuscitate children of different ages and weights. Cuffed tracheal tubes are not used in small children. Small intravenous cannulae may be necessary and intraosseous needles can be used for resuscitation in children under six years of age. Different sized cervical collars, oxygen face masks, laryngoscopes and other equipment should be readily available in any resuscitation room receiving children.

Notwithstanding the above, the *ABCD* sequence of resuscitation that is followed in the child is the same as that followed in the adult; *A*irway with cervical spine control, *B*reathing with oxygen, *C*irculation with control of bleeding, *D*isability.

The choice of fluids for the replacement of traumatic blood loss is controversial and poorly understood. Intravenous volume replacement is begun with infusion of an isotonic crystalloid such as 0.9% saline or Ringer's lactate. In the UK, after 1000–2000 mL of crystalloid, a colloid is commonly given prior to, or together with, blood. Theoretically, colloids (such as gelatins, starches or dextrans) might be expected to be beneficial, but there is no good evidence to suggest this in clinical practice, and recent analyses suggest that even albumin solutions (the body's 'natural' colloid) are less suitable for volume replacement than are crystalloids.

Irrespective of the fluid chosen, it must be warmed to 37–38°C before infusion to prevent hypothermia and aggravating coagulation deficits. This is achieved by in-line warming devices that infuse the fluid at the required temperature, regardless of flow rate.

SUMMARY BOX

Initial blood samples in the trauma patient

- Blood grouping and cross-matching
- Full blood count and haematocrit
- Urea and electrolytes
- Plasma glucose
- Arterial blood gases
- Kleihauer–Betke analysis (in pregnant patients)

Intravenous iv fluid administration is initially dictated by the nature of the patient's injuries, an estimate of the current volume deficit, and the clinical and haemodynamic responses to treatment. Failure to respond to the first 1–2 L of volume replacement suggests that the volume deficit is great (> 40% of circulating volume). It is, however, inappropriate to correct haemodynamic measurements in isolation, and there are situations where, in the presence of an uncontrolled bleeding site (for example in the pelvis or peritoneum), increasing blood pressure will simply exacerbate blood losses.

SUMMARY BOX

Situations where blood loss may be misappreciated

- The elderly
- Patients on concurrent drug therapy (e.g. β-blockers, antihypertensives, antianginals)
- Patients with a pacemaker
- Athletes
- Pregnancy
- Hypothermia

Blood transfusion requirements depend upon the magnitude of blood loss and the physiological response. It is usual to replace losses with the aim of maintaining the patient's haematocrit at ~30%. Where there is immediately life-threatening haemorrhage group O Rh negative blood is given, but more usually fully cross-matched or type-specific blood can be supplied. Most transfusion services supply packed red cells. There is no evidence that 'fresh' whole blood is preferable. In situations of massive blood loss, where replacement of more than the equivalent of one circulating blood volume is needed, then coagulation problems should be anticipated. Close liaison with the Blood Transfusion Service and haematology laboratories is essential, and platelet concentrates and coagulation factors are given on their guidance rather than purely on an empirical basis.

Measurement of urine output (> 1 mL/kg body weight/h normally implies adequate renal perfusion), continuous intra-arterial blood pressure monitoring and serial lactate levels assist in monitoring the response to infusion. In this situation intra-arterial blood pressure monitoring is significantly more accurate than standard cuff methods, and has the additional advantage that the indwelling cannula permits regular arterial blood sampling without additional patient discomfort. Continuous ECG monitoring, oxygen saturation (by pulse oximetry) core temperature and serial blood pressure measurements are standard requirements and augment clinical judgement. A low or falling GCS may

---

SUMMARY BOX

Monitoring the trauma patient

- Heart rate
- Blood pressure (cuff and intra-arterial)
- Capillary refill
- Respiratory rate
- Glasgow Coma Scale
- Urine output
- Core temperature
- ECG
- Pulse oximetry

---

indicate cerebral hypoperfusion due to hypovolaemia. More sophisticated means of cardiovascular assessment can provide additional information and should be used at an early stage, but techniques such as central venous and pulmonary artery wedge pressure and cardiac output measurement are usually impracticable in the immediate resuscitative phase. They will be used later, particularly if vasoactive agents such as inotropes are used.

Analgesia and splinting

A calm, gentle and reassuring approach does much to relieve anxiety and is the first step in pain relief. Adequate analgesia is often neglected – or worse, thought to be unnecessary or hazardous in trauma patients. Physiological responses to pain produce adverse effects – for example by increasing intracranial and arterial pressure – and so analgesia is essential. Further, it must be given according to the patient's individual requirements, rather than as a rigid process.

In cooperative, fully conscious patients without respiratory problems, Entonox (50% nitrous oxide, 50% oxygen) is useful for short-duration procedures such as manipulations. Its value is limited by the need for patient cooperation (the euphoric effect may be associated with confusion and disorientation), its short duration of action and its limited analgesic effect.

Opioid drugs such as morphine or diamorphine, given i.v. (*never* i.m.) with an antiemetic remain unsurpassed for analgesia. In this situation the newer synthetic opioids have no advantages and non-steroidal analgesics are contraindicated. The drug is given by titration in 1–2 mg aliquots until the pain is relieved. Provided the drug is given like this, haemodynamic disturbance or respiratory depression is rare.

Head injury or suspected head injury is not an *absolute* contraindication to opioid administration, provided that the agent is given as above and that the patient's airway, ventilation and haemodynamic status are carefully monitored. If necessary, naloxone can be given if there is doubt as to whether alterations in conscious level are due to the opioid or to the head injury and its effects.

Local anaesthetic techniques are generally of limited value in major trauma, but an exception is the use of a femoral nerve block for patients with femoral shaft fractures. Long-bone fractures need to be immobilized to reduce pain and blood loss from the fracture site, facilitate the taking of X-rays, patient movement and transfer, and reduce the chances of fat embolism syndrome. Inflatable or foam-cushioned splints are suitable for upper-limb or below-knee injuries; adjustable traction splints are best for femoral shaft fractures.

Patients with major pelvic fractures cause difficult management problems in that conventional splintage is impossible and massive and uncontrollable blood loss may result. The optimal approach is the application of external fixator devices in the resuscitation phase, followed, if required, by angiographic embolization. MAST (medical anti-shock trouser) devices may have a role in providing temporary splintage in these patients if more sophisticated techniques are not available.

The next phase

The above assessments and interventions represent only the immediately life-saving procedures and should occupy just the first 10 minutes after arrival in the Accident and Emergency department. Then, provided the patient's condition permits, a more detailed history and examination is undertaken, with appropriate laboratory and imaging investigations to determine the full extent of the patient's injuries and the requirement for surgery or other care.

This review, or secondary survey, should enable a definitive management plan to be formulated. Throughout, the continuing priorities of *Airway*, *Breathing* and *Circulation* must be constantly reviewed and corrected as necessary.

The patient is examined from top to toe to ensure that no wound, bruise or swelling is missed. The back and spine are examined with the patient 'log-rolled', looking specifically for localized tenderness, swelling, bruising or a 'step'. The perineum is examined and a rectal examination performed.

Rectal examination in the trauma patient includes:

- Anal sphincter tone
- Prostate: position, bogginess
- Blood in the rectum
- Pelvic fractures
- Perineal injury.

The neurological status of the patient is recorded regularly, including the GCS, pupil sizes and reactions, and any focal deficit. The ears, nose and mastoid areas are carefully exam-

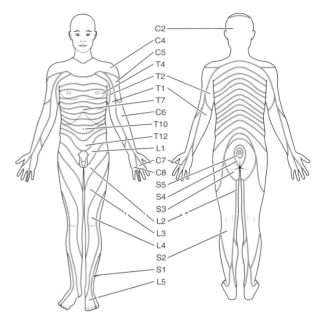

Fig. 9.4 Mannikin with sensory dermatomes illustrated.

ined for evidence of skull-base injury, such as blood/CSF oto- or rhinorrhoea, or bruising. Muscle power should be tested and recorded using the MRC scale, and the tendon reflexes examined. It is vital to test sensation in a methodical fashion (Fig. 9.4). The perineal area must be included (this is most easily achieved at the time of rectal examination) as the lowest (sacral) dermatomes are in this area.

Any decrease in the patient's conscious level (i.e. a numerical fall in GCS) must prompt an immediate search for, and correction of, a primary cause, such as intracranial haematoma, or secondary factors such as hypoxia, hypercarbia, hypotension or hypoglycaemia.

SUMMARY BOX

*Causes of **early** neurological deterioration in the trauma patient*

Intracranial	**Extracranial**
Haematoma	Hypoxia
Cerebral oedema	Hypotension
Fitting	Hyper/hypocarbia
Impaired cerebral venous drainage, e.g. neck collar applied too tightly, head-down tilt, tapes around neck etc.	Hyper/hypoglycaemia

---

Table 9.1   The Glasgow Coma Scale

Eye opening	
Spontaneously	4
To speech	3
To pain	2
None	1
Verbal response	
Orientated	5
Confused	4
Inappropriate words	3
Incomprehensible sounds	2
None	1
Motor response	
Obeys commands	6
Localizes to pain	5
Flexion (withdraws) to pain	4
Abnormal flexion to pain	3
Extension to pain	2
None	1
Total	/15

Confounding factors may render the assessment of the GCS difficult, especially if the patient has taken alcohol or other drugs, but altered consciousness or other neurological deficit should never be assumed to be due solely to alcohol or other drugs alone until proven otherwise (see Glasgow Coma Scale, Table 9.1, and MRC scale Table 9.2).

Table 9.2   Assessing muscle power – the MRC scale

No flicker of movement	0
A flicker of contraction, but no movement	1
Movement, with gravity neutralized	2
Movement against gravity	3
Movement against added resistance	4
Normal power	5

IMAGING AND OTHER DIAGNOSTIC AIDS

The radiological investigations needed in the initial phase of the management of a major trauma patient are limited but important. It is important to obtain the best-quality views and fixed overhead X-ray facilities in the resuscitation room itself are invaluable, as transfer of the patient to a main X-ray department can be hazardous. A portable machine brought to the resuscitation room is preferable to transfer although the images obtained will be of poorer quality.

SUMMARY BOX

Initial X-rays in the patient with blunt trauma

- Chest (an *erect* film, provided that this can be performed safely)
- Cervical spine
- Pelvis
- Thoracic/lumbar spine views are indicated in patients with:
  - A mechanism of injury consistent with spinal injury, altered consciousness, distal neurological abnormality, or where other injuries or conditions, e.g. alcohol/drug use, may prevent the identification of spinal injury

---

There are three primary X-ray views in the blunt trauma patient, but these do have limitations:

- The *chest X-ray* may demonstrate thoracic injuries previously unrecognized on clinical examination, but even on a good-quality erect view over half of the rib fractures actually present will be missed (Fig. 9.5). The patient's condition often precludes an erect film, and on a supine view pneumothoraces and/or haemothoraces are difficult to detect; even in the absence of pathology the mediastinal contours are displaced and widened.
- The *lateral view of the cervical spine* should be a cross-table film and must include *all* of the vertebrae from C1 to T1. This provides valuable information on acute bony injury (Fig. 9.6), but a 'normal' neck X-ray does not exclude significant injury to soft tissues, including the cervical cord.
- On a *plain AP view of the pelvis* injuries to the posterior elements (especially around the sacroiliac regions which may lead to significant occult haemorrhage) are difficult to see.

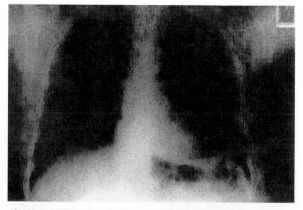

Fig. 9.5   Chest X-ray showing rib fractures and subcutaneous emphysema.

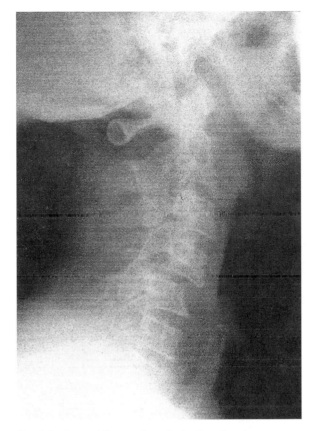

Fig. 9.6 Lateral X-ray of cervical spine showing C4/5 subluxation.

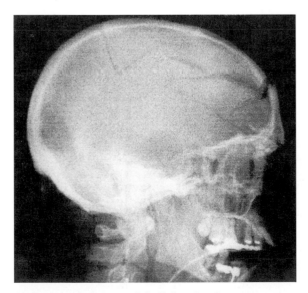

Fig. 9.7 Lateral X-ray of skull showing fracture.

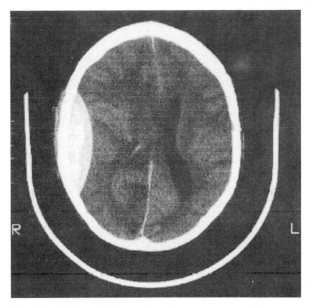

Fig. 9.8 Right-sided extradural haematoma with midline shift.

The use of additional imaging techniques depends upon their availability and the clinical state of the patient. For head, spinal and pelvic injury CT is unsurpassed and rapid. In contrast to the information provided by conventional skull X-rays (Fig. 9.7), CT defines the nature and magnitude of the intracranial insult (Fig. 9.8). It is therefore invaluable in providing the information needed to decide the requirement for neurosurgical intervention.

In experienced hands, ultrasound examination of the abdomen is a quick, non-invasive and accurate method of detecting free intraperitoneal fluid. It can be performed in the resuscitation room and has largely supplanted diagnostic peritoneal lavage, although this technique remains a simple and rapid method for establishing the presence of intraperitoneal bleeding. Injury to some solid organs, the retroperitoneum and hollow viscera is less easily demonstrated on ultrasound, and CT scanning – with contrast as necessary – is preferable, provided that the patient is stable and can be transferred to the CT suite.

AFTER THE RESUSCITATION ROOM

The immediate aim of the resuscitation team is to assess and treat life-threatening injuries. There is no absolute guide as to the length of time this process will take, but the procedures and referral must be performed expediently without compromising patient care. The result should be a patient with a patent airway, with adequate gas exchange, and whose circulatory status is normal or in the process of being adequately corrected. Long-bone fractures should have been splinted appropriately and cervical spine control maintained throughout.

Continuing care then involves identifying the correct destination for the patient. The nature and extent of the injuries and the patient's physiological response to treatment dictate this. In some situations it is impossible to 'stabilize' the patient without immediate surgical intervention. Examples include patients with exanguinating intra-abdominal or intrathoracic haemorrhage in whom immediate laparotomy or thoracotomy is mandated.

More commonly the patient is, at least temporarily, stable such that further investigation can be undertaken beyond the resuscitation room prior to definitive surgical or intensive care unit admission. Senior anaesthetic and surgical staff must accompany the patient in these situations, so that if sudden deterioration occurs the patient can be transferred directly to theatre. Full monitoring and resuscitation equipment is mandatory for the transfer.

The subsequent destination of the patient then depends upon their overall condition and the findings of these investigations. Intensive care admission is required if ventilation is needed or anticipated, if there are multiple injuries involving main systems, or if the patient needs invasive monitoring. Stable, self-ventilating patients with less severe injuries may be managed in a high-dependency unit, but the attending staff must be familiar with multiple trauma assessment and the relevant specialties must liaise closely to ensure a multidisciplinary approach.

It may be necessary to transfer the patient to another hospital for emergency investigation not available in the receiving hospital, or as part of definitive treatment by a specialist service. Interhospital transfer – or indeed intrahospital transfer – is hazardous and must be performed by experienced anaesthetic and nursing staff with relevant monitoring and resuscitation equipment. The aspects of airway, ventilation and circulation control must be secured prior to transfer. The receiving unit must be informed of the relevant patient details, allowing them to prepare effectively for his or her arrival. The type of transport used will depend upon the distance and geography of the journey involved, but may involve air transportation with all its attendant specific considerations. Regular updates should be supplied to the receiving specialist.

SUMMARY BOX

Information required by the receiving unit or hospital

- Patient's name, age and sex
- Previous health status and medications (if known)
- Pulse, blood pressure, respiratory rate (at scene, on arrival, and current)
- Glasgow Coma Scale (at scene, on arrival, and at present)
- Summary of injuries: include signs of head injury, and any lateralizing signs
- Summary of i.v. fluids (including blood) and the haemodynamic and urine output responses
- X-ray, CT or other imaging results
- Blood grouping/cross-matching, haematology and biochemistry results
- Tetanus status/cover provided, antibiotics and other drugs given (include doses and timing)

SECTION 2
THE OPERATION

Preoperative assessment and investigations

T.S. Walsh, A.J. Pollok

This chapter describes the preoperative assessment of patients undergoing surgery. The first part is a general description of the process of assessment, the most relevant features of the history, and the specific questions relevant to anaesthesia. The second part reviews in detail the relevance to surgery and anaesthesia of specific diseases, and their management in the perioperative period.

ASSESSMENT OF FITNESS FOR OPERATION

Assessment takes place at several points. A preliminary assessment of fitness may be given by the GP in the referral letter. Thereafter, the surgeon will evaluate the patient at the outpatient clinic, when specific investigations may be organized. The surgeon may request an anaesthetic review prior to admission to hospital, particularly in patients considered to have a high perioperative risk. In some hospitals patients are seen at a preadmission clinic several days before surgery, where a history is taken and relevant examination and investigations performed. An anaesthetist may review patients at the preadmission clinic, but in most cases they are not seen until after admission to hospital. After admission, a further assessment of fitness for surgery and anaesthesia is made. Increasing numbers of patients are admitted 24 hours before surgery; it is therefore important that essential investigations are performed on an outpatient basis or immediately following admission. It is also important to recognize potential problems early in order to avoid delays and patient distress.

The decision regarding fitness for surgery is made by the anaesthetist. The recognition of patients with significantly increased perioperative risk is a fundamental part of preoperative assessment. In these cases, liaison with the anaesthetist prior to admission will reduce unnecessary delays before surgery. Very few patients require admission to hospital more than 24–48 hours before surgery if the appropriate investigations have been anticipated and performed.

Following the patient's hospital admission the house surgeon will document a full history and clinical examination. He or she should confirm the availability of the patient's old notes and organize outstanding investigations such as ECG, urea and electrolytes, full blood count and chest X-ray. The requirement for additional investigations will be dictated by comorbidity identified from the history and clinical examination, drug therapy, the nature of the surgical procedure, and the interval between the outpatient visit and hospital admission. These are discussed later in this chapter. The anaesthetist should be consulted when there is uncertainty about the need for additional investigations. It is important to ensure that the patient and relatives are informed about the diagnosis and understand the nature and implications of the operation that is proposed. A more detailed explanation and discussion of the operation, and its associated risks and benefits, is undertaken by the surgeon prior to completion of the operation consent form.

The anaesthetist usually visits the patient on the evening before or on the day of surgery. He or she will undertake a systemic enquiry and clinical examination, with an emphasis on the cardiovascular and respiratory systems. An examination of the upper respiratory tract, teeth and neck will alert them to potential airway problems. An explanation of the proposed anaesthetic, along with the plan for early post-operative care and analgesia, is given. At this point the patient should have the opportunity to voice any concerns and obtain reassurance. When appropriate, the various options for anaesthesia and postoperative analgesia can be discussed and the patient's preferences taken into account.

Perioperative risk

The aim of preoperative assessment is to ensure the patient's physical condition is optimal in order to minimize risk. Patients require both physical and psychological preparation, and need to be fully informed about the procedure and its risks. For emergency surgery compromises may have to be made for some aspects of preparation, and balanced against the risks of delaying surgery. Perioperative risk can be considered to have several components.

- The risks directly attributable to the surgery itself. These include technical problems with surgery and anaesthesia, and complications such as wound infection. To quantify these risks the surgeon and anaesthetist can give a patient estimates from audit of their own practice or from published data.
- The risk from the physiological stress surgery places on the individual. This is often difficult to quantify because it depends on the nature of the surgery, the technical success of surgery in that individual, complications that occur (such as infection), and the physiological fitness or reserve of the patient. The majority of physiological complications of surgery involve the cardiovascular and respiratory systems. Cardiorespiratory disease is common in patients presenting for surgery, and these are therefore the most important systems to consider during preoperative assessment.
- The psychological risks of surgery. Almost all patients will suffer some anxiety in relation to proposed surgery and anaesthesia. Part of the role of both surgeon and anaesthetist is to identify sources of concern for individual patients and use explanation to minimize anxiety. The source of anxiety may be unexpected; for example, a patient may have little concern about the surgery itself but be terrified of postoperative nausea, or of being 'aware' during the operation.

The logical sequence for assessment of fitness for surgery and anaesthesia is as follows:

1. Identify known health problems, assess their current severity from the history, examination and relevant investigations, and whether these conditions can be improved prior to surgery.
2. Screen the patient for common conditions that may be undiagnosed, such as hypertension and diabetes.

3. Identify other factors that increase risk, such as smoking, alcohol intake and obesity.
4. Document the patient's drug therapy and any modifications that may be required in the perioperative period.
5. Identify allergies to drugs.
6. Document problems with previous anaesthetics.

These factors are considered in detail below. Once an assessment of risk has been made by the surgeon and anaesthetist, this needs to be balanced against the indication for and urgency of surgery, and discussed with the patient. For example, it is usual to accept a higher risk for a patient requiring urgent cancer surgery than for one requiring elective varicose vein surgery.

In children, the co-existence of a congenital or genetic abnormality or the long-term effects of prematurity (including respiratory disease and cerebral palsy), may have a major impact on the safe provision of general anaesthesia.

Coexisting chronic health problems

Oxygen transport to tissues

The reason that cardiovascular and respiratory diseases are the most relevant in assessing risk is that the most serious complications of anaesthesia result from inadequate supply of oxygen to tissues, resulting in hypoxia and organ damage. In its most extreme form a patient suffering a reduction in oxygen supply to the brain during the perioperative period can suffer irreversible hypoxic brain damage.

The delivery of oxygen to tissues requires the efficient transfer of oxygen from the lungs into blood, an adequate concentration of functioning haemoglobin to transport oxygen, and satisfactory cardiac output and blood pressure to transport oxygen from the lungs to the tissues. The **tissue oxygen delivery** of an individual can be calculated from the product of the cardiac output and oxygen content of arterial blood. The oxygen content of arterial blood is dependent on the haemoglobin concentration and arterial oxygen saturation. An average resting awake adult requires approximately 250 mL oxygen per minute. During anaesthesia this decreases to about 175 mL. Oxygen delivery is normally approximately 1000 mL/min, so there is a considerable safety margin. A reduction in one parameter alone may not significantly reduce the oxygen delivery, but a reduction in all three can result in a profound decrease in oxygen delivery and cause critical organ ischaemia. The response of tissues to decreasing oxygen delivery is to compensate by increasing the amount of oxygen removed during the passage of blood through the organ (increasing **oxygen extraction**). Most organs can extract up to about 50–60% of the oxygen in arterial blood, but this **critical oxygen extraction ratio** varies widely from organ to organ. If the critical oxygen extraction ratio is exceeded tissue hypoxia occurs, and cells must switch to anaerobic metabolism to generate energy.

SUMMARY BOX

Transport of oxygen to tissues

Oxygen delivery =
cardiac output × (%saturation of
haemoglobin × haemoglobin concentration × 1.34)

For an average 70 kg man:
Oxygen delivery or DO_2 is about 1000 mL/min
Cardiac output is about 5000 mL/min
Haemoglobin concentration is 14 g/dL
1.34 represents the amount of oxygen in mL that
1 g of haemoglobin can carry when
100% saturated
The oxygen consumption of the body is about
250 mL/min

SUMMARY BOX

*Factors that can compromise oxygen
supply to tissues during the
perioperative period.*

Lungs	Chronic lung disease
	● COPD
	● Asthma
	● Fibrotic lung disease
	Acute lung disease
	● Upper or lower respiratory tract infection
	● Acute respiratory distress syndrome
	● Pleural effusion
	● Pulmonary embolus
	● Pneumothorax
Cardiovascular system	Chronic conditions
	● Ischaemic heart disease
	● Cardiac failure
	● Valvular heart disease
	● Arrhythmias
	Acute conditions
	● Shock
	● Myocardial infarction
	● Acute dysrhythmias
Haematological system	Chronic conditions
	● Anaemias
	Acute conditions
	● Haemorrhage
	● Disseminated intravascular coagulation

Many factors alter the transport of oxygen to tissues during the perioperative period. Some cannot be anticipated, but factors such as chronic cardiovascular and respiratory disease or severe anaemia increase the likelihood of reduced oxygen delivery, particularly if these diseases are not optimally managed prior to surgery. Anaesthetic agents and techniques can alter cardiovascular function and gas exchange, and so preoperative assessment enables the anaesthetist to choose the technique best suited to the patient.

The following section describes important factors in the initial assessment of patients.

Cardiovascular system

History and examination

Angina indicates significant coronary artery disease. Exertional dyspnoea, orthopnoea and paroxysmal nocturnal dyspnoea suggest left ventricular failure, particularly if associated with ankle oedema. A history of blackouts or faints may indicate dysrhythmias, valvular heart disease or postural hypotension. Recent myocardial infarction is very important (see later). Routine examination should detect undiagnosed dysrhythmia (for example atrial fibrillation), heart murmurs or hypertension.

Patients with valvular heart disease, septal defects (whether surgically repaired or not) or prosthetic valves are at added risk of developing bacterial endocarditis following any surgical or dental procedure, including endoscopy of the gastrointestinal, respiratory and genitourinary tracts. They should all receive prophylactic antibiotics preoperatively.

SUMMARY BOX

*Recommended antibiotic prophylaxis
for patients with valvular heart
disease*

Amoxycillin (1 g intravenously/intramuscularly prior to induction, with 500 mg orally 6 hours later)

Prosthetic heart valve or previous endocarditis
Amoxycillin plus gentamicin (120 mg intramuscularly/intravenously prior to induction).

Penicillin-allergic patients
Vancomycin (1 g intravenously over 60 min) substituted for amoxycillin

---

Investigations

Patients with known cardiovascular disease should have a preoperative ECG. ECG is worthwhile in patients at risk from cardiac disease, for example the elderly, diabetics, or patients with renal failure. The chance of detecting an important abnormality is low, but the preoperative ECG provides a baseline against which to compare any subsequent tracings. There is little value in performing routine ECG examinations in other groups of patients.

In patients with symptoms of left ventricular or congestive cardiac failure an erect posteroanterior chest X-ray (CXR) will detect cardiomegaly and left ventricular failure. Occasionally a transthoracic echocardiogram may be indicated to assess valve function and myocardial contractility. Cardiac dysrhythmias which are identified on the systemic enquiry, clinical examination or by ECG should be fully investigated prior to surgery, and may require a cardiologist's opinion. The significance of some common dysrhythmias is listed in Table 10.1. The perioperative management of the patient with a pacemaker is discussed later.

Table 10.1 Significance of common arrhythmias in the perioperative period

Arrhythmia	Significance
Uncontrolled atrial fibrillation	Exclude metabolic causes, e.g. electrolyte abnormality, thyrotoxicosis May compromise cardiovascular function Ventricular rate should be controlled prior to surgery
Controlled atrial fibrillation	Rarely causes severe perioperative problems unless associated with other significant heart disease Patient may be on anticoagulants; if not, consider thromboprophylaxis.
Ventricular extrasystoles	Usually of little significance. May indicate ischaemia in patients with IHD
First-degree heart block	Little significance
Asymptomatic bi- or trifascicular block or asymptomatic second-degree heart block	Previously considered an indication for temporary pacemaker insertion. Now usually managed by careful monitoring in the perioperative period
Third-degree heart block	Requires pacemaker insertion prior to anaesthesia

Respiratory system

History and examination

The recent onset or a change in severity of cough, sputum, wheeze or breathlessness suggest acute respiratory disease or a change in the severity of a chronic condition. In patients with known COPD (chronic obstructive pulmonary disease), asthma or fibrotic lung disease a productive cough, increased and/or purulent sputum or fever suggests chest infection. Asthmatic patients can usually compare their current to their optimum status in terms of wheeze, dyspnoea and limitations in daily activity. It is useful to document whether patients have ever required oral steroid therapy, admission to hospital or mechanical ventilation, as these indicate more severe disease.

The severity of dyspnoea is one of the best indicators of the functional reserve of the patient's lungs. The simplest way of assessing dyspnoea is to relate it to everyday activities. It is useful to document how far patients can walk on the flat, up hills or up stairs. In patients who report significant exercise limitation it should be confirmed that this is due to dyspnoea rather than other disease, such as angina or peripheral vascular disease. Where the history suggests significant exercise limitation due to dyspnoea, investigations of respiratory function are indicated.

Patients in the acute phase of a viral infection should have their surgical procedure delayed if possible, particularly if pyrexia, chest signs or an elevated white cell count are present. Acute viral illness is associated with an increased risk of bronchospasm in the perioperative period, and of postoperative chest infection. Chest infection is more likely because pulmonary epithelium already affected by viral infection is more susceptible to secondary bacterial infection. The majority of general anaesthetic drugs inhibit the ciliary action of the airways, predisposing the patient to postoperative pulmonary complications.

Investigations

Clear or white sputum suggests the absence of pus cells or infection, but yellow or green sputum is suspicious and should be sent for bacteriological examination. Patients are often aware themselves if sputum production is increased or more purulent. Acute exacerbations merit appropriate antibiotic therapy, chest physiotherapy and rescheduling of surgery.

In patients with known pulmonary disease a chest X-ray will exclude potentially serious complications such as consolidation, collapse or pleural effusion. In this situation the preoperative CXR also provides a useful baseline against which to compare postoperative changes. In patients without pre-existing pulmonary disease the routine preoperative chest X-ray is of no value for assessing pulmonary function and rarely gives additional information. Its sensitivity for detecting undiagnosed lung conditions is also very low.

Pulmonary function tests give information about the severity of lung disease and the reversibility of any obstructive component. There is no indication for pulmonary function tests in patients without lung disease or significant pulmonary symptoms, except in some specific situations, such as before thoracic surgery. The commonly performed respiratory function tests and their meaning are listed in Table 10.2. Although frequently used, the predictive value of respiratory function tests for postoperative complications is low.

A simple non-invasive method of assessing hypoxaemia is to measure the oxygen saturation by pulse oximetry. Because of the shape of the haemoglobin oxygen dissociation curve, the Pao_2 is unlikely to be less than 8 kPa if the haemoglobin oxygen saturation is >92%. Arterial blood gases are useful for assessing some patients. Modern blood gas analysers measure the partial pressure of oxygen and carbon dioxide, and the hydrogen ion concentration. Other variables are calculated or derived (Table 10.3). Some indications for blood gas analysis in the preoperative period are shown in Table 10.4. Perioperative risk increases with the severity of hypoxaemia. Following major surgery to the abdomen or thorax, Pao_2 decreases even in normal individuals unless supplemental oxygen is administered. Hypoxaemia is also more severe when postoperative analgesia is inadequate. The importance of adequate postoperative analgesia is discussed later in the chapter.

Patients with respiratory failure are at particular risk from anaesthesia and surgery. A minority of these patients rely on hypoxic drive rather than $Paco_2$ for ventilation, and increased concentrations of inspired oxygen may result in hypoventilation and worsening respiratory failure. These patients have a very high risk of severe postoperative pulmonary complications such as pneumonia and respiratory

Table 10.2 Common respiratory function tests carried out prior to surgery

Test	Meaning
FEV_1 (forced expiratory volume in 1 s)	Integrated measure of airflow limitation and respiratory muscle strength If <50% predicted or FEV_1 <1 L, indicates severe pulmonary disease
FVC (forced vital capacity)	Integrated measure of lung volume and respiratory muscle strength <50% predicted values indicate severe pulmonary disease
FEV_1/FVC ratio	A measure of airway obstruction (normal value >75%) If less than 75%, reversibility to bronchodilator therapy should be tested
PEFR (peak expiratory flow rate)	Assesses airway obstruction If <70% predicted, suggests significant lung disease
Gas transfer factor (usually with carbon monoxide; Tco and Kco)	An estimate of the lungs' overall ability to exchange gases Any reduction over predicted values indicates reduced lung reserve

Table 10.3 Blood gas parameters

	Normal range	Meaning
Measured variables		
Pao_2	12–15 kPa	Partial pressure of oxygen in arterial blood
$Paco_2$	4.4–6.1 kPa	Partial pressure of carbon dioxide in arterial blood
H^+ concentration	36–44 nmol/L	Degree of acidaemia or alkalaemia
Derived variables		
Bicarbonate concentration (HCO_3)	21–28 mmol/L	Bicarbonate concentration in arterial plasma. Reflects respiratory *and* metabolic factors
Standard bicarbonate concentration (SBC) and	21–28 mmol/L	Bicarbonate concentration corrected to normal $Paco_2$.
base excess (BE)	–2 to +2 mmol/L	Only reflects *metabolic* factors

Table 10.4 Indications for blood gas analysis in the preoperative period	
	Useful features
Elective surgery Moderate–severe chronic obstructive pulmonary disease Fibrotic lung disease Severe chest wall deformities, e.g. ankylosing spondylitis, scoliosis Severe asthma Bronchiectasis/cystic fibrosis Lung tumour (prior to surgery)	Document the severity of hypoxaemia (Pao_2) Distinguish patients with type I failure (normal $Paco_2$) from patients with type II failure (elevated $Paco_2$) Distinguish patients with compensated hypercapnia (H^+ normal) from those with decompensated hypercapnia (H^+ elevated, respiratory acidosis)
Emergency surgery Known chronic lung disease Dyspnoea Shock (any form) Acute lung disease, e.g. pneumonia, pneumothorax, ARDS	Document the severity of underlying lung disease (above) Document the magnitude of acute hypoxia and acid–base disturbance

failure and frequently require ventilatory support and intensive care.

Smoking

All patients should be informed of the risks associated with smoking and advised to stop prior to surgery, preferably at the initial clinic visit. Many patients are unwilling or unable to stop simply because a decision to operate has been made. However, there are significant benefits for the patient from even short-term cessation in the preoperative period:

- The airway may become less hyperreactive, reducing the incidence of bronchospasm.
- Sputum production may decrease if the patient stops smoking several weeks before surgery, reducing the risk of postoperative pulmonary collapse and infection.
- The ciliary function of pulmonary epithelium improves within 1–2 days, increasing sputum clearance.
- The carboxyhaemoglobin concentration of blood falls within several hours, increasing the oxygen-carrying and -unloading capacity of blood.
- The circulating concentration of nicotine, which can cause systemic and coronary vasoconstriction, decreases within hours of stopping smoking.

Alcohol

An assessment of alcohol intake is important in all patients presenting for surgery. The relevance of chronic high alcohol intake is as follows:

- Chronic alcohol excess results in the induction of liver enzymes. These enzymes are involved in the metabolism of many anaesthetic drugs. As a result, patients may have

an apparent resistance to general anaesthetic agents and require larger than expected doses for the induction and maintenance of anaesthesia.
- Patients may develop an acute alcohol withdrawal syndrome in the early postoperative period (see Chapter 13).
- Patients may have alcohol-related chronic liver disease or cardiac disease.

Patients requiring emergency surgery who are intoxicated generally require reduced doses of anaesthetic. They are at increased risk of perioperative aspiration and may require close monitoring in the postoperative period.

Obesity

Obese patients are at increased risk from anaesthesia and surgery. This results from the technical problems caused by obesity itself, and from the increased incidence of chronic diseases and perioperative complications (Table 10.5). Obese patients require careful assessment. If the perioperative risk is considered too great, the patient should be advised to lose weight before surgery can be considered. In these cases referral to a dietitian is helpful.

Drug therapy

All prescribed drugs being taken by the patient on admission should be recorded. In general, preadmission drug therapy should not be stopped prior to surgery. This is particularly important for cardiovascular and respiratory medications (see later sections). The perioperative management of diabetic patients is described later. Some drug therapies which have specific relevance to the perioperative period are as follows:

Table 10.5   Significance of obesity in the perioperative period

Cardiovascular system
  Increased cardiac work
  Hypertension and ischaemic heart disease more common
  Accurate measurement of blood pressure difficult

Respiratory system
  Airway management often difficult
  Lung volumes reduced
  Postoperative pulmonary collapse, pneumonia and pulmonary embolism more likely
  Increased risk of perioperative hypoxia

Surgical
  Access for surgery difficult
  Increased wound infection and dehiscence

Miscellaneous
  Venous access difficult
  Increased incidence of diabetes and cardiovascular disease
  Increased incidence of hiatus hernia and aspiration

- Long-term steroid therapy may have resulted in adrenocortical suppression. For most surgery, continuation of the patient's normal dose, or an equipotent dose of hydrocortisone intravenously (5 mg prednisolone = 20 mg hydrocortisone), is adequate. For major surgery a moderate increase in the normal dose may be given, although many anaesthetists continue the patient's normal dose, or equivalent, even for major surgery. In all patients on long-term steroids it is important to monitor for signs of postoperative hypoadrenalism, such as hypotension/shock, hyperkalaemia and hyponatraemia. This is more likely if the patient develops other complications, notably infection.
- Anticoagulants. These are considered later in the chapter.
- The oral contraceptive pill. Oestrogen-containing medication increases the risk of venous thrombosis and should be stopped about 6 weeks prior to surgery. Progesterone-only pills do not significantly increase risk.
- Antidepressant drugs of the monoamine oxidase inhibitor class (MAOI) can interact with opioids or pressor agents, resulting in neurological and cardiovascular complications. These reactions are not universal, but ideally the drugs should be stopped 2–3 weeks prior to surgery and another agent substituted. The use of MAOIs is decreasing with the advent of newer classes of antidepressants. In an emergency surgery can proceed, but opioids and pressor agents should be avoided.

Allergies

Adverse or idiosyncratic responses to drugs or other agents (eg. iodine, elastoplast) must be recorded, as failure to avoid a second exposure may result in a life-threatening hypersensitivity reaction. Latex allergy is increasingly recognized and is important because exposure is extremely common in the perioperative period unless special precautions are taken.

Previous operations and anaesthetics

It is important to enquire into previous anaesthetics and document unexpected complications or distressing side-effects. If possible the anaesthetic charts from previous admissions should be available for review. These will document problems such as difficult intubation and reactions to anaesthetic drugs. Major complications from previous anaesthetics or a family history of anaesthetic reactions raise the possibility of rare genetically inherited abnormalities. These are usually one of two types:

- **Pseudocholinesterase deficiency ('scoline apnoea')** Prolonged apnoea following the administration of the short-acting depolarizing muscle relaxant suxamethonium chloride suggests a deficiency in the circulating enzyme pseudocholinesterase. The patient may have required mechanical ventilation for several hours after previous surgery. Usually patients should have been investigated to confirm the diagnosis. In these cases the use of suxamethonium should be avoided.
- **Malignant hyperpyrexia** An abnormality in muscle metabolism predisposes patients to the life-threatening condition malignant hyperpyrexia when they are exposed to powerful triggers such as volatile anaesthetics and suxamethonium. Patients with the condition or a family history should have been investigated in a specialist centre.

Postoperative nausea and vomiting following anaesthesia can be particularly distressing for some patients. By using short-acting agents, avoiding parenteral opiates and prescribing an antiemetic the anaesthetist can reduce the incidence and/or severity of this side-effect. Minor complications of anaesthesia are common, but may cause significant distress to patients. The risk of many of these occurring again can often be reduced by modifying the anaesthetic technique.

Preoperative investigations

The aim of preoperative investigations is to provide the surgeon and anaesthetist with the information necessary to assess fitness for operation, and to decide whether further improvement can be made prior to surgery. Special investigations relevant to specific chronic diseases have already been considered, and some are discussed in more detail later. Laboratory blood testing is the other type of preoperative investigation frequently undertaken.

Blood biochemistry

In patients with renal dysfunction, fluid balance problems, cardiovascular disease, or those who are receiving diuretic therapy, analysis of plasma urea and electrolytes is indicated. There is little value in checking these indices in fit patients presenting for minor elective surgery, although it is useful in the elderly or in patients undergoing major procedures. Disorders of potassium balance are the most relevant finding because both hypo- and hyperkalaemia can be associated with intraoperative dysrhythmias. Major abnormalities in electrolyte concentrations should be corrected preoperatively. For a full description of the causes and management of water and electrolyte disorders see Chapter 5 of *Davidson's Principles and Practice of Medicine* (Haslett et al 1999 Davidson's Principles and Practice of Medicine 18 edn. Churchill Livingstone, Edinburgh).

Liver function tests

Any patient with a history of liver disease, high alcohol intake or who on clinical examination is found to have signs of liver disease, such as jaundice, hepatomegaly or splenomegaly, should have liver function tests and a coagulation screen performed.

Full blood count

Patients with a history of chronic ingestion of non-steroidal anti-inflammatory agents, upper or lower gastrointestinal tract symptoms, menorrhagia or clinical signs of anaemia should have a full blood count. The importance of functioning haemoglobin in the carriage of oxygen to tissues has

already been stressed. In patients with coexisting diseases that might compromise oxygen supply to tissues it is important to check and if necessary, increase the haemoglobin concentration prior to surgery. In addition, patients undergoing surgery with the potential for significant blood loss should be tested.

The lowest acceptable level of haemoglobin for elective surgery is a subject of debate. Most surgeons and anaesthetists accept stable haemoglobin concentrations as low as 8 g/dL unless the patient has significant cardiorespiratory comorbidity, or is undergoing surgery for which significant blood loss is anticipated. The most important factor suggesting a higher haemoglobin concentration should be present (>10 g/dL) is the presence of ischaemic heart disease. In the case of the anaemia of chronic disease, e.g. patients with chronic renal failure, compensatory mechanisms increase tissue oxygen delivery at reduced haemoglobin concentrations. For example, the viscosity of blood is reduced and the efficiency of oxygen unloading to tissues is increased because 2,3 diphosphoglycerate (DPG) concentrations increase in red cells. There is no proven value in transfusing these patients preoperatively.

An increased white cell count is suggestive of infection, which requires further investigation. The platelet count may be elevated in patients with chronic inflammatory or some haematological conditions. These patients are at increased risk of thromboembolic complications and thromboprophylaxis should be administered perioperatively. Platelet counts below 100×10^9/L may increase the risk of perioperative bleeding and are a relative contraindication to some regional anaesthetic techniques such as epidural anaesthesia. In addition to informing the anaesthetist, advice from a haematologist may be necessary.

Coagulation screen

The patient's coagulation function is usually tested by measuring the prothrombin time (PTT) and 'activated partial thromboplastin time (APTT)'. If disseminated intravascular coagulation (DIC) is suspected fibrinogen concentration, fibrin degradation products or D-dimers can be measured. Coagulation should only be measured when there is a clinical suspicion of an abnormality, or when the proposed surgery may alter coagulation. Some specific disorders of coagulation are considered later.

Blood cross-matching

The need to group and screen a patient's blood or cross-match blood is dependent on the nature of the surgery. Most hospitals will have policies regarding the number of red cell units that should be available prior to particular types of surgery. For more information regarding blood and blood products see Chapter 4.

> **SUMMARY BOX**
>
> *Indications for measuring coagulation in the preoperative patient*
>
> *Patient factors*
> - Liver disease
> - Haematological disease affecting coagulation
> - Patient on heparin or warfarin
> - Patient shocked or has other risk factors for DIC, e.g. severe infection
> - Patient gives a history of excessive bleeding after minor trauma (may have undiagnosed disorder)
> - Patient has a history of thrombotic events, e.g. multiple deep vein thromboses (may have prothrombotic disorder)
> - Hypersplenism (causes thrombocytopenia)
>
> *Surgical factors*
> - Major hepatobiliary surgery
> - Surgery involving anticoagulation, e.g. cardiopulmonary bypass
> - Surgery in which major blood loss is anticipated

The high-risk patient

Patients with hepatitis B or C infection and those with HIV infection represent an additional risk to medical and nursing staff. In these cases it is essential to alert theatre staff in advance of surgery to enable appropriate precautions to be taken. In addition, laboratory staff who may receive samples taken from the patient should also be informed, and samples clearly labelled as high risk.

Some patients may be at increased risk of infection but may not have been tested, for example patients known to abuse intravenous drugs or who have partners known to be infected. In these cases preoperative testing should be considered after discussion with and consent from the patient. When hepatitis virus or HIV status is unknown, patients should be treated as high risk. Precautionary measures include the use of goggles to protect eyes, covering areas of broken skin, using disposable anaesthetic circuits and filters, and double-layering gloves and gowns.

Assessment of the patient for emergency surgery

The principles of assessment already discussed apply equally to the patient presenting for emergency surgery. The main difference from an elective procedure is that there is little time for investigations and less information may be available. Patients requiring emergency surgery may be very sick and may require basic resuscitation prior to anaesthesia and surgery. The principles of resuscitation – airway, breathing and circulation – should be followed (see Chapters 3 and 9). The correction of hypovolaemia is particularly important prior to anaesthesia because the induction of anaesthesia is associated with a significant attenuation of the normal cardiovascular compensatory mechanisms. In the hypovolaemic or inadequately resuscitated patient, in whom subclinical hypovolaemia has not been appreciated, induction may be followed by severe hypotension. Unless there is life-threatening uncontrollable haemorrhage an adequate blood volume must be restored before anaesthesia commences.

THE PREOPERATIVE WARD ROUND

The purpose of the preoperative ward round is to check that the patient has been adequately assessed and prepared. Both surgeon and anaesthetist should ensure that the patient has had a full explanation of the procedures and techniques that are planned, and has no further questions or concerns. It is important that the patient knows what to expect postoperatively, for example which ward they will be in and what surgical drains or intravascular catheters will be present. They should also be clear how analgesia will be maintained, and if necessary have had instruction in the use of patient-controlled analgesia devices.

Premedication

The requirement for premedication will be decided by the anaesthetist during the preoperative visit. The aim is for the patient to arrive in the anaesthetic room in a relaxed and pain-free state. This can often be achieved non-pharmacologically by explanation and reassurance. Where premedication is considered appropriate a benzodiazepine has the advantages of oral administration and does not require accurate timing in relation to anaesthetic induction. Where parenteral administration is the only option, and/or the patient requires a drug with analgesic properties, an opiate such as intramuscular morphine is commonly prescribed.

Fasting

To minimize the risk of regurgitation and aspiration at induction of anaesthesia the patient presenting for an elective procedure should have no food for 4 hours or fluids for 2 hours before the procedure. These recommendations will result in the majority of patients arriving in the anaesthetic room with an empty stomach. However, in patients with upper gastrointestinal pathology, such as hiatus hernia, gastric outlet obstruction, delayed gastric emptying, autonomic neuropathy (e.g. long-standing diabetes mellitus), and in the emergency situation, an empty stomach cannot be guaranteed irrespective of the duration of fasting. This is also true of patients in acute pain and who have received opiates, both of which reduce gastric emptying. In these situations the anaesthetist should assume the patient has a full stomach and modify the anaesthetic induction technique in order to reduce the risk of regurgitation, and quickly secure the airway to avoid aspiration.

IMPLICATIONS OF CHRONIC DISEASE IN THE PERIOPERATIVE PERIOD

Cardiovascular disease

Ischaemic heart disease

The incidence of ischaemic heart disease is high in western cultures, increases with age, and is more prevalent in some geographic areas than others. It is increased in patients with risk factors (Table 10.6) and may be asymptomatic. Patient assessment should therefore include not only documentation of known disease, but consideration of the likelihood of undiagnosed disease.

Myocardial infarction The incidence of perioperative myocardial infarction in previously healthy patients is approximately 0.2%. This contrasts with an incidence of about 5% (25 times higher) in patients with previous

Table 10.6   Risk factors for ischaemic heart disease
Family history
Smoking
Hypertension
Diabetes mellitus
Obesity
Hypercholesterolaemia

Table 10.7 Risk of postoperative myocardial infarction in patients with a previous history of myocardial infarction	
Time from myocardial infarction	Incidence of postoperative myocardial
	infarction (%)
< 6 months	50
6–12 months	25
1–2 years	20
2–3 years	8
>3 years	2
No previous history	0.2

myocardial infarction. The time from the last myocardial infarction has a major influence on the risk of reinfarction and should be clearly documented (Table 10.7). The mortality from postoperative myocardial infarction is higher (up to 50%) than myocardial infarction occurring outside the perioperative period. Postoperative myocardial infarction is more difficult to diagnose because the symptoms are often not typical (for example, there may be no chest pain). In addition, thrombolytic treatment is frequently contraindicated. If possible, elective surgery should be delayed for at least 6 months following myocardial infarction unless the risk of delay (for example cancer surgery) is greater than that of another cardiac event. If surgery is carried out invasive cardiovascular monitoring can reduce the risk of cardiac events (see later).

Angina The risk of perioperative myocardial infarction in patients with angina is related to the severity of symptoms. It is important to establish and document the frequency and severity of pain, precipitating factors, and the response to antianginal treatment. A change in symptoms over recent months is also significant. The extent to which a patient's everyday activities are limited (for example shopping or leisure activities) is a good indication to the overall severity of disease. Many patients may have been investigated by a cardiologist and had coronary angiography. In these cases it is important to document the time from when these investigations were performed and the results.

A patient with stable angina occurring once or twice weekly when climbing steep hills, whose pain resolves within minutes of resting, and who requires a single antianginal drug for symptom control is at low risk. However, a patient on maximum antianginal therapy, with nitrate-resistant pain occurring at rest or on minimal exertion, is at high risk of perioperative cardiovascular complications. In these cases investigation by a cardiologist should be performed prior to surgery, as symptoms may be improved by angioplasty or even coronary artery bypass surgery prior to elective surgery. In cases such as these the surgeon and anaesthetist must balance the risk of anaesthesia and surgery against the benefits.

Coronary artery bypass graft (CABG) Patients may present for surgery with a history of ischaemic heart disease treated by CABG surgery. The cardiovascular risk in these patients relates to the success of their surgery and whether they have developed recurrent disease. These patients should be assessed in a similar manner to those with angina.

Congestive cardiac failure

The commonest cause of cardiac failure is ischaemic heart disease, but the exact cause should be identified prior to surgery. Cardiac failure is associated with increased perioperative risk via several mechanisms (Table 10.8). The

Table 10.8 Increased perioperative risk in patients with cardiac failure

Mechanism	Complication
Poor 'pump function'	Pulmonary oedema Cardiogenic shock Renal failure Organ ischaemia, e.g. bowel ischaemia Venous thrombosis
Cardiac disease	Arrythmias Myocardial infarction Thromboembolism

risk associated with cardiac failure is linked closely to how well it is controlled prior to surgery. The presence of a third heart sound indicates poorly compensated left ventricular failure and is associated with a very high perioperative risk. The presence of peripheral oedema, dyspnoea or orthopnoea also suggest inadequately treated cardiac failure. The investigation, aetiology and medical management of cardiac failure are described in Chapter 3 of Davidson's *Principles and Practice of Medicine*.

Valvular heart disease

For a detailed description of the aetiology and management of valvular heart disease see Chapter 3 of Davidson's *Principles and Practice of Medicine*. In the perioperative patient it is important to know the severity of valvular lesions and whether the patient suffers from associated arrythmias or ventricular dysfunction. This information is

Table 10.9 Perioperative considerations in patients with valvular heart disease

Arrhythmia	Optimize antiarrhythmic therapy prior to surgery Avoid precipitating factors, e.g. electrolyte abnormalities
Endocarditis	Prophylactic antibiotics for all invasive procedures
Anticoagulation	Stop warfarin prior to surgery Substitute heparin if necessary
Valve dysfunction	
Native valves	Document pattern and severity to enable optimum haemodynamic management
Artificial valves	Investigate change in patient symptoms, new murmurs or new arrhythmias

usually available from recent echocardiography or cardiac catheterization. The risks specifically associated with valvular heart disease, and factors specifically to be considered in these patients, are listed in Table 10.9.

Pacemakers

In the past the function of some pacemakers was affected by intraoperative monitoring devices and diathermy, but this is now rarely a problem. It is important to document the reason for pacemaker insertion, when it was inserted, what type of device is in place, and when it was last checked by a cardiologist. Cardiological review prior to surgery may be indicated, particularly if the device has not been checked in the recent past.

Hypertension

Untreated hypertension increases perioperative risk, particularly for cerebrovascular accident and myocardial infarction. The risk relates mostly to the degree of elevation of the diastolic rather than the systolic blood pressure. The normal range for blood pressure increases with age. In a patient not known to be hypertensive it is first important to establish the resting blood pressure unaffected by anxiety and stress. Repeated measurements over time, reference to recent medical notes, contacting the GP, or examination for the complications of hypertensive disease (such as retinopathy) are useful. Once an accurate resting blood pressure has been established it must be interpreted with reference to the patient's age. A detailed description of the investigation and management of hypertension is given in Davidson's *Principles and Practice of Medicine*, Chapter 3.

The blood flow to organs is normally tightly regulated over a range of arterial blood pressures, in order to maintain adequate oxygen supply to cells (see later). In untreated hypertensive patients these autoregulatory mechanisms become 'reset' to higher levels. This means that organ perfusion may be compromised during periods of modest hypotension. Perioperative risk can be reduced by ensuring that blood pressure has been adequately controlled for several weeks prior to surgery, because with time autoregulatory mechanisms return towards normal limits. As a general rule, if the resting diastolic pressure is ≥110 mmHg elective surgery should be delayed.

When surgery is urgent, blood pressure should be controlled acutely using drugs that can be titrated until an appropriate diastolic pressure is achieved. As the autoregulatory mechanisms that control organ blood flow take several days to normalize, the anaesthetist will administer sufficient drugs to achieve a moderate reduction in blood pressure, rather than completely normal values.

<table>
<tr><td colspan="2">SUMMARY BOX</td></tr>
</table>

SUMMARY BOX

History, symptoms and signs associated with high cardiovascular risk

High risk	Myocardial infarction in the past 6 months
	Poor left ventricular function
	Presence of third heart sound (poorly controlled cardiac failure)
	Resting diastolic blood pressure >110 mmHg
Moderate risk	Poorly controlled/untreated arrhythmia
	Age >70
	Significant aortic stenosis

Table 10.10   Monitors of cardiovascular status during the perioperative period

Monitor	Information given
Arterial catheter	Continuous measurement of blood pressure
Central venous catheter	Central venous pressure (a measure of cardiac preload)
Pulmonary artery catheter	Pulmonary artery pressure
	Pulmonary capillary wedge pressure (a measure of left atrial pressure)
	Cardiac output (by thermodilution)
Oesophageal doppler	Cardiac output

Perioperative management of patients with cardiovascular disease

Drug therapy In most patients normal cardiac drug therapy should be continued until the morning of surgery. When possible, patients should continue oral medication postoperatively. If oral intake is not possible, cardiac or antihypertensive medication can be administered intravenously if necessary. As hypotension occurs relatively frequently following major surgery, the need for intravenous therapy and the timing of reintroduction of oral medication is decided on an individual basis. The following two classes of cardiac drugs merit special consideration:

β-Blockers The perioperative use of β-blockers in patients with ischaemic heart disease has been associated with a significant reduction in cardiovascular morbidity, even if the patients were not taking these drugs prior to surgery. This probably occurs by maintaining a slow heart rate, thereby maximizing myocardial oxygen supply during diastole (see below).

Angiotensin-converting enzyme (ACE) inhibitors These agents are widely used to treat cardiac failure and hypertension. However, in patients taking these drugs up to the time of surgery intra- and postoperative hypotension is common. The decision to continue or omit an ACE inhibitor in the perioperative period is usually made by the anaesthetist at the time of the preoperative visit.

Cardiovascular status In patients at risk from myocardial ischaemia and/or with poor cardiac function, there are two principles of management for the intra- and postoperative periods:

1. *Minimize myocardial oxygen demand* Cardiac output can be increased via four mechanisms: increased preload, heart rate, contractility or decreased afterload. The oxygen 'cost' for each of these mechanisms differs considerably. The most efficient method of generating

adequate cardiac output is to optimize preload with fluids. Tachycardia, sympathetic activation or excessive peripheral vasoconstriction all have a high oxygen 'cost' and should be avoided.

2. *Maximize myocardial oxygen supply* Blood flow to the myocardium of the left ventricle, which has the highest myocardial oxygen demand, occurs only during diastole. It depends on the coronary perfusion pressure, which is the difference between the diastolic and the left ventricular end-diastolic pressures. Myocardial oxygen supply is therefore optimal when the heart rate is slow (when diastole is long relative to systole) and the diastolic blood pressure is high.

In order to optimize and closely monitor myocardial oxygen supply and demand patients with severe cardiovascular disease benefit from invasive haemodynamic monitoring during the perioperative period, particularly for major surgery. The various possible monitors, and the information they give, are listed in Table 10.10. For a fuller description of haemodynamic monitoring see Chapter 15 of Davidson's *Principles and Practice of Medicine*.

Respiratory disease

The assessment of respiratory disease has already been considered. The aim is to ensure that lung function is optimal prior to surgery. Patients with poor respiratory function require close monitoring, particularly after abdominal or thoracic surgery. They are ideally managed in a high-dependency or intensive care unit. Principles of perioperative management for the patient with chronic respiratory disease are as follows:

Anaesthetic technique

General anaesthesia causes significant alterations in pulmonary function that place patients with respiratory disease at increased risk of postoperative pulmonary complications. Regional anaesthetic techniques should therefore be used whenever possible. This usually involves spinal or epidural anaesthesia or the use of nerve blocks (for example ilio-inguinal block for hernia repair). Regional anaesthesia is discussed in Chapter 11.

Postoperative analgesia

Wound pain impairs ventilation and coughing, and may result in pulmonary collapse/atelectasis, hypoxia and sputum retention. This increases the risk of postoperative infection. Effective analgesia is particularly important in the patient with respiratory disease. Systemic opiates can be used, but result in sedation and impaired coughing. Regional techniques have minimal central effects and should be considered whenever possible.

Physiotherapy

Pre- and postoperative physiotherapy is extremely important for patients with chest disease. A physiotherapist should see the patient regularly throughout the perioperative period.

Postoperative ventilation

Some patients will have insufficient reserves following surgery, or require ventilation because of complications such as pneumonia. Postoperative ventilation of patients with respiratory disease can often be avoided by close attention to the factors described above. It is better to avoid ventilation if possible, because prolonged tracheal intubation results in an increased risk of respiratory infection. The principles of ventilation and intensive care are described in Davidson's *Principles and Practice of Medicine*, Chapter 15.

Jaundice

Patients with jaundice preoperatively most commonly present for biliary or hepatic surgery. However, it is important to clearly define the aetiology of jaundice prior to surgery. Perioperative risk related to jaundice is attributable to the following:

- *Hepatitis* Patients with clinical jaundice or biochemical evidence of liver inflammation (elevated aminotransferases) should be screened preoperatively for hepatitis A, B and C viruses. The presence of hepatitis B or C carries the risk of transmission to medical and nursing staff. The incidence of asymptomatic hepatitis C infection is increasing in western cultures.
- *Coagulation* Intestinal bile salts are necessary for the absorption of fat-soluble vitamins (A, D, E and K). Patients with obstructive jaundice therefore have reduced absorption of vitamin K, which is an essential cofactor for the synthesis of coagulation factors II, VII, IX and X. Vitamin K-related coagulopathy is associated with prolongation of the prothrombin time. In jaundiced patients with abnormal coagulation surgery is best deferred until the jaundice has resolved and coagulopathy corrected. This is aided by relief of biliary obstruction by stenting or drainage (see Chapter 9) and the administration of synthetic vitamin K for several days prior to surgery.
- *Acute renal failure* Jaundice is associated with an increased risk of perioperative renal failure for several reasons:
  1. Dehydration commonly accompanies jaundice.
  2. Sepsis, particularly biliary sepsis, is common.
  3. A high concentration of conjugated bilirubin is toxic to renal tubular cells.

  The single most important intervention to prevent renal failure in jaundiced patients is adequate hydration. Diuretic agents such as mannitol, frusemide and dopamine have been used, but there is little evidence that any agent is more effective than a volume load of 0.9% NaCl solution adequate to maintain a urine output of at least 0.5–1 mL/kg/h. Central venous pressure monitoring can assist fluid management.

Table 10.11 Common indications for surgery in the diabetic patient	
Ophthalmic disease	Proliferative retinopathy Cataract
Cardiovascular Disease	Peripheral vascular surgery Diabetic feet Coronary artery bypass surgery
Renal Disease	Vascular access for haemodialysis Renal transplantation
Infection	Abscess drainage

Diabetes mellitus

About 50% of diabetic patients will require surgery at some time during their life, often for complications of their disease (Table 10.11). Perioperative risk associated with diabetes mellitus is attributable to the comorbidity associated with diabetes or to the effect of surgical stress on diabetic control.

Diabetic comorbidity

Vascular disease Diabetics have an increased incidence of microvascular and major vessel disease. The risk of myocardial infarction, hypertension, cerebrovascular accident and thromboembolic disease is increased. Vascular disease may significantly impair wound healing.

Renal disease Renal failure is common in diabetics and increases in frequency and severity with duration of disease, particularly if associated with hypertension. Reduced renal reserve increases the risk of perioperative acute renal failure. These patients are more likely to develop acute renal failure in response to hypotension, sepsis or nephrotoxic drugs.

Neuropathy Patients with peripheral neuropathy are at increased risk from trivial trauma, for example from positioning during surgery. Autonomic neuropathy may cause cardiovascular instability during and following surgery. Delayed gastric emptying increases the risk of regurgitation and aspiration during and after anaesthesia.

Infection Infective complications are increased in diabetic patients, particularly if diabetic control is poor.

Effect of surgical stress on diabetic control

The metabolic responses to surgery, trauma and infection are described in Chapter 1. Many of the neuroendocrine responses increase glucose mobilization and lipolysis, resulting in hyperglycaemia and increased circulating free fatty acids. In addition, increased insulin release is part of the normal response to stress. In diabetic patients with decreased endogenous insulin secretion, or reduced peripheral insulin sensitivity, surgery results in hyperglycaemia. Ketoacidosis may occur if insulin deficiency is severe and/or there is a major stress response. It is normal for diabetic patients to suffer increased hyperglycaemia following surgery and for insulin requirements to increase.

SUMMARY BOX

Perioperative risks in patients with diabetes mellitus

Risk	Possible complication
Hyperglycaemia	Infection
Hypoglycaemia	Reduced conscious level Brain injury
Ketosis	Diabetic ketoacidosis
Hypovolaemia	Shock Renal failure
Comorbidity	Myocardial infarction Thromboembolism Acute renal failure

Principles of managing the diabetic patient

Patients with diabetes mellitus require sufficient circulating insulin and glucose to ensure an adequate supply of glucose to cells. As insulin-mediated glucose transfer into cells is linked to potassium influx, an adequate potassium supply to prevent hypokalaemia is also necessary. In general the risk to the patient from hypoglcaemia is greater than that of mild hyperglycaemia. A blood glucose concentration of 6–10 mmol/L is the usual target during the perioperative period. The approach used to achieve this depends on:

- Whether the patient is normally managed by diet alone, oral hypoglycaemics or insulin
- The magnitude of the surgery (which relates to the anticipated stress response)
- The likely period during which the patient will be unable to take oral calories and drugs
- Whether surgery is elective or emergency, and particularly if infection is present.

Typical scenarios for patients presenting for surgery are presented in Table 10.12. In practice an appropriate regimen is best tailored to the individual patient. It is usual for diabetic patients to be placed first on an operating list, to minimize the duration of fasting.

Table 10.12   Some typical scenarios for diabetic patients presenting for surgery

Patient	Procedure	Management
Diet-controlled diabetic	Elective laparoscopic cholecystectomy (moderate stress response)	Monitor blood glucose until eating
Patient on oral hypoglycaemics	Hernia repair (minor stress response)	Omit oral hypoglycaemic on morning of surgery Monitor preoperatively for hypoglycaemia Monitor postoperatively until eating normally Restart oral hypoglycaemics when on normal diet
Patient on oral hypoglycaemics Normally well controlled	Elective aortofemoral bypass (major stress response)	Omit oral hypoglycaemic on morning of surgery Monitor peroperatively for hypo- or hyperglycaemia If blood glucose >10 mmol/L commence glucose/insulin/potassium infusion
Patient on oral hypoglycaemics Normally poorly controlled Blood sugar >10 mmol/L	Emergency aortofemoral bypass (major stress response)	Commence glucose/insulin/potassium infusion prior to surgery Stop oral hypoglycaemics peroperatively
Insulin-dependent diabetic Well controlled	Cataract surgery (minor stress response)	Omit morning insulin Monitor blood sugar for hypoglycaemia Restart regular insulin when eating
Insulin-dependent diabetic Normally well controlled	Elective CABG (major stress response)	Convert to glucose/insulin/dextrose prior to surgery Monitor blood sugar peroperatively Convert to subcutaneous short-acting insulin and then regular insulin as diet reintroduced
Insulin-dependent diabetic Blood sugar >20 mmol/L Ketones in urine	Emergency laparotomy for diverticular abscess (major stress response)	Treat as diabetic ketoacidosis and stabilize *prior* to surgery. Ensure adequate volume resuscitation Continue glucose/insulin/potassium infusion peroperatively Convert to intermittent short-acting and then normal insulin as diet reintroduced

Methods of administering insulin

Insulin, dextrose and potassium can be delivered either as a mixture or as separate infusions. Generally, in straightforward cases a mixture of dextrose, insulin and potassium (often termed the Alberti regimen) is simplest and safest (Table 10.13). For more complex and less well controlled patients, such as those with sepsis, separate infusions allow more flexibility but require more frequent monitoring of blood sugar and electrolytes.

Chronic renal failure

Patients with chronic renal failure frequently present for elective or emergency surgery, and are at increased risk of

Table 10.13   The Alberti regimen
500 mL 10% dextrose *plus* 10 iu short-acting soluble insulin *plus* 10 mmol KCl
Run 500 mL every 4–6 hours via a controlled infusion pump
Check blood glucose every 2–6 hours (depending on stability) and potassium 1–2 times daily
On average give 250 g glucose daily (1000 kcal) and 50 iu insulin
Adjust insulin and potassium according to results

Table 10.14   Risk factors in patients with renal failure undergoing surgery
Cardiovascular Frequently have ischaemic heart disease Hypertension Left ventricular dysfunction
Respiratory Pulmonary oedema and fluid overload (impaired water clearance)
Gastrointestinal Delayed gastric emptying
Biochemical Electrolyte disturbance (especially hyperkalaemia)
Haematological Anaemia Impaired coagulation (platelet dysfunction)
Miscellaneous Malnutrition Multiple drug therapies Abnormal drug metabolism Vascular access

perioperative complications for the reasons listed in Table 10.14.

Special consideration should be given to whether patients are established on dialysis or not.

Patients not requiring dialysis

In the perioperative period these patients are at risk of acute deterioration in renal function. This is relevant because they

may become permanently dialysis dependent. Factors that reduce the risk of deteriorating renal function are:

- Optimizing fluid balance. These patients are at risk from hyper- and hypovolaemia. Central venous pressure monitoring is useful, particularly for major surgery or trauma.
- Avoiding nephrotoxic drugs. These include NSAIDs for analgesia, and some antibiotics such as gentamicin.
- Avoiding hypotension. Hypotension may be related to fluid status, cardiovascular drug therapy, anaesthetic drugs or regional anaesthesia. Complications can be avoided by close monitoring and regular review.
- Caution with drugs that are renally excreted. Some drugs used in the perioperative period will accumulate in patients with renal dysfunction not receiving dialysis. For example, morphine metabolites can accumulate, causing excessive sedation and respiratory depression.

Patients on dialysis

Particular considerations in these patients are:

- Patients often pass very little urine and rely on dialysis for fluid removal. Fluids should be administered very cautiously, preferably guided by central venous monitoring in complex cases.
- Patients have access devices for dialysis, such as peritoneal dialysis catheters or fistulae. A limb with a fistula should be protected during surgery to prevent thrombosis, and should never be used for vascular access or blood sampling.

SUMMARY BOX

Advantages and disadvantages of different methods of administering insulin and dextrose

Combined dextrose/insulin/potassium infusions

Advantages	Disadvantages
Simple	Bags may require frequent changes
Cheap	Less flexibility in poorly controlled patients
Decreased risk of hypoglycaemia	
Single infusion	
Only requires single dedicated cannula	

Separate infusions of dextrose and insulin

Advantages	Disadvantages
Flexible	Multiple pumps and cannulae needed
	Frequent blood sugar measurement required
	Increased risk of hypoglycaemia
	Expensive

- Electrolyte abnormalities are common. In particular, hyperkalaemia may develop rapidly and should be checked in the immediate preoperative period.
- Patients often require dialysis prior to surgery. This requires close communication with the nephrologist and dialysis unit.

Haematological disease

The significance of anaemia has already been considered. Abnormal coagulation has major implications in the perioperative period. Haemostatic disorders fall broadly into three categories: patients on anticoagulant therapy, those with inherited disorders of coagulation, and patients with acute coagulopathy:

Anticoagulant therapy

Patients receiving warfarin anticoagulation should usually stop medication 2–4 days prior to surgery to allow some correction of the anticoagulant effect. The amount required depends on the nature of the surgery and the risk to the patient from reversal of the effect. Generally speaking, a prothrombin ratio of 1.5–2:1 is acceptable for major surgery. If the warfarin effect is more completely reversed, or a greater degree of anticoagulation is required (for example patients with an artificial heart valve), parenteral heparin anticoagulation is substituted for warfarin during the perioperative period. When warfarin effect requires rapid reversal, for example when emergency surgery is needed, several options are available. Intravenous vitamin K reverses warfarin effects in most patients in 24–48 hours. In more urgent cases fresh-frozen plasma can be administered, after discussion with a haematologist. Heparin has a relatively short half-life and coagulation returns to normal within 4–6 hours of discontinuation. In rare situations where rapid reversal is required the drug protamine can be used. This is usually only done in the setting of major vascular or cardiac surgery. Haemostasis is considered in more detail in Chapter 11 of Davidson's *Principles and Practice of Medicine*.

Inherited disorders of coagulation

The most important inherited disorder of coagulation is haemophilia, an inherited impairment of factor VIII production. For major surgery factor VIII levels should be maintained at 30–40% of normal levels by transfusion of factor concentrates. This is usually monitored by serial measurement of factor VIII concentrations in plasma. Haemophiliacs presenting for surgery must be managed in close collaboration with a haematologist. A significant number of haemophiliacs have been infected with hepatitis C and HIV (considered earlier).

Acute coagulopathy

Acute coagulopathy is most commonly thrombocytopenia and/or disseminated intravascular coagulation (DIC). These conditions are often associated with life-threatening illnesses such as shock, multiple trauma, transfusion reactions and sepsis. Microvascular coagulation and activated fibrinolysis result in tissue ischaemia and simultaneous depletion of coagulation factors and platelets. The coagulation screen typically shows prolonged prothrombin and activated partial thromboplastin times, thrombocytopenia, low fibrinogen concentration, and elevated D-dimers or fibrin degradation products. The management is complex and should involve a haematologist.

Pregnancy

Surgery should be avoided during pregnancy. The fetus is particularly sensitive to drugs, hypoxia, hypotension and infection during the first trimester. Surgery during pregnancy is usually an emergency or related to delivery itself. Many of the perioperative risks of pregnancy relate to anaesthesia, and early communication with an anaesthetist is essential when pregnant women require surgery.

SUMMARY BOX

Perioperative risks associated with surgery in pregnant patients

- Spontaneous abortion or premature labour
- Hypotension lying supine (inferior vena caval compression in second and third trimesters)
- Gastro-oesophageal reflux (increased risk of aspiration)
- Hypoxia (due to high metabolic rate, and reduced lung functional residual capacity)
- Teratogenic effects of drugs (particularly in first trimester)
- Peripartum:
  - massive blood loss
  - pre-eclampsia/eclampsia
  - amniotic fluid embolism

Miscellaneous conditions

There are many diseases that have particular relevance in the perioperative period. A detailed description is beyond the scope of this chapter, but some of those encountered most frequently are listed in Table 10.15. For a detailed description of the individual conditions the reader should refer to Davidson's *Principles and Practice of Medicine*.

Table 10.15   Relevance of some medical conditions in the perioperative period

Condition	Considerations
Rheumatoid arthritis	Neck may be 'unstable'; careful positioning necessary; complex drug therapy; associated chronic diseases, e.g. renal failure, lung disease
Multiple sclerosis	Reduced respiratory reserve; stress of surgery can cause relapse or worsening of disease
Epilepsy	Drugs may interact with anaesthetics; surgical stress and some drugs may precipitate seizures
Scoliosis or spondylitis	Can significantly reduce respiratory reserve; difficult endotracheal intubation
Myasthenia gravis	Risk of respiratory failure or aspiration; anaesthetic technique needs modifying
Sickle cell anaemia	Stress of surgery, hypoxia, hypothermia can all precipitate sickle cell crisis

11 Anaesthesia and the operation
A.J. Pollok, T. Walsh

A successful preoperative visit from the anaesthetist, supplemented with appropriate premedication, should result in a patient arriving in the anaesthetic room in a relaxed state. Theatre staff and the ward nurse will check that the patient's clinical notes, a completed operation consent form, drug chart and results from preoperative investigations are available. A preoperative checklist is followed that includes patient identification, the procedure to be undertaken, appropriate marking of the operation site, allergies, and the presence of pacemakers or other relevant unusual factors. Anaesthesia should only be started when the checklist has been satisfactorily completed.

GENERAL ANAESTHESIA

The overall aims of general anaesthesia are to produce a reversible and safe loss of consciousness, an attenuation of the major physiological responses to surgical stimulation (such as reflex skeletal muscle movement, tachycardia, hypertension and sweating), and optimal operating conditions. Anaesthesia is often considered to have three major components:

- *Hypnosis*: the loss of consciousness and awareness
- *Analgesia*: the provision of pain relief
- *Relaxation*: muscle relaxation to enable surgery to take place.

When anaesthesia was introduced in 1846–47 the limited drugs available dictated that the above conditions had to be achieved with a single volatile agent, either ether or chloroform, which was inhaled and absorbed via the lungs. All of the effects of these volatile agents were via direct action on the central nervous system. As a result, high concentrations were required that caused cardiorespiratory side-effects, significant morbidity and occasionally death.

There are now many different types of anaesthetic agent. The mechanisms by which drugs bring about analgesia and muscle relaxation are relatively well understood, but the way in which anaesthetics cause hypnosis and loss of consciousness are not known. It is therefore important to be able to describe the potency of an agent in order to judge how much to administer to individual patients. For volatile and gaseous anaesthetics this is done by calculating the 'minimum alveolar concentration' (MAC). This is the minimum alveolar concentration at atmospheric pressure that prevents 50% of the population from moving in response to a painful stimulus. The MAC of an individual agent is an indication of its potency. In general, if more than one agent is used their effects are additive. For example, 0.5 MAC of one agent and 0.5 MAC of another have the combined effect of 1 MAC.

In addition to their potency, clinically important properties of anaesthetics are the rate of onset and offset of their action. For gaseous agents this depends on factors such as the solubility of the agent in blood and adipose tissue. For intravenous agents, solubility in tissues and the rates of metabolism in the body are important.

Phases of anaesthesia

It is useful to consider the anaesthetic in several phases:

1. *Induction* The aim of induction is to achieve a rapid and smooth loss of consciousness. This is most commonly done using rapidly acting intravenous agents (e.g. propofol or thiopentone), but occasionally using a rapidly acting gaseous agent (e.g. sevoflurane). In addition, the anaesthetist will administer muscle relaxants and analgesics, depending on the requirements for the individual patient and the surgery planned. Some local anaesthetic techniques, such as epidural catheter placement, may be done prior to induction. Others, such as peripheral nerve block, may be done immediately afterwards before surgery commences.

2. *Maintenance* The aim of maintenance is to keep adequate hypnosis, analgesia and muscle relaxation during surgery. This is usually achieved by administering gaseous and volatile agents via an anaesthetic machine. Relaxation and analgesia can be achieved by administering supplemental doses of intravenous agents intravenously.

3. *Recovery* Recovery of consciousness is achieved by discontinuing hypnotic agents such as volatile anaesthetics. When the patient has been mechanically ventilated muscle relaxants are reversed to enable spontaneous breathing. The aim of recovery is a rapid smooth return to consciousness without pain or complications.

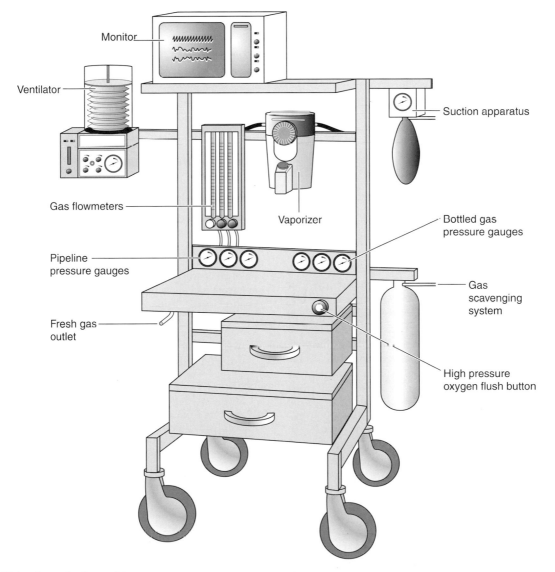

Fig. 11.1 Anaesthetic machine.

The anaesthetic machine

The anaesthetic machine is designed to deliver and accurately monitor gases (oxygen, nitrous oxide and medical air) from anaesthetic gas pipelines (Fig. 11.1). In addition, bottled reserves of oxygen and nitrous oxide attached to the machine are available in case of pipeline failure. One or more vaporizers mounted on the machine enable the accurate administration of volatile anaesthetics. A breathing system connects the gas outlet from the machine to the patient and carries the gas mixture set by the anaesthetist.

The features of the breathing circuit are:

1. A reservoir of gas (usually a 2 L bag) of sufficient size to contain the largest tidal volume that a patient might take during spontaneous breathing;
2. Tubing of sufficient diameter to cause minimal resistance to gas flows during normal breathing (maximum flows are approximately 25 L/min during quiet respiration);
3. Valves to direct gas flow and vent expired gases;
4. The ability to give intermittent positive-pressure ventilation. This is usually done by partially closing expiratory valves and squeezing the reservoir bag to force gas into the lungs.

There are different types of breathing system. The individual system used is dictated by the anaesthetist's preference and whether the patient is breathing spontaneously or being mechanically ventilated. Expired gas from the patient contains carbon dioxide that needs to be removed to avoid rebreathing. Carbon dioxide can either be flushed from the system between breaths by setting an appropriate gas flow, or removed by absorption. The necessary gas flow to flush out carbon dioxide between breaths can be predicted for each kind of breathing system from the estimated total minute volume of the patient. It will differ depending on whether the patient breathes spontaneously during the anaesthetic or is ventilated. Generally speaking, this is an inefficient way of administering anaesthetic because high gas flows are needed (6–12 L/min) and anaesthetic gas is wasted as it is vented from the system. If the carbon dioxide excreted by the patient is absorbed in the circuit (by an incorporated soda lime absorber) exhaled gas can be rebreathed. This is the principle behind *circle breathing systems*, which enable reduced fresh gas flows. These systems are extremely efficient and, when correctly used, allow gas flows from the machine of <1 L/min to be safely administered.

Irrespective of the breathing circuit used all expired gas and anaesthetic agent vented from the circuit has to be removed and discharged safely from the operating theatre to minimize the exposure of staff. This is done via *scavenging systems* which collect the gas leaving the breathing system.

The anaesthetic machine has a *ventilator* for automatic intermittent positive-pressure ventilation of the lung. The ventilator is either electrically operated or powered by the high pressure in the oxygen pipeline. The design and complexity of ventilators vary widely, but the basic features are the ability to set the number of breaths per minute and the volume of each breath (the tidal volume). High-pressure suction apparatus should always be available throughout an anaesthetic for clearing the patient's airway. This is commonly an integral part of the anaesthetic machine. There are also usually a number of drawers for additional equipment, and a work surface for chart recording and drug dispensing.

All anaesthetic machines have integrated alarm systems, although the complexity varies between individual models. Some alarms relate to measured physiological variables from the monitoring systems, such as oxygen saturation and blood pressure. Others relate directly to the function of the machine, such as oxygen delivery failure and ventilator disconnection. Before using an anaesthetic machine the anaesthetist will carry out a specified check to ensure satisfactory operation of all aspects of the machine's function.

Patient monitoring is an essential part of the anaesthetic, and is becoming increasingly complex (Table 11.1). In modern machines patient monitors are fully incorporated.

Induction of anaesthesia

After preoperative checks have been completed the patient is connected to ECG, blood pressure and pulse oximetry monitoring systems and baseline measurements are obtained. The anaesthetist obtains reliable venous access by placing an intravenous cannula, usually in the non-dominant arm. Anaesthesia is commonly induced by the injection of an appropriate dose of intravenous anaesthetic drug, but inhalational induction is occasionally used, for example in children or patients with needle phobia. As the administered dose of any anaesthetic agent increases, central

Table 11.1 Monitoring during anaesthesia
Essential monitors
Inspired oxygen fraction (FiO_2)
Electrocardiograph (ECG)
Non-invasive blood pressure (NIBP)
Oxygen saturation (pulse oximetry)
End-tidal carbon dioxide pressure (ET-CO_2)
Desirable monitors
Airway pressure (Paw)
Tidal volume (V_T)
Inspired/expired anaesthetic gas partial pressure
Body temperature
Invasive intravascular pressures (when clinically indicated)

Table 11.2   Guedel's stages of anaesthesia (originally described for ether administration)
Stage 1 'analgesia': spans full consciousness to loss of consciousness
Stage 2 'excitement': an unpleasant stage characterized by reflex hyperexcitability, breath-holding, large pupils, risk of regurgitation and bladder emptying
Stage 3 'surgical anaesthesia': characterized by a return of a regular breathing pattern. As anaesthesia continues to deepen the respiratory muscles increasingly fail, starting with the accessory muscles and finally the diaphragm. This stage can be divided into four planes
Stage 4 'overdose': is respiratory arrest, which will quickly lead to cardiac arrest unless oxygenation is maintained. The pupils become dilated and fixed

nervous system depression occurs in a predictable manner. These 'stages of anaesthesia' were originally described by Guedel during ether anaesthesia, which was slow in onset. They remain useful in judging the depth of anaesthesia of individual patients (Table 11.2). However, with modern rapidly acting intravenous agents it is unusual to distinguish the different stages during induction. The signs of ideal depth of anaesthesia for surgery (stage 3) are regular breathing, central midpoint pupils and loss of eyelash reflexes. This is usually achieved within 1–2 minutes of intravenous anaesthetic administration.

Anaesthetic induction agents

The anaesthetist has a choice of intravenous anaesthetic induction agents. The drug used depends on the procedure performed, patient characteristics, and the preference of the individual anaesthetist. Some features of the commonly used agents are shown in Table 11.3.

Muscle relaxants

It is possible to use a single volatile anaesthetic agent to produce the anaesthetic triad of loss of consciousness, analgesia and muscle relaxation, but this requires large doses that cause significant side-effects. Patients can be maintained at lighter and safer levels of anaesthesia by administering a separate drug to produce muscle paralysis. The first drug to produce reversible neuromuscular blockade was D-tubocurarine (introduced in the 1940s), although this has since been superseded by newer agents. The introduction of muscle relaxants, together with an understanding of artificial ventilation, heralded the arrival of safe, modern anaesthetic.

Muscle relaxants act by temporarily blocking transmission at the neuromuscular junction. They are usually classified as depolarizing or non depolarizing:

- *Depolarizing agents* Suxamethonium is the only muscle relaxant that stimulates the neuromuscular junction before blocking it, which is seen as muscle fasciculation immediately before the onset of block. It has very rapid onset (30–60 seconds) and a short duration of action

Table 11.3 Commonly used anaesthetic induction agents			
Agent	**Typical dose (mg/kg)**	**Advantages**	**Disadvantages**
Propofol	2–3	Smooth onset Short-acting (5–10 minutes) No 'hangover' Can be used by infusion	Hypotension Pain on injection Can cause excitory movements
Thiopentone	3–5	Smooth onset Inexpensive	Hangover effect Rarely allergic reactions or bronchospasm Hypotension Postoperative nausea/vomiting
Etomidate	0.3	Haemodynamic stability Rapid recovery	Pain on injection (common) Excitatory movements Postoperative nausea/vomiting
Ketamine	1–2 i.v. 5–10 i.m.	Haemodynamic stability Can be given i.m. Potent analgesic Useful in difficult situations (e.g. battlefields)	Slow onset and recovery 'Emergence' phenomena (nightmares, hallucinations) Increases airway secretions

Table 11.4   Commonly used non-depolarizing muscle relaxants

Drug	Initial dose (mg/kg)	Duration of action (min)	Advantages	Disadvantages
Pancuronium	0.1	20–40	Cardiovascular stability	Unpredictable duration of action Tachycardia
Atracurium	0.5	20	Predictable duration of action	Histamine release
Vecuronium	0.1	20	No histamine release	
Rocuronium	0.6	30	Rapid onset (60–90 seconds) No histamine release	Expensive

(5–10 minutes). Its short duration of action is due to hydrolysis by circulating plasma pseudocholinesterase. Deficient or abnormal cholinesterase is occasionally found and is most commonly an inherited abnormality. This results in a variable prolongation of action of up to 8 hours. Suxamethonium is most widely used when the anaesthetist needs to achieve rapid control and protection of the patient's airway (see rapid-sequence induction).

- *Non-depolarizing agents* The majority of muscle relaxants are non-depolarizing blockers. These act by competitive inhibition of the action of acetylcholine at the neuromuscular junction, and in general onset of action is slow (2–3 minutes). The main differences between the available agents are in rate of onset, duration of action, route of elimination and side-effect profile (Table 11.4).

Reversal of non-depolarizing neuromuscular blockade

Blockade can be reversed by the administration of the anticholinesterase neostigmine. The inhibition of cholinesterase at the neuromuscular junction results in a local increase in the concentration of acetylcholine. This competes with any residual muscle relaxant molecules present and restores normal transmission. Neostigmine is not specific for the neuromuscular acetylcholine receptor (nicotinic), and acts also at muscarinic receptors of the parasympathetic nervous system. Neostigmine alone therefore can cause bradycardia and increased secretions, and should only be administered with an anticholinergic agent such as atropine or glyco-pyrolate. The type of block, its intensity and the adequacy of reversal can be monitored by the anaesthetist using a peripheral nerve stimulator.

The airway under anaesthesia

Any unconscious patient should be considered unable to maintain or protect their airway. General anaesthesia reduces tone in the pharyngeal muscles, and in muscles related to the hyoid bone in the neck. As a result, the support that normally maintains the position of the tongue is lost and it tends to fall back towards the posterior pharyngeal wall. This, together with the loss of pharyngeal muscle tone, can lead to partial or complete obstruction to gas flow, particularly when the patient is in the supine position. The airway is most likely to remain patent if the head is placed in the 'sniffing the morning air' position, namely neck flexed on a pillow and head extended on the neck. In patients who remain obstructed in this position, a jaw thrust and/or insertion of an oral (Geudel) or nasopharyngeal airway usually relieves airway obstruction.

Patients are routinely fasted prior to anaesthesia and elective surgery in order to reduce the risk from aspiration of gastric contents. Most anaesthetists consider 4 hours for solid food and 2 hours for liquids a sufficient period of fasting. Some conditions are associated with an increased risk of incomplete gastric emptying and/or an increased chance of regurgitation and aspiration during anaesthesia (Table 11.5). The most reliable technique for protecting the airway from aspiration is endotracheal intubation, because a cuff forms a physical barrier against lung contamination. For routine surgery during which muscle paralysis and mechanical ventilation is necessary, a dose of non-depolar-

Table 11.5   Risk factor for gastric aspiration

Very high risk
   Intestinal obstruction
   Late pregnancy
   Acute abdomen
   Ileus (any cause)
   Shock

High risk
   Hiatus hernia
   Obesity
   Autonomic neuropathy
   Acute pain and/or large doses of opiates
   Any emergency surgery inside the abdomen

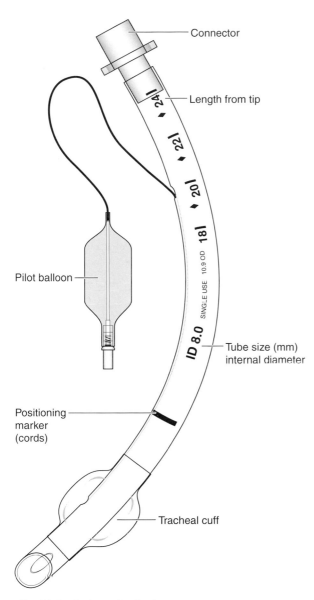

Connector

Length from tip

Pilot balloon

Tube size (mm) internal diameter

Positioning marker (cords)

Tracheal cuff

Fig. 11.2 Endotracheal tube.

Table 11.6   Steps in a rapid-sequence induction

1. Check that the patient is on a tipping trolley or table, and that aids to difficult intubation are available.
2. Ensure suction apparatus is available and switched on.
3. Preoxygenate the patient with 100% oxygen for 3 minutes via a tightly fitting mask. This washes out nitrogen from the lungs and delays the onset of hypoxaemia if intubation is difficult.
4. Administer a predetermined dose of intravenous induction agent and a rapidly acting muscle relaxant (usually suxamethonium).
5. A trained assistant should apply cricoid pressure to prevent regurgitation into the pharynx.
6. As soon as the patient's muscles have stopped fasciculation intubate the trachea and inflate the tube cuff.
7. Ventilate the patient's lungs and ensure the tube is correctly positioned by listening over both lung fields and stomach, and checking the capnograph for expiratory carbon dioxide.
8. Release cricoid pressure.

The laryngeal mask

The laryngeal mask comprises a cylindrical oropharyngeal airway with an elliptical opening which sits over the laryngeal inlet (Fig. 11.3). A cuff surrounding the ellipse is inflated with air once the device is in place and forms a seal with the pharyngeal muscles. The airway provided is more dependable than an oropharyngeal airway, but unlike the endotracheal tube it does *not reliably protect the lungs from aspiration*. It is easy to insert and frees the anaesthetist from holding a mask. Pharyngeal reflexes are sufficiently

izing muscle relaxant is given with the induction agent and the patient is ventilated via a mask until relaxation is achieved. An endotracheal tube (Fig. 11.2) can then be inserted using a laryngoscope and connected to the breathing circuit and ventilator. If the patient is at very high risk of regurgitation a 'rapid-sequence induction' should be used to minimize the time between induction of anaesthesia and protection of the airway with the endotracheal tube (Table 11.6).

In patients at low risk of gastric aspiration alternative methods of maintaining the airway can be used.

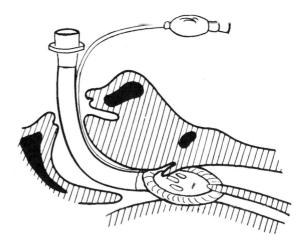

Fig. 11.3   The laryngeal mask airway.

obtunded by intravenous and volatile agents that muscle relaxation is not required for placement, unlike an endotracheal tube. The laryngeal mask is used predominantly during spontaneous ventilation, but the effective seal produced by the pharyngeal cuff does allow it to be used in selected cases where artificial ventilation is undertaken. In patients who are difficult to intubate the laryngeal mask has been shown to be very useful, both as an alternative and as an aid to intubation.

Maintenance of anaesthesia

After the induction of anaesthesia maintenance of hypnosis, analgesia and muscle relaxation can be achieved in a number of ways.

Hypnosis

For most anaesthetics, hypnosis is maintained after intravenous induction agents by gaseous and/or volatile agents delivered in an oxygen or air/oxygen mixture by the anaesthetic machine. Occasionally, anaesthesia is maintained using infusions of rapidly cleared intravenous agents (usually propofol).

Nitrous oxide Nitrous oxide was one of the first anaesthetic agents discovered and is still the most frequently used gaseous anaesthetic agent. It is a gas at room temperature and is poorly soluble in blood and tissues. These properties mean that high partial pressures are achieved rapidly in the body, so that the onset and offset of anaesthetic action is rapid. The main disadvantage of nitrous oxide is low potency, as the MAC value is 105 kPa (i.e. approximately atmospheric pressure at sea level). The highest partial pressure that can be safely administered to a patient is approximately 70 kPa, because at least 30 kPa partial pressures of oxygen need to be added to any gas mixture. Effective anaesthesia cannot therefore be achieved with nitrous oxide alone. Nitrous oxide is used for the following purposes in modern anaesthesia:

- To reduce the concentration of volatile anaesthetic required to achieve adequate anaesthesia. This is possible because the fractions of MACs of different agents have additive effects (see earlier). This decreases the incidence of concentration-related side effects from volatile agents;
- As an analgesic for use during labour or in other ward situations (e.g. changing dressings). A 50% mixture of nitrous oxide and oxygen (Entonox) can be delivered via specialized inhalation devices.

Volatile anaesthetics Volatile anaesthetics are more potent than nitrous oxide (Table 11.7). Hypnosis is usually maintained by a mixture of volatile anaesthetic and nitrous oxide, or by volatile anaesthetic alone delivered in an air/oxygen mixture. The different volatile anaesthetics differ in their potency, rate of onset and recovery, side-effect profile and expense. These factors, together with the preference of the anaesthetist, influence which agent is used for a particular patient.

Analgesia and muscle relaxation

During the anaesthetic, analgesia and muscle relaxation can be maintained by giving boluses of drugs intermittently, or by using infusions of short-acting agents. When local anaesthetic techniques have been used (see below) intravenous analgesia may not be required. The intensity and nature of the neuromuscular block can be monitored by using a nerve stimulator.

LOCAL ANAESTHESIA

Local anaesthetic agents such as lignocaine and bupivacaine act by altering membrane sodium permeability, resulting in a block to the transmission of impulses along the nerve fibre. They are non-specific and therefore block all three groups of nerves (autonomic, sensory and motor). The sensitivity of an individual nerve depends on its physical properties. Size, which relates to the number of cover-

Table 11.7	Volatile anaesthetic agents		
Agent	**MAC (kPa)**	**Advantages**	**Disadvantages**
Halothane	0.8	Cheap Non-irritant	Bradycardia and ventricular ectopics Rarely liver failure
Enflurane	1.7		Low potency Pro-convulsive (contraindicated in epilepsy)
Isoflurane	1.2	Low metabolism Little cardiac depressant effect	Too irritant for gas induction
Sevoflurane	2.0	Very rapid onset/recovery	Expensive

ings and degree of myelination, is a major factor. Small unmyelinated nerves, such as sympathetic neurons, are sensitive and are blocked early, whereas large myelinated nerves such as motor neurons are blocked last and recover first. The duration and intensity of the block depends on the local anaesthetic agent used (bupivacaine lasts longer than lignocaine), the total dose administered, the proximity of the injection to the nerve and the presence of a vasoconstrictor (usually adrenaline 1:200 000). Adrenaline prolongs block by producing local vasoconstriction, thereby slowing systemic uptake of local anaesthetic, which is the main mechanism of the offset of action. The most important complication of local anaesthetic injection is systemic toxicity due to high plasma concentrations. Patients should therefore have ECG, non-invasive blood pressure and pulse oximetry monitoring during the injection of large doses of local anaesthetic. In addition, there are recommended safe maximum doses of drug that should not be exceeded (Table 11.8). Major blocks using large doses of local anaesthetic should only be performed by personnel fully trained in cardiopulmonary resuscitation within an area where resuscitation equipment and drugs are readily available. Signs of local anaesthetic toxicity are given in Table 11.9. If toxicity occurs the patient's airway and breathing should be secured, and cardiovascular collapse treated with adrenergic agents such as ephedrine. Convulsions may be controlled with small increments of benzodiazepines or thiopentone.

Table 11.8 Safe maximum doses of commonly used local anaesthetics		
Drug	**With adrenaline (mg/kg)**	**Without adrenaline (mg/kg)**
Lignocaine	6	2
Bupivacaine	2	2
Prilocaine	maximum 600 mg	

Table 11.9 Signs of local anaesthetic toxicity
Early
Numbness/tingling of the tongue
Perioral tingling
Anxiety
Light-headedness
Tinnitus
Late
Loss of consciousness
Convulsions
Cardiovascular collapse
Apnoea

Local anaesthetics are used to block sensory nerves, allowing surgery to be performed painlessly within the area supplied by the nerve. They can be used as the sole anaesthetic (especially in operations on the arms and below the umbilicus) where a general anaesthetic is contraindicated, or combined with general anaesthesia. Local anaesthetic techniques are also an important component of postoperative analgesic regimens.

Topical anaesthesia

Satisfactory mucosal absorption allows lignocaine (0.5–4%)-containing solutions, gels and creams to be used to anaesthetize the conjunctiva, and the mucosa of the mouth, pharynx, larynx and urethra. These can be applied as lozenges, sprays, gargles, and on soaked pledgets of cotton wool. Anaesthesia is rapid and usually lasts 30–60 minutes. A mixture of lignocaine and prilocaine (EMLA cream) is an effective topical anaesthetic for the skin if applied 1 hour prior to venous cannulation. It is particularly useful in children and in adults with a needle phobia.

Local infiltration

Local anaesthetic can be infiltrated directly into the surgical field. Injection into inflamed tissues should be avoided because alterations to drug pharmocokinetics occur. Local vasodilatation can result in rapid systemic absorption and toxicity, but the decreased local tissue pH can reduce the local anaesthetic action. The addition of a vasoconstrictor such as adrenaline (1:200 000) can prolong the duration of local infiltration anaesthesia. Adrenaline-containing solutions should be avoided where there are end-arteries present (digits and appendages), as arterial vasoconstriction can result in a critical impairment of blood flow and ischaemia.

Regional intravenous anaesthesia (Bier's block)

Minor procedures on the limbs (e.g. reduction of closed fractures or median nerve decompression) which usually take less than 30 minutes can be performed under intravenous regional anaesthesia (Fig. 11.4). Anaesthesia is produced by the intravenous injection of a large volume of dilute solution (40 mL 0.5% or 0.75% prilocaine) into the limb. Prior to injection the limb requires to be exsanguinated (by the application of an elastic bandage, or simply elevation with occlusion of the main arterial pulse) and isolated from the circulation by the application of a pneumatic tourniquet inflated to 100 mmHg above the patient's systolic blood pressure (usually about 250 mmHg). The principle behind the technique is that the venous compartment of the occluded limb is filled with local anaesthetic solution, which tracks into the vasa nervosum to

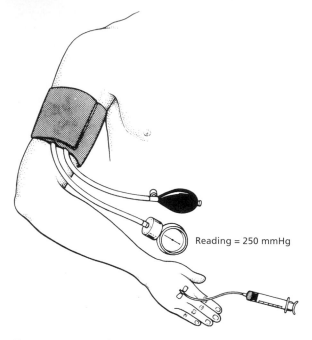

Fig. 11.4   Regional intravenous anaesthesia.

Table 11.10 Commonly performed peripheral nerve blocks	
Block	**Indication**
Axillary or supraclavicular	Upper limb surgery
Interscalene	Shoulder and upper limb
Femoral	Lower limb surgery
Sciatic	Lower limb surgery
Intercostal nerves	Thoracotomy Fractured ribs Cholecystectomy
Ilioinguinal/iliohypogastric	Inguinal hernia
Penile	Circumcision

block the nerves. Patients may not lose all modalities of sensation: the larger nerves transmitting touch and pressure sensation may continue conducting, whereas the smaller fibres transmitting pain sensation are adequately blocked. Anaesthesia remains as long as the cuff is inflated, but in practice conscious patients can rarely tolerate the discomfort of the cuff for more than 30–40 minutes. The cuff must not be deflated until at least 15 minutes have elapsed since the injection, to reduce the risk of systemic toxicity.

Peripheral nerve block

A detailed knowledge of the course of a nerve with respect to surface anatomy, its relationship to important surrounding structures and the area of body supplied allows the anaesthetist to inject local anaesthetic around the nerve in order to achieve a block. By using a nerve stimulator and insulated regional block needles, the anaesthetist can locate the nerve accurately before injection and improve the chances of a successful block. For large nerve trunks (e.g. sciatic and brachial plexus blocks) a large dose of local anaesthetic may be needed and there can be a delay of 30–40 minutes before the onset of a dense block. Commonly performed nerve blocks, and their indications, are shown in Table 11.10.

When multiple superficial nerves supply an area (e.g. groin or scalp), a 'field block' can be achieved by a series of injections to block the nerves. During injection, *atten-*

tion should be given to the total dose of drug administered in relation to the maximum recommended dose, and to the avoidance of accidental intravascular injection by repeated aspiration before injecting.

Spinal anaesthesia

Local anaesthetic can be administered into the subarachnoid (spinal) or extradural (epidural) spaces blocking the nerves within the vertebral canal before they exit from the intervertebral foramina. In order to avoid the possibility of damaging the spinal cord spinal anaesthesia is performed below the level at which the cord ends (L2). Similar to a lumbar puncture, a spinal needle is inserted between L3/4 or L4/5 and the subarachnoid space is identified by the free aspiration of clear CSF (Fig. 11.5).

As the nerves of the cauda equina only receive their perineural coverings and myelin sheaths as they exit through the dura, they are very sensitive to the effects of local anaesthetics. A small volume of lignocaine or bupivacaine (2–4 mL) will usually block all the spinal nerves below T10. The addition of 6% dextrose to the local anaesthetic will render it hyperbaric with respect to CSF. The spread of this 'heavy' solution can be influenced by gravity, which gives the anaesthetist additional control over the height of the resultant block. Spinal anaesthesia results in a reliable, rapid onset and dense block using a small dose of local anaesthetic. With hyperbaric solutions a reliable block to a level of T6 is usually achieved. The single injection usually gives 2–3 hours of surgical anaesthesia before sensation begins to return.

Epidural anaesthesia

In epidural anaesthesia a 'loss of resistance' technique is used to position the tip of the needle in the epidural space between the ligamentum flavum and the dura–arachnoid membrane (Fig. 11.6). This space runs the whole length of

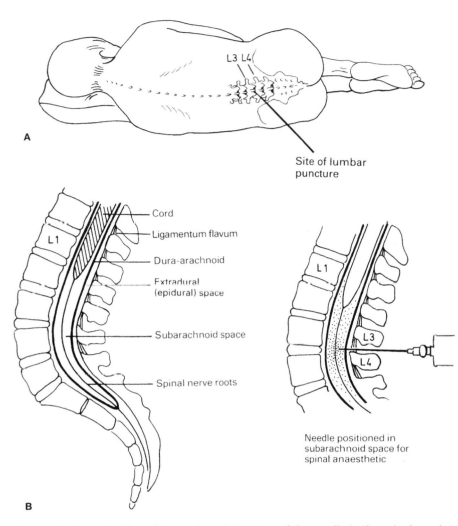

A

Site of lumbar
puncture

Cord

Ligamentum flavum

Dura-arachnoid

Extradural
(epidural) space

Subarachnoid space

Spinal nerve roots

Needle positioned in
subarachnoid space for
spinal anaesthetic

B

Fig. 11.5 Spinal anaesthesia. **A** Position of the patient. **B** Position of the needle in the spinal canal.

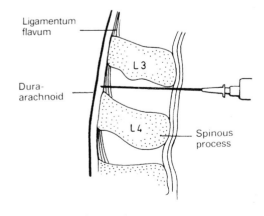

Ligamentum
flavum

Dura-
arachnoid

Spinous
process

Fig. 11.6 Epidural anaesthesia.

the vertebral canal and can be approached at any level from the cervical spine to the sacrum (caudal canal). The level of injection is dictated by the spinal nerves requiring blockade. Unlike nerve roots in the subarachnoid space, the nerves in the epidural space have their full complement of coverings and myelin. As a result, much larger doses of local anaesthetic are required than for spinal anaesthesia. A volume of 10–20 mL will spread upwards and downwards from the point of injection to create a band of anaesthesia that spreads several dermatomes on either side of the level of injection. Commonly a fine catheter is passed through the needle and is left in the epidural space, allowing for multiple injections or infusions of local anaesthetic solutions. Using this technique the anaesthesia produced for the surgical procedure (either alone or in combination with a light general anaesthetic) can be continued to produce high-quality analgesia in the post-operative period (considered later).

Spinal and epidural anaesthesia also block the sympathetic outflow within the anterior nerve roots. Rapid vasomotor paralysis reflects the small unmyelinated nature of the nerves and is an early indication of a successful block. Frequently the patient comments on warm feet, owing to cutaneous vasodilatation and an increase in blood flow through the skin. The same mechanism explains the common complication of hypotension seen with these techniques, which requires the judicious administration of intravenous fluids and/or vasoconstrictors (ephedrine, phenylephrine).

Many types of surgery can be performed using local anaesthetic techniques alone, with or without sedation. However, patients should always be fasted as for general anaesthesia, and monitoring and facilities for resuscitation should always be present.

RECOVERY AND THE RECOVERY ROOM

Prior to the completion of surgery the dose of anaesthetic will have already been reduced, paralleling the progressive reduction in surgical stimulation. At the point of skin suturing any residual neuromuscular blockade is reversed, and following the return of neuromuscular function and spontaneous ventilation the anaesthetic agents are switched off and the patient is allowed to breathe 100% oxygen. This speeds up recovery by accelerating the excretion of anaesthetic agents via the lungs. Transfer to the recovery room only occurs when the anaesthetist is satisfied that the patient is cardiovascularly stable, with a satisfactory ventilatory pattern and acceptable oxygen saturation. Upon arrival in the recovery room the patient is monitored with continuous ECG and pulse oximetry, together with regular blood pressure measurements. The anaesthetist is responsible for maintaining and protecting the airway until the patient has woken up from the anaesthetic. The recovery room nurse is trained in the care of the unconscious patient, and monitors them during this period. If the patient has been intubated the endotracheal tube can be left in situ until the effects of the anaesthetic have worn off sufficiently for the patient to be aware of the tube and object to its presence. At this point the laryngeal reflexes have returned sufficiently to protect the airway and the tube can be safely removed, after aspiration of the pharynx and deflation of the cuff. Recovery from anaesthesia is safest in the lateral position with the patient slightly head down, as this reduces the risk of aspiration. If a nasogastric tube is in place the stomach should be emptied by applying gentle suction and the tube left on free drainage to reduce the risk of accumulated gastric secretions being regurgitated and aspirated. These precautions are of particular importance in situations where the patient may have a full stomach (see earlier). The recovery room nurse will pay particular attention to:

- Careful monitoring of cardiorespiratory parameters (pulse, blood pressure, oxygen saturation, respiratory rate) and conscious level;
- Instituting the prescribed analgesic regimen and assessing its effectiveness through regular scoring of sedation, pain and nausea;
- The postoperative intravenous fluid regimen and monitoring output from urine, nasogastric tubes and surgical drains;
- Recording all the above, either as part of the anaesthetic record or on a dedicated postoperative chart.

Patients are ready for discharge to the ward when they are able to obey commands, are cardiovascularly stable and have satisfactory pain control.

THE HIGH-DEPENDENCY UNIT (HDU)

The HDU is used for the awake and spontaneously breathing patient who requires a level of postoperative monitoring and nursing care that is not available on the general surgical ward. It is an appropriate location for patients who have undergone major surgery with prolonged anaesthesia, have significant preoperative cardiorespiratory disease, or who are receiving complex analgesic techniques such as a continuous epidural infusion of local anaesthetic. Acute surgical emergencies may be admitted preoperatively for resuscitation and optimization prior to surgery.

Close attention is paid to fluid balance and analgesic requirements. Bedside monitors allow continuous display of cardiovascular parameters such as ECG, invasive and non-invasive blood pressure and CVP measurement. Pulse oximetry is a monitor of *oxygenation* but is a poor guide to *ventilation*, especially when supplemental oxygen is given. Regular recording of respiratory rate and sedation is therefore important. The increasing availability and sophistication of modern ward-based blood gas analysers means that blood biochemistry and arterial gas analysis are often available to assist in the management of the sick patient.

THE INTENSIVE THERAPY UNIT (ITU)

The ITU differs from the HDU in a number of respects. The continuity of medical care is delivered by personnel (intensivists) with a special interest in treating the very sick patient. A ratio of one nurse to each patient allows for uninterrupted clinical monitoring and care of the acutely ill patient. In many patients the underlying pathophysiological process is so severe that their clinical condition is continuously changing. The instability that characterizes the ITU patient necessitates a level of monitoring not available anywhere else outside the operating theatre. In addition to clinical examination at the bedside and simple non-invasive monitoring such as blood pressure, ECG and pulse oximetry, more invasive monitoring is available to help the bedside nurse and the physician identify sudden changes in the patient's clinical condition. Cardiovascular monitoring may include placing a catheter into the radial artery for continuous blood pressure monitoring and access for regular arterial blood gas estimations. Central venous pressure can be measured if a 10–15 cm long catheter is passed via the internal jugular or subclavian vein into the superior vena cava. Severe myocardial dysfunction or shock may require a pulmonary artery catheter (pulmonary artery flotation or Swan–Ganz catheter), inserted via the superior vena cava, left atrium and ventricle. This can measure pulmonary artery pressure and pulmonary artery wedge venous pressure as an indirect measurement of left atrial filling pressure. Modern catheters can continuously measure the mixed venous oxygen saturation and cardiac output.

The other major aspect to the work of an ITU is to manage the organ failure that often accompanies severe illness. Respiratory failure is managed with sophisticated assisted ventilation, but many of these patients require additional support for other organ dysfunction. These include renal replacement therapy for acute renal failure (haemofiltration or haemodialysis), total parenteral nutrition for gastrointestinal tract failure, and intravenous infusions of inotropic drugs for cardiovascular failure. To assist in patient management the modern ITU will have a dedicated laboratory machine that can measure arterial blood gases, electrolytes, glucose, lactate and haemoglobin. The goal is to support the failing organs until the pathophysiological process responsible has been identified, treated and/or reversed, allowing for organ and patient recovery. Depending on the underlying pathological process many specialties may be involved in the patient's management, including general, orthopaedic and neurosurgeons, renal physicians, microbiologists, radiologists and haematologists.

POSTOPERATIVE ANALGESIA

Pain relief is an essential component of perioperative care. Inadequate analgesia is associated with an increased incidence of chest infection and thromboembolism because patient mobility is decreased. Effective analgesia can decrease the magnitude of the stress response to surgery (see Chapter 1). Many factors influence the amount of pain experienced by patients in the postoperative period (Table 11.11). Some of these relate to the surgery itself, but patient-related factors are also important. Planning the methods for achieving pain relief, and explaining these to

Table 11.11 Factors influencing postoperative pain perception

Surgical factors		
Type of surgery	Thoracotomy Upper abdominal	
	Lower abdominal Limbs Hips Faciomaxillary Perineum	increasing pain
	Inguinal Craniotomy	
Amount of tissue injury	Surgical technique, e.g. excessive use of diathermy increases pain	

Patient factors associated with increased perception of pain
Neurotic and extrovert personality types
Anxiety (acute or chronic)
Low motivation of patient
Cultural and social background
Previous bad experiences
Younger > older patients

the patient, should be done prior to surgery. This is usually done by the anaesthetist who initiates analgesia during surgery. Many hospitals have a dedicated acute pain team, composed of anaesthetists and specialist nurses who regularly review patients postoperatively to ensure pain relief is adequate.

The pain pathway

Acute postoperative pain results from the transmission of nerve impulses from the site of tissue injury to the sensory cortex of the brain (Fig. 11.7). This pathway can be modulated at various points to modify the conscious perception of pain by the individual. The effect of drugs or techniques that alter the transmission of acute pain impulses at different sites in the pain pathway may be additive or synergistic (a combined effect greater than the sum of individual effects). This *multimodal* approach to treating postoperative pain is often more effective than using single agents or techniques.

Pain fibres Pain is transmitted by two types of nerve fibre. Unmyelinated *C fibres* conduct slowly (1–2 m/s) and characterististically give rise to slow burning pain. Myelinated Aδ fibres conduct faster (5–20 m/s) and give rise to a sharper pain sensation. Fibres are carried in peripheral nerves and enter the spinal cord through the dorsal routes, crossing the epidural space prior to penetrating the dura

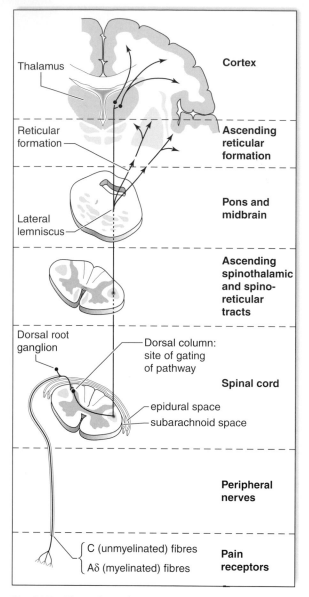

Fig. 11.7 The pain pathway.

Spinal cord transmission Long fibres arise from the neurons of the dorsal horn. These transmit the net signal resulting from the interaction of pain impulses and gating mechanisms to the brain. These fibres cross the midline immediately via the anterior commissure and pass to the brain in the *spinothalamic* and *spinoreticular* tracts.

The brain In the brain there are two major routes of pain transmission. The Aδ fibres terminate in the ventrobasal portion of the thalamus, from which signals are transmitted to other parts of the thalamus and to the somatic sensory area of the cortex. The C fibres terminate in the reticular area of the brain stem and in the intralaminar nuclei of the thalamus. These fibres form part of the reticular formation, which communicates with most parts of the brain. As a result the perception of pain is influenced by many different 'higher' functions of the brain.

Techniques for postoperative analgesia

Epidural analgesia

Epidural analgesia is particularly suited to thoracotomy, major abdominal and lower limb surgery. The epidural is usually placed prior to surgery and continued into the postoperative period for 1–5 days. The epidural catheter is best placed at a level close to the midpoint of the dermatomes involved in surgery (Fig. 11.8). Epidural analgesia is usually maintained by a continuous infusion of local anaesthetic solution, to which additional drugs with analgesic properties at the spinal level can be added. The concentration of local anaesthetic solution may vary according to the preference of the individual anaesthetist or hospital protocol. The commonest drugs added to local anaesthetic solutions are opiates, for example diamorphine or fentanyl. Local anaesthetics and opiates have synergistic analgesic properties at the spinal level. Some commonly used epidural infusion mixtures are:

- Bupivacaine 0.125% plus 30 μg/mL diamorphine running at 8–12 mL/h
- Bupivacaine 0.125% plus 2 μg/mL fentanyl running at 8–12 mL/h.

Complications of epidural analgesia

Hypotension This occurs frequently in postoperative patients receiving epidural analgesia, and is more likely than with other analgesic techniques because of sympathetic blockade. Hypotension has several possible causes, as follows:

- *Hypovolaemia* Patients with an epidural block are less able to respond to hypovolaemia by vasoconstriction. The patient's lower limbs are usually warm because of

mater. After entering the cord fibres ascend one or two segments and synapse in the dorsal horns of the grey matter.

Dorsal horns The dorsal horns are an important site of pain modulation. C and Aδ fibres synapse with neurons in the *substantia gelatinosa* of the dorsal horn. Transmission of impulses via these neurons can be modulated by other impulses arriving from peripheral or descending tracts. Inhibition of these neurons by stimulation of these tracts, or by drugs acting on receptors in the dorsal horn, can decrease the transmission of pain impulses to the brain. This is the basis of the *gating* theory of pain transmission.

sympathetic blockade. A useful clinical sign is vasoconstriction and cold in the upper limbs, where sympathetic blockade is absent.

- *Excessive epidural blockade* This can be detected by regularly testing the dermatomes for which analgesia is present. Ideally the epidural block should involve only the dermatomes involved in surgery. Excessively high thoracic block can affect the cardiac sympathetic nerves and cause inappropriate bradycardia. If excessive block is present the rate of infusion should be decreased or stopped temporarily. Very rarely, an epidural catheter can migrate to the subarachnoid space, causing excessive block.

- *Haemorrhage* Occult haemorrhage should always be considered in patients with severe hypotension in the absence of excessive epidural blockade.

- *Sepsis* In the absence of other explanations for hypotension, sepsis should be considered. Classic signs such as fever and leukocytosis may not always be present. When sepsis is secondary to intra-abdominal complications, such as anastomotic breakdown, clinical signs may be masked by the epidural block.

Inadequate analgesia This can result from:

- *Epidural catheter displacement* If the catheter has not been well secured, or is pulled out as a result of patient

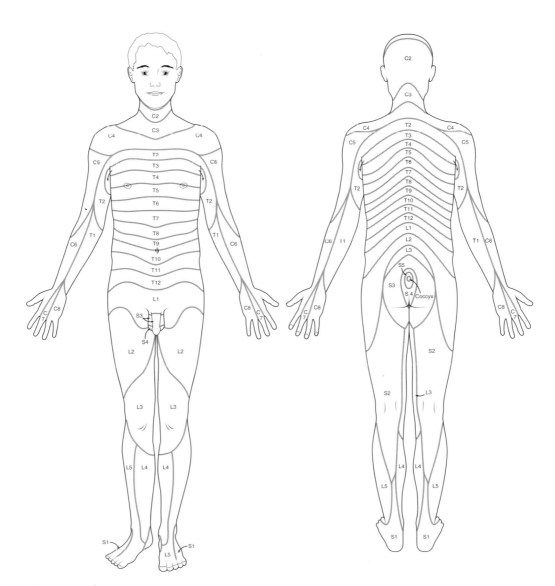

Fig. 11.8 Cutaneous dermatomes.

movement, the block will be absent or inadequate and not improve after a top-up anaesthetic dose.

- *Inadequate block* This is usually easily detected by testing the dermatomes blocked using cold or pinprick. Inadequate block is usually because the dose of anaesthetic solution is inadequate. In the latter case this can be treated by giving a bolus dose of local anaesthetic and/or increasing the infusion rate of the analgesic solution.
- *Unilateral block* Some patients develop a unilateral block during epidural analgesia. This can be due to anatomical variation of the epidural space, or to migration of the epidural catheter. The anaesthetist can sometimes correct unilateral block by pulling the catheteter 1–2 cm out at the skin and resecuring it.

Headache Headache is common following anaesthesia and surgery, but a *postdural puncture headache* has special implications. This occurs if the dura is punctured by accident during epidural catheter placement and is usually, but not always, apparent to the anaesthetist at the time. Postdural puncture headache can also occur after spinal anaesthesia, but is relatively rare because modern spinal needles are narrow and blunt-ended. A postdural puncture headache usually occurs within 2 days of the anaesthetic and is often severe, frontal, and can be associated with meningism and photophobia. The patient will complain that the pain is worse sitting than when lying. If bed-rest and simple analgesics are inadequate, the headache will usually resolve if an epidural blood patch is performed by the anaesthetist.

Patients with epidural infusions require adequate monitoring to prevent complications, and are ideally managed in a high-dependency unit. The time that the epidural is continued postoperatively depends on several factors:

- Adequacy of epidural block
- Facilities for monitoring
- Magnitude of pain associated with surgery
- If patient comorbidity warrants prolonged regional blockade. This is particularly important for patients with significant respiratory disease (see chapter on preoperative assessment).

Peripheral nerve blockade (see earlier)

This is usually carried out at the time of surgery, but provides analgesia for a variable time during the postoperative period depending on the nerve(s) involved and the type and dose of local anaesthetic used. In some situations peripheral nerve blockade can be repeated during the postoperative period, for example intercostal blockade for thoracotomy. Occasionally the anaesthetist may place a catheter close to the nerve at the time of surgery to enable continuous infusion of local anaesthetic.

Peripheral opiate administration

There are several methods for administering postoperative opiate drugs (Table 11.12). When relatively little postoperative pain is anticipated intramuscular opioids can be prescribed 'as required' to supplement simple analgesics.

Table 11.12   Methods of administering opioids during the postoperative period

Method	Advantages	Disadvantages
Intermittent intramuscular injection	Simple and cheap Respiratory depression unlikely Less need for close patient monitoring	Relies on nurse administration Unpredictable analgesic effects Variable rates of drug absorption No patient control
Continuous intravenous infusion	Effective Does not rely on patient cooperation Individual titration to patient requirement	Highest risk of side-effects Requires close monitoring Requires dedicated infusion system
Patient-controlled analgesia (PCA)	Effective Patient benefits from 'feeling in control' Accommodates variability in requirement	Requires close monitoring Risk of side-effects Specialized administration system
Transdermal (patches)	Simple Relatively safe	Expensive No flexibility Unpredictable analgesia

Table 11.13 Complications of opioid administration	
Respiratory depression	Results in hypercapnia Usually clinically significant if respiratory rate < 8 breaths per minute Rarely causes hypoxia if patient is receiving supplemental oxygen
Cough suppression	May impair clearance of secretions
Sedation	Slows mobility
Confusion	Particularly in elderly patients
Nausea and vomiting	
Decreased intestinal motility	May contribute to postoperative ileus

SUMMARY BOX

Patient-controlled analgesia

Setting up
- Infusion — Usually morphine (1 mg/mL or 2 mg/mL concentration)
- Additives — Some anaesthetists add antiemetics
- Bolus dose — 1 or 2 mg morphine, or equivalent if other drugs used
- Lockout period — Usually 5 minutes

Connection
- Pump should be placed below the level of the patient (reduces risk of accidental infusion)
- One-way valve should always be placed on the accompanying intravenous fluid infusion
- Ensure functioning intravenous cannula

Monitoring
- Regular monitoring of vital signs, especially respiratory rate, essential

Charting
- A standard chart with guidelines should be used

For major surgery, intramuscular opioids are only effective if the nurse is available to administer analgesia frequently. The most effective method of administering intravenous opioids is the patient-controlled analgesia pump (PCA). With this technique the patient self-administers an intravenous dose of drug by pressing a hand held button. A bolus dose is set as well as a lockout period, which is the minimum time period between drug administrations by the machine. If the patient presses the button more often this registers as an unsuccessful demand. Excessive sedation should not occur if an appropriate bolus dose and lock-out time have been set on the infusion system, because the patient will stop pressing the button if they become excessively sedated. Patient-controlled analgesia is a very safe technique as long as simple guidelines are followed and medical and nursing staff are aware of possible complications.

If significant opioid side-effects occur (Table 11.13) these should be managed as follows:

1. Assess airway, breathing and circulation (ABC).
2. Discontinue opioid administration until side-effects are reversed.
3. When more urgent intervention is required (e.g. hypoxaemia) administer naloxone slowly in small doses (e.g. 50 µg every 1–2 minutes) until the desired effect is achieved. Avoid excessive doses because this will cause pain, anxiety and hypertension. Naloxone effects diminish after 20–30 minutes, so the patient should be monitored for further respiratory depression.

Peripherally administered opioids should be used with caution in patients receiving epidural opioids because the additive effects can be unpredictable.

Mild/moderate analgesics

Analgesic drugs with mild/moderate efficacy are effective in the following postoperative situations:

- As the only analgesic therapy after minor surgery;
- As analgesia late in the recovery from major surgery after regional analgesia or potent opioids have been discontinued;
- As an adjunct to epidural analgesia or potent opioids to decrease the dose requirement for these drugs and potentially reduce the severity of side-effects.

Paracetamol Paracetamol is an effective simple analgesic drug with few side-effects. It can be administered orally or by suppository.

Non-steroidal anti-inflammatory drugs (NSAIDs) This class of drugs act by inhibiting prostaglandin production and are very effective for mild/moderate postoperative pain. They are a useful adjunct to more potent techniques, for example in reducing pleuritic pain from chest drains after thoracotomy. A large number of different drugs exist with differing potencies and pharmacokinetics. Commonly used agents in the postoperative setting are diclofenac, ketorolac, ibuprofen and piroxicam. In addition to oral administration, some agents can be administered by suppository (e.g. diclofenac), buccally (e.g. piroxicam) or intravenously (e.g. diclofenac and ketorolac). Using NSAIDs in addition to patient-controlled analgesia can significantly reduce the total dose of opiates used by patients. NSAIDs can have

Table 11.14   Cases in which NSAIDs are relatively contraindicated for postoperative analgesia

Peptic ulcer disease
Acute or chronic renal failure
Platelet disorders
Coagulopathies
Dehydration
Hypovolaemia

significant side-effects and should be used with caution in certain patients (Table 11.14).

Tramadol This drug has analgesic potency between strong opiates and simple analgesics. It is a partial opioid agonist with fewer of the side-effects of full agonists such as morphine. In addition, it is thought to inhibit the transmission of pain signals to the brain by blocking reuptake of neurotransmitters (serotonin and adrenaline) at the dorsal horn of the spinal cord (see above). Tramadol can be administered orally, intravenously or intramuscularly.

Oral opiates Oral opiate drugs, such as codeine phosphate and dihydrocodeine, are potent analgesics that are useful for moderate postoperative pain. They have potential

to cause the same side-effects as potent opiates. In the late postoperative period constipation and delayed bowel function can be a particular problem.

Combination preparations These are popular and effective analgesics for moderate postoperative pain. Their potency depends largely on the dose of the opiate drug component.

POSTOPERATIVE NAUSEA AND VOMITING (PONV)

Nausea and vomiting are common after surgery and result from many factors (Table 11.15). For patients at high risk of PONV prophylactic antiemetics are effective, particularly if administered before or during surgery. PONV is an extremely unpleasant complication of surgery and all at-risk patients should be prescribed antiemetics 'as required'.

SUMMARY BOX

Postoperative analgesic drugs and techniques

Severe pain
- Intravenous opiates
- Epidural analgesia
- Peripheral nerve block(s)

Moderate pain
- NSAIDs
- Intramuscular opiates
- Potent oral opiate-based analgesics
- Combination preparations
- Tramadol

Mild pain
- NSAIDs
- Paracetamol

Table 11.15   Factors increasing the risk of postoperative nausea and vomiting (PONV)

Patient factors
   Past history of PONV
   Susceptibility to travel sickness
   More common in women
   Decreases with advancing age

Perioperative drugs
   Opioids

Anaesthetic techniques
   Etomidate use for induction of anaesthesia
   Volatile anaesthetic agents (less important with modern agents)
   Nitrous oxide (relatively small effect)

Operation site
Particularly common for surgery to:
   Abdomen
   Middle ear
   Extraocular surgery (squints)
   Gynaecological

Other factors
   Nasogastric tubes
   Prolonged surgery
   Hypotension (particularly during regional anaesthesia)

12 Practical procedures and patient investigation

R.W. Parks

INTRODUCTION

Every practical procedure performed on a conscious patient should be preceded by an explanation, which should include the reasons for the procedure and what it will entail. Appropriate reassurance should always be given. Many patients find comfort in continuing reassurance throughout the procedure, and most are helped by a description of sensations they are likely to experience before these occur. Where appropriate, informed written consent should be obtained.

GENERAL PRECAUTIONS

It is important to be aware of the risk of infection or trauma to patient, operator and assistant during any practical procedure. These risks are minimized by following a few simple rules:

- Needles should not be resheathed and all disposable sharp instruments discarded by the operator should be placed in an appropriate container. These measures minimize the risk of needle-stick injury to operator and assistant.
- Drapes and other soiled equipment should be placed in appropriate containers.
- Gloves and gown should only be removed after all used instruments and disposable equipment have been placed in appropriate containers.

ASEPTIC TECHNIQUE

Transmission of infection is an ever-present problem, and the risk of spread should be minimized. As a minimum precaution the skin should be cleansed with an antiseptic solution before all procedures, and sterile instruments should be used. For some procedures, such as central venous catheterization, bladder catheterization, insertion of chest drains and lumbar puncture, a full aseptic technique must be used. The steps required are outlined in the box (below).

LOCAL ANAESTHESIA

Local anaesthetic agents inhibit membrane depolarization and hence block the transmission of nerve impulses. They may be used topically, i.e. painted or sprayed on mucous membranes and wound surfaces, so that they are absorbed locally to produce analgesia. Areas suitable for topical analgesia include the urethra, eye, nose, throat and bronchial tree. Local anaesthesia may also be administered by local infiltration, and this is used widely for minor surgical procedures. Local anaesthetic drugs are potentially toxic and care must be taken to avoid inadvertent intravascular injection. The first sign of toxicity is often numbness or tingling of the tongue or around the mouth, followed by lightheadedness and tinnitus. At higher blood levels there is loss of consciousness, convulsions and apnoea. Cardiovascular collapse eventually occurs as a result of myocardial depression, vasodilation and hypoxia. In general, efficacy is related to correct placement and toxicity to total dose. Where there is doubt about placement or a wide area of infiltration is anticipated, it is safer to calculate the maximum recommended dose and dilute it to the desired volume with 0.9% saline.

Lignocaine is the most widely used local anaesthetic agent and is available in 0.5–2% solutions. The maximum recommended dose is 3 mg/kg. Lignocaine is a short-acting anaesthetic (lasting up to 2 hours), whereas bupivacaine is longer acting (up to 8 hours). A mixture of the two can be administered.

Solutions of local anaesthetic mixed with a 1:200 000 concentration of adrenaline are also available. Adrenaline acts as a vasoconstrictor. It minimizes bleeding and reduces redistribution of the anaesthetic agent, thereby increasing its efficacy and duration of action. Local anaesthetic agents with adrenaline should not be used in anatomical areas supplied by an end-artery, such as the digits, because of the risk of vasoconstriction, ischaemia and gangrene developing.

WOUND SUTURE

The purpose of suturing is to approximate wound edges in such a manner as to allow optimum primary healing to take place. Wounds are sutured under as near-sterile conditions as possible using a strict aseptic technique. A few basic principles underlie good wound care:

- Tissue should be handled gently. The wound should not be rubbed with swabs. Blood in a wound is removed by pressing a swab on to it.
- Haemostasis should be meticulous to prevent wound haematoma.
- All foreign material and devitalized tissues should be removed. Where this is prevented by heavy contamination, delayed primary suture or secondary suture should be considered.
- Potential spaces (dead space) in the wound should be closed using adsorbable suture material such as Vicryl. Where this is not possible, a suction drain is led from the potential space before more superficial layers are closed.
- The tension on knots is critical. If they are tied too tightly the suture line may become ischaemic, leading to delayed healing or non-healing and an increased risk of wound infection. Equally, insufficient tension on the suture may result in failure to appose the wound edges or inadequate haemostasis.

Suturing the skin

Cutting needles are used to suture skin. Non-absorbable sutures (see below) are generally preferred, but require subsequent removal. Interrupted sutures have the advantage over continuous sutures that the removal of one or two appropriately sited stitches may allow adequate drainage if the wound becomes infected. The sutures should be placed equidistant from one another, taking equal 'bites' on either side of the wound. A sufficient number should be inserted to maintain apposition without the skin edges gaping. The

Table 12.1 Times recommended for removal of sutures	
Face and neck	4 days
Scalp	7 days
Abdomen and chest	7–10 days
Limbs	7 days
Feet	10–14 days

size of bite is determined by the amount of subcutaneous fat and by whether or not the fat has been separately sutured. In the abdomen the bite is approximately 5 mm on either side of the wound, whereas on the face a 1–2 mm bite is preferred. The wound edge is picked up with toothed dissecting forceps, and the needle is introduced through the skin at an angle as close to vertical as possible and brought out on the other side at a similar angle.

Similar principles apply when using a continuous suture. A subcuticular continuous suture is preferred by some surgeons and avoids the small pinpoint scars at the site of entry and exit of the traditional suture, or the ugly cross-hatching that results if sutures are tied too tightly or left in too long. Table 12.1 gives the suggested times for removal of sutures.

Cosmetic results as good as those achieved by subcuticular suturing can be obtained by removing sutures in half the times listed in Table 12.1 and replacing them with adhesive strips (e.g. Steristrip). Skin stapling or clipping is being increasingly used for scalp wounds, but can be used for closure at any site. Skin clips are supplied in disposable cartridges for single patient use.

Suture materials

Non-absorbable

Non-absorbable sutures may be classified into three groups:

1. Natural braided sutures (e.g. silk, linen) have good handling qualities and knot easily and securely. Their disadvantage is increased tissue reaction and suture line sepsis, caused by the capillary action of the braided material drawing microorganisms into the suture track. Such materials also lose tensile strength quickly with time, or when wet.
2. Synthetic braided materials (e.g. Nurolon, Ethibond, Mersilene) cause less tissue reaction than natural materials. They have good handling qualities and knot easily and securely.
3. Synthetic monofilament materials (e.g. nylon, polypropylene) have less drag through the tissues and cause little tissue reaction. They are free from the capillary effect of braided sutures and cause less suture track sepsis. However, they handle less well because of

increased 'memory' (i.e. they retain the configuration in which they were packaged). Knots in monofilament sutures are less secure than those in braided or natural sutures, requiring multiple throws on each one.

Absorbable sutures

Absorbable sutures are generally made from synthetic materials. They cause relatively little tissue reaction, retain their tensile strength and are absorbed slowly. They can be multifilament, such as Dexon (polyglycolic acid) and Vicryl (polyglycolic plus polylactic acid), or monofilament, such as Maxon (polyglyconate) and PDS (polydioxonone). These synthetic sutures are commonly used for subcuticular wound closure. In small wounds this may mean interrupted sutures with each knot buried, whereas in longer wounds a continuous subcuticular suture is used.

> **SUMMARY BOX**
>
> *Suggested gauge of suture material for skin suture*
>
> - Around the eyes: 6/0 sutures
> - Elsewhere on the face: 5/0 sutures
> - Neck, hands and digits: 4/0 sutures
> - Other sites: 3/0 or even 2/0 sutures
> - Subcuticular wound closure 4/0 sutures

ABDOMINAL PROCEDURES

Nasogastric tube insertion

A nasogastric tube is inserted to drain stomach contents in conditions such as intestinal obstruction, or to administer enteral nutrition. In most situations a 14–16 Fr single-lumen radio-opaque nasogastric tube with multiple distal openings will suffice. Double-lumen tubes are occasionally used to allow continuous low-pressure suction without the lumen becoming blocked by gastric mucosa.

Procedure

The nose is inspected for any deformity and the more patent nasal passage is chosen for insertion. The patient is placed in the sitting position and a local anaesthetic spray may be used to anaesthetize the nasal passage. The tube is well lubricated with gel and passed backwards along the floor of the nasal passage (Fig. 12.1). A slight resistance may be felt as the tube passes from the nasopharynx to the oropharynx, and the patient should be warned that a retching sensation may be experienced at this point.

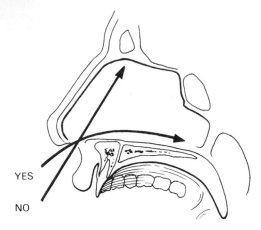

Fig. 12.1 Nasogastric intubation. Note the correct direction for inserting the tube.

The patient is now asked to swallow, and with each swallow the tube is advanced down the oesophagus. It is important not to push the tube rapidly and force its insertion in a patient who is retching: rather, slow and steady progress should be sought, with small advancements made during each act of swallowing. Ideally about 10–15 cm of the tube should be placed into the stomach. The oesophagogastric junction is about 40 cm from the incisor teeth. Most nasogastric tubes have markings to allow measurement of the length inserted. Correct placement of the tube is confirmed by free aspiration of gastric contents, and by auscultation in the epigastrium while 20 ml of air is insufflated. Once in place, the tube is fixed to the nose with adhesive tape.

In patients with head injuries the nasal route is avoided because of the risk of introducing infection – or even the nasogastric tube itself – into the central nervous system through an open fracture of the skull base. The oral route is also considered in patients with serious coagulopathy, as passage of the tube through the nose may result in significant haemorrhage. Finally, blind passage of a tube in the early period following oesophagectomy should never be attempted as this may disrupt the anastomosis.

Fine-bore nasogastric tubes

Elemental diets tend to have an unpleasant taste and are poorly tolerated when swallowed normally. Such diets are therefore best given by infusion through a fine-bore nasogastric tube, which are more comfortable and less likely to cause oesophageal erosions than a standard nasogastric tube. They do, however, require great care in insertion, as they can easily pass into the respiratory tract.

Procedure

Fine-bore nasogastric tubes have a wire stylet to facilitate passage. The tube is passed in the same way as a standard nasogastric tube. Again, it is important not to force the tube but to advance it slowly and steadily with each swallowing action made by the patient. The position of the tube is confirmed by X-ray, and only then is the stylet removed. Once removed, it must never be reintroduced while the tube remains in place. as there is a significant risk of perforating both the tube and the oesophagus. The tube tends to collapse if aspirated, so that aspiration cannot be used to check its position.

It is often advantageous to position the fine-bore feeding tube in the jejunum. This can be achieved using a radiological imaging technique or by the use of enteral feeding tubes, which have a mercury-filled tip and are 'self-propelled' into the jejunum.

Gastric lavage

The commonest indication for gastric lavage is the removal of ingested poisons or drugs. Much less commonly it is used to lower or raise the core body temperature.

Aspiration of gastric contents is a serious risk. If there is any doubt about the patient's ability to maintain the airway, expert assistance must be sought and endotracheal intubation considered prior to the procedure. The patient's level of consciousness, the presence of a gag reflex and their ability to cough are the most useful guides to the need for endotracheal intubation.

Procedure

After assessing the need for endotracheal intubation, the patient is placed on the left side in the recovery position, with a 15° head-down tilt of the trolley. A large-bore gastric tube is introduced into the mouth. A mouth gag is useful to prevent the patient biting the tube. As the tube is passed into the oropharynx and upper oesophagus the patient is likely to gag, and even to vomit. The tube is advanced into the stomach and its correct position confirmed by the free flow of gastric contents. If there is doubt, ausculation of the epigastrium during injection of air down the tube will confirm correct placement. About 100–200 mL of warm water are passed down the tube into the stomach. The end of the tube is then lowered below the level of the stomach into a collecting bucket, and gastric contents allowed to syphon out. The manoeuvre is repeated until the returned water becomes clear. It is important to avoid overdistension of the stomach. Activated charcoal can be instilled into the stomach to act as an absorbent if this is appropriate. On completion of lavage the tube is removed.

Oesophageal tamponade

The Sengstaken tube is a gastric aspiration tube with inflatable gastric and oesophageal balloons, which may be used for emergency treatment of bleeding oesophageal varices. A modification, the Sengstaken–Blakemore or Minnesota tube (Fig. 12.2), has an additional channel to allow the aspiration of saliva from the oesophagus above the level of the oesophageal ballon.

Procedure

The Sengstaken–Blakemore tube should be stored in a refrigerator, as this renders it less pliable and thus facilitates insertion. The oesophageal and gastric balloons are checked for leaks and then completely deflated using an aspiration syringe prior to insertion. The tube is inserted in the same way as a normal nasogastric tube. However, it is much more uncomfortable and local anaesthesia is recommended for nasal passage. A patient with bleeding varices is unlikely to cooperate fully and the tube may have to be passed with the patient on their side. If there is difficulty inserting the tube via the nasal route, the oral route may be used.

The tube is advanced approximately 60 cm and the gastric balloon inflated with 150–200 mL of air or water. The tube is then drawn back until this lower balloon impacts at the cardia. An assistant holds the tube in this position under slight tension, and the oesophageal balloon is inflated with air to a pressure of approximately 40 mmHg, checked by attaching a sphygmomanometer. The tube is secured in position with tape, but no additional traction is necessary.

The stomach is aspirated regularly through the main lumen of the tube to check for further bleeding. This lumen may also be used for the administration of medication, such as lactulose and neomycin. A fourth lumen allows aspiration of the upper oesophagus and pharynx and reduces the risk of bronchial aspiration. In patients who are stuporose or comatose, the airway should be protected by an endotracheal tube.

The use of a Sengstaken–Blakemore tube is generally a temporary measure to control haemorrhage prior to definitive treatment, or to allow transfer of the patient to a specialist centre. It is advisable to deflate the oesophageal balloon for 5 minutes every 6 hours to avoid the risk of ischaemic necrosis and ulceration of the oesophageal mucosa. The tube is not normally kept in place for more than 24 hours.

Abdominal paracentesis

Abdominal paracentesis is performed to relieve the discomfort caused by distension with ascitic fluid, or to obtain fluid for cytological examination. The bladder must be emptied, if necessary by preliminary catheterization. A 'Trocath' peritoneal dialysis catheter with multiple side perforations over a length of 8 cm is inserted under sterile conditions.

Procedure

The operator scrubs up and wears a grown and gloves. Local anaesthetic is infiltrated through all layers of the abdominal wall. This can be done either in the midline (one-third of the way from the umbilicus to the pubic symphysis), or in the right or left iliac fossa (at the junction of the outer and middle thirds of a line drawn from the anterior superior spine to the umbilicus) (Fig. 12.3). The depth at which the peritoneum is entered is determined by aspiration with the syringe. The vicinity of scars should be avoided, as adhesions increase the risk of bowel perforation.

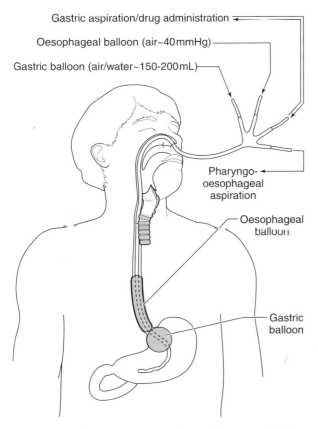

Gastric aspiration/drug administration

Oesophageal balloon (air~40mmHg)

Gastric balloon (air/water~150-200mL)

Pharyngo-oesophageal aspiration

Oesophageal balloon

Gastric balloon

Fig. 12.2 A four-lumen Sengstaken–Blakemore tube in position for oesophageal tamponade.

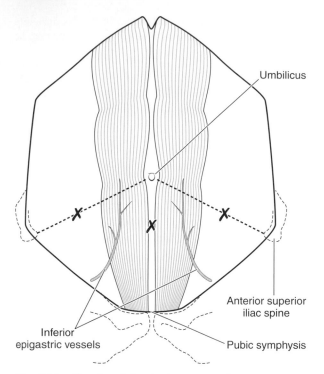

Fig. 12.3 Sites for abdominal paracentesis.

A 3-mm stab incision is made in the skin with a scalpel. The trocar is introduced into the catheter and the shaft of the catheter is held firmly between left thumb and index finger some 4–5 cm higher than the estimated depth of the peritoneum. This prevents 'overshoot' as the right hand thrusts the trocar and catheter through the abdominal wall into the peritoneum (Fig. 12.4).

The catheter is now advanced further with the left hand while the trocar is withdrawn with the right. If any resistance is noted the catheter is withdrawn 2–3 cm, rotated

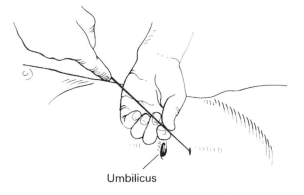

Fig. 12.4 Insertion of peritoneal dialysis catheter.

180°C and then advanced again. The minimum final length of catheter within the peritoneal cavity must be 10 cm. If this position is not obtained, the side perforations of the catheter may lie within the abdominal wall and allow troublesome extravasation of ascitic fluid into the subcutaneous tissues. The one-way metal disc is slid down the catheter to make contact with the skin and secured to it with adhesive tape. The catheter is divided some 4 cm above the disc and attached via a connection tube with a flow-control clamp to a sterile drainage bag.

Drainage of large volumes of ascitic fluid must be accompanied with intravenous infusion of albumin in order to avoid precipitating a marked shift of fluid from the intravascular compartment into the peritoneal cavity. This prevents significant changes in haemodynamics and reduces the risk of developing cardiovascular instability, renal impairment or hepatic encephalopathy.

Diagnostic peritoneal lavage

This procedure may be undertaken to look for the presence of blood or intestinal contents following blunt abdominal trauma. If the patient is stable a CT scan of the abdomen is the investigation of choice; however, diagnostic peritoneal lavage (DPL) is indicated in unconscious trauma patients, in patients with multiple injuries and unexplained shock, or in patients with equivocal physical signs. The patient should have a nasogastric tube and a urethral or suprapubic catheter inserted prior to DPL, to reduce the risk of injury to the stomach or bladder.

Procedure

This procedure can be performed using a closed or open technique, the latter being favoured to minimize the risk of intra-abdominal injury. Under sterile conditions and following the instillation of local anaesthesia, a 5 cm vertical subumbilical incision is made and dissection continued through the subcutaneous tissue and linea alba. The peritoneum is opened and a cannula inserted into the peritoneal cavity and advanced into the pelvis. A syringe is connected to the dialysis catheter, and if frank blood is immediately aspirated this is a positive DPL result. If gross blood is not obtained, 1 L of warm sterile isotonic saline is infused and allowed to distribute evenly throughout the peritoneal cavity. The fluid is then retrieved by placing the infusion bag on the floor and allowing the effluent to drain from the abdomen by gravity. An unequivocal test will reveal gross evidence of blood, bile or faeces. If necessary, fluid can be sent to the laboratory for analysis. A positive result is obtained if the red cell count is >100 000/mm^3, the white cell count is >55 mm^3 or the amylase is >175 units/mL.

AIRWAY PROCEDURES

Maintaining the airway

The ability to maintain the airway is a basic skill which every doctor, nurse, paramedic and indeed member of the general public should have. Its simplicity belies its importance, but it is a life-saving skill which must be learnt through practice.

In the unconscious patient, muscles which normally maintain a clear airway become lax. The tongue and soft tissue fall backwards, particularly in the supine patient, occluding the airway. Maintaining a clear airway allows the patient to breathe or allows the lungs to be ventilated.

Procedure

The simplest manoeuvre is to place the patient on their side with the neck extended in the so-called 'recovery position'. This allows the tongue and soft tissues to fall clear of the larynx and provide a patent airway. The mouth and pharynx should be checked and cleared of debris such as dentures, vomit or food.

Where the patient has to be kept supine, the neck should be extended. The mouth is opened slightly and the mandible pulled firmly forward by pressure applied behind both angles of the jaw. The mandible is held in this position by closing the mouth and using the teeth as a splint. Forward pressure is maintained behind the angles of the jaw (jaw-thrust manoeuvre) or submentally (chin-lift manoeuvre), avoiding pressure on the soft tissues (Fig. 12.5). In some cases, particularly in edentulous patients, an oropharyngeal airway helps to maintain patent airway.

Ventilation by mask

The lungs may be ventilated by mask and bag using one of two systems. The first is a rebreathing bag with an adjustable valve and fresh gas supply (which should be present in each anaesthetic room, intensive therapy unit and resuscitation room). The second and more widespread is the self-reinflating type of bag such as the 'Ambu' or 'Laerdel' bags, which do not rely on a gas supply but to which supplemental oxygen can be added. For the inexperienced, this technique is best performed with the help of an assistant.

Procedure

The airway is held patent with the patient supine as described above. A mask is applied to the face and held in position using the thumb and index fingers of both hands. The little fingers of each hand are placed behind the angles of the jaw and used to lift the mandible forward. The ring and middle fingers are placed on the mandible to help

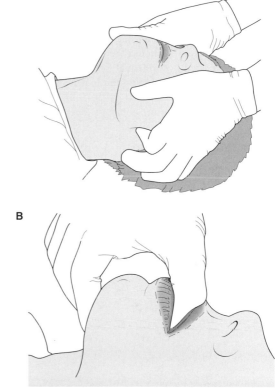

A

B

Fig. 12.5 **A** The jaw-thrust manoeuvre. **B** The chin-lift manoeuvre.

maintain this position. The assistant squeezes the bag to ventilate the lungs. The adequacy of ventilation is assessed by observing the patient's chest movement.

With more experience it is possible to maintain a patent airway and hold the mask on with one hand, and squeeze the bag with the other.

The laryngeal mask airway

This recently introduced airway is designed to be inserted into the pharynx, and has a cuff which when inflated forms a cup around the larynx. It is not a replacement for endotracheal intubation and does not protect the airway from aspiration. It does, however, provide a patent airway when positioned correctly, and allows effective ventilation of the lungs. As with other procedures, insertion should be learned under supervision.

Procedure

The cuff should be deflated and lubricated with gel. The patient's head and neck are positioned as for intubation.

The mask is held in the right hand and introduced into the mouth, and the left hand is used to maintain the head in the extended position (Fig. 12.6). For women a size 3 is suitable and for men a size 4. Smaller sizes are available for children. The mask is passed backwards over the tongue until resistance is felt. It should then be at the level of the larynx at the upper oesophageal sphincter. The cuff is inflated and the mask should be seen to rise slightly out of the mouth. Position is confirmed by the ability to ventilate the lungs with gentle pressure on a bag system.

Endotracheal intubation

Endotracheal intubation can be life-saving: it can maintain a patent airway, facilitate oxygenation and prevent aspiration. The student is advised to take every opportunity to acquire this skill in the elective situation in the anaesthetic room.

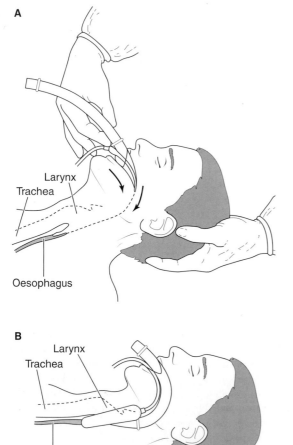

Procedure

The patient's neck is flexed and the head extended at the atlanto-occipital joint. Retaining a pillow under the head but free from beneath the shoulders will usually help to attain this position. Failure to position the patient correctly is one of the commonest causes of difficulty in intubation.

The laryngoscope is held in the left hand and its blade is inserted into the right side of the patient's mouth and passed backwards along the side of the tongue into the oropharynx. The blade is designed to push the tongue over to the left side of the mouth. Care is taken to avoid damage to the lips and teeth. The laryngoscope is *pulled* upwards and forwards, *not* used as a lever, to lift the tongue and jaw and reveal the epiglottis (Fig. 12.7). The blade is then advanced to the base of the epiglottis.

Failure to visualize the epiglottis usually reflects the fact that the blade has not been inserted far enough, in which case only the base of the tongue will be seen. Alternatively, it may mean that it has been inserted too far, in which case the upper oesophagus will be seen. The appropriate adjustment in posi-

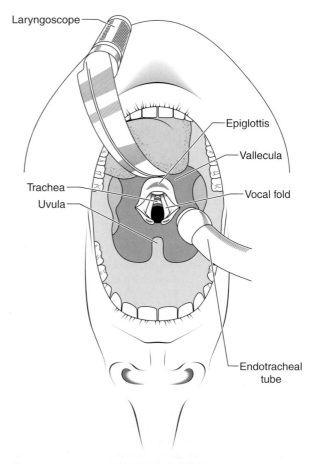

Fig. 12.6 Insertion of a laryngeal mask airway.

Fig. 12.7 Oral endotracheal intubation.

tion should be made. The laryngoscope is pulled further upwards and forwards to reveal the vocal cords.

For women an 8-mm cuffed tube is usually appropriate and for men a 9-mm tube. For children a rough rule of thumb to gauge tube size is age divided by 4 + 4.5 mm. Normally an uncuffed tube is used in children.

The endotracheal tube is passed through the vocal cords into the trachea and advanced until its cuff is about 1 cm through. Many endotracheal tubes have a mark to indicate this position. The laryngoscope blade is then withdrawn and the cuff inflated to provide an airtight seal in the trachea.

The most serious complication of endotracheal intubation is failure to recognize misplacement of the tube, particularly in the oesophagus or, to a lesser degree, in the right main bronchus. Misplacement is best avoided by direct visualization of passage of the tube between the vocal cords, inspection of the chest wall for equal movement of both sides of the chest, and auscultation for breath sounds bilaterally in the midaxillary line. Absence of or the presence of only quiet breath sounds in the epigastrium is a further reassuring sign. If there is any doubt about the position of the tube, it should be removed and ventilation instituted by mask.

Surgical airway

Inability to intubate the trachea is an indication for creating a surgical airway. In the emergency situation, such as in patients with severe facial trauma or pharyngeal oedema secondary to burns, the insertion of a large-caliber plastic cannula through the cricothyroid membrane (**needle cricothyroidotomy**) below the level of the obstruction can be life-saving. Intermittent jet insufflation of oxygen at 15 L/min (1 s inspiration and 4 s to allow expiration) can provide oxygenation for a limited period (30–45 minutes) until a more definitive procedure can be undertaken.

Surgical cricothyroidotomy is performed by making a incision that extends through the cricothyroid membrane and inserting a tracheostomy tube.

In children care must be taken to avoid damage to the cricoid cartilage, which is the only circumferential support to the upper trachea. Surgical cricothyroidotomy is therefore not recommended for children under 12 years of age.

Procedure

It is important to check all the equipment and connections before starting. With the patient in the supine position and the neck in a neutral position, the thyroid cartilage (Adam's apple) and cricoid cartilage are palpated. The cricothyroid membrane lies between the lower border of the thyroid car-

tilage and the upper border of the cricoid cartilage. The skin is cleansed with antiseptic solution and local anaesthetic infiltrated into the skin if the patient is conscious. The thyroid cartilage is stabilized with the left hand and a small transverse skin incision made over the cricothyroid membrane. The blade of the scalpel is inserted through the membrane and then rotated through 90° to open the airway. An artery clip or tracheal spreader may be inserted to enlarge the opening enough to admit a cuffed endotracheal or tracheostomy tube (Fig. 12.8). The central trocar of the tube is removed and the tube connected to a bag-valve or ventilator circuit. The cuff is then inflated and air entry to each side of the chest is checked. The tube is secured to prevent dislodgement.

Formal **open tracheostomy** may be performed as an emergency procedure but is more commonly undertaken to wean critically ill patients from long-term ventilation. It is a procedure for an experienced clinician and involves making an inverted U-shaped opening through the second, third and fourth tracheal rings.

Changing a tracheostomy tube

It is common practice to change a tracheostomy tube every 7 days. Suction must be available.

Procedure

If a cuffed tube is to be inserted the integrity of the cuff is checked and it is then fully deflated. Lubricant gel is applied to both the cuff and tube. The patient is placed semirecumbent with the neck extended. If replacement is likely to be difficult, a suction catheter inserted into the old tracheostomy tube can be used as an introducer for the new tube.

The cuff of the old tube is deflated. Secretions often collect above the cuff and enter the trachea when it is deflated, causing the patient to cough: both patient and operator should be alert to this. Because the tube is curved it should be removed with an 'arc-like' movement. The site is then cleansed and any secretions removed. In the spontaneously breathing stable patient there is no need for undue haste. The new tube is inserted with a similar movement to that employed for removal, and its cuff inflated.

Any signs of respiratory distress should alert one to the possibility of misplacement or occlusion of the tube. The tube and trachea are immediately checked for patency by passing a suction catheter through the tube. If the catheter passes easily into the respiratory tract, usually signified by the patient coughing as the catheter touches the carina, other causes for respiratory distress should be sought.

When the tracheostomy is no longer needed, an airtight dressing is applied over the site after removing the tube. There is no need for formal surgical closure at this stage, as in most instances the wound will close and heal sponta-

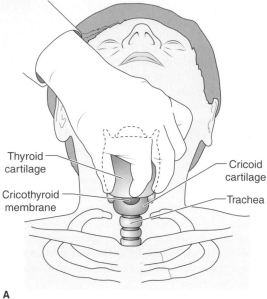

A

Thyroid cartilage

Cricothyroid membrane

Cricoid cartilage

Trachea

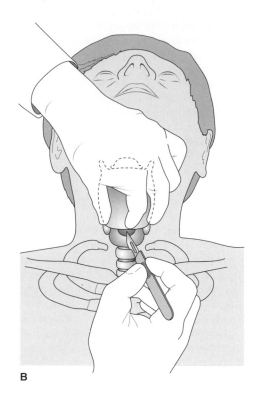

B

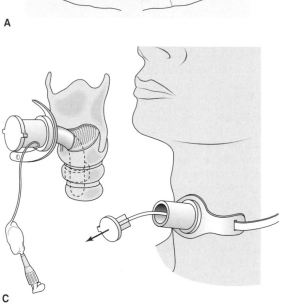

C

Fig. 12.8 Surgical cricothyroidotomy.

neously. For the first few days, the patient should be encouraged to press firmly on the dressing when he or she wishes to cough, so as to avoid air leakage through the tracheostomy site.

THORACIC PROCEDURES

Intercostal tube drainage

Intercostal intubation is used to drain a large pneumothorax, haemothorax or pleural effusion. To drain a pneumothorax, a size 14–16 Fr catheter is inserted using a lateral approach in the midaxillary line of the sixth intercostal space. Drainage of an effusion or haemothorax requires a larger drain (20–26 Fr), which should be inserted in the seventh, eighth or ninth intercostal space in the posterior axillary line. A slightly higher insertion in the midaxillary line may be technically easier in supine, acutely ill patients.

Procedure

If a low lateral approach is to be used, reference should be made to the chest X-ray to ensure that the drain will not be inserted subdiaphragmatically. A strict aseptic technique must be used. The skin, intercostal muscles and pleura are infiltrated with local anaesthetic. If a rib is encountered by the needle the tip is 'walked' up the rib to enter the pleura above the rib edge. The depth at which the pleural space is entered is determined by aspiration with the syringe. A 3-cm horizontal incision is now made in the skin. A tract is developed by blunt dissection through the subcutaneous tissues and the intercostal muscles are separated just superior to the top of the rib to avoid damage to the neurovascular bundle. The parietal pleura is punctured with the tip of a pair of artery forceps and a gloved finger is inserted into the pleural cavity (Fig. 12.9). This ensures the incision is correctly placed, prevents injury to other organs, and permits any adhesions or clots to be cleared. The trocar is removed from the thoracostomy tube, the proximal end is clamped, and then the tube is advanced into the pleural space to the desired length. The tube is sutured to the skin with a heavy suture to prevent accidental dislodgement. A 'Z' suture is placed around the incision, wrapped tightly around the drainage tube and tied, thus securing the tube. A sterile dressing and an adhesive bandage are applied to form an airtight seal and prevent aspiration of air around the tube. The drainage tube is attached to an underwater drainage system and a chest X-ray is then obtained. Low-pressure suction may be applied to the drainage bottle to assist drainage or re-expansion of the lung.

Removal of an intercostal drainage tube

The drainage tube may be removed 12–24 hours after cessation of drainage. As a precaution in the case of pneumothorax, the tube is first clamped for several hours and a chest X-ray taken to ensure that there has been no recurrence.

Procedure

The 'Z' suture is freed from the tube and can be used to close the wound. Where this is not possible, the suture should be removed totally and a new one inserted around the wound. The patient is asked to hold their breath and an assistant withdraws the tube, after which the skin is firmly closed with the previously inserted suture. A sterile dressing is firmly applied over the wound and the chest X-ray repeated to confirm that there is no pneumothorax.

Pleural aspiration

Aspiration of fluid from the pleural cavity is performed for diagnostic or therapeutic purposes. Protein or amylase content, and cytological or bacteriological examination may be diagnostic. Complete aspiration of large effusions allows fuller expansion of the lungs and may improve ventilation.

Procedure

Where aspiration is to be undertaken for diagnostic purposes only, a 21-gauge needle and syringe are adequate. In therapeutic aspiration a larger-bore needle, 50 mL syringe and three-way tap system should be used. The procedure is carried out using a strict aseptic technique.

The patient is positioned sitting up, resting the arms and elbows on a table. The position and size of the effusion should be outlined by percussion and chest X-ray. The lower border of the effusion is determined, particularly on the right to avoid puncturing the liver. In the case of small effusions, ultrasound guidance is helpful.

The skin, intercostal muscles and pleura are infiltrated with local anaesthetic in the seventh or eighth space, in line with the inferior angle of the scapula. A 2-mm stab incision is made in the skin and the needle advanced over the upper

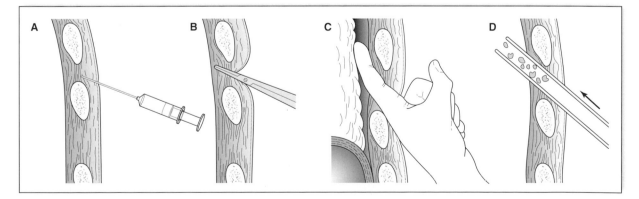

Fig. 12.9 Chest drain insertion. **A** Infiltration of local anaesthesia. **B** Blunt dissection of tissues. **C** Exploration of pleural cavity with gloved finger. **D** Chest drain inserted without the use of a trocar.

border of the rib to avoid damage to the neurovascular bundle. Continuous suction should be applied to the syringe and the needle advanced no further than is required to aspirate fluid freely, thereby avoiding damage to the underlying lung.

If the volume of fluid to be removed is greater than the volume of the syringe being used, a three-way tap greatly reduces the risk of air entry and allows the syringe to be emptied into a collection vessel (Fig. 12.10); this avoids having to disconnect the syringe each time it is filled. It is normally recommended that no more than 1–1.5 L of fluid be removed at any one time. This reduces the risk of sudden mediastinal shift or the development of pulmonary oedema associated with rapid re-expansion of a collapsed lung. Coughing or pain on aspiration is an indication that visceral pleura is in close contact with the end of the cannula, which should be repositioned or withdrawn.

At the end of the procedure the needle is withdrawn and a sterile dressing applied. A chest X-ray is taken to assess the amount of residual fluid present and to exclude a pneumothorax.

VASCULAR PROCEDURES

Venepuncture

The antecubital fossa is the most convenient site as the median cubital vein, median vein of the forearm and the cephalic vein are all easily accessible. Care must be taken

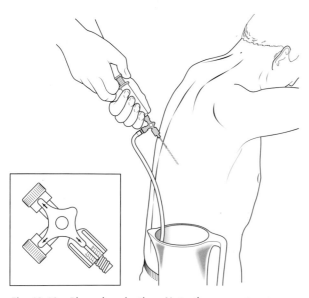

Fig. 12.10 Pleural aspiration. Note three-way tap on needle to enable larger volumes to be aspirated without withdrawing needle.

to avoid the brachial artery. Sampling from smaller veins on the forearm or the back of the hand may at first sight appear more attractive, but these veins collapse easily on aspiration and adequate samples are difficult to obtain. In cases of extreme difficulty the femoral vein should be considered. This vessel lies medial to the femoral artery, which is used as a landmark. In adults a 21-gauge needle is used and in children a 23-gauge or 25-gauge will suffice.

Procedure

A venous tourniquet is applied to the upper arm and the patient encouraged to clench the fist several times to increase venous filling. The position of the vein is identified and the skin cleansed. The needle is advanced through the skin and into the vein, with the needle bevel facing upwards. This manoeuvre is carried out in a 'two-step' fashion, first through the skin and then through the vein wall. Entry through the skin with a decisive action causes much less discomfort than a slow hesitant movement. The needle is advanced 2–3 mm into the vein and the position of the needle and syringe stabilized with one hand. The plunger of the syringe is slowly withdrawn with the other hand until the required amount of blood is obtained. The tourniquet is then released, the needle withdrawn and pressure immediately applied over the site of entry into the vein to prevent haematoma formation, which is painful for the patient and makes subsequent sampling more difficult.

The blood is placed into the appropriate sample tubes after removal of the needle from the syringe. With pre-vacuumed sample tubes the needle should be left on the syringe in order to fill the tubes. Haemolysis invalidates some results, for example potassium and phosphate levels, and is more likely to occur when smaller needles are used. It can be minimized by slow withdrawal of blood into the syringe.

Safety measures

Used needles and syringes should be placed in specially reinforced carriers – 'cin-bins' – to avoid the risk of needle-stick injury or blood contamination to portering or other staff. To further reduce the risk of blood spillage or contamination to medical and laboratory staff, systems have now been introduced in which the sample tubes themselves are modified so that they may be used as syringes, and sent to the laboratory without the need to transfer blood from syringe to tube (e.g. Sarstedt Monovette®).

Venepuncture for blood culture

This procedure is carried out for microbiological culture and identification of organisms that may be present in the blood. The procedure is similar to venepuncture but particular care must be taken to avoid contamination. The skin must be thoroughly cleansed and a strict 'no-touch' technique used.

Procedure

A venous tourniquet is applied as before. The patient's skin is thoroughly cleansed using an appropriate solution and a sterile swab or cottonwool ball. Venepuncture is performed without the operator touching the skin around the site of entry of the needle. After withdrawal the needle is removed from the syringe and a second sterile needle substituted. This is then used to introduce the appropriate aliquot of blood into the culture bottles (both aerobic and anaerobic culture bottles should be used). Exact volumes of blood required and the number of bottles filled will depend on local laboratory policies. All blood culture bottles should be sent immediately to the laboratory or, if this is not possible, placed in an incubator at 37°C until transport is available.

Peripheral venous cannulation

Most intravenous infusions are given into the forearm. The veins of the leg are generally avoided because of the greater risk of thrombosis. Intravenous cannulae should not be sited over joints, if possible, as this necessitates splinting and reduces the free use of the arm by the patient. Even with splinting, cannulae are subject to more movement in these positions and are prone to more complications.

A wide range of cannulae are commercially available but all consist essentially of an outer flexible sheath and an inner metal needle. A 16-gauge or 18-gauge cannula will suffice for most purposes in adults. Where rapid infusions of large quantities of fluid are required, a larger cannula should be used.

Procedure

A venous tourniquet is applied and the site of insertion chosen. The skin is cleansed and local anaesthetic infiltrated intradermally at the insertion site. Venepuncture is made in the 'two-step' fashion described above and confirmed by a 'flashback' of blood into the cannula. The cannula is then advanced 2–3 mm into the vein. The cannula sheath is then advanced into the vein with one hand while the metal needle is partially withdrawn with the other.

Once the cannula sheath is fully inserted into the vein, the tourniquet is released and gentle pressure applied over the vein at the tip of the cannula. The metal needle is then fully withdrawn from the cannula and the giving set, previously primed with normal saline, is connected. The cannula and distal 10–15 cm of the giving set are securely fixed to the skin with adhesive tape.

Cannulation sites should be inspected regularly for signs of swelling, erythema or tenderness, which may indicate extravasation, thrombophlebitis or infection. If any of these is present, or the patient complains of pain at the site, the infusion must be stopped and the cannula resited.

Extravasation may cause tissue necrosis. Thrombophlebitis occurs more readily when small veins are used, or when the pH of the infusate differs significantly from blood pH. The chances of infection increase the longer a cannula is left in situ, and infusion sites must be changed regularly.

Bolus injections through an intravenous cannula should not be made without first ensuring that the cannula is patent and that there is no extravasation.

Venous cutdown

This may be carried out for access for fluid replacement or for access to the central veins for long-term parenteral nutrition or drug administration.

Venous cutdown for fluid replacement is rarely required except in seriously hypovolaemic patients, usually following trauma. The most common site is the long saphenous vein at the ankle (Fig. 12.11). Other sites include the

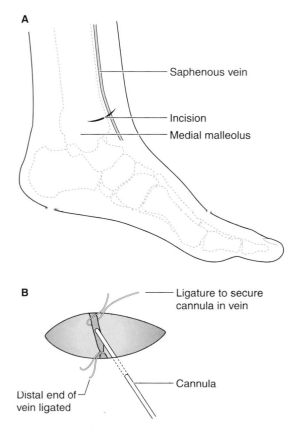

Fig. 12.11 Saphenous venous cutdown.

basilic vein in the antecubital fossa and the cephalic vein in the deltopectoral groove. It should only be regarded as a temporary measure for resuscitation.

Procedure

Venous cutdown is performed with an aseptic technique. Local anaesthetic is infiltrated over the site and a transverse incision is made in the skin over the vein, which is then identified by blunt dissection. At the ankle, the site of cutdown is 2–3 cm anterior to the medial malleolus. The vein should be cleared for a distance of 1–2 cm. The distal end of the vein is ligated with an absorbable ligature. The proximal end of the exposed vein is elevated to prevent backflow of blood, using a second absorbable ligature.

A transverse incision is then made in the vein. A large-bore cannula is passed through the skin 2 cm below the skin incision and guided into the vein. The cannula is advanced beyond the proximal ligature, which is then tied securely. The intravenous infusion is then commenced.

The wound is closed with non-absorbable sutures and the cannula sutured to the skin to prevent accidental displacement. A sterile dressing is applied.

Central venous catheter insertion

Placement of a central venous catheter is indicated for monitoring of the central venous pressure (CVP) and for prolonged drug administration or parenteral nutrition.

Insertion is carried out using a strict aseptic technique, as infection is one of the commonest complications of this procedure. If the catheter is to be used for drug therapy or parenteral nutrition, the procedure should be carried out in the operating theatre. The common sites of insertion of catheters into the superior vena cava are from the internal jugular vein in the neck, from the subclavian vein, or occasionally from a peripheral vein in the antecubital fossa. A variety of cannulae and catheters are available, but in general they are one of three types: (1) an extra-long intravenous cannula; (2) a catheter inserted through a large cannula; and (3) a catheter inserted over a wire (Seldinger technique). Each has advantages and disadvantages.

Internal jugular vein cannulation

Several approaches are described, but the high approach at the level of the thyroid cartilage carries the least risk. The right internal jugular vein is preferred, as this provides a straighter route into the superior vena cava and avoids the risk of damaging the thoracic duct on the left. In general the Seldinger technique is used and several commercial kits are available with the necessary equipment.

Procedure

The patient is placed in a supine position with at least 15° head-down tilt to distend the neck veins and reduce the risk of air embolism. The patient's head is turned to the left unless there is a potential of a cervical spine injury following trauma. A wide area around the right side of the neck is cleansed and draped using an aseptic technique.

The carotid artery is identified at the level of the thyroid cartilage using the index and middle fingers of the left hand. The internal jugular vein lies just lateral and parallel to it. A bleb of 1% lignocaine is injected into the skin at the proposed puncture site.

Using an 18-gauge needle on a 10-ml syringe held in the right hand, the needle is advanced through the skin just lateral to the carotid pulsation, at an angle of 60° to the skin and in the line of the vein (Fig. 12.12). Free aspiration of blood confirms the position of the vein. This manoeuvre is repeated to place a larger (16-gauge) needle in the vein. The flexible 'J' end of the guidewire is now passed through this needle into the vein, and the needle removed over it. This leaves the guidewire in the internal jugular vein. A dilator is now passed over the wire into the vein and then withdrawn. The catheter is then advanced over the wire and then the wire is removed, leaving the catheter in situ. In most adults no more than 15 cm of catheter need be advanced into the vein to ensure correct placement. Blood is then aspirated from the catheter to confirm its position in the major vein. Heparinized saline (5 ml) is injected and the catheter is sutured to the skin to fix it in position. A chest X-ray is taken to check the position of the catheter and to exclude the presence of a pneumothorax, which is a recognized complication.

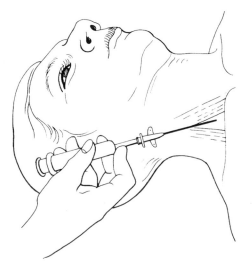

Fig. 12.12 Cannulation of the internal jugular vein. Note the triangle between the sternal and clavicular heads of the sternocleidomastoid muscle.

Subclavian vein cannulation

Several approaches to the subclavian vein are described, but usually a subclavicular one is used. Any approach to the subclavian vein carries a significant risk of causing a pneumothorax or puncturing the subclavian artery. Like all procedures, this one in particular should be learnt under close supervision by an experienced operator. The Seldinger technique is generally used to insert a subclavian catheter. The patient should be placed in a supine position with head-down tilt of at least 15°. A small pad is placed between the shoulder blades to allow the shoulders to drop backwards. Local anaesthetic is infiltrated into the skin and subcutaneous tissue. Under aseptic conditions a large-calibre needle attached to a 10-ml syringe is introduced 1 cm below the junction of the middle and medial thirds of the clavicle. The needle is directed medially, slightly cephalad and posteriorly behind the clavicle towards the tip of a finger placed in the suprasternal notch (Fig. 12.13). Applying suction, the needle is advanced until blood is withdrawn into the syringe. The syringe is then disconnected, a flexible guidewire inserted through the needle and the needle removed. The catheter is subsequently passed over the guidewire and the latter is withdrawn. The catheter is flushed with heparinized saline and fixed in position. A chest X-ray is taken to check the position and exclude a pneumothorax.

Peripheral venous catheterization

In theory this is the safest approach as it avoids the risk of pneumothorax. Haemorrhage from accidental arterial puncture or as a result of a coagulopathy can be controlled by pressure. Thrombosis and thrombophlebitis are, however, more frequent than when either the subclavian or the internal jugular route is used. Normally the long catheter is placed through a large cannula.

Procedure

A venous tourniquet is applied to the arm and a suitable vein in the antecubital fossa through which the catheter can be passed is selected. The area is prepared using an aseptic technique and local anaesthetic is infiltrated into the skin at an appropriate site. The cannula is inserted into the vein as for normal intravenous cannulation, and the needle withdrawn. The long catheter is passed through the cannula into the vein and the venous tourniquet is then released.

The catheter is advanced up the basilic vein and into the superior vena cava. A guide is often provided to gauge the length of catheter inserted. Difficulty is often experienced in advancing the catheter past the axilla, and extension of the arm may help overcome this.

The insertion cannula is then withdrawn from the vein, leaving the long catheter in place. A chest X-ray is taken to confirm placement.

Measurement of central venous pressure (CVP)

The CVP is the pressure in the superior vena cava as it enters the right atrium. The zero point is taken as the level

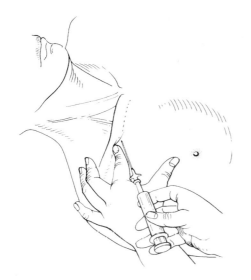

Fig. 12.13 Cannulation of the subclavian vein.

> **SUMMARY BOX**
>
> *Central venous cannulation*
>
> - Air embolism is always a risk, even in the head-down position.
>
> - When using a guidewire, always hold it at some point along its length while it remains in the patient.
>
> - Blood should be easily aspirated from the catheter if it is correctly positioned.
>
> - A chest X-ray should always be taken to confirm the absence of a pneumothorax and correct positioning. A rough guide to position is that the tip of the catheter should lie at the level of the carina on X-ray.
>
> - Cannulae inserted for intravenous nutrition are tunnelled in the subcutaneous tissue to emerge on the chest wall at a distance from the site of entry into the vein (Fig. 12.14). This minimizes the risk of sepsis spreading down the tract into the vein.

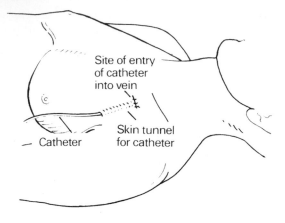

Fig. 12.14 Skin tunnel for central venous catheter.

of the right atrium. With the patient lying supine, the midaxillary line is the surface marking to use as the reference point and is assumed to represent zero or the level of the right atrium (Fig. 12.15). It is often convenient to mark the skin position to provide consistency in the recordings. An alternative surface reference point is the junction of the second rib and the sternum. In the supine patient this is considered to lie 5 cm above the right atrium. Whichever reference point is used, confusion is avoided by remembering that the pressure being measured is in relation to the level of the right atrium. Consistency of recording is achieved by always using the same reference point with the patient in the supine position. A water manometer is normally used to measure this pressure.

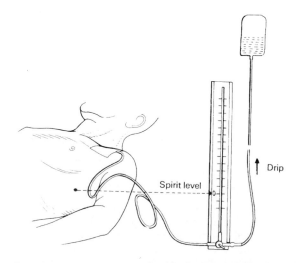

Fig. 12.15 Measurement of central venous pressure. Note the midthoracic point (marked by a black dot), which is used as the zero reference point.

Procedure

The water manometer system is primed with 5% dextrose prior to connection to the central venous catheter. The zero point on the manometer scale is levelled with the chosen reference point. The column is then filled to a higher level than the expected pressure and opened to the central venous catheter. The water column is allowed to fall and equilibrate. Fluctuation of the column with respiration is a reassuring sign of patency and correct positioning. The CVP is the level of the column at end-expiration.

Arterial blood sampling

Arterial blood sampling is undertaken to measure arterial Po_2, Pco_2, $[H^+]$ and standard $[HCO_3^-]$. The radial artery at the wrist is the site of choice. The brachial artery at the elbow and the femoral artery may also be used.

A heparinized sample is required to prevent blockage in the blood gas analyser as a result of coagulation of the sample. There are several commercially available preheparinized syringes, but an ordinary 2-ml syringe which has been preheparinized as described below will suffice.

Procedure

If the syringe is not preheparinized, draw up to 0.5 mL of 1000 units/mL heparin into the syringe. The plunger is then fully withdrawn, following which the air and excess heparin are expelled from the syringe. The residual heparin will be sufficient to anticoagulate the sample. A 23-gauge needle is suitable for arterial puncture.

The course of the artery is defined by palpating the pulse between the index and middle fingers held 2 cm apart. The skin is cleansed and the needle, with its bevel upwards, introduced through the skin at an angle of about 60°. The needle is then advanced into the artery. Correct positioning is confirmed by blood pulsating into the syringe under pressure; 1–1.5 mL is normally sufficient.

The needle is withdrawn and firm pressure applied by an assistant over the puncture site for 3 minutes to avoid haematoma formation. The needle is removed from the syringe and any air bubbles expelled before capping the syringe. The syringe is gently inverted several times to ensure mixing of the heparin. The sample is sent immediately for analysis. Where delay is anticipated it should be transported in ice.

Needle pericardiocentesis

Cardiac tamponade may result from penetrating or blunt trauma to the chest. Cardiac function may be significantly impaired by a minimal amount of blood within the fixed, fibrous pericardium. The classic signs are elevated CVP, hypotension and muffled heart sounds (Beck's triad). Immediate pericardiocentesis may be life-saving.

Procedure

The patient should be monitored throughout this procedure, with particular reference to the vital signs, CVP and ECG. An aseptic technique is used and the skin in the subxiphoid region is infiltrated with local anaesthetic. The skin is punctured 1–2 cm inferior to the left xiphochondral junction with a wide-bore plastic-sheathed needle (at least 15 cm in length) with a syringe attached. The needle is angled at 45° and aimed towards the tip of the left scapula (Fig. 12.16). The syringe is aspirated as the needle is advanced, until it easily fills with blood. ECG changes suggest the needle has been advanced too far. Positive pericardiocentesis must be followed by surgical exploration.

URINARY PROCEDURES

Urethral catheterization

This procedure may be carried out to relieve urinary retention or to determine urine output when it needs to be closely monitored. Occasionally, catheterization is necessary to facilitate nursing the incontinent patient. Anatomical obstruction may often be the cause of urinary retention in the male. It is particularly important to avoid forcing the passage of the catheter in this procedure, and if difficulty is experienced assistance should be sought. A full aseptic technique is required for both male and female catheterization.

Procedure in the male

The shaft of the penis is held with a sterile swab and the urethral orifice cleansed with a non-alcoholic, non-iodine-containing solution. The foreskin, if present, is retracted. The shaft of the penis is held erect with a sterile swab in the left hand and traction applied to elongate the urethra. Lignocaine gel is instilled into the urethra slowly and carefully, with light but steady pressure. It is important to leave the local anaesthetic agent a sufficient length of time before proceeding with catheterization, as difficulty in male catheterization is often caused by poor analgesia.

The urinary catheter is introduced into the urethra with a 'no-touch' technique and advanced to its full length (Fig. 12.17). Correct placement is confirmed by the passage of urine down the catheter. If this does not occur, suprapubic pressure may help. Alternatively, a bladder syringe can be attached to the catheter and aspiration used. With the passage of urine the balloon on the catheter is inflated with the recommended volume of sterile water (generally 10–30 mL). The catheter is gently withdrawn until the balloon engages the bladder neck, and it is then connected to the drainage tubing. The foreskin, where present, should be replaced over the glans to prevent paraphimosis.

Procedure in the female

A 16–18 Fr catheter is suitable for this procedure. The labia minora are separated with the thumb and fingers of the left hand to expose the urethral meatus on the anterior vaginal wall. The pudenda are now swabbed with antiseptic solution. Two swabs are used, each being swept once across the pudenda from anterior to posterior and then discarded.

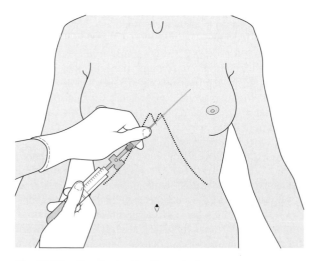

Fig. 12.16   Needle pericardiocentesis.

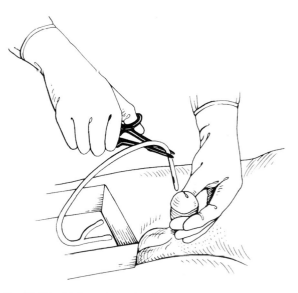

Fig. 12.17   Male catheterization.

In general, the catheter need only be inserted for half its length before the passage of urine confirms correct placement. The balloon is inflated and the catheter withdrawn until the balloon impacts in the bladder neck.

Suprapubic catheterization

This procedure is only appropriate when the bladder is distended and urethral catheterization has failed or is contraindicated. It is carried out with a full aseptic technique.

Procedure

The position of the bladder is determined by percussion. Where available, ultrasound guidance is helpful. Generally the point of insertion lies two finger-breadths above the pubic symphysis in the midline.

The area is cleansed and draped. Local anaesthetic is then infiltrated through all layers of the anterior abdominal wall using an 18-gauge needle. The depth and position of the bladder can be gauged by the free aspiration of urine through this needle. The needle is withdrawn and a stab incision made in the skin. The trocar and catheter are advanced through the incision, into the bladder (Fig. 12.18). Entry into the bladder is confirmed by the loss of resistance, at which point the catheter is advanced as the trocar is withdrawn. Free passage of urine confirms correct placement. The catheter must be advanced far enough into

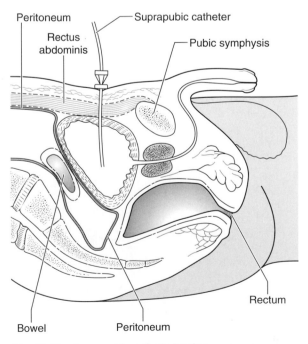

Fig. 12.18 Suprapubic catheterization.

the bladder so that the balloon, when inflated, is well within the bladder. The balloon is then filled with 10 mL of water and a sterile dressing applied.

CENTRAL NERVOUS SYSTEM PROCEDURES

Lumbar puncture

Lumbar puncture is carried out to obtain a sample of cerebrospinal fluid (CSF) for diagnostic purposes, to measure the CSF pressure or to introduce materials into the CSF. It is important to examine the patient beforehand for evidence of raised intracranial pressure, examining in particular the fundi for evidence of papilloedema. Lumbar puncture is contraindicated if there is any suggestion of raised intracranial pressure, as it may result in 'coning' in such patients. The advent of CT scanning has provided a non-invasive aid to the detection of raised intracranial pressure, and in some conditions, such as subarachnoid haemorrhage, has removed the need for lumbar puncture.

Procedure

Lumbar puncture is carried out using a strict aseptic technique. The patient is placed on one side (usually the left) with their back at the edge of the bed or trolley. They are then asked to curl up as much as possible to flex the lumbar spine and open up the interspinous spaces.

The skin is thoroughly cleansed and drapes applied. The space between the spinous processes of the third and fourth lumbar vertebrae is identified by the point at which a vertical line dropped from the highest point of the iliac crest crosses the spine. Local anaesthetic is infiltrated into the skin and subcutaneous tissues to a depth of about 2 cm. A small stab incision is made in the midline, midway between the two spinous processes.

For most purposes a 22-gauge spinal needle is adequate. The needle is inserted through the stab incision and advanced in the midline in a slightly headward direction. Entry into the subarachnoid space is felt with a distinct loss of resistance, and will occur in most adults at a depth of 4–6 cm from the skin.

The stylet is withdrawn from the needle and the position confirmed by the free flow of CSF. If the subarachnoid space is not entered, or bone is encountered, check that the needle has been advanced in the midline. This is best done by observing (from the side) the angle of the needle in relation to the patient's back. If the needle is in the midline, withdraw it and reinsert it in a slightly more headward direction. If the patient experiences pain, a nerve has been touched. The needle should be immediately withdrawn and repositioned.

Once the procedure is complete the needle is withdrawn and a sterile dressing applied. The patient is usually advised to remain supine for at least 12 hours to minimize the risk of developing a 'spinal' headache. Persistent headache may be a result of continued CSF leakage through the puncture in the dura. In these circumstances an anaesthetist should be asked to advise on an epidural 'blood patch'. With modern needles the risk of CSF leakage is lessened and the advice to remain supine for 12–24 hours may be unnecessary.

DRUG ADMINISTRATION

The importance of correct prescription and administration of drugs cannot be overemphasized. Drugs once administered can rarely be retrieved, particularly when they are administered intravenously or intramuscularly. Very few drugs have specific antagonists, with the important exceptions of opiates and benzodiazepines. It is good clinical practice to check drugs with an assistant, particularly where dilutions are involved. Important and useful sources of information include the manufacturer's data sheet, national formulae, hospital formulae and hospital pharmacy drug information services.

SUMMARY BOX

Practice points for drug administration

- Use generic names wherever possible.
- Print generic and, if indicated, proprietary names clearly on the prescription card.
- Check that the correct drug is to be administered.
- Check the patient's identity, particularly if you do not know them.
- Label syringes clearly with the drug, the concentration, and the time and date drawn up.
- Check the compatibility of the diluent.
- Check calculations when diluting drugs or administering on a body-weight basis.
- Check that the correct route of administration in the correct concentration is being used, and that the time over which the drug should be given is correct.
- Carry out checks with an assistant.
- It is good practice to administer only drugs you have drawn up yourself and checked with an assistant, or drugs that have been prepared under conditions which you are satisfied will result in the patient receiving the correct therapy.

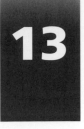

13 Postoperative care and complications

R.W. Parks

INTRODUCTION

Following an operation there are three phases of patient care. After a short period of **immediate postoperative care** in a recovery room to ensure the full return of consciousness, the patient is returned to **surgical ward care** unless there are indications for transfer to a high-dependency unit or intensive therapy unit. On discharge from ward care, the patient may still require **rehabilitation and convalescence** before they are ready to resume domestic or other activities. This chapter discusses the first two phases, during which attention focuses on the regulation of homeostasis and the prevention, detection and management of complications.

The major life-threatening complications that may arise in the recovery room are airway obstruction, myocardial infarction, cardiac arrest, haemorrhage and respiratory failure. These complications can also arise during ward care, but except for haemorrhage and cardiopulmonary catastrophe, many of the problems arising in this phase do not threaten life and are often specific to the operation performed.

IMMEDIATE POSTOPERATIVE CARE

Patients who have received a general anaesthetic should be observed in the recovery room until they are conscious and their vital signs are stable. Acute pulmonary, cardiovascular and fluid derangements are the major causes of life-threatening complications in the early postoperative period, and the recovery room provides specially trained personnel and equipment for the observation and treatment of these problems.

In general, the anaesthetist exercises primary responsibility for the patient's cardiopulmonary function and the surgeon is responsible for the operative site, the wound, and any surgically placed drains. Clinical notes should accompany the patient. These include an operation note describing the procedure performed, an anaesthetic record of the patient's progress during surgery, a postoperative instruction sheet with regard to the administration of drugs and intravenous fluids, and a fluid balance sheet.

Monitoring of airway, breathing and circulation is the main priority in the immediate postoperative period. The nature of the surgery and the patient's premorbid medical condition will determine the intensity of postoperative monitoring required; however, the patient's colour, pulse, blood pressure, respiratory rate, oxygen saturation and level of consciousness will be routinely observed. The nature and volume of drainage into collecting bags or wound dressings, and urinary output are also monitored, if appropriate. Continuous ECG monitoring is undertaken and oxygenation is assessed by the use of a pulse oximeter. Monitoring of central venous pressure (CVP) may be indicated if the patient is hypotensive, has borderline cardiac or respiratory function, or requires large amounts of intravenous fluids.

The patient may initially remain intubated, but following extubation should receive supplemental oxygen by face mask or nasal prongs and should be encouraged to take frequent deep breaths. The patient must breathe adequately and maintain a good colour. Shallow breathing may mean that the patient is still partially paralysed. A dose of neostigmine can reverse the residual effects of curariform agents. Cyanosis is an ominous sign indicating hypoxaemia due to inadequate oxygenation, and may be due to airway obstruction or impaired ventilation.

Airway obstruction

The main causes of airway obstruction are as follows:

- *Obstruction by the tongue* may occur with a depressed level of consciousness. Loss of muscle tone causes the tongue to fall back against the posterior pharyngeal wall, and may be aggravated by masseter spasm during emergence from anaesthesia. Bleeding into the tongue or soft tissues of the mouth or pharynx may be a complicating factor after operations involving these areas.
- *Obstruction by foreign bodies*, such as dentures, crowns and loose teeth. Dentures must be removed before operation and precautions taken to guard against displacement of crowns or teeth.
- *Laryngeal spasm* can occur at light levels of unconsciousness and is aggravated by stimulation.
- *Laryngeal oedema* may occur in small children after traumatic attempts at intubation, or when there is infection (epiglottitis).
- *Tracheal compression* may follow operations in the neck, and compression by haemorrhage is a particular anxiety after thyroidectomy.
- *Bronchospasm or bronchial obstruction* may follow inhalation of a foreign body or the aspiration of irritant material, such as gastric contents. It may also occur as an idiosyncratic reaction to drugs and as a complication of asthma.

Attention is directed at defining and rectifying the cause of airway obstruction as a matter of extreme urgency. Airway maintenance techniques include the chin-lift or jaw-thrust manoeuvres, which lift the mandible anteriorly and displace the tongue forward (Chapter 12). The pharynx is then sucked out, an oropharyngeal airway is inserted to maintain the airway, and supplemental oxygen is administered. If cyanosis does not improve, or if stridor persists, reintubation may be necessary.

Haemorrhage

Significant blood loss via a surgical drain, particularly if associated with hypovolaemic shock, is an indication for immediate transfer of the patient from the recovery room back to the operating theatre for re-exploration and control of the bleeding source. Reactive bleeding is usually caused by a slipped ligature or dislodgement of a diathermy coagulum as the blood pressure recovers from the operation. Superficial bleeding into the surgical wound rarely requires immediate action; however, patients who have undergone neck surgery must be observed for the accumulation of blood in the wound. If necessary the wound can be reopened in the recovery room to prevent airway compression and asphyxia.

Late secondary haemorrhage typically occurs 7–10 days after an operation and is due to infection eroding a blood vessel. Rigid drain tubes may also occasionally erode a large vessel and cause dramatic late postoperative bleeding. Secondary haemorrhage associated with infection is often difficult to control. Interventional radiological techniques may achieve temporary control, but surgical re-exploration is usually indicated.

SUMMARY BOX

Immediate postoperative monitoring

Airway – attention to maintenance of airway
Breathing – ensure adequate ventilation
Circulation – monitor for evidence of blood loss
Assess the patient's
   Colour
   Pulse
   Blood pressure
   Respiratory rate
   Oxygen saturation
   Level of consciousness

SURGICAL WARD CARE

General

Monitoring of vital signs, including temperature, continues on return to the ward. In addition, output from the urinary catheter, nasogastric tube and surgical drains is monitored. The frequency of recordings or measurements can be reduced as the patient stabilizes.

Patients are normally visited morning and evening by the medical staff to ensure that there is steady progress. Anxiety, disorientation and minor changes in personality, behaviour or appearance are often the earliest manifestation of complications. The general circulatory state and adequacy of oxygenation are noted, and vital signs recorded on the nursing chart are checked. Temperature readings provide vital information regarding progress and may give early indication of potentially serious postoperative complications.

The chest is examined and all sputum inspected. Full chest expansion and coughing is encouraged. Following abdominal surgery the abdomen is examined for evidence of excessive distension or tenderness. The return of bowel sounds and the free passage of flatus reflects recovery of gut peristalsis. The legs are checked for swelling, discoloration or calf tenderness.

Tubes, drains and catheters

If a nasogastric tube is in place it is kept open at all times to serve as a vent for swallowed air. Free drainage of gastric contents may be supplemented by intermittent manual aspiration. Nasogastric tubes are removed once the volume of aspirate diminishes. It is not always necessary to wait until bowel sounds have returned or flatus has been passed. Nasogastric tubes are uncomfortable and may prevent coughing with expectoration, and so they should not be retained for longer than necessary. Surgical drains are generally removed when the volume of effluent diminishes. If a urinary catheter has been placed, it should be removed once the patient is mobile.

Fluid balance

Fluid balance is reviewed regularly. The standard intravenous fluid requirement for an adult is 3 L/day, of which 1 L should ordinarily be normal (isotonic) saline and 2 L should be 5% dextrose; however, this should be judged according to the patient's general circulatory status, the observed fluid losses and the daily measurement of serum urea and electrolyte levels. It is not necessary to replace potassium within the first 24–48 hours after surgery as the body's store is sufficient. Potassium supplements (60–80 mmol daily) can subsequently be added to intravenous fluids provided urinary output is adequate. Intravenous fluid therapy is discontinued once oral fluid intake has been established.

Blood transfusion

Haemoglobin measurement will be a guide to the need for postoperative blood transfusion. A full blood count should be undertaken within 24 hours of surgery and, as a general rule, blood administered if the Hb is less than 8 g/dL. Above this level patients can be prescribed oral iron, unless they have cardiovascular instability or are symptomatic from their anaemia. If a blood transfusion is given, pulse, blood pressure and temperature should be recorded to detect a transfusion reaction. Major ABO incompatibility can result in an anaphylactic hypersensitivity reaction, with severe bronchospasm and hypotension, whereas incompatibility of minor factors may result in tachycardia, pyrexia and rash. Other potential complications of blood transfusion are hypothermia (if the blood has not been adequately warmed), hyperkalaemia (due to leakage of potassium from the red blood cells), acidosis (if the blood has been stored for a long period) and coagulation abnormalities (as stored blood is deficient in clotting factors).

Nutrition

Nutrition in postoperative patients is frequently poorly managed. A few days of starvation may cause little harm, but enteral or parenteral nutrition is essential if starvation is prolonged. Enteral nutrition is preferred as it is associated with fewer complications and is believed to augment gut barrier function. If a prolonged period of starvation is anticipated in the postoperative period, a feeding jejunostomy tube can be inserted at the time of abdominal surgery. Alternatively, a fine-bore nasogastric or nasojejunal feeding tube can be passed (Chapter 12). If the enteral route cannot be used, total parenteral nutrition can be prescribed. Dietary intake should be monitored in all patients in the postoperative period, and oral high-calorie supplements given if appropriate.

COMPLICATIONS OF ANAESTHESIA AND SURGERY

General complications

Nausea and vomiting can be caused by surgery and/or anaesthesia, and an antiemetic can prove useful. If nausea has been associated with previous anaesthetics, antiemetic drugs should be administered prophylactically. Transient hiccups in the first few postoperative days are usually no more than a nuisance. Persistent hiccups can be a serious complication, exhausting the patient and interfering with sleep, and may be due to diaphragmatic irritation, gastric distension or metabolic causes, such as renal failure. If no precipitating cause can be found, small doses (25 mg) of intravenous chlorpromazine may be helpful.

Spinal anaesthesia may cause headache as a result of leakage of cerebrospinal fluid, and patients should remain recumbent for 12 hours after this form of anaesthesia. If headache persists it may be necessary to seal the injection site in the dura–arachnoid by a 'blood patch' (i.e. an extradural injection of the patient's blood, which clots and so seals the leak). Myalgia affecting the chest, abdomen and neck is a specific complication of suxamethonium administration, and may last for up to a week.

Intravenous administration of irritant drugs or solutions can cause bruising, haematoma, phlebitis and venous thrombosis. Intravenous cannulae, particularly those placed in large veins, should be securely sealed to guard against air embolism. Sites of cannula insertion should be checked regularly for signs of infection, and the cannula replaced if necessary. Arterial cannulae and needle punctures are the commonest cause of arterial injury, and may rarely lead to arterial occlusion and gangrene.

Pulmonary complications

Respiratory complications remain the largest single cause of postoperative morbidity and the second most common cause of postoperative death in patients over 60 years of age. Pulmonary complications are more common after emergency operations. Special hazards are posed by pre-existing chronic obstructive airways disease (COAD). Once a patient has fully recovered from anaesthesia the main respiratory problems are pulmonary collapse and pulmonary infection. Pleural effusion and pneumothorax occur less commonly. Pulmonary embolism is a major complication of deep venous thrombosis, which is considered later.

Pulmonary collapse

Inability to breathe deeply and cough up bronchial secretions is the primary cause of pulmonary collapse after surgery. Contributory factors include paralysis of cilia by anaesthetic agents, impairment of diaphragmatic movement, oversedation, abdominal distension and wound pain. When there is complete obstruction of a bronchus or bronchiole, air in the lung distal to the obstruction is absorbed, the alveolar spaces close (atelectasis) and the affected portion of the lung contracts and becomes solid. Small bronchioles (1 mm or less) are prone to close when lung volume reaches a critical point (closing volume). The closing volume is higher in older patients and in smokers, owing to the loss of elastic recoil of the lung, which increases the risk of atelectasis. The extent of collapse varies from closure of a small segment to collapse of a lobe or, when a main bronchus is obstructed, the entire lung. Atelectasis is a very common complication of surgery and usually occurs within 24 hours. It is of clinical relevance because it leads to increased work of breathing, impaired gas exchange and a predisposition to infection.

The clinical signs of pulmonary collapse include rapid respiration, tachycardia and mild pyrexia, with diminished breath sounds and dullness to percussion over the affected segment. Arterial PaO_2 is low and the chest X-ray shows areas of increased opacification.

Postoperative pulmonary collapse is prevented by encouraging the patient to breathe deeply, cough and mobilize. Adequate analgesia and regular chest physiotherapy are of great importance in the postoperative period. Placement of an epidural catheter in patients undergoing major abdominal surgery may help alleviate postoperative wound pain. Hypoxia is treated by giving oxygen by mask or nasal prongs, and bronchospasm is relieved by inhalation of salbutamol.

When hypoxia is severe, endotracheal intubation, assisted ventilation and repeated bronchial aspiration may be needed. Posture is important and the patient should be placed initially on the unaffected side to aid expansion of the collapsed lung. Bronchoscopy may be needed to suck out a plug of inspissated secretion.

Pulmonary infection

Pulmonary infection commonly follows pulmonary collapse or the aspiration of gastric secretions. Pyrexia, tachypnoea and green sputum are typical. The chest signs are those of collapse with absent or diminished breath sounds, often in association with bronchial breathing and coarse crepitations from surrounding areas of partial bronchial occlusion. Chest X-ray usually demonstrates patchy fluffy opacities.

The patient is encouraged to cough, and antibiotics are prescribed after sending sputum for bacteriological examination. Most pulmonary infections are caused by the respiratory commensals *Streptococcus pneumoniae* and *Haemophilus influenzae*, but many postoperative pulmonary infections are caused by Gram-negative bacilli acquired by aspiration of oropharyngeal secretions. Antibiotics provide the mainstay of treatment. Oxygen is given if there is hypoxia, and more intensive measures, including bronchoscopy and assisted ventilation, are instituted if respiratory function continues to deteriorate.

Respiratory failure

Respiratory failure is defined as an inability to maintain normal partial pressures of oxygen and carbon dioxide (PaO_2 and $PaCO_2$) in arterial blood. Blood gas determinations are the key to its early recognition and should be repeated frequently in patients with previous respiratory problems. The normal PaO_2 is >13 kPa at the age of 20 years, falling to around 11.6 kPa at 60 years; respiratory failure is denoted by a value of less than 6.7 kPa. Severe hypoxaemia may result in visible central cyanosis.

Acute respiratory distress syndrome (ARDS)

ARDS is characterized by impaired oxygenation, diffuse lung opacification on chest X-ray and an increasing 'stiffness' of the lungs (decreased compliance). It may result from pulmonary or systemic sepsis, following massive blood transfusion, or as a consequence of aspiration of gastric contents. The syndrome displays a wide spectrum of severity. Many minor and transient cases recover spontaneously, whereas in a proportion of cases progressive respiratory insufficiency occurs. Tachypnoea with increasing ventilatory effort, restlessness and confusion develop. Hypoxia initially responds to increasing the oxygen content of inspired air, but progressively increasing concentrations are required to prevent the PaO_2 from falling. The pathophysiology is unclear, but endotoxin-activated leukocytes are thought to be deposited in the pulmonary capillaries, releasing oxygen-derived free radicals, cytokines and other chemical mediators. Damage to the vascular endothelium results in increased capillary permeability and leakage of fluid, causing widespread interstitial and alveolar oedema. This is seen as bilateral diffuse fluffy opacities on chest X-ray. The lungs become increasingly stiff and difficult to ventilate. Management includes supportive measures in the form of ventilation with positive end-expiratory pressure (PEEP) and treatment of the underlying condition, i.e. control of infection by antibiotics, drainage of any source of pus, correction of hypovolaemia. The mortality rate of severe ARDS is approximately 50%.

Pleural effusion

Small pleural effusions are not uncommon following upper abdominal surgery, but are usually of no clinical significance. They may be secondary to other pulmonary pathology, such as collapse/consolidation, pulmonary infarction or secondary tumour deposits. The appearance of a pleural effusion 2–3 weeks after an abdominal operation may suggest the presence of a subphrenic abscess. Small effusions may be left alone to reabsorb if they do not interfere with respiration. Alternatively, pleural aspiration is performed and the fluid sent for bacteriological culture.

Pneumothorax

The most common cause of postoperative pneumothorax is the insertion of a central venous line, and a chest X-ray is necessary after this procedure to exclude this potential complication. There is also an enhanced risk of pneumothorax in patients on positive-pressure ventilation, presumably owing to rupture of pre-existing bullae. The insertion of an underwater seal drain is usually followed by rapid expansion of the lung.

Cardiac complications

The risks of anaesthesia and surgery are increased in patients suffering from cardiovascular disease. Whenever possible, arrhythmias, unstable angina, heart failure or hypertension should be corrected before surgery. Valvular disease, especially aortic stenosis, impairs the ability of the heart to respond to the increased demand of the postoperative period. The administration of fluids to patients with severe aortic or mitral valve disease should be carefully monitored.

Myocardial ischaemia/infarction

Although in most cases there is a history of preceding cardiac disease, myocardial ischaemia or cardiac arrest can occur in an otherwise fit patient. Patients with ischaemia may complain of gripping chest pain, but this is not invariable (particularly in the elderly diabetic patient, or in the early postoperative period) and hypotension may be the only sign. The absence of symptoms after operation is thought to be due to the residual effects of anaesthesia and to the administration of postoperative analgesia. If ischaemia is suspected, an ECG is performed urgently and arrangements are made for cardiac monitoring. A sample of

blood is withdrawn to estimate concentrations of cardiac enzymes. One-third of postoperative myocardial infarctions are fatal.

Cardiac failure

Although acute cardiac failure occurs most often in the immediate postoperative period, patients with ischaemic or valvular heart disease, arrhythmias or major surgical insult can also go into failure in the subsequent recovery period. Clinical manifestations are progressive dyspnoea, hypoxaemia and diffuse congestion on chest X-ray. Excessive administration of fluid in the early postoperative period in patients with limited myocardial reserve is a common cause, which can be avoided by monitoring central venous pressure. Treatment consists of avoiding further fluid overload, and the administration of diuretics and cardiac inotropes.

Arrhythmias

Sinus tachycardia is common and may be a physiological response to hypovolaemia or hypotension. It is also caused by pain, fever, shivering or restlessness. Tachycardia increases myocardial oxygen consumption and may decrease coronary artery perfusion. Sinus bradycardia may be due to vagal stimulation by neostigmine, pharyngeal irritation during suction, or the residual effects of anaesthetic agents.

Atrial fibrillation is the commonest postoperative arrythmia. Fast atrial fibrillation may result in haemodynamic disturbances and may require pharmacological intervention. Refractory cases may require cardioversion.

Urinary complications
Postoperative urinary retention

Inability to void postoperatively is common, especially after groin, pelvic or perineal operations, or following operations under spinal/epidural anaesthesia. Postoperative pain, the effects of anaesthesia and drugs, and difficulties in initiating micturition while lying or sitting in bed may all contribute. Males tend to be more commonly affected than females. When its normal capacity of approximately 500 mL is exceeded, the bladder may be unable to contract and empty itself. Frequent dribbling or the passage of small volumes of urine may indicate overflow incontinence, and examination may reveal a distended bladder. The management of acute urinary retention is catheterization of the bladder, with removal of the catheter after 2–3 days (Chapter 12).

Urinary tract infection

Urinary tract infections are most common after urological or gynaecological operations. Pre-existing contamination of the urinary tract, urinary retention and instrumentation are the principal factors contributing to postoperative urinary infection. Cystitis is manifested by frequency, dysuria and mild fever, and pyelonephritis by high fever and flank tenderness. Treatment involves adequate hydration, proper drainage of the bladder and appropriate antibiotics.

Renal failure

Acute renal failure after surgery results from protracted inadequate perfusion of the kidneys. The commonest cause of postoperative oliguria is prerenal vascular insufficiency from hypovolaemia, water depletion or extracellular fluid depletion. Hypoperfusion of the kidney may be aggravated by hypoxia, sepsis and nephrotoxic drugs. Patients with pre-existing renal disease and jaundice are particularly susceptible to hypoperfusion, and are more likely to develop acute renal failure.

The complication can largely be prevented by adequate fluid replacement before, during and after surgery, so that urine output is maintained at 0.5 mL/kg/h or more. The importance of monitoring hourly urine output means that bladder catheterization is needed in all patients undergoing major surgery, and in those at risk of renal failure. Early recognition and treatment of bacterial and fungal infections is also important in the prevention of renal failure.

Urine output below 700 mL in 24 hours (or less than 0.5 mL/kg/h for several hours on catheter drainage) should be considered pathological oliguria. Management involves the restoration of an adequate circulating intravascular compartment by the administration of intravenous fluids. A CVP line is usually required to measure circulating blood volume. Diuretics may be administered only if the patient is well hydrated; however, they should not be continually prescribed if the patient remains oliguric. Low-dose dopamine may increase renal blood flow.

Acute postoperative renal failure occurs when the reversible stage of acute renal insufficiency progresses to acute tubular necrosis. Volume loading becomes potentially dangerous with established renal failure, and the mainstays of treatment at this stage are the replacement of observed fluid loss, plus an allowance of approximately 500 mL/day for insensible loss and restriction of dietary protein intake to less than 20 g/day. Biochemical status is checked by frequent estimations of serum urea and electrolytes. Hyperkalaemia can be treated by intravenous administration of insulin and glucose or cation exchange resins. Haemofiltration or haemodialysis may be indicated if conservative measures fail to prevent rapid rises in serum concentrations of urea and potassium. Recovery from acute tubular necrosis can be anticipated in survivors after 2–4 weeks. The patient will then enter a polyuric phase, in which fluid and electrolyte balance requires careful monitoring. The mortality rate in patients who develop postoperative renal failure is 50%.

Cerebral complications

Cerebrovascular accidents (CVA)

These are usually precipitated by sudden hypotension during or after surgery in elderly hypertensive patients with severe atherosclerosis. They are a specific complication of carotid endarterectomy, occurring in 1–3% of cases, but may also complicate cardiac surgery.

Neuropsychiatric disturbances

These occur frequently and cover a wide spectrum of disorders. The most common is mental confusion with agitation, restlessness and disorientation, and is known as delirium. It usually occurs in the elderly and may arise on a background of dementia due to cerebral atrophy, but is often precipitated by the use of sedative or hypnotic drugs.

Acute toxic confusion state is a well recognized acute psychiatric disorder that occurs in some patients during a serious illness or after a major surgical intervention. Many factors can contribute, and it is important to look for a treatable cause, such as hypoxia, sepsis, or a metabolic disturbance such as uraemia or electrolyte imbalance. Sleep deprivation, particularly in intensive care units, can also cause severe mental disturbance.

Delirium tremens (acute alcohol withdrawal syndrome)

Delirium tremens occurs in alcoholics who stop drinking suddenly. In most instances this can be predicted from a detailed history. Prodromal symptoms include personality changes, anxiety and tremors. The fully developed condition is characterized by extreme agitation, visual hallucinations, restlessness, confusion and, rarely, convulsions and hyperthermia. If symptoms are mild, treatment involves the prescription of oral diazepam and vitamin B. Control of extreme agitation may require intravenous administration of diazemuls, droperidol or haloperidol.

Venous thrombosis and pulmonary embolism

These complications are discussed in detail in Chapter 27, but the essential details are summarized here for convenience.

Deep venous thrombosis (DVT)

The incidence of deep venous thrombosis varies with the type of operation and the associated risk factors, which include increasing age, obesity, prolonged operations, pelvic and hip surgery, malignant disease, previous DVT or PE (pulmonary embolism), varicose veins, pregnancy, and use of the oral contraceptive pill.

Measures to prevent DVT include taking care to avoid prolonged compression of the leg veins during and after the operation; the use of graded compression support stockings (TED stockings); mechanical or electrical compression of the calf muscles during surgery; and subcutaneous heparin (5000 units 12-hourly). Many surgeons use low molecular weight heparin (at doses recommended by the manufacturer) in all patients over 40 who require a general anaesthetic.

DVT is frequently asymptomatic, but may give rise to calf tenderness and swelling of the foot and leg. Duplex ultrasonography is now the investigation of choice for diagnosing DVT. Ascending venography may be used to confirm the presence and extent of thrombosis, and is particularly useful for iliofemoral thrombosis. Radiolabelled fibrinogen uptake can also be used to detect DVT, but at present its use is limited to patients being screened for DVT.

If the thrombosis is confined to the calf and is less than 5 cm long, anticoagulation may not be indicated. Thrombosis affecting the iliofemoral segment of the deep veins carries a significant risk of embolism, particularly when the clot is non-occlusive, and the patient should be anticoagulated. If there is suspicion of pulmonary embolism or the venogram shows a tail of non-occlusive thrombus, consideration should be given to inserting a filter into the vena cava.

Anticoagulation is commenced with an intravenous bolus of heparin (5000 units) followed by a continuous intravenous infusion of 1000–2000 units/h, the dose being adjusted to maintain a whole-blood clotting time of two to three times the normal value. Heparinization is normally continued for 7–10 days and then gradually substituted by long-term oral anticoagulation using warfarin. The induction dose of warfarin is 10 mg/day, the dose being adjusted to maintain a prothrombin time (now reported as the International Normalized Ratio [INR]) at two to three times normal. The INR is measured daily until the ratio stabilizes.

Tinzaparin is a low molecular weight heparin which has been shown to be as effective as dose-adjusted unfractionated heparin for the treatment of DVT. The dose is calculated in relation to the weight of the patient and no monitoring of the clotting time is required; 175 iu/kg body weight is administered subcutaneously once daily for at least 6 days and until the INR is within the therapeutic range.

Pulmonary embolism

Massive pulmonary embolus with severe chest pain, pallor and shock demands immediate cardiopulmonary resuscitation, heparinization and urgent CT pulmonary angiography. Fibrinolytic agents such as streptokinase or urokinase can be infused intravenously to encourage clot lysis if the patient is at least 6 days post surgical intervention, or in extreme cases the clot can be removed at open pulmonary embolectomy under cardiopulmonary bypass.

If a small embolus is suspected in a patient complaining of chest pain, sometimes in association with tachypnoea, haemoptysis and a pleural rub and effusion, a radioisotope perfusion–ventilation lung scan (V/Q scan) is the key investigation. A chest X-ray and electrocardiogram (ECG) are advisable, mainly to rule out alternative causes of pain and collapse. If the V/Q scan reveals lobar or segmental perfusion defects, the patient is heparinized and monitored carefully. In such cases it is also important to search for the source of the embolus; if phlebography reveals thrombus in the iliofemoral segments then a filter can be inserted into the inferior vena cava to prevent further pulmonary emboli.

SUMMARY BOX

Complications of anaesthesia and surgery

General complications
  Nausea and vomiting
  Hiccups
  Headache

Pulmonary complications
  Pulmonary collapse
  Pulmonary infection
  Respiratory failure
  Acute respiratory distress syndrome (ARDS)
  Pleural effusion
  Pneumothorax

Cardiac complications
  Myocardial ischaemia/infarction
  Cardiac failure
  Arrhythmias

Urinary complications
  Urinary retention
  Urinary tract infection
  Renal failure

Cerebral complications
  Cerebrovascular accidents (CVA)
  Neuropsychiatric disturbances
  Delirium tremens

Venous thromboembolism
  Deep venous thrombosis
  Pulmonary embolism

Wound complications
  Wound infection
  Wound dehiscence

Warfarin therapy is recommended in all patients who have sustained a pulmonary embolus, and therapy is normally continued for 3–6 months.

Wound complications

Infection

This is the commonest complication in surgery. The incidence varies from less than 1% in clean operations to 20–30% in dirty cases. Subcutaneous haematoma is a common prelude to a wound infection, and large haematomas may require evacuation. The onset is usually within 7 days of operation. Symptoms include malaise, anorexia, and pain or discomfort at the operation site. Signs include local erythema, tenderness, swelling, cellulitis, wound discharge or frank abscess formation, as well as an elevated temperature and pulse rate. If a wound becomes infected it may be necessary to remove one or more sutures or staples prematurely to allow the egress of infected material. The wound is then allowed to heal by secondary intention. Antibiotics are only required if there is evidence of associated cellulitis or septicaemia. If the wound infection is chronic the presence of a suture sinus or an entero-cutaneous fistula must be excluded.

Dehiscence

The incidence of abdominal wound dehiscence should be less than 1%. Wound dehiscence may be partial (deep layers only) or complete (all layers, including skin). A serosanguinous discharge is characteristic of partial wound dehiscence. The extrusion of abdominal viscera through a complete abdominal wound dehiscence is known as evisceration. This rare complication usually occurs within the first 2 weeks after operation. Risk factors include obesity, smoking, respiratory disease, obstructive jaundice, nutritional deficiencies, renal failure, malignancy, diabetes and steroid therapy; however, the most important causes are poor surgical technique, persistently increased intra-abdominal pressure, and local tissue necrosis due to infection. The wound should be resutured under general anaesthesia. Incisional herniation complicates approximately 25% of cases.

14 Day-case surgery
A.S. Evans, S. Paterson-Brown

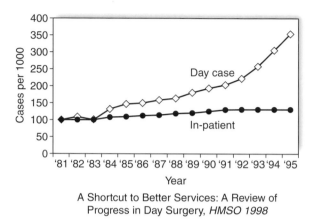

A Shortcut to Better Services: A Review of Progress in Day Surgery, *HMSO 1998*

Fig. 14.1   Changes in the number of patients treated as inpatients and day cases.

INTRODUCTION

Although day-case surgery has been performed for over 50 years it has taken the increasing economic constraints on healthcare over the last 10 years to produce the changes in culture that have resulted in the increase we see today (Fig. 14.1). This chapter will attempt to outline some of the reasons behind these changes and describe the type of patients and procedures suitable for day-case surgery, along with the process involved in the delivery of surgical care.

The Royal College of Surgeons of England published guidelines on day-case surgery in 1985, and subsequent support from the government followed in 1990. The definition of a surgical day case, according to these guidelines, is a patient who is admitted for investigation or operation on a planned, non-resident basis (i.e. goes home in the evening), and occupies, for a period, a bed or unit set aside for this purpose. This should exclude those patients who can be dealt with competently on an ambulatory basis in A&E or outpatients.

REASONS FOR DAY-CASE SURGERY

It is clear that the ability to perform a procedure as a day case has many advantages. These are highlighted in Table 14.1 along with some of the disadvantages.

Cost efficiency

In terms of cost efficiency, many factors must be taken into consideration. Day surgery is not cheap and the emphasis should be put on efficiency of expenditure rather than overall cost. Day surgery should aim to provide an intensive, efficient service with high turnover and minimal disruption to patients. For these reasons day surgery units should be well equipped with up-to-date facilities, and also be diverse enough to allow utilization by many specialties for a wide spectrum of patients. Many hospitals have now decided to invest in independent day surgery units, which prevent beds from being used by emergency patients.

Major cost-saving areas have been identified, including the reduction in routine, inappropriate preoperative investigations and excessive and repetitive documentation. As

Table 14.1 Advantages and disadvantages of day surgery

Advantages	Disadvantages
More cost efficient	Less immediate follow-up
Reduction of waiting lists for certain procedures	Unexpected need for inpatient care postoperatively
Consultant-based service	Dependence on other services, e.g. A&E, GP if problems occur
Reduced patient stress of being in hospital	Not all patients suitable
Quicker, e.g. GP fast-tracking	Not all specialties available

the majority of units run on a 5-day basis this also allows a reduction in nursing and medical staffing costs overnight and at weekends. Although it is difficult to quantify the added expenditure in terms of reliance on other services (such as A&E, GP and district nurses) in the event of a problem outside the hospital setting, it is generally agreed that this adds up to considerably less than inpatient hospital care.

Accommodation factors

Patients utilize a bed for only a short period of time, and when procedures are performed in specialist day surgery units beds in the general hospital wards are left available for others who require more specialist input. This has the advantage of improved continuity of care for the inpatient, but also allows the continuation of elective surgery in times of inpatient bed shortage. Some units are now able to sustain a rate of service that allows two patients to use a bed in the same day. All this has a significant impact on inpatient waiting lists, and allows both groups of patients to be treated more quickly.

The other main advantage of short-term care is early mobilization and a reduction in the subsequent risk of thromboembolic disease, as patients are increasingly encouraged to begin mobilizing as early as possible following their surgery.

Psychological aspects

The psychological benefits of day-case surgery are apparent from patient questionnaires, which have consistently revealed that the majority of patients prefer day care to inpatient care. This is particularly relevant in children, for whom the stresses of being in hospital can be overwhelming. The ambience of a specialist day unit and the ability to

return home to a familiar environment quickly after surgery goes a long way to alleviating these stresses, and also reduces any anxieties regarding future hospital visits. Another positive feature from the patients' viewpoint is the fact that services are generally consultant led, although nurse run, and any contact is usually with a specialist. The majority of patients are given a date for their surgery on the day of their clinic visit, allowing planning around the procedure. Patients with certain conditions, particularly lesions amenable to local anaesthetic removal, do not require clinic review and can be added straight to a list, thereby reducing the clinic waiting list and inconvenience to the patient.

Disadvantages

Unfortunately, day-case surgery does have certain disadvantages. Not all procedures are suitable for the day-case unit and not all patients are suitable for day-case surgery. Some considered suitable may turn out to require ongoing investigation or care after surgery. Furthermore, because patients come in on the morning of surgery, some may have to be cancelled for a number of reasons, including uncontrolled hypertension, new-onset disease, such as diabetes, or abnormal results of investigations performed at booking which have not been reviewed before admission. However careful preoperative assessment and efficient planning should keep these cancellations to a minimum.

REFERRAL FOR DAY-CASE SURGERY

Referral for day surgery can come about in a number of ways and the common methods will be discussed (Fig. 14.2).

Referral from clinic

This is the most conventional method of referral and occurs when the patient is seen in the outpatient clinic, considered

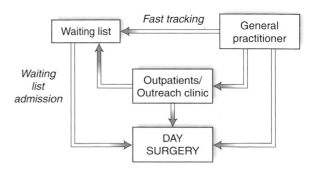

Fig. 14.2 Flowchart for day-surgery referral.

suitable for day-case surgery and referred directly to the day unit for preassessment. This is advantageous as it allows all the necessary details to be discussed and planned in a single trip, and means that if the strict criteria for suitability are not met the patient can be referred back to the surgeon for alternative arrangements to be made. It also allows for any investigations required to be performed that day, so that the results can be reviewed in time for surgery.

Waiting-list admission

This occurs when patients requiring a procedure suitable to be performed as a day case are added to a day-case surgery waiting list. Following discussion with the appropriate clinicians, the bed manager takes patients from this list and invites them for preassessment. Patients are given a date for surgery and an appointment for preassessment.

This produces a structured operating list using the 'first come, first served' principle. However, this system has inherent flaws. Patients are invited for preassessment with little knowledge of their pre-existing medical and social circumstances. This often means that they are unsuitable for day-case surgery, thus wasting valuable preassessment time as well as inconveniencing the patient. Patients may also fail to attend their preassessment appointment.

Outreach clinics

Many consultants provide clinics in peripheral settings such as local cottage hospitals or health centres, and many of the patients seen in these clinics are suitable for day surgery. These patients can then be referred to the day surgery unit for preassessment, or can be seen in these outreach clinics by preassessment nurses.

Direct GP referral

This is a relatively new method of referring patients for a day-case procedure and is usually reserved for the more minor procedures carried out under local anaesthesia. It is the process whereby patients visit their GP with a problem remediable by day-case surgery and are added directly to a day-case list following discussion with the unit manager. These patients will not meet their consultant until the day of operation, and will only have received postal or telephone information regarding their procedure and the unit. No formal preassessment is usually required.

With increasing demand for integrated care pathways this method of referral might become increasingly popular for other procedures, such as hernia repair, provided clear protocols are established between GPs and surgeons.

PREASSESSMENT

Preassessment is one of the most important aspects of day-case surgery. It will identify concurrent diseases, and therefore the appropriate preoperative investigations, and at the same time provide time for explaining the procedure to the patient.

All patients having general anaesthesia require preassessment, and it may also be necessary for patients undergoing certain local anaesthetic procedures, when additional investigations might be required, such as for liver biopsy. Patients undergoing most local anaesthetic procedures do not require a detailed preassessment.

The interview

Patients deemed suitable by the surgeon for a day-case procedure undergo an interview with the preassessment nurse. This usually takes the form of a sit-down discussion in the same outpatient clinic or in the day-surgery unit, but can often be conducted at another mutually convenient time or over the telephone. At this interview a number of important points are covered; some of these are outlined in Table 14.2.

The interview is usually led by a senior member of the nursing staff with experience in day-case surgery, and is conducted according to protocols and a unit operational policy. These protocols should be agreed on and reviewed regularly by managers, anaesthetists, surgeons, physicians and nurses.

Ideally all details are kept in a unitary record that will follow the patient through their surgery, acting as a quick and easy reference and avoiding unnecessary replication. An example of this is given in Figure 14.3.

At the beginning of the interview a patient's personal details are taken, including a telephone number in case of a short-notice cancellation. Details of past medical history and previous surgery are obtained, as well as a list of medications and any allergies. All patients have their height,

Table 14.2 Important points covered at preassessment
Date of procedure
Attendance details and transport arrangements
Unit procedure
Detailed explanation of surgery, including patient information sheets
Description of likely postoperative experiences
Procedure specific postoperative instructions
Questions outside outpatient clinic setting

DAY CASE SURGERY ASSESSMENT FORM
PATIENT SELF-ASSESSMENT (please answer the following questions)

Have you ever had: **Yes/No**

1. Any surgical operations? ☐/☐
Please list:

2. Any anaesthetic or surgical problems? ☐/☐
Please list:

3. Is there a family history of ☐/☐
anaesthetic problems?
Please list:

4. Any other serious illnesses? ☐/☐
Please list:

Social History: **Yes/No**

1. Can someone accompany you home ☐/☐
in a car or taxi?
2. Does/can someone responsible stay ☐/☐
in the house with you post-surgery?
3. Do you have a telephone? ☐/☐
4. Do you have easy access to a toilet? ☐/☐
5. How many flights of stairs do you have
to climb to get to your front door? ☐ ☐
6. Do you smoke?
   1 = never;
   2 = stopped > 6 months;
   3 = stopped < 6 months;
   4 = current
      (How many per day?) ☐ / day
7. Do you drink alcohol? ☐/☐
If you answered yes, how much per week?

Please tick the box if you suffer from any of the following conditions:

1. Chest pain on exercise or at night ☐
2. Asthma, bronchitis or significant breathing problems ☐
3. High blood pressure ☐
4. Heart murmur ☐
5. Fits or faints ☐
6. Yellow jaundice ☐
7. Indigestion, heartburn or acid reflux ☐
8. Diabetes ☐
9. Arthritis or neck problems ☐
10. Anaemia or other blood problems ☐
11. Excessive bleeding or bruising ☐
12. Kidney or waterwork problems ☐
13. Weakness of muscles ☐
14. Do you have a pacemaker? ☐

What medicines do you take?
Please list:

Do you have any allergies?
Please give details:

SURGEON'S ASSESSMENT

1. Diagnosis?

2. Proposed prcedure?

3. Anaesthetic proposed?

4. Pre-operative investigations required?
Please tick those required:

ECG ☐
(over 60 years old or ischaemic heart disease)
U & E's ☐
(on diuretic therapy)
FBC ☐
(history of anaemia/menorrhagia)
Sickle ☐
(Afro-Caribbean)
Other (please specify) ☐

Considered suitable for day case procedure? ☐/☐

Fig. 14.3 Day-case surgery assessment form.

weight, pulse and blood pressure recorded, along with a urinalysis. Their body mass index (BMI) is then calculated using the following equation:

$$\text{Body mass index} = \frac{\text{Weight (kg)}}{\text{Height (m}^2)}$$

Key: *26–32* Overweight
32–40 Obese
>41 Grossly obese

The values and answers obtained are then checked against the protocols and anyone not fulfilling the desired criteria is returned to the referring surgeon with an explanation. The surgeon can then add that patient to their inpatient waiting list or contact the GP to arrange treatment prior to reassessment.

Investigations

If the criteria are fulfilled the patient then undergoes any appropriate investigations as per protocol. These should be minimal, and a possible protocol is suggested below:

- Electrocardiogram – all patients over 60 years old + those with heart disease, hypertension or long-term diabetes
- Urea and electrolyte estimations – all patients taking diuretics
- Sickle test – all Afro-Caribbean patients.

Other preoperative investigations should be performed as clinically indicated, but should again be kept to a minimum.

Information

One of the keys to a successful preassessment interview is the transfer of information to the patient. This should be done in a relaxed atmosphere, so that on the day of their operation patients will understand what is happening and why. Patients will often take little away from their consultation with the doctor owing to a combination of anxiety and pressure on time. The preassessment interview should cover all the relevant points relating to the patient's procedure and anticipated experience, in addition to allowing them time to ask any questions. Relatives should be encouraged to participate in this process. Invariably people will forget what has been discussed, or be unable to explain to relatives what is wrong with them. For this reason many units provide patient information sheets, which give a brief description of the procedure and the postoperative instructions (Fig. 14.4). A number to call in case of emergencies or should further questions arise, should also be included in this document. Informed consent should be obtained by the surgeon undertaking the procedure, either in the clinic or on the day of surgery, depending on whether there is likely to be a significant delay.

Patient selection

Day surgery is expanding in terms of the procedures available and the spectrum of patients on whom they can be performed, and this growth is expected to continue. The decision to refer a patient for a day-case procedure ultimately lies with the surgeon who reviews the patient in the outpatient clinic and who will be performing the operation. Certain standards should be met to ensure that the patients will undergo their procedure with minimal upset, and ultimately that the procedure will be safe. A number of social and medical factors influence this decision, and a few of these are outlined in Table 14.3. Many of these will directly influence (a) suitability for a day-case procedure, (b) the type of operation performed, (c) the type of anaesthetic undertaken and (d) the need for special precautions.

Coutraindications to day surgery

It is generally accepted that the following are considered contraindications to day surgery:

- Patients with unstable/significant medical conditions which will usually make them ASA 3 and 4 (see Table 14.4)
- Gross obesity (BMI >41)
- Operation likely to exceed 2 hours
- Type of procedure unsuitable (as defined by each specialty)
- Hypertension (diastolic >100 mmHg)
- Severe gastro-oesophageal reflux disease (lying flat or bending)
- Poorly controlled diabetes
- History of anaesthetic complications and certain drugs, e.g. warfarin
- Poorly controlled asthma
- Sickle-positive (sickle trait is OK)
- Cervical spine or mandible problems
- Lives >1 hour's travelling time/does not have someone responsible to take them home

Table 14.3 Patient factors influencing suitability for day-case surgery
Age
Demographics
Past medical history
Medications
Convenience and patient preference
Transport availability
Home circumstances
Anaesthetic considerations and ASA status

DAY CASE SURGERY ~ PATIENT INFORMATION SHEET

HERNIA

A hernia is a bulge in the abdominal wall due to a weakness in the muscle wall. At your operation the weakness will be identified and repaired using either stitches or a nylon mesh. This procedure is often carried out as a day case, but even when you go home there will still be discomfort in your groin for five to seven days. You may go back to normal activities as soon as you feel able, and this will usually depend on pain. There is a small incidence of recurrent hernias (i.e. the same hernia returning over the following years). This only occurs in approximately 2% of patients and if this does occur you should contact your GP.

Wound/stitches/dressings

The skin will have been closed with either a long continuous stitch visible only at either end of the wound, or with separate individual stitches or dissolvable stitches. We will let you know if and when they are to be removed. The wound may bleed a little and if so press firmly over the wound for 5 minutes. If the wound becomes hot, red, swollen or painful, go to your GP or Accident and Emergency.

Pain

We will give you a supply of pain killers. Take these regularly for the first 24-48 hours then take as necessary thereafter. Do not wait until you have pain.

Work/driving/exercise

You should plan to take the first 2 weeks after surgery relatively quietly. The amount of exercise is limited by discomfort but once this has settled normal activities including lifting can be resumed. You should not drive until you are able to do an emergency stop comfortably - practise this before driving!

Bathing/showering

Avoid bathing/showering for a couple of days. Your dressing may come off the first time you bath - this is all right and does not need to be replaced.

Follow-up

A follow up appointment will not normally be made to see the surgeon again but this can be arranged via your GP or the Day Surgery Unit. There is a small incidence of recurrent hernias i.e. a hernia reappearing over the following years. This only occurs in approximately 2-5% of cases. There is a small chance of a degree of numbness below the wound. This should not cause undue concern and usually settles in time.

Fig. 14.4 Day-case surgery patient information sheet: hernia.

- No-one responsible living in the same house
- No access to telephone
- Difficult access to house (too many stairs to front door).

Social factors Social problems are the most common reason for a patient being deemed unsuitable for day-case surgery. Conditions in the patient's home should be suitable to allow a speedy and comfortable recovery, and the absence of a responsible adult at home in case of problems, an accessible toilet and access to a telephone in case of an emergency are all contraindications to day-case surgery.

Age Age should not be an absolute discriminating factor and no age at present signals a cut-off in most units. However, elderly patients are more likely to have social and medical issues that will exclude them from consideration. Recovery of fine motor skills and cognitive functions is slowed with increasing age, and this necessitates a longer period of postoperative supervision. At the other end of the spectrum the very young (less than 6 months) are reported to have an increased incidence of postoperative apnoeic episodes and should be observed overnight.

Demographics The distance a patient lives from the day-surgery unit is very important. It is recommended that the journey home take no more than 1 hour and that their house is accessible to emergency services should these be required. For this reason people living in isolated areas cannot be considered.

Patients' demographic details are also relevant in terms of where their surgery is carried out. This may ultimately influence their waiting time for surgery owing to the difference in waiting-list size between units.

Medications It is important to identify those drugs that might have an adverse effect on the outcome of the anaesthetic or the procedure itself. It is essential that, in conjunction with the anaesthetists, protocols be drawn up highlighting any drugs of particular concern so that appropriate action can be taken at an early stage. The use of anticoagulants will most often exclude someone from day-case surgery involving incision or biopsy, and aspirin should be stopped 10 days prior to surgery. For certain procedures women taking the oral contraceptive pill are recommended to stop this 6 weeks before surgery to reduce the risk of thromboembolic disease. Those taking oral hypoglycaemics should be told to omit them on the morning of surgery, but otherwise patients should be instructed to take all regular medications as normal, unless contraindicated.

The use of certain medications, such as diuretics and lithium, will necessitate the patient undergoing certain preoperative investigations. Provided the results are normal this should not serve to exclude them from a day-case procedure.

Past medical history Clues from the patient's past medical history should become apparent at the initial consultation as to their suitability for day surgery. If something is missed there are safety nets further down the line to prevent unsuitable patients being referred, and this will be discussed in a later section. Insulin-dependent diabetics are not generally considered suitable for day-case surgery unless they are very well controlled. Most other comorbid conditions should not serve to exclude someone, provided control of these conditions is satisfactory and, if necessary, a decision can be made following discussion with appropriate specialists (e.g. cardiologist, respiratory physician, endocrinologist and anaesthetist) before the day of surgery. However the anaesthetist will have the final say.

Anaesthetic considerations It is generally agreed that those patients not falling into classes 1 or 2 of the American Association of Anesthesiologists (ASA) classification of physical status should not be considered for day surgery (Table 14.4). Some units allow certain ASA class 3 patients to undergo day surgery provided their condition is not maintained by medication. Past anaesthetic reactions are also very important for obvious reasons, and if anaesthetic complications are suspected, inpatient facilities should be easily available.

Special considerations Other important points to pick up on which may influence decisions regarding the suitability for and nature of surgery performed are listed in Table 14.5. As discussed earlier, day-case surgery may be ideal for children provided parents are willing to accept the responsibility of aftercare. The provision of the service for children should allow for the fact that nurses with paediatric training are required, and that the ward area has facilities for the accommodation of both child *and* parent. The unit must also have facilities available for paediatric anaesthesia and cardiopulmonary resuscitation.

Table 14.4 American Society of Anesthesiologists (ASA) new classification of physical status

Class 1 The patient has no organic, physiological, biochemical or psychiatric disturbance. The pathological process for which operation is to be performed is localized and does not entail a systemic disturbance.

Class 2 Mild to moderate systemic disturbance, caused either by the condition to be treated surgically or by other pathophysiological processes.

Class 3 Severe systemic disturbance or disease, from whatever cause, even though it may not be possible to define the degree of disability with finality.

Class 4 Severe systemic disorders that are already life-threatening, not always correctable by operation

Class 5 The morbid patient who has little chance of survival but is submitted to operation in desperation.

Table 14.5 Factors that might influence day-case surgery – special considerations
Previous anaesthetic problems
Previous surgery
Children
Infections, e.g. HIV, hepatitis B or C, MRSA
Religious beliefs, e.g. Jehovah's Witness
Sickle-cell disease
Cardiac pacemakers and use of bipolar diathermy
Psychiatric conditions

Table 14.7 General surgical procedures performed as day cases
Minor anal procedures, e.g. lateral sphincterotomy
Laparoscopy – diagnostic and therapeutic
Hernia – unilateral or bilateral laparoscopically
Varicose veins
Minor oral surgery, e.g. release tongue tie, biopsies
Family planning – vasectomy, female sterilization
Excision of skin lesions
Minor breast surgery
Endoscopy

Finally, it is important to remember that patient preference should be one of the most important discriminatory factors. Following a careful explanation of procedure at preassessment the patient should be allowed to make an informed decision. The other advantage of this process is that the patient has the opportunity to broadly select a date that is convenient for them in terms of work or travel, and which allows them to make early preparations for their surgery.

PROCEDURES

The Royal College of Surgeons of England in their guidelines on day-case surgery suggest a number of procedures that should be suitable. However, the final choice will depend on clinical judgement and the facilities available. Some of the principles to be considered when carrying out an operation as a day case are shown in Table 14.6.) Table 14.7 gives examples of general surgical procedures that are currently carried out as day cases.

Certain general surgical procedures merit further discussion owing to the increasing trend to perform them as day cases. Laparoscopic cholecystectomy, one of the more common operations performed in general surgical units, is currently under review regarding its feasibility as a day-case procedure. Early studies are encouraging and there is no doubt that it is feasible; however, some studies have reported a high (20% or higher) rate of planned day cases requiring overnight care owing to postoperative nausea, vomiting and pain, or because of conversion to an open procedure. There are also a small number of patients who will require readmission following complications, but it has been shown that this is no more frequent than those operated on as an inpatient. Laparoscopic hernia repair is also feasible as a day-case procedure, particularly for bilateral or recurrent hernias, which usually require an overnight stay. Although more expensive than conventional open surgery it has been shown to result in an earlier return to normal activities and less postoperative pain.

Another common general surgical procedure worthy of mention is day-case haemorrhoidectomy. Previous practice has been to monitor these patients as inpatients until their bowels have opened, before discharge home. Recent studies have now shown that haemorrhoidectomy is feasible and safe when performed as a day case, with little difference in postoperative pain or complication rates compared with inpatient care. A small readmission rate is to be expected, usually secondary to bleeding or pain, and some series have shown that a minority of patients said that if they had to undergo a subsequent haemorrhoidectomy they would prefer inpatient care.

Many other specialities utilize day-surgery facilities and they each have their own recommended procedures. Some of these merit mention because they are common procedures that until recently would have placed a large strain on inpatient facilities. They include:

Table 14.6 Principles applied when considering a procedure for day surgery
Duration (not absolute)
Minimal risk
Low complication rate
Possibility of early mobilization
Minimal postoperative pain
Experience of surgeon
Facilities available
Type of anaesthetic

Ophthalmology – Cataract correctional surgery
                    – Correction of strabismus
Orthopaedics – Arthroscopy
                    – Carpal tunnel release
                    – Dupuytren's contracture release
                    – Manipulations and plaster changes

Gynaecology	– Surgical termination of pregnancy
	– Hysteroscopy
	– Diagnostic laparoscopy
	– Laparoscopic sterilization
ENT	– Removal of foreign bodies and EUA
	– Insertion of grommets
	– Nasal polypectomy
	– Manipulation of nasal fractures
	– Diagnostic laryngoscopy, pharyngoscopy and oesophagoscopy – rigid and flexible
	– Removal of vocal cord lesions.

Recent attention has also been directed towards the possibility of day-case tonsillectomy. As one of the most common childhood operations, day-case tonsillectomy is already popular in the USA. Some early UK studies suggest that this is feasible in children, with no increase in reactionary haemorrhage rates or postoperative pain compared with inpatients. However, studies carried out on adult populations have shown that a high proportion of patients preferred to stay overnight for analgesia and control of nausea and vomiting.

Decision for surgery

The decision to undertake a procedure as a day case should involve a number of factors, of which the length of time the procedure will take is important. The Royal College of Surgeons' of England guidelines suggest no more than 30 minutes per case, although with recent advances in day-case anaesthesia and antiemetics this can be extended, in some units to 2 hours. In order to maximize cost-effectiveness a number of procedures should be undertaken on each list. The complexity of the procedure should be appropriate to the experience of the surgeon and the facilities of the unit, as well as the experience of the nursing staff. The likelihood of complications should be seriously considered, as those that require other specialists or facilities not on site should lead to that procedure not being performed as a day-case.

Training opportunities

For the above reasons many of the procedures are for common conditions and so provide excellent training opportunities for junior staff. As a lot of day surgery is consultant led this provides an opportunity for intensive one-on-one teaching and demonstration of basic skills. Day surgery provides a setting for a sound practical education, with expert assistance should problems be encountered.

DAY-CASE ANAESTHESIA AND POSTOPERATIVE CARE

Anaesthetic considerations and the anticipated degree of postoperative pain and nausea are important factors that make a procedure suitable for day-case operation.

For all procedures the patient should be fasted from the previous night, or early on the morning of operation for afternoon procedures. The anaesthetist reviews all patients, as well as the results of any preoperative investigations, before surgery, and at this time any previous anaesthetic problems can be discussed and premedication prescribed.

Day-case anaesthesia should ideally include (a) a rapid smooth onset of action, particularly in the absence of pre-medication; (b) rapid recovery without residual side-effects and active metabolites; and (c) absence of adverse effects, such as nausea and vomiting.

Day-case surgery can be conducted under general, regional or local anaesthesia (with or without sedation). The choice of anaesthetic depends on the patient and surgical factors, including previous anaesthetic reactions and any requirement for paralysis.

General anaesthesia

General anaesthesia remains the most popular technique, especially with the newer agents that cause less of a 'hang over' effect. Intravenous agents are generally used for induction, and maintenance is usually performed with an inhalational agent, although for some cases intravenous maintenance is used. The risks of day-case general anaesthesia are the same as for any general anaesthetic.

Airway control is secured with an endotracheal tube or laryngeal mask. The latter has a lower incidence of postoperative sore throat and fewer requirements for muscle relaxation, as well as avoiding some of the haemodynamic responses encountered when inserting endotracheal tubes. There is, however, an increased risk of gastric aspiration with laryngeal masks compared with endotracheal intubation. For other procedures, especially those that are very short, some anaesthetists use only a face mask and an oropharyngeal airway.

Local and regional anaesthesia

Many day-case procedures are performed under local anaesthesia. This avoids the potential hazards and side-effects of general anaesthesia while at the same time resulting in fewer requirements for postoperative nursing and a faster return home.

Simple procedures may be performed using only local infiltration, whereas others may require a field block. Epidural and spinal anaesthesia are occasionally used for lower-extremity operations, but their use is limited by persisting sympathetic blockade requiring longer post-operative observation.

Pain

The minimization of postoperative pain is of paramount importance in day-case surgery. Ideally pain should be controllable using conventional oral analgesia *before* discharge. Potent opioid analgesics, e.g. fentanyl, alfentanyl and morphine, are still used but cause a significant increase in nausea and vomiting. Another technique employed to reduce postoperative pain is the infiltration of the wound with local anaesthetic, or a regional block while the patient is still under general anaesthesia. This means that the patient is comfortable on coming round from the anaesthetic, and works on the basis that preventing pain is superior to treating it.

Patients should be discharged with a small supply of take-home medication, usually combining a paracetamol-based compound with a potent non-steroidal anti-inflammatory agent.

Nausea and vomiting

Nausea and vomiting remain the most troublesome side-effects following day-case anaesthesia and are a common cause of unexpected overnight admission. A variety of agents, used both prophylactically and therapeutically, have been used to combat nausea, including metoclopramide and droperidol, but these unfortunately have significant psycho-motor side-effects. Use of the newer agent ondansetron has improved the treatment of drug-induced postoperative vom-

iting, and also has fewer side-effects. However, it is significantly more expensive than other, more conventional agents.

Discharge arrangements

All patients are seen after surgery by both anaesthetist and surgeon. Once they are fully recovered the procedure is explained to them and instructions given regarding further follow-up, including arrangements for removal of sutures, wound review, and what to do if there are any problems. Although these should all have been covered in the preoperative assessment and patient information sheet, it is best to go over it again with each patient before discharge.

Day case surgery has been well established in paediatric practice for longer than in adult practice. Children requiring minor operative procedures under general anaesthetic recover well at home in a familiar and friendly environment. The provision of local anaesthetic regional blocks using long-acting local anaesthetic agents has had a major impact on the acceptability of such surgery in children. Home visits by suitably trained paediatric nursing staff in the post-operative period provide both patients and parents with the necessary reassurance and support to allow such surgery to be undertaken successfully.

Conditions which are suitable for day case surgery in children include inguinal herniotomy, ligation of a patent processus vaginalis (hydrocele), release of tongue tie, umbilical herniorraphy, circumcision, orchidopexy, minor plastic surgery procedures (including laser therapy for pig-

Procedure	Management executive targets for 1997 (%)	Accounts Commission proposed targets (%)
Inguinal hernia – adults	10	20
Inguinal hernia – children	60	80
Breast lumpectomy	60	65
Anal fissure operation	70	75
Varicose veins	20	40
Cystoscopy	80	80
Circumcision	60	80
Dupuytren's contracture	20	50
Carpal tunnel release	80	85
Arthroscopy	65	75
Ganglion	85	90
Orchidopexy	25	60
Cataracts	1	80
Squint correction	25	80

Table 14.8   Areas where day surgery is underutilized

mented skin lesions), upper gastrointestinal endoscopy, diagnostic cystoscopy and surgery to correct bat ears.

THE FUTURE

The Accounts Commission undertook an audit of day-case surgical services in 1998. This revealed that a higher percentage of elective surgery was being performed as day cases (Fig. 14.1) and that more dedicated day-surgery units had been set up since 1991. However, areas were identified where day-case surgery was still underutilized and recommendations made to the different health authorities and trusts to review and implement changes (Table 14.8).

With the increase of minimally invasive surgery and superior anaesthesic techniques there may come a time when the majority of operations will be performed on a day-case, ambulatory or 23-hour basis.

Ambulatory surgery

Ambulatory surgery, if the American definition is used, includes all patients who leave hospital within 23 hours. It is more than 'day surgery' and represents an approach to healthcare that capitalizes on technological developments and which optimizes the service delivered to patients. It encompasses the patient's journey from GP consultation through treatment and care on a 23-hour basis to discharge, or ongoing care in a primary care setting. Care packages are run according to strictly tailored protocols understood by all and agreed with GPs to ensure appropriate referral and levels of treatment.

The aims of ambulatory care are (a) to maximize one-stop, minimal-stop and locally accessible services wherever possible; (b) to increase day surgery and direct access to secondary care services from primary care and (c) to utilize advances in medical and information technology to promote flexibility in service provision and accessibility.

SUMMARY BOX

- The use of day-case surgery has been dramatically increasing over recent years.

- Not all patients are suitable for day-case surgery and carefully designed protocols are required to prevent late cancellations.

- An increasing number of procedures are now being performed on a day-case basis, in particular minimally invasive procedures.

- Facilities must be available for inpatient care if required.

- There are still opportunities to increase the provision of day-case surgery in order to come in line with recent government recommendations.

- Ambulatory or 23-hour surgery is one way to increase the provision of current day surgical services.

SECTION 3
UPPER GASTROINTESTINAL SURGERY

15 Abdomen, abdominal wall and hernia

R.W. Parks

THE ABDOMINAL CAVITY AND THE PERITONEUM

Surgical anatomy

The abdominal cavity extends from the level of the nipples above to the level of the gluteal crease below. It is lined by the parietal peritoneum, a thin sheet of smooth glistening mesothelium which also covers the abdominal viscera (visceral peritoneum). The peritoneal cavity has a greater and a lesser sac, the two being connected by the epiploic foramen. The omentum (Fig. 15.1) is a double fold of peritoneum which connects the liver to the stomach (lesser omentum) and the stomach to the transverse colon (greater omentum). The greater omentum is folded back on itself, but the potential extension of the lesser sac is normally obliterated by adhesions. The peritoneum is relatively resistant to infection, but contamination in conditions such as the perforation of a hollow viscus leads readily to peritonitis.

Ascites

Ascites, or the accumulation of free fluid within the peritoneal cavity, can occur in many diseases (Table 15.1). The fluid is frequently clear and straw-coloured, as in chronic liver disease; bloodstained fluid suggests malignancy, cloudy fluid suggests infection, and white milky fluid suggests chylous ascites due to blockage of the thoracic duct. Protein concentration is often used to determine whether ascitic fluid is a transudate (< 25 g/L) or an exudate (> 25 g/L), although this division is of limited value in that protein concentrations show wide variations in different diseases. Particularly high protein concentrations are found in tuberculous peritonitis, hepatic venous congestion and pancreatic ascites (leakage of pancreatic juice associated with pancreatic duct disruption due to acute pancreatitis or trauma, producing ascitic fluid with a very high amylase content).

Clinical features

Ascites is characterized by dullness to percussion in the flanks when the patient is lying supine. 'Shifting dullness' may be demonstrated if the patient lies on one side, resulting in a shift of the level at which resonance on percussion gives way to dullness owing to fluid gravitating to the

Table 15.1   Common causes of ascites
Transudates
Hypoalbuminaemia
Nephrotic syndrome
Malnutrition
Raised central venous pressure
Congestive cardiac failure
Hepatic vein obstruction
Chronic liver disease
Liver malignancy
Portal vein obstruction
Exudates
Inflammatory disease
Malignancy
Chylous ascites
Miscellaneous causes

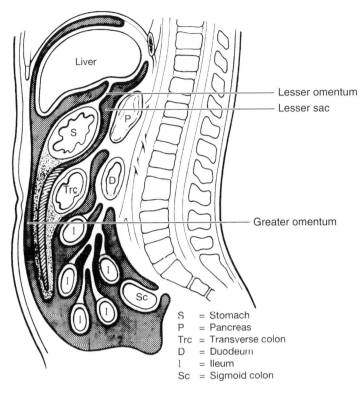

S = Stomach
P = Pancreas
Trc = Transverse colon
D = Duodeum
I = Ileum
Sc = Sigmoid colon

Fig. 15.1 Sagittal section through the abdomen showing the arrangement of peritoneal folds which form the lesser and greater omentum.

dependent part of the peritoneal cavity. A 'fluid thrill' can also be elicited in patients with ascites. One hand is placed flat on the flank while the opposite flank is tapped or flicked with the other hand. If a thrill is felt, transmission through the anterior abdominal wall must be prevented by placing the hand of the patient or an assistant in the midline of the abdomen (Fig. 15.2).

Investigations

On plain films of the abdomen, when there is a large amount of free fluid, ascites produces a ground-glass appearance. Ultrasonography can detect as little as 50 mL of free fluid, and may be used to confirm the diagnosis.

Paracentesis carried out under local anaesthesia (Ch. 11) can be used to relieve discomfort and obtain samples of ascitic fluid for bacteriology, cytology and biochemistry (protein and amylase concentration). Peritoneal biopsy may also be helpful if tuberculous peritonitis is suspected.

Treatment

Treatment is directed at the cause of ascites where possible. Bed rest, restriction of sodium intake (and in some cases

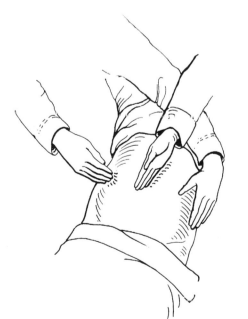

Fig. 15.2 Clinical detection of fluid thrill due to ascites.

water intake) and diuretic therapy are the mainstays of treatment of non-malignant ascites. Intractable ascites may be an indication for peritoneovenous shunting (using a Le Veen or Denver shunt) or a transjugular intrahepatic porto-systemic stent shunt (TIPSS) procedure. The instillation of chemotherapeutic drugs (e.g. bleomycin) may be considered for malignant symptomatic ascites.

SUMMARY BOX

Ascites

- Free peritoneal fluid may be detected by shifting dullness or eliciting a fluid thrill; ultrasonography will detect as little as 50 mL of fluid.

- The commonest causes of ascites are liver disease and intraperitoneal malignancy.

- High protein concentrations (> 25 g/L) are found in tuberculous peritonitis, hepatic venous obstruction and pancreatic ascites.

- Pancreatic ascites is due to leakage of fluid from the pancreatic duct system, and the amylase content of the peritoneal fluid exceeds that of the serum.

- Bed rest, restriction of salt intake and diuretics (e.g. spironolactone) are the mainstays of treatment if the underlying cause cannot be rectified.

- Intractable ascites may justify the insertion of a peritoneovenous shunt or TIPSS insertion; in malignant ascites peritoneal instillation of chemotherapy (e.g. bleomycin) may be worthwhile.

Peritonitis

Inflammation of the peritoneum is a common feature of the acute abdomen. Peritonitis can be classified as acute or chronic, septic or aseptic, and primary or secondary. Acute suppurative peritonitis secondary to visceral disease is the commonest form of peritonitis in surgical practice (Table 15.2), but primary peritonitis is rare. Chronic peritonitis due to tuberculosis is now rare, but can cause abdominal pain, ascites or obstruction due to matting of the bowel by dense adhesions. Aseptic peritonitis is generally due to chemical (e.g. bile, urine, blood, gastric contents, meconium) or foreign-body irritants (e.g. starch, talc, cellulose), and is frequently followed by secondary bacterial peritonitis.

Secondary acute peritonitis

Irritation of the peritoneum by leaking bile, gastric juice, pancreatic enzymes or urine produces an exudate which is

---

Table 15.2 Causes of peritonitis

Acute suppurative peritonitis
  Primary peritonitis
  Secondary peritonitis
    Inflammatory disease of viscera
    Perforation of bowel or biliary tree
    Infection of the female genital tract
    Penetrating injury of abdominal wall
    Rupture of intra-abdominal abscess
    Strangulation of gut

Tuberculous peritonitis
    Ascitic tuberulous peritonitis
  Plastic tuberculous peritonitis

Aseptic peritonitis
Granulomatous peritonitis
Postoperative peritonitis

---

initially sterile but which invariably becomes infected within 6–12 hours. In other cases (e.g. perforated diverticular disease) there is infection from the outset. As peritonitis develops, inflammation of the visceral and parietal peritoneum produces a purulent exudate. In some conditions (e.g. acute cholecystitis or acute appendicitis) peritonitis may remain localized for some time, whereas in others (e.g. perforated peptic ulcer) it may rapidly disseminate (Fig. 15.3). Localization depends on adhesions forming between viscera and the capacity of the omentum to 'wall off' infection. When localization fails, the peritoneal cavity fills with foul-smelling purulent fluid and the intestine becomes flaccid and dilated and covered with fibrinous plaques that form adhesions between bowel loops.

In small children, secondary acute peritonitis can present late. Most frequently, a non-specific illness comprising anorexia, fever, vomiting and diarrhoea followed by abdominal pain and abdominal distension is seen. Abdominal X-rays will show distended loops of small and large bowel with or without gas/fluid levels on the erect or decubitus film. The specific underlying cause of the peritonitis is often not obvious but acute appendicitis is usually the explanation.

Clinical features

The symptoms associated with secondary acute peritonitis depend on the nature of the underlying primary condition. Inflammation of the parietal peritoneum produces somatic pain which is localized to the site of infection. As infection spreads throughout the peritoneum the pain becomes diffuse. Irritation of the diaphragm may be accompanied by pain referred to the shoulder tip. Movement and coughing tenderness. The abdomen becomes silent as paralytic ileus supervenes and the pulse rate and temperature rise.

In advanced peritonitis vomiting becomes more profuse and faeculent. Sequestration of fluid and electrolytes in the peritoneal cavity and in the dilated loops of small intestine results in hypovolaemia, dehydration and electrolyte imbalance. Pain often abates at this stage, and the abdomen becomes less rigid but more distended. The pulse is rapid and there is often a combination of hypovolaemic and septic shock. Without adequate treatment, respiratory, renal and cardiac failure ensues.

Investigations

Leukocytosis and haemoconcentration are common laboratory findings. Serum electrolytes often vary, but the urea concentration is usually elevated. Serum amylase may help to differentiate acute pancreatitis. Blood gas analysis may show a metabolic acidosis. Plain abdominal films may point to the cause of the peritonitis, but often merely reveal dilated flaccid loops of bowel. Free air may be seen under the diaphragm on an erect chest X-ray when perforation of a hollow viscus has occurred.

Management

The primary objective is to deal promptly and effectively with the underlying cause. For example, perforation of a viscus must be repaired, infarcted bowel must be resected, and infective foci should be removed or drained. Operation is undertaken with minimal delay. The only time which should be spent before operation is that needed to resuscitate an ill patient. It is imperative that extracellular fluid volume is replaced adequately, and central venous pressure monitoring is essential in critically ill and elderly patients. A nasogastric tube should be inserted to empty the stomach and prevent further vomiting, and a urinary catheter should also be placed to monitor urinary output. Antibiotic cover is indicated in all patients with established secondary peritonitis and is directed against gut flora in the first instance (e.g. a third-generation cephalosporin and metronidazole). Thorough peritoneal lavage is an essential adjunct to operation, and some surgeons employ an antibiotic-containing solution.

Primary acute peritonitis

Primary peritonitis is uncommon, although in childhood it can account for up to 15% of acute abdominal emergencies. The condition used to be common in young girls following the ascent of pneumococcal or streptococcal infection from the genital tract.

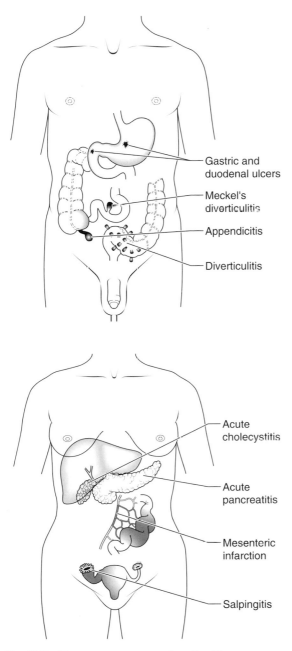

Gastric and duodenal ulcers

Meckel's diverticulitis

Appendicitis

Diverticulitis

Acute cholecystitis

Acute pancreatitis

Mesenteric infarction

Salpingitis

Fig. 15.3 The common causes of peritonitis.

exacerbate the pain. Vomiting is common but is usually not a marked early feature.

The patient usually lies still and is afraid to move. Respiration is shallow, and in the early stages the abdomen is scaphoid. The most important clinical sign is tenderness on palpation, the extent depending on whether the inflammation is localized or generalized within the abdominal cavity. There is associated rigidity, guarding and rebound

Escherichia coli is now the predominant causal organism and probably gains access through the gut wall, or rarely by bloodborne spread from a distant focus. In adults, spontaneous bacterial peritonitis (SBP) may occur in patients with the nephrotic syndrome, but is more frequently seen with liver cirrhosis or chronic renal failure (particularly in those on chronic peritoneal dialysis). The mortality rate for patients with primary bacterial peritonitis varies from 20 to 80%.

Classically, diffuse peritonitis with generalized abdominal tenderness and rigidity develops within 24 hours. Fever and leukocytosis occur early. Abdominal rigidity is relatively uncommon. A sample of peritoneal fluid, which is usually turbid, is sent for Gram staining and bacterial culture. Antibiotic therapy is the mainstay of treatment, but laparotomy may be needed to rule out a surgical cause if this is suggested by the culture of enteric organisms.

Postoperative peritonitis

Peritonitis after abdominal surgery may be a residual effect of the original disease or a direct complication of its operative management (e.g. anastomotic leakage). Diagnosis is difficult, as:

1. The patient is usually receiving analgesia and/or sedation, and may not complain of pain
2. Any pain and tenderness may be attributed to the wound
3. There is often a 24–48 hour period after abdominal surgery when bowel sounds are absent and the abdomen is distended.

Persisting abdominal distension or the development of vomiting and distension after an initial return to normality should raise the suspicion of peritoneal infection. Suspicion is heightened if the patient looks unwell and has fever, tachycardia and an altered mental state. Plain abdominal films may merely show dilatation of the intestine, but ultrasonography can be used to detect collections. Anastomotic leakage can be demonstrated radiologically using water-soluble contrast.

Fluid and electrolyte replacement, nasogastric suction and broad-spectrum antibiotic therapy are instituted, and the need for reoperation is considered. In those patients managed conservatively intraperitoneal collections may form or abscesses develop, but operation can sometimes be avoided by percutaneous drainage under radiological guidance.

Intra-abdominal abscess

An intra-abdominal abscess may develop in conjunction with an underlying inflammatory process or be a complication of peritonitis or intra-abdominal surgery. The abscess gives rise to pyrexia, tachycardia and clinical signs of toxic-

---

SUMMARY BOX

Peritonitis

- Acute suppurative peritonitis secondary to visceral disease is the commonest type of peritonitis seen in surgical practice. Common causes include perforated peptic ulcer, perforated diverticular disease and acute cholecystitis.

- Postoperative peritonitis may represent persistence of the infection that led to surgery or result from a complication, notably anastomotic leakage.

- Intraperitoneal abscesses are a common complication of peritonitis and frequently occur in the subphrenic and subhepatic spaces, the pelvis, and between loops of bowel. Ultrasonography and CT scanning allow diagnosis and percutaneous drainage, so that surgical drainage can often be avoided.

- Primary acute peritonitis is now rare but was once common in young girls following ascent of the genital tract by pneumococcal or streptococcal infection. Spontaneous bacterial peritonitis in adults may complicate ascites in cirrhosis or the nephrotic syndrome.

- Chronic infective peritonitis (tuberculosis) and granulomatous peritonitis (e.g. following the use of starch as surgical glove powder) are now rare.

---

ity. Leukocytosis is usual. Common sites for abscess formation are the subphrenic and subhepatic spaces, the pelvis, and between loops of bowel (Fig. 15.4). Complications include rupture with generalized peritonitis, the erosion of blood vessels with potentially catastrophic bleeding, and septicaemia. Occasionally, subphrenic abscesses rupture into the pleural cavity, and pelvic abscesses sometimes discharge spontaneously through the rectum.

The site of the abscess may be suspected from the history and clinical examination, but localizing signs can be surprisingly few (particularly with subphrenic abscess, hence the expression 'pus somewhere, pus nowhere else, pus under the diaphragm'). Unexplained fever after peritoneal infection or operation should always raise the suspicion of abscess formation. Tachycardia is usual. Pain and tenderness over the ribcage, shoulder-tip pain and a 'sympathetic' pleural effusion strengthen the suspicion of subphrenic abscess, whereas urgency of defaecation, diarrhoea and a boggy swelling in the pouch of Douglas on rectal examination are features of a pelvic abscess (Fig. 15.5).

Ultrasound and/or CT scans are of immense value in diagnosis (Fig. 15.6). Isotope scans following injection of

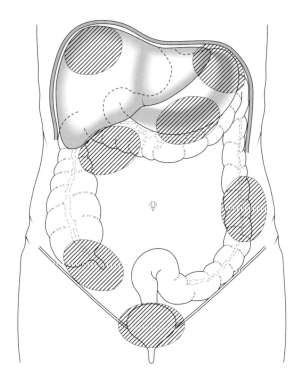

Fig. 15.4 Common locations of peritoneal abscess formation.

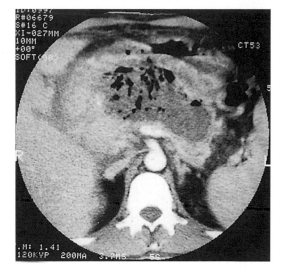

Fig. 15.6 CT scan of upper abdomen showing pancreatic abscess containing streaks of gas.

[111]In-labelled leukocytes are now used infrequently. Ultrasonography or CT scanning may also be used to guide percutaneous drain insertion and to obtain material for bacteriological culture. However, surgical drainage may still be needed to ensure effective drainage, particularly if the collection is loculated. Pelvic abscesses frequently rupture spontaneously into the rectum, but may require incision and drainage through the anterior rectal wall. Antibiotic therapy is used in conjunction with drainage of the abscess. Signs usually resolve rapidly following effective drainage, but female patients may be left infertile if the ostia of the fallopian tubes have been involved in a large pelvic collection.

Tumours of the peritoneum and retroperitoneum

Primary peritoneal tumours

Such tumours are rare. **Mesotheliomas** in asbestos workers may produce a bulky mass or diffuse peritoneal involvement with ascites. **Pseudomyxoma peritonei** is an uncommon low-grade malignant tumour that arises from the ovary or from rupture of a mucocele of the appendix. Lobulated peritoneal deposits give rise to copious secretion of mucus and abdominal distension. Intermittent intestinal obstruction may occur. Repeated operations may be needed to debulk the tumour, but can prolong survival.

Secondary peritoneal tumours

These tumours are common, the stomach, pancreas and ovary being the main primary sites. Seedlings may stud the peritoneal cavity and produce malignant ascites and a mass in the pouch of Douglas which is palpable rectally.

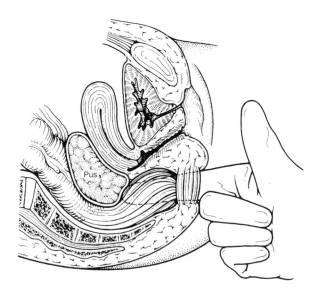

Fig. 15.5 Rectal examination for pelvic abscess.

Retroperitoneal tumours

Arising from connective tissue, these occasionally produce an abdominal mass. CT scanning is helpful and a tissue diagnosis must be obtained by radiologically guided sampling or, if need be, by laparotomy. The majority of these tumours are malignant. They tend to be locally aggressive but rarely metastasize. Occasionally such tumours turn out to be lesions with a relatively good prognosis (e.g. lymphomas), provided appropriate treatment is instituted.

THE ABDOMINAL WALL

Umbilicus

Development abnormalities

Persistent vitellointestinal duct

The vitellointestinal duct runs in intra-uterine life from the apex of the midgut loop to the yolk sac. It is normally obliterated long before birth, but part of it may persist as a Meckel's diverticulum on the antimesenteric border of the ileum. Rarer abnormalities include persistence of a band attaching the umbilicus to a Meckel's diverticulum or a loop of ileum; a patent communication (fistula) between the ileum and umbilicus; an encysted

portion of the duct which does not connect with the ileum (enterocystoma); an umbilical sinus; and a persistent umbilical portion of the duct which forms a polypoidal raspberry-like tumour of the umbilicus (enteroteratoma) (Fig. 15.7).

Symptomatic remnants may have to be excised, although a broad-based Meckel's diverticulum is usually left alone if found incidentally at laparotomy. Persisting bands can cause intestinal obstruction.

Urachus

The urachus runs from the apex of the bladder to the umbilicus. It is normally obliterated at birth but may give rise to cysts, a urinary fistula, or a discharging umbilical sinus if parts of it remain patent. Symptomatic remnants require excision.

Umbilical sepsis

Umbilical sepsis in neonates may give rise to portal thrombophlebitis, liver abscess formation, jaundice and portal vein thrombosis, which may result in portal hypertension. Tetanus can follow the application of cow dung to the umbilicus, as was once practised in some primitive societies.

In adults, sepsis can result from retention of inspissated sebum within the folds of the umbilicus, and from infection

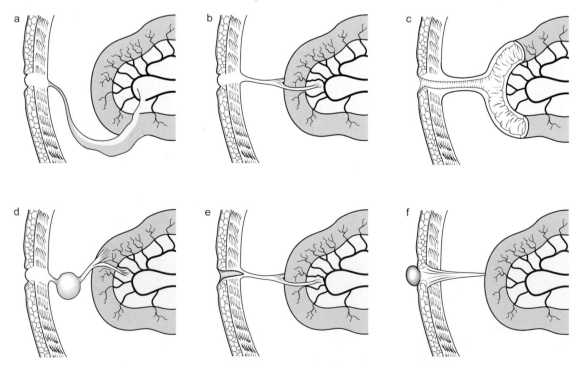

Fig. 15.7 Persistence of the vitellointestinal duct giving rise to **A** a Meckel's diverticulum, **B** a fibrous cord to the ileum, **C** an umbilical intestinal fistula, **D** an enterocystoma, **E** an umbilical sinus, and **F** an enteroteratoma.

of a pilonidal sinus of the umbilicus. Infection is usually mixed staphylococcal and streptococcal, characterized by erythema, tenderness and swelling. Treatment involves drainage of any pus and the prescription of systemic antibiotics.

Umbilical tumours

The umbilicus may rarely be involved by primary neoplasms (e.g. squamous carcinoma or melanoma) or secondary tumour which has tracked along the ligamentum teres from the liver or lymph nodes in the porta hepatis. Neoplasia is an occasional unexpected finding in an umbilicus which has been excised because of persistent discharge.

Afflictions of the rectus muscle

Haematoma of the rectus sheath

Spontaneous or traumatic rupture of a branch of the inferior epigastric artery occasionally produces a painful swelling of the rectus sheath in association with rigidity. This condition is not commonly diagnosed, but may represent an unusual presentation of acute abdominal pain in the elderly patient. A history of excessive physical exertion may precede the onset of symptoms. Ultrasonography can be used to confirm the diagnosis, and ligation of the bleeding artery with evacuation of clot may be indicated.

Desmoid tumour

This rare tumour is thought to arise from fibrous intramuscular septa in the lower rectus abdominis muscle. It is commoner in women of childbearing age and can be associated with intestinal polyposis in Gardner's syndrome. The lesion must be excised widely as it is prone to recur and can become malignant (fibrosarcoma).

ABDOMINAL HERNIA

A hernia is an abnormal protrusion of an organ (e.g. intestine, brain) or tissue (e.g. muscle, fat) outside its normal body cavity or constraining sheath. Hernia of the abdominal wall are common. They may exploit natural openings such as the inguinal and femoral canals, umbilicus, obturator canal or oesophageal hiatus, or protrude through areas weakened by stretching (e.g. epigastric hernia) or surgical incision. The hernia is immediately invested by a peritoneal sac drawn from the lining of the abdominal wall (Fig. 15.8). The sac is covered in turn by those tissues which are stretched in front of it as the hernia enlarges (i.e. the coverings). The neck of the sac is the constriction formed by the orifice in the abdominal wall through which the hernia passes. A hernia may contain any intra-abdominal structure

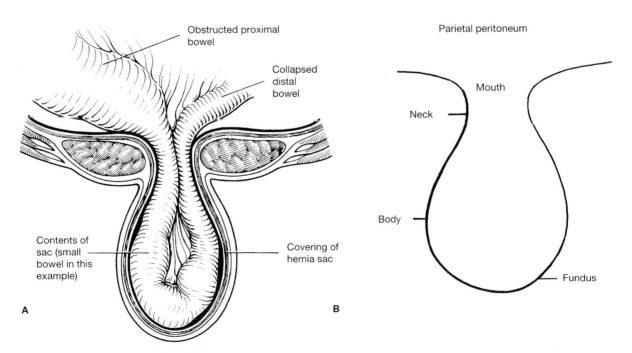

Fig. 15.8   Hernia. **A** Anatomical structure; **B** parts of the hernial sac.

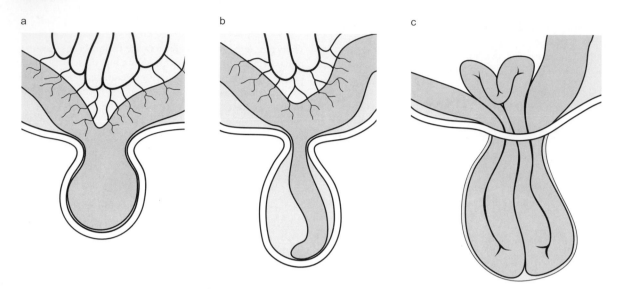

Fig. 15.9 Unusual inguinal hernias. **A** Richter's hernia; **B** Littre's hernia; **C** Maydl's hernia.

but most commonly contains omentum and/or small bowel. A hernia may involve only part of the circumference of the bowel (Richter's hernia), a Meckel's diverticulum (Littre's hernia) or two involved loops of bowel (Maydl's hernia) (Fig. 15.9). A sliding inguinal hernia is defined as one in which a viscus forms a portion of the wall of the hernia sac. Most commonly, the viscus involved is caecum, sigmoid colon or urinary bladder.

Inguinal hernia

Groin herniae account for three-quarters of all abdominal wall herniae, and inguinal herniorrhaphy is one of the most common minor operative procedures. The commonest types of groin hernia are indirect inguinal (60%), direct inguinal (25%) and femoral (15%). Most (85%) groin herniae occur in males. In early life an indirect inguinal hernia is by far the most common variety. After middle age, weakness of the abdominal musculature leads to an increasing incidence of direct inguinal herniae. Femoral herniae are relatively more common in females (possibly because of stretching of ligaments and widening of the femoral ring in pregnancy), but an indirect inguinal hernia is still the commonest type of groin hernia in women.

Inguinal herniae occur in one to three percent of all newborn males. The incidence in premature infants is 30 times that seen at term. All of these herniae are indirect and are caused by a failure of closure of the processus vaginalis. Inguinal herniae can also, less commonly, affect girls; the hernial sac can contain the ovary.

The diagnosis is usually obvious, but sometimes, where the groin swelling cannot be reproduced, a decision to operate can be made on the basis of a reliable history from the parents and the presence of thickening of the spermatic cord on the affected side.

SUMMARY BOX

Hernia

- A hernia is an abnormal protrusion of an organ or tissue outside its normal body cavity or restraining sheath.

- Hernia of the abdominal wall are common and may exploit natural openings (inguinal, femoral and obturator canals, umbilicus and oesophageal hiatus) or weak areas caused by stretching or surgical incisions.

- Abdominal hernia have a peritoneal sac, the neck of which is often unyielding and a potential source of compression of the hernial contents.

- Hernia may be classified as reducible or irreducible, and the contents (e.g. bowel) may become obstructed or strangulated.

- Strangulation denotes compromise of the blood supply of the contents and its development significantly increases morbidity and mortality. The low-pressure venous drainage is occluded first and then the arterial supply becomes occluded, with the development of gangrene.

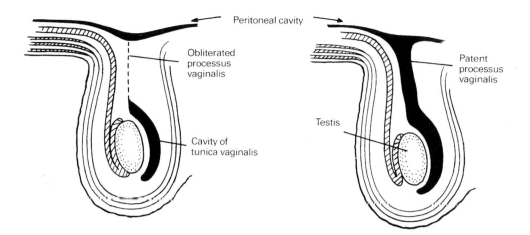

Fig. 15.10 Processus vaginalis testis. **A** Normal obliteration of processus vaginalis testis; **B** persistence of patent processus.

The deep inguinal ring lies immediately behind the superficial inguinal ring at this age. As such, the operation to correct the problem is a simple inguinal herniotomy without any need to strengthen the posterior wall of the inguinal canal. In older children this procedure is usually undertaken as a day-case with liberal use of local anaesthetic blocks for post-operative pain relief. In neonates and premature infants, the incidence of irreducibility and strangulation is much higher than that seen in older children. Surgery in this group is therefore undertaken more urgently. In very premature infants, the procedure may need to be done under regional block alone and where general anaesthesia is used, elective post-operative ventilation may be required.

Surgical anatomy

The inguinal canal is an oblique passage in the lower anterior abdominal wall through which the spermatic cord passes to the testis, or in the female the round ligament to the labium majus. The processus vaginalis traversing the canal is normally obliterated at birth (Fig. 15.10), but persistence in whole or in part presents an anatomical predisposition to an indirect inguinal hernia. The openings of the canal are formed by the internal and external rings. The internal (deep) inguinal ring is an opening in the transversalis fascia which lies 1 cm above the midinguinal point (midway between the public tubercle and the anterior superior iliac spine). The internal inguinal ring is bounded medi-

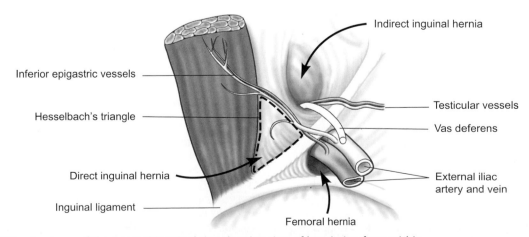

Fig. 15.11 Anatomy of the internal inguinal ring showing sites of herniation from within.

ally by the inferior epigastric artery (Fig. 15.11). The inguinal canal ends at the external (superficial) inguinal ring, which is an opening in the aponeurosis of the external oblique muscle just above and medial to the pubic tubercle. At birth, the internal and external rings lie on top of each other so that the inguinal canal is short and straight; with growth, the two rings move apart so that the canal becomes longer and oblique.

The testis and spermatic cord receive a covering from each of the layers as they pass through the abdominal wall. The innermost layer is derived from the transversalis fascia (the internal spermatic fascia), the middle layer from the internal oblique muscle (the cremasteric muscle and fascia), and the outer layer from the external oblique aponeurosis (the external spermatic fascia). Within the inguinal canal the spermatic cord is covered only by the cremasteric and internal spermatic fasciae. The spermatic cord consists of the vas deferens, the artery of the vas (branch of the inferior vesical artery), the testicular artery (branch of the aorta on the right and renal artery on the left), the cremasteric artery (branch of the inferior epigastric artery), the pampiniform plexus of veins, the ilioinguinal nerve, the genital branch of the genitofemoral nerve and lymphatics.

Indirect inguinal hernia

Many indirect inguinal hernias are probably the result of failure of obliteration of the processus vaginalis. An indirect inguinal hernia enters the internal (deep) inguinal ring and descends within the coverings of the spermatic cord so that it can pass on down into the scrotum. The hernia may remain within the inguinal canal (bubonocele), protrude through the external (superficial) inguinal ring (funicular) or extend into the scrotum (complete or scrotal) (Fig. 15.12). Very occasionally it enlarges between the muscle layers of the abdominal wall to form an interstitial hernia.

Clinical features

The moment of herniation (or rupture) may be associated with sudden groin pain, or may pass unnoticed. Thereafter

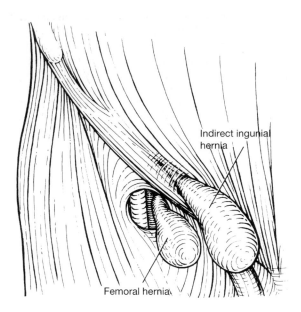

Fig. 15.13   Exit of femoral and inguinal hernias.

there may be a dragging discomfort in the groin, particularly during lifting or straining, but in the absence of strangulation further pain is unusual.

The hernia forms a swelling in the inguinal canal which may extend into the scrotum. It is often readily visible when the patient stands or is asked to cough. An inguinal hernia, which passes into the scrotum, passes above and medial to the public tubercle, in contrast to a femoral hernia, which bulges below and lateral to the tubercle (Fig. 15.13). A cough impulse is normally palpable, and bowel sounds can often be heard within the hernia on auscultation. If there is no visible swelling a cough impulse is sought with the patient standing.

The hernia often reduces spontaneously when the patient lies down, or it may be reduced by gentle pressure applied in an upward and lateral direction. Once reduced, it may be possible to control the hernia by placing a finger over the internal (deep) inguinal ring.

Direct inguinal hernia

Direct herniae are due to weakness of the abdominal wall and may be precipitated by increases in intra-abdominal pressure (e.g. obstructive airways disease, prostatism or chronic constipation). The hernia protrudes through the transversalis fascia in the posterior wall of the inguinal canal. The defect is bounded above by the conjoint tendon, below by the inguinal ligament, and laterally by the inferior epigastric vessels (Fig. 15.11). These boundaries mark the area known as Hesselbech's triangle. The hernia occasion-

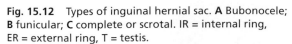

Fig. 15.12   Types of inguinal hernial sac. **A** Bubonocele; **B** funicular; **C** complete or scrotal. IR = internal ring, ER = external ring, T = testis.

ally bulges through the external (superficial) inguinal ring, but the transversalis fascia cannot stretch sufficiently to allow it to descend down into the scrotum. The sac has a wide neck so that the hernia seldom becomes irreducible, obstructs or strangulates. As shown in Figure 15.11, the neck of the sac of a direct inguinal hernia lies medial to the inferior epigastric vessels, whereas that of an indirect hernia lies lateral to them. Both indirect and direct hernias may occur on the same side (pantaloon or saddle-bag hernia), with sacs straddling the inferior epigastric vessels.

Clinical features

The hernia forms a diffuse bulge in the region of the medial part of the inguinal canal. It is usually readily reduced by backward pressure and the edges of the defect may then be palpable. Clinically, it is frequently impossible to determine whether a hernia confined to the inguinal canal is of the direct or the indirect variety.

Treatment of uncomplicated inguinal hernia

The identification of an inguinal hernia in any child is *always* an indication to operate. In newborns the procedure must be carried out with some urgency because of the risk of incarceration. In older children, elective surgery is indicated.

Adult inguinal herniae can be controlled by a truss, but this is uncomfortable and is now seldom indicated, given that the hernia can be repaired under local anaesthesia. Groin herniae can be repaired by an open or laparoscopic surgical approach.

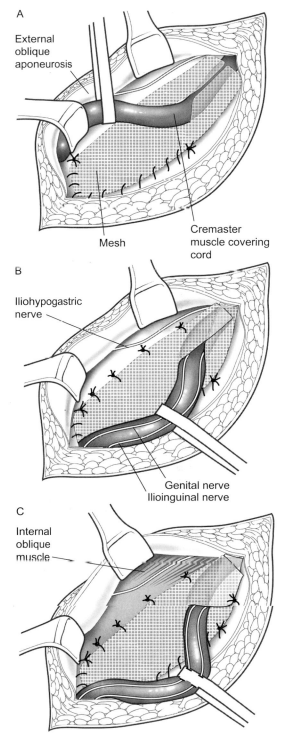

Fig. 15.15 Lichtenstein repair.

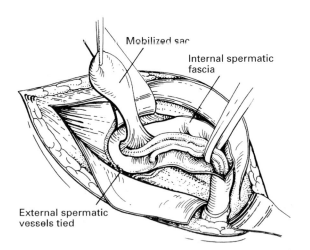

Fig. 15.14 Principle of dissection in the repair of an inguinal hernia.

Indirect inguinal hernia

The first step in the open approach is to open the inguinal canal, free the hernial sac from the spermatic cord (Fig. 15.14) and excise it after transfixing and ligating its neck. Simple excision of the sac (**herniotomy**) is all that is needed in young children. In older children and adults the internal ring is usually stretched and widened, and therefore after herniotomy it is necessary to tighten the deep ring and strengthen the posterior wall (**herniorrhaphy**). The simplest and most common surgical procedure now performed is the Lichtenstein tension-free repair, which involves the insertion of a synthetic mesh underneath the spermatic cord (Fig. 15.15). The mesh is secured to the aponeurotic tissue

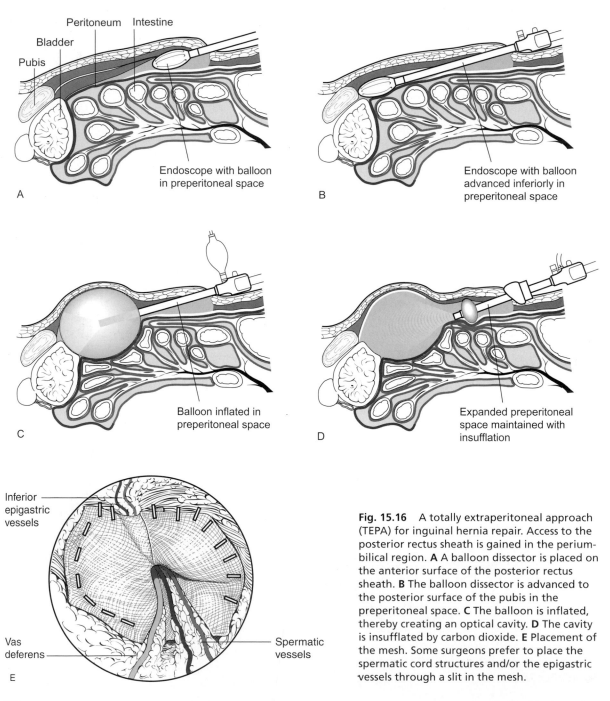

Fig. 15.16 A totally extraperitoneal approach (TEPA) for inguinal hernia repair. Access to the posterior rectus sheath is gained in the periumbilical region. **A** A balloon dissector is placed on the anterior surface of the posterior rectus sheath. **B** The balloon dissector is advanced to the posterior surface of the pubis in the preperitoneal space. **C** The balloon is inflated, thereby creating an optical cavity. **D** The cavity is insufflated by carbon dioxide. **E** Placement of the mesh. Some surgeons prefer to place the spermatic cord structures and/or the epigastric vessels through a slit in the mesh.

overlying the pubic bone medially, the inguinal ligament inferiorly, and the internal oblique aponeurosis and conjoint tendon superiorly. Laterally the mesh is divided and its two sides wrapped around the spermatic cord and sutured in place. The darn operation (using non-absorbable mono-filament sutures) is rarely performed now as it is associated with high recurrence rates and significant postoperative pain. The Shouldice operation (division of the transversalis fascia and reconstitution by a double-breasting technique) is a more complex procedure but is associated with low recurrence rates (<1%) in expert hands.

Direct hernia

In a direct hernia the sac is not normally excised and it is simply invaginated by sutures placed in the transversalis fascia. Insertion of a synthetic mesh is currently used to reinforce the posterior wall of the inguinal canal.

In all hernia repairs it is important to avoid constricting the spermatic cord by making the deep inguinal ring too tight. This may compromise repair, particularly in large or recurrent herniae, and in older patients removal of the testis may be considered so that the inguinal canal can be completely obliterated.

Laparoscopic hernia repair can be undertaken using a trans-abdominal preperitoneal (TAPP) repair or a totally extraperitoneal approach (TEPA). The actual hernia repair is similar in both these techniques, the main difference being in the manner in which access to the preperitoneal space is achieved. TAPP uses intraperitoneal trocars and creates a peritoneal flap over the posterior inguinal area, whereas TEPA provides access to the preperitoneal space without entering the peritoneal cavity (Fig. 15.16). The technique involves excising or reducing the hernia sac and inserting a mesh, which is stapled or sutured in position.

The indications for a laparoscopic approach remain controversial. Proponents of these techniques emphasize minimal pain, a more rapid return to normal activities, improved cosmesis and fewer infective complications; however, critics emphasize the necessity for a general anaesthetic, the violation of the peritoneal cavity (with the TAPP repair), increased costs and lack of long-term follow-up. It is generally accepted that the laparoscopic approach is particularly useful for patients with recurrent inguinal hernias or bilateral inguinal hernias.

Sportsman's hernia

Groin injury leading to chronic groin pain is often referred to as the sportman's hernia. However, the definition, investigation and treatment of this condition remains controversial. The differential diagnosis includes musculotendinous injuries, osteitis pubis, nerve entrapment, urological pathology or bone and joint disease. In many cases clinical signs are lacking, despite the patient's symptoms. Herniography studies have demonstrated a significant incidence of symptomatic impalpable hernia in patients presenting with obscure groin pain. A deficiency of the posterior inguinal wall is the commonest operative finding in patients with chronic groin pain. Some authors have described a tear in the conjoint tendon as the cause of the pain, whereas in

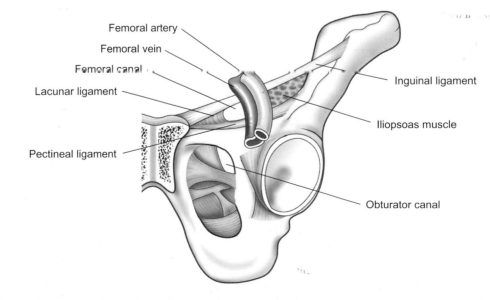

Fig. 15.17 Anatomy of the femoral ring.

Gilmore's description a tear in the external oblique aponeurosis causing dilatation of the external (superficial) inguinal ring was implicated. Surgical intervention is recommended only when conservative management has failed. Appropriate repair of the posterior wall of the inguinal canal has proved to be of therapeutic benefit in selected patients.

Femoral hernia

A femoral hernia projects through the femoral ring and passes down the femoral canal. The ring is bounded laterally by the femoral vein, anteriorly by the inguinal ligament, medially by the lacunar ligament, and posteriorly by the superior ramus of the pubis and the reflected part of the inguinal ligament (pectineal ligament of Astley Cooper) (Fig. 15.17). As the hernia enlarges it passes through the saphenous opening in the deep fascia of the thigh (the site of penetration of the long saphenous vein to join the femoral vein) and then turns upwards to lie in front of the inguinal ligament. The hernia has many coverings and may be deceptively small, sometimes escaping detection. It frequently contains omentum or small bowel, but the urinary bladder can 'slide' into the medial wall of the sac.

Clinical features

The hernia forms a bulge in the upper inner aspect of the thigh. It can sometimes be difficult to differentiate between an inguinal and a femoral hernia, but as indicated earlier, the former passes above and medial to the pubic tubercle as it enters the groin, whereas the latter passes below and lateral to it. Tracing the tendon of adductor longus upwards to its insertion is a useful guide to the position of the pubic tubercle.

A femoral hernia is frequently difficult or impossible to reduce because of its *J*-shaped course. As well as differentiation from inguinal hernia, it can be confused with an inguinal lymph node (no cough impulse, irreducible), saphenous varix (positive cough impulse or 'saphenous thrill', which is prominent on standing but which disappears on elevating the leg), ectopic testis, psoas abscess, hydrocele of the spermatic cord or a lipoma.

Surgical repair of femoral hernia

A femoral hernia is particularly likely to obstruct and strangulate, and therefore surgical intervention is indicated. As with inguinal hernia, repair can be carried out under local or general anaesthesia.

The aim of operation is to excise the sac and obliterate the femoral ring by suturing the inguinal ligament to the pectineal ligament. The femoral canal can be approached from below the inguinal ligament, through the inguinal canal, or from above by entering the rectus sheath and displacing the rectus abdominis medially. The approach from above (McEvedy approach) gives the best access and is particularly useful if the hernia contains strangulated bowel and intestinal resection is required.

SUMMARY BOX

Groin herniae

- Indirect inguinal herniae comprise 60% of all groin herniae and commence at the deep inguinal ring, lateral to the inferior epigastric vessels.

- Direct inguinal herniae account for 25% of all groin hernias and bulge through a weakness in the back wall of the inguinal canal, medial to the inferior epigastric vessels. They rarely obstruct or strangulate.

- Indirect inguinal herniae may pass down within the coverings of the spermatic cord to the scrotum; direct herniae do not descend into the scrotum.

- Femoral herniae account for 15% of all groin herniae and pass through the femoral canal, emerging below and lateral to the pubic tubercle (in contrast to inguinal herniae descending to the scrotum, which pass medial to the tubercle).

- Femoral herniae are often small and easy to miss on clinical examination, but are prone to obstruct and strangulate.

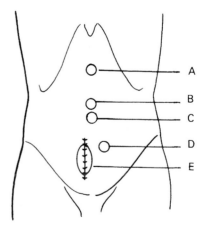

Fig. 15.18 Types of ventral hernia. **A** Epigastric (through the linea alba); **B** umbilical (through umbilical scar); **C** paraumbilical (above or below the umbilicus); **D** Spigelian (adjacent to rectus sheath); **E** incisional (anywhere).

Ventral hernia

Ventral herniae occur through areas of weakness in the anterior abdominal wall (Fig. 15.18), namely the linea alba (epigastric hernia), the umbilicus (umbilical and para-umbilical hernia), the lateral border of the rectus sheath (Spigelian hernia), and the scar tissue of surgical incisions (incisional hernia).

Epigastric hernia

Epigastric herniae protrude through the linea alba above the level of the umbilicus. The herniation may be of extraperitoneal fat or be a protrusion of peritoneum containing omentum. The hernia is common in thin individuals and can cause local discomfort. It is repaired by closing the defect with interrupted non-absorbable sutures.

Umbilical hernia

 A true umbilical hernia occurs in infants. The small sac protrudes through the umbilicus, particularly as the child cries, but is easily reduced. Over 95% of these herniae close spontaneously in the first 3 years of life. Persistence after the third birthday is an indication for elective repair. Surgery involves excision of the hernial sac and closure of the defect in the fascia of the abdominal wall.

Paraumbilical hernia

This hernia is caused by gradual weakening of the tissues around the umbilicus. It most often affects obese multiparous women, and passes through the attenuated linea alba just above or below the umbilicus. The peritoneal sac is often preceded by the extrusion of a small knuckle of extraperitoneal fat through the linea alba. The hernia gradually enlarges, the covering tissues become stretched and thin, and eventually loops of bowel may become visible under parchment-like skin. The sac is often multilocular and may be irreducible because of adhesions forming between omentum and loops of bowel. The skin may become reddened, excoriated and ulcerated, and rarely an intestinal fistula may even develop.

Operation is advised because of the risk of obstruction and strangulation. Unless there is a large protrusion of the umbilicus itself, most surgical repairs can be performed

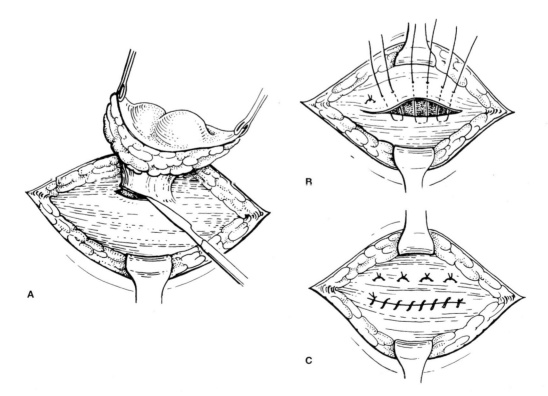

Fig. 15.19   Mayo repair of adult paraumbilical hernia. **A** Excision of sac after reduction of its contents; **B** insertion of overlapping sutures into rectus sheath; **C** final appearance.

preserving the umbilicus. Through a transverse subumbilical incision, the anterior layer of the rectus sheath is exposed. The sac is opened and the contents reduced. The classic Mayo repair involves the development of a flap of rectus sheath and linea alba above and below the hernia defect. The defect is closed by overlapping the layers using mattress sutures of non-absorbable material in a 'double-breasted' fashion (Fig. 15.19). Alternatively, the defect can be closed using interrupted transverse sutures. If apposition of the hernia edges is not possible, a non-absorbable mesh can be used.

Incisional hernia

Incisional herniae occur after 3–5% of all abdominal operations. Midline vertical incisions are most often affected, and poor technique, wound infection, obesity and chest infection are important predisposing factors. The diffuse bulge in the wound is best seen when the patient coughs or raises the head and shoulders from a pillow, thereby contracting the abdominal muscles. Strangulation is rare, but surgical repair is usually advised. Some patients prefer to wear an abdominal support to control the hernia.

The skin wound is excised and flaps are elevated to expose the aponeurosis. The sac can be invaginated or excised, and the edges of the defect are then repaired with overlapping sutures or the insertion of a synthetic mesh.

Rare external hernia

A **Spigelian hernia** occurs through the linea semilunaris at the outer border of the rectus abdominis muscle. Treatment is surgical, as the hernia is liable to strangulate.

A **lumbar hernia** forms a diffuse bulge above the iliac crest between the posterior borders of the external oblique and latissimus dorsi muscles. It seldom requires treatment.

An **obturator hernia** is a rare hernia which is commoner in women and which passes through the obturator canal. Patients may present with knee pain owing to pressure on the obturator nerve; however, the diagnosis is frequently only made when the hernia has strangulated and is discovered at laparotomy.

Internal hernia

Herniation of the stomach through the oesophageal hiatus in the diaphragm (hiatus hernia) is a common cause of internal herniation which is considered in Chapter 18. A variety of cul-de-sacs and peritoneal defects resulting from rotation of the bowel and other abnormalities of development may be responsible for the entrapment of bowel and acute intestinal obstruction. For example, herniation may occur through the foramen of Winslow (opening of the

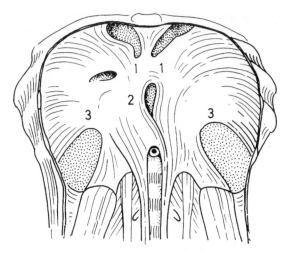

Fig. 15.20 Sites of diaphragmatic herniation. (1) Parasternal, between the sternal and costal slips of the diaphragm (foramen of Morgagni). (2) Oesophageal hiatus. (3) Pleuroperitoneal canal (foramen of Bochdalek).

lesser sac) into various fossae around the duodenum and through various openings in the diaphragm, including the oesophageal hiatus (Fig. 15.20).

Complications of hernia

Irreducibility

An irreducible hernia is one in which the contents cannot be manipulated back into the abdominal cavity. This may be due to narrowing of the neck of the sac by fibrosis, distension of the contained bowel, or adhesions to the walls of the sac.

Obstruction

An irreducible hernia may progress to intestinal obstruction. Abdominal pain, vomiting and distension signal the need for urgent operation *before* strangulation supervenes.

Strangulation

The vessels supplying the bowel within a hernia may be compressed by the neck of the sac or the constricting ring through which the hernia passes. The contents initially become swollen as a result of venous congestion, and there is exudation of a bloodstained fluid. The arterial supply is subsequently compromised and gangrene follows. Organisms and toxins pass out through the bowel wall, causing local peritonitis.

The patient complains of pain in the hernia and usually has features of intestinal obstruction. The hernia is tender, the cough impulse is lost, and there may be increasing evidence of circulatory collapse and sepsis. In a Richter's hernia only part of the circumference of the bowel is strangulated, and there may be no evidence of intestinal obstruction.

Treatment

If there is no evidence of strangulation an attempt can be made to reduce an apparently irreducible hernia by giving analgesia, putting the patient to bed with the foot of the bed elevated, and applying gentle pressure. Undue force must never be used for fear of rupturing the bowel or returning the entire hernia to the abdomen with the bowel still trapped within it (reduction en masse). If the hernia does not reduce readily, surgery is advised to avoid further complications.

Urgent operation is indicated for all obstructed herniae as one can never be certain that strangulation is not present. The hernial sac is opened and the contents inspected carefully. If they are viable they can be returned to the abdominal cavity and the hernia repaired. If there is doubt about the viability of a loop of bowel or omentum, the devitalized tissue must be resected before proceeding to repair.

In infants and children, the majority of irreducible inguinal herniae can be safely reduced by a suitably trained clinician. Small doses of intravenous opiate analgesia administered in the presence of suitably trained paediatric nursing staff can relax the child and assist with the reduction process. The hernia can then be repaired within 72 hours on the next available operating list. The child should be detained in hospital pending repair to allow early detection of further episodes of incarceration. Failure to reduce a hernia in this manner necessitates emergency surgery. This is usually extremely difficult and should only be attempted by experienced surgeons.

The acute abdomen and intestinal obstruction

G.C.S. Smith, S. Paterson-Brown

INTRODUCTION

The 'acute abdomen' is a term used to encompass a spectrum of surgical, medical and gynaecological conditions, ranging from the trivial to the life-threatening, which require hospital admission, investigation and treatment. The primary symptom of the condition is abdominal pain.

For the purposes of multicentre studies looking at acute abdominal pain, the definition is taken as 'abdominal pain of less than 1 week's duration requiring admission to hospital, which has not been previously investigated or treated'. Acute abdominal pain following trauma is usually considered separately.

The acute abdomen is a very common clinical entity. It has been estimated that at least 50% of general surgical admissions are emergencies, and of these 50% present with acute abdominal pain. The acute abdomen therefore represents a significant part of the general surgical workload. Furthermore, patients with acute abdominal pain have a significant morbidity and mortality. Studies have shown a 30-day mortality of 4% among patients admitted with acute abdominal pain, rising to 8% in those who undergo operative treatment. Not surprisingly, the mortality rate varies with age, being the highest at the extremes of age. The highest mortality rates are associated with laparotomy for unresectable cancer, ruptured abdominal aortic aneurysm and perforated peptic ulcer.

Individual conditions presenting with acute abdominal pain will not be dealt with in depth in this chapter, but will be covered elsewhere.

AETIOLOGY

The causes of the acute abdomen may be subdivided into surgical, medical and gynaecological disorders. Surgical causes may be classified according to the organ involved, as well as the underlying pathological process. The most common causes in any population will vary according to age, sex and race, as well as genetic and environmental factors (Tables 16.1–16.3).

The remainder of this chapter will be concerned principally with surgical conditions although it should be borne in mind that medical and gynaecological conditions may present with acute abdominal pain.

PATHOPHYSIOLOGY OF ABDOMINAL PAIN

To be able to make an accurate clinical assessment of the patient presenting with acute abdominal pain, it is necessary to understand the pathophysiology. Abdominal pain can be divided into visceral and somatic types.

Table 16.1 Possible causes of acute abdominal pain

Surgical	Medical	Gynaecological
Inflammation	*Cardiovascular*	Ectopic pregnancy
Inflammatory bowel disease	Myocardial ischaemia	Ovarian cyst
Acute appendicitis	Myocardial infarction	Torsion
Acute diverticulitis	(inferior)	Rupture
Acute pancreatitis		Haemorrhage
Acute cholecystitis	*Gastrointestinal*	Infarction
Acute cholangitis	Gastritis	Infection
Meckel's diverticulitis	Gastroenteritis	Pelvic inflammatory
	Mesenteric adenitis	disease
Obstruction	Hepatitis	Fibroid degeneration
Intestinal obstruction	Hepatic abscess	Salpingitis
Biliary colic	Curtis–FitzHugh	Mittelschmerz
Ureteric colic	syndrome	Endometriosis
Acute retention of urine	Primary peritonitis	
Ischaemia	*Abdominal wall conditions*	
Mesenteric ischaemia	Rectus sheath haematoma	
Torsion of a viscus		
	Genitourinary	
Perforation	Urinary tract infection	
Perforated peptic ulcer disease	Pyelonephritis	
Perforated diverticular disease		
Perforated appendix	*Neurological*	
Toxic megacolon with perforation	Tabes dorsalis	
Acute cholecystitis and perforation		
Perforated oesophagus	*Haematological*	
Perforated bladder	Sickle cell disease	
Perforation of a length of strangulated	Malaria	
bowel	Hereditary spherocytosis	
Ruptured abdominal aortic aneurysm		
	Endocrine	
	Diabetes mellitus	
	Thyrotoxicosis	
	Addison's disease	
	Metabolic	
	Uraemia	
	Hypercalcaemia	
	Porphyria	
	Infective	
	Herpes zoster	

Somatic pain

The parietal peritoneum covers the anterior and posterior abdominal walls, the undersurface of the diaphragm and the pelvic cavity. It develops from the somatopleural layer of the lateral plate mesoderm and its nerve supply is therefore derived from somatic nerves supplying the abdominal wall musculature and the skin (T5–L2). The exception to this is the diaphragmatic portion, which is supplied centrally by afferent nerves in the phrenic nerve (C3–C5), and peripherally in the lower six intercostal and subcostal nerves

The parietal peritoneum is sensitive to mechanical, thermal or chemical stimulation, and cannot be handled, cut or cauterized painlessly. As a result of its innervation, when the parietal peritoneum is irritated there is reflex contraction of the corresponding segmental area of muscle, causing rigidity of the abdominal wall (guarding) and hyperaesthesia of the overlying skin.

Table 16.2   Common causes of acute abdominal pain requiring admission to hospital in UK adults

Condition	Approximate incidence (%)
Non-specific abdominal pain	35
Acute appendicitis	30
Acute cholecystitis and biliary colic	10
Peptic ulcer disease	5
Small bowel obstruction	5
Gynaecological disorders	5
Acute pancreatitis	2
Renal and ureteric colic	2
Malignant disease	2
Acute diverticulitis	2
Dyspepsia	1
Miscellaneous	5

Table 16.3   Common causes of acute abdominal pain in UK children

Acute appendicitis
Urinary tract infection
Mesenteric adenitis
Gastroenteritis

When the diaphragmatic portion of the parietal peritoneum is irritated peripherally there will be pain, tenderness and rigidity in the distribution of the lower spinal nerves, but when it is irritated centrally, pain is referred to the cutaneous distribution of C3, 4 and 5 (i.e. the shoulder area (Fig. 16.1). Somatic pain is classically described as sharp or knife-like in nature, and is usually well localized to the affected area.

Visceral pain

The visceral peritoneum forms a partial or complete investment of the intra-abdominal viscera. It is derived from the splanchnopleural layer of the lateral plate mesoderm, and shares its nerve supply with the viscera (i.e. the autonomic nerves). Visceral pain is mediated through the sympathetic branches of the autonomic nervous system, with afferent nerves joining the presacral and splanchnic nerves, which eventually join thoracic (T6–T12) and lumbar (L1–L2) segments of the spinal cord. The visceral peritoneum and the viscera are insensitive to mechanical, thermal or chemical stimulation, and can therefore be handled, cut or cauterized painlessly. However, they are sensitive to tension, when applied by overdistension or traction on mesenteries, visceral muscle spasm and ischaemia.

Visceral pain is described typically as dull and deep-seated. It is usually localized vaguely to the area occupied by the viscus during development, and is referred to the overlying skin of the abdominal wall according to the dermatome level with the sympathetic supply as mentioned above. Therefore, pain arising from the intestine and its outgrowths (the liver, biliary system and pancreas) is usually felt in the midline. Irritation of foregut structures (the lower oesophagus to the second part of the duodenum) is usually felt in the epigastric area. Pain from midgut structures (the second part of the duodenum to the splenic flexure) is felt around the umbilicus. Pain from hindgut structures (the splenic flexure to the rectum) is felt in the hypogastrium. Although the division of abdominal pain into visceral and somatic pain is useful, it is important to realize that some pathological conditions will result in a mixed picture. For example, acute appendicitis classically presents with acute abdominal pain that is initially felt in the umbilical area resulting from appendicular obstruction, which gradually localizes to the right iliac fossa and becomes sharper in nature as the overlying parietal peritoneum becomes inflamed.

PATHOGENESIS

As one can see from the list of surgical conditions that may present with acute abdominal pain (Table 16.1), there are two main underlying pathological processes involved: inflammation and obstruction. These processes may be triggered by a variety of underlying abnormalities. It is important to realize that in any one patient a combination of abnormalities and processes may be involved.

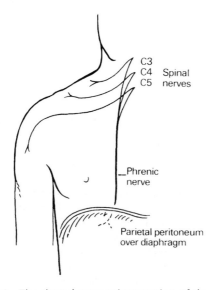

C3
C4   Spinal
C5   nerves

Phrenic nerve

Parietal peritoneum over diaphragm

Fig. 16.1 The shared sensory innervation of the shoulder and diaphragm.

Table 16.4	Injurious agents causing inflammation
Infective	Non-infective
Bacterial	Chemical
Viral	Ischaemia
Fungal	Physical
Parasites	Trauma
	Heat
	Cold
	Radiation
	Immune mechanisms

Inflammation

Acute inflammation of an intra-abdominal organ or the peritoneum may occur as a result of a variety of irritants. These may be broadly classified into infective or non-infective in nature (Table 16.4).

No matter what the trigger of the inflammation, the subsequent pathological process is the same. There is reactive hyperaemia of the injured tissue as a result of capillary and arteriolar dilatation; exudation of fluid into the tissues as a result of an increase in the permeability of the vascular endothelium; and an increase in filtration pressure. Finally, there is emigration of leukocytes from the vessels into the inflamed tissues.

Table 16.5   Classification of peritonitis

Generalized peritonitis
Primary
Infection of the peritoneal fluid without intra-abdominal disease:
  Haematogenous spread
  Lymphatic spread
  Direct spread: usually associated with CAPD catheters
  Ascending infection: from the female genital tract

Secondary
Inflammation of the peritoneum arising from an intra-abdominal source:
  Infectious
  Non-infectious
    Blood
    Ischaemia
    Bile
    Chemical
    Foreign body
  Perforation
Localized peritonitis
Usually due to spreading inflammation across the wall of an intra-abdominal viscus

The clinical consequences of the inflammatory process depend upon a multitude of factors, the most important being the underlying condition, its severity and duration, the organ involved, the patient's age and comorbidity. In general, the patient will complain of abdominal pain and tenderness, which occurs as a result of tissue stretching and distortion and is due to the release of inflammatory mediators, some of which also mediate pain. On general examination the patient may be pyrexial and have a tachycardia; investigations may reveal a raised white cell count. Examination of the abdomen will reveal tenderness in the affected area, with guarding and rigidity if the parietal peritoneum is involved.

Peritonitis

Inflammation of the peritoneum may result from a variety of injuries and, as described in Table 16.4, they may be divided into infective or non-infective in nature. Peritonitis may be classified according to extent (either localized or generalized) and aetiology (Table 16.5). In a surgical setting the most common cause of generalized peritonitis is perforation of an intra-abdominal viscus. Inflammation of the peritoneum results in an increase in its blood supply and local oedema formation. There is transudation of fluid into the peritoneal cavity, followed by the accumulation of a protein-rich fibrinous exudate. In the normal state the greater omentum constantly alters its position within the abdominal cavity as a result of intestinal peristalsis and abdominal muscle contraction. In the presence of an inflammation, the greater omentum will adhere to and surround the abnormal organ. The fibrinous exudate effectively glues the omentum to the inflamed viscus, walling it off and preventing the further spread of inflammation. In addition, the exudate inhibits intestinal peristalsis, resulting in a paralytic ileus which also limits the spread of the inflammation and infection. As a result of the ileus, fluid accumulates within the lumen of the intestine and, along with the formation of large volumes of intraperitoneal transudate and exudate, this will lead to a decrease in the intravascular volume, producing the clinical features of hypovolaemia.

The clinical features of peritonitis will again vary according to a wide variety of factors. The most common symptom is abdominal pain, which is constant and often described as sharp. The pain is usually well localized if it is secondary to inflammation of an intra-abdominal viscus, but may spread to involve the whole peritoneal cavity. Primary peritonitis can present rather more subtly, and as many as 30% of affected individuals may be asymptomatic.

The term 'peritonitis or peritonism' detected on clinical examination is used to describe the collection of signs associated with inflammation of the parietal peritoneum, and includes 'guarding' and 'rebound' tenderness. Evidence of inflammation of the parietal peritoneum in association with inflammation of an intra-abdominal viscus is often a strong indication that the patient requires some form of surgical intervention.

Infarction

An infarct is an area of ischaemic necrosis caused either by an occlusion of the arterial supply or the venous drainage in a particular tissue, or by a generalized hypoperfusion in the context of shock (Table 16.6). The typical histological feature of infarction is ischaemic coagulative necrosis. An inflammatory response begins to develop along the margins of an infarct within a few hours, stimulated by the presence of the necrotic tissue.

The consequences of decreased perfusion of a tissue depend on several factors: the availability of an alternative vascular supply, the rate of development of the hypo-perfusion, the vulnerability of the tissue to hypoxia, and the blood oxygen content. In the context of acute abdominal pain, intestinal infarction is the commonest cause. Other organs that may infarct include the ovaries, kidneys, testes, liver, spleen and pancreas.

In general the patient will complain of severe abdominal pain and the onset will depend on the nature of the under-lying process. Embolization will result in a sudden onset of pain, whereas the onset in thrombosis is likely to be more gradual. Infarction or ischaemia are potent triggers of inflammation of the affected structure, and the clinical features reflect this.

Perforation

Spontaneous perforation of an intra-abdominal viscus may be the result of a range of pathological processes. Weaken-ing of the wall of the viscus, which might follow degenera-tion, inflammation, infection or ischaemia, will predispose

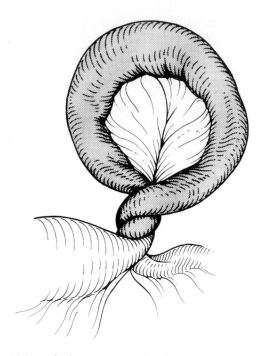

Fig. 16.2 Volvulus – an example of closed-looped obstruction. Three-stage resection of large bowel.

to perforation. An increase in the intraluminal pressure of a viscus, such as occurs in a closed loop obstruction (Fig. 16.2), will predispose to perforation, as will peptic ulceration, acute appendicitis and acute diverticulitis. Other less common causes are carcinoma of the colon, inflam-matory bowel disease and acute cholecystitis.

Perforation can also be iatrogenic, and may occur during the insertion of a Verress needle at laparoscopy, because of a careless cut or suture placement during surgery, and during the course of an endoscopic procedure.

Spontaneous perforation of a viscus usually results in the sudden onset of severe abdominal pain, which is usually well localized to the affected area. The resultant clinical picture depends on the nature of the perforated viscus and the relative sterility and toxicity of the material that is spilt into the abdominal cavity, in addition to the speed with which the perforation is surrounded and sealed (if at all) by the adjacent structures and omentum. The inevitable peri-toneal contamination will lead to either localized or gener-alized peritonitis, and the associated symptoms and signs as already discussed.

Obstruction

The term obstruction refers to impedance of the normal flow of material through a hollow viscus. It may be caused by the presence of a lesion within the lumen of the viscus,

Table 16.6	Aetiology of infarction
Occlusive	
Arterial:	
Embolism	
Thrombosis	
Extrinsic compression	
Venous:	
Thrombosis	
Extrinsic compression	
Non-occlusive	
Shock:	
Hypovolaemia	
Cardiogenic	
Sepsis	
Vasoconstrictor drugs	

an abnormality in its wall, or a lesion outside be viscus causing extrinsic compression.

The smooth muscle in the wall of the obstructed viscus will contract reflexly in an effort to overcome the impedance. This reflex contraction produces colicky abdominal pain. The exception to this rule is 'biliary colic'. The gall-bladder and biliary system has little smooth muscle in its wall and attempts at contraction tend to be more continuous than 'colicky'.

If the obstruction is not overcome, there will be an increase in intraluminal presure and proximal dilatation. The end result depends on the anatomical location of the obstruction, whether it is partial or complete, and whether the blood supply to the organ is compromised. For example, a urinary bladder calculus causing partial urinary outflow obstruction may result in a dilatation of the ureter and renal pelvis, and subsequent 'postrenal' renal failure. An obstructed inguinal hernia, on the other hand, will not only produce proximal dilatation of the intestine (usually associated with vomiting) but may also result in ischaemia of the bowel wall, leading to infarction and perforation.

CLINICAL ASSESSMENT

The ability to make an accurate assessment by taking a good history and performing an appropriate examination is a vital skill in the management of the patient with acute abdominal pain. Although an exact diagnosis is often impossible to make after the initial assessment, and often relies on further investigations, it is the formulation of an appropriate, safe and effective management plan that is the most important issue. In most cases it is possible to take a full history and perform a thorough examination, but this is not always so, and occasionally a rapid evaluation followed by immediate resuscitation is required.

History

The main presenting complaint of patients with an acute abdomen is pain. The characteristics of the pain (Table

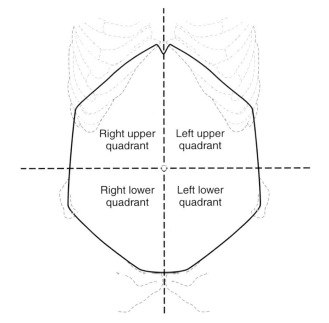

Fig. 16.3   The four quadrants of the abdomen.

16.7) give important clues to the likely underlying diagnosis, and these should be explored in depth. However, the importance of a full history cannot be overemphasized and is essential in all patients.

Site of pain

The site of abdominal pain is perhaps the most valuable pointer to the underlying diagnosis. In order to describe the site of pain, the abdomen is traditionally either divided into quarters or ninths (Figs 16.3 and 16.4).

Nature of pain

There are two main pathological mechanisms in the development of abdominal pain; obstruction and inflammation. Inflammation produces a constant pain made worse by local or general disturbance, and pain which is made worse by movement or coughing suggests inflammation of the parietal peritoneum. In this situation the patient will often be seen to lie very still in order not to exacerbate the pain.

Obstruction of a muscular viscus produces a colicky pain. This pain comes and goes in 'spasm', often only lasting a few minutes at a time but returning at frequent intervals. It may be described as 'gripping' in nature, and between spasms the patient is usually pain free. The pain itself is severe and may be helped by moving around or drawing the knees up towards the chest. Underlying inflammation must be suspected when a colicky pain does not disappear between spasms, or becomes continuous. In the case

Table 16.7	Characteristics of abdominal pain
Site	
Time and mode of onset	
Severity	
Nature	
Progression	
Duration	
Exacerbating/relieving factors	
Radiation	

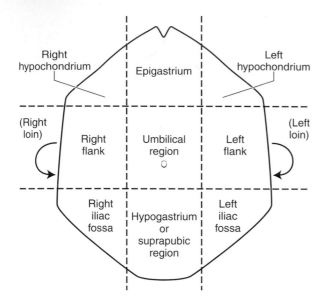

Fig. 16.4   The abdomen divided into ninths.

of intestinal obstruction this might mean strangulation and urgent surgery is required.

Radiation of pain

Radiation is the site to which the pain extends while the initial pain persists. When a pain radiates, it signifies that other structures are becoming involved. For example, pain from a duodenal ulcer may radiate through to the back, indicating that inflammation through the wall of the duodenum to involve structures of the posterior abdominal wall, such as the pancreas, has occurred. Ureteric pain radiates to the tip of the penis in men and to the labium majoris in women.

Onset of pain

The onset of pain can be sudden or gradual. Typically, pain from a perforation is sudden and that from inflammation is gradual. Patients with the former can usually remember exactly what they were doing at the time of onset, whereas in the latter localization of time is more difficult.

Severity of pain

A patient's description of the severity of pain is very subjective. Every individual has a different reaction to pain, and this is often more reflective of the patient's personality than of the underlying pathology. A better indication is to assess the affect of the pain on the patient's life. For example, did they call their GP? Were they unable to attend

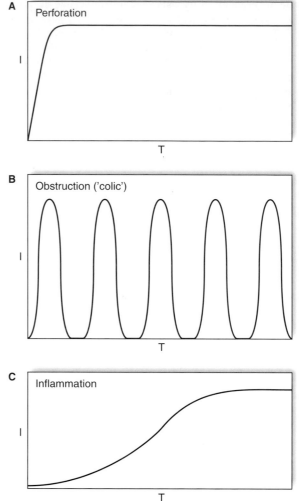

Fig. 16.5   Time vs intensity graphs for acute abdominal pain.

work? Did the pain interfere with their sleep? Furthermore, it is often useful to ask the patient to give the severity of the pain as a score on a numerical or pictorial scale.

Progression of pain

Once a pain has occurred it may remain exactly the same, gradually improve or worsen, or may fluctuate.

Movement of pain

It is also useful to note whether the pain moves. The classic example of this is acute appendicitis, which starts as a vague central 'referred' pain and then moves to the right iliac fossa as the adjacent parietal peritoneum becomes inflamed.

The various characteristics of abdominal pain, as shown in Figure 16.5, are essential in helping the clinician formulate a differential diagnosis.

Examination

During the course of taking a history it is possible to get a general impression of the state of the patient. The unwell patient with acute abdominal pain may look pale and sweaty, lie flat on the bed, be cerebrally obtunded and unable to move without experiencing pain. Others, however, may look surprisingly well, have a good colour, sit up in bed, talk normally and be able to move freely. All these observations should be noted and recorded along with the temperature, pulse, blood pressure and respiratory rate.

Other important features to look for on general examination include clinical evidence of anaemia, jaundice,

cyanosis and dehydration. It is important to bear in mind that physical signs are often less obvious than might be expected in the elderly, the obese, the generally unwell, and those taking steroids. As in every emergency patient a full examination, including the cardiovascular, respiratory and neurological systems, in addition to the abdomen and pelvis, must be carried out and the results documented. Specific details relating to the abdominal examination are described below and in Table 16.8.

In small children with abdominal pain, it is useful to ask the child to 'blow out' and 'suck in' their abdomen and to cough. These three movements will usually elicit pain in the presence of peritonism without laying a hand on the child's abdomen. Rebound tenderness should *never* be elicited in children. Gentle tapping with the percussing finger will elicit the same information (tap tenderness) in a much less cruel way.

Table 16.8 Checklist for examination of the acute abdomen

Method	Question	Significance
Inspection		
	What is the abdominal contour?	Distension – intestinal obstruction or ascites
	Does the abdomen move with respiration?	Rigid abdomen – peritonitis
	Can the patient blow out/suck in the abdomen?	Rigid abdomen – peritonitis
	Does the patient lie still or writhe about?	Fear of movement – peritonitis
		Writhe about – colic
	Are there visible abnormalities?	Scars – relevant previous illness, adhesions
		Hernia – intestinal obstruction
		Visible peristalsis – intestinal obstruction
		Visible masses – relevant pathology
Gentle palpation		
	Is there tenderness, guarding or rigidity?	Tenderness/guarding – inflamed parietal peritoneum
		Rigidity – peritonitis
Deep palpation		
	Are there abnormal masses/palpable organs?	Palpable organs/masses – relevant pathology
	(Is there rebound tenderness?)	Rebound tenderness – peritonitis
Percussion		
	Is the percussion note abnormal?	Resonance – intestinal obstruction
		Loss of liver dullness – gastrointestinal perforation
		Dullness – free fluid, full bladder
		Shifting dullness – free fluid
Auscultation		
	Are bowel sounds present/abnormal?	Absent sounds – paralytic ileus
		Hyperactive sounds – mechanical obstruction – gastroenteritis
	Is there a bruit?	Bruit – vascular disease
Do not forget to:		
	Examine the groin	
	Do a digital rectal examination	
	Do a vaginal examination when appropriate	
	Examine the chest	

Inspection of the abdomen

In order to examine the abdomen the patient must be adequately exposed and positioned. The full extent of the abdomen should be visible, and by convention the patient should be exposed from 'nipples to knees'. This prevents the common mistake of not examining the breasts, groins and external genitalia. Patient dignity should be maintained and the breasts and genitalia covered once assessed. The patient should be positioned supine on a couch with a single pillow behind the head and shoulders and the arms resting by their side.

Inspection of the abdomen may reveal a wealth of information. Abdominal swellings due to abnormal enlargement of the liver, kidneys or spleen, tumours of the bowel, ovaries or other intra-abdominal or retroperitoneal structures may be visible. Scars from previous abdominal or pelvic surgery may be observed, and are of importance in the presence of bowel obstruction which may be secondary to adhesions. All scars should be tested for the presence of herniation. Distended veins on the abdominal wall may be secondary to portal hypertension or occlusion of the inferior vena cava. The abdomen may be generally distended by intra-abdominal blood or fluid, or as a result of intestinal obstruction. In cases of obstruction, intestinal peristalsis may be visible if the patient is thin.

Palpation

Palpation of the abdomen should be carried out in a systematic manner, beginning with gentle superficial examination of the whole abdomen looking for tenderness. This should start away from the site of maximum pain and move towards the tender site, encompassing all areas as shown in Figures 16.3 and 16.4. Palpation over an area of tenderness will cause pain, which in turn will stimulate the patient to contract the overlying muscles (**voluntary guarding**). If the pain is due to inflammation, the approximation of the parietal peritoneum on to the inflammatory area will result in a reflex contraction of the overlying muscles (**involuntary guarding**). If the whole peritoneal cavity is inflamed then there will be generalized peritonitis and the abdominal wall will be rigid (**board-like rigidity**). When the palpating hand, which has been pushing the parietal peritoneum against the inflamed viscus, is suddenly released, the viscus will bounce back and hit the parietal peritoneum, causing an additional sharp pain (**rebound tenderness**). This is an excellent indication of underlying peritoneal inflammation (peritonism) but is very painful and is better tested by light percussion. A history of pain on coughing is also a good indication of peritoneal inflammation.

If light palpation of the whole abdomen elicits no pain, the process is repeated pressing more firmly to detect deep tenderness. This will allow for the detection of organomegaly and the presence of any masses.

In the past the administration of opiate analgesia was traditionally withheld from patients with acute abdominal pain on the assumption that it might mask important clinical signs, particularly of localized tenderness. This has now been shown not to be the case, and analgesia should never be withheld from a patient pending formal examination. Indeed, the administration of analgesia relaxes the patient and may often help the examination. However, repeated administration of opiate analgesia to a patient with abdominal pain in whom a definite diagnosis has not been made cannot be supported without regular reassessment, as this suggests progression of the disease process and that surgical intervention may be indicated.

During the general examination particular attention should be paid to the supraclavicular fossae, axillae and cervical regions for the presence of lymphadenopathy. The hernial orifices must also be specifically examined, as must the male external genitalia, looking for tenderness and masses within the scrotum.

Percussion

Percussion is useful in the localization and assessment of tenderness, particularly in the assessment of rebound tenderness, in addition to determining the presence of fluid within the peritoneal cavity. The normal abdomen is universally resonant because of the presence of gas-containing bowel lying in front of the solid retroperitoneal structures, and because the normal pelvic viscera lie entirely within the bony pelvis.

The liver gives a dull note to percussion anteriorly from the level of the right fifth rib to the right costal margin, and loss of liver dullness to percussion may represent free intraperitoneal gas. The presence of suprapubic dullness may indicate a full bladder due to urinary retention. If there is free intraperitoneal fluid the percussion note will be dull in the flanks. The site of the dullness moves as the patient rolls on to their side (**shifting dullness**). One litre or more of fluid is required before this sign can be elicited.

Auscultation

Bowel will only produce gurgling noises if it contains a mixture of fluid and gas. Normal bowel sounds are low-pitched and occur every few seconds. Their absence over a 30-s period suggests that peristalsis has ceased, a condition termed **ileus**. This may be due to generalized peritonitis or atony of the bowel smooth muscle, such as might follow a prolonged period of obstruction. Increased peristalsis produces a higher volume, pitch and frequency of the bowel sounds and can be heard in mechanical obstruction (often described as 'tinkling'), in addition to conditions such as gastroenteritis. In general bowel sounds should be described as present and normal; present and abnormal; or absent.

Auscultation should continue over the course of the aorta and the iliac arteries, listening for the presence of bruits, which are indicative of turbulent flow.

If gastric outlet obstruction is clinically suspected, the patient's abdomen may be shaken from side to side in an attempt to elicit a **succussion splash**.

Finally, a rectal examination is performed to assess the pelvis and, if a gynaecological disorder is suspected, a vaginal examination is indicated. Examination of the rectum is 'routine' but may be omitted, particularly in young patients, when a diagnosis and management plan have already been made and are unlikely to be influenced by any information obtained. Useful information which might be obtained from a rectal examination include the presence of masses, tenderness and blood.

Specific clinical signs in acute abdominal pain

- **Murphy's sign** In acute cholecystitis a deep breath taken by the patient elicits acute pain when the examiner presses downwards into the right upper quadrant. This is

---

SUMMARY BOX

Abdominal pain

- Visceral abdominal pain is mediated by the sympathetic nervous system and is typically deep-seated and ill-localized to the area originally occupied by the viscus during intrauterine life.

- Colic is a form of visceral pain which arises from a hollow viscus with muscle in its walls (e.g. gut, gallbladder, ureter), and results from excessive muscle contraction, often against an obstructing agent.

- Patients experiencing colic are usually unable to remain still during the bout of pain but are pain-free between attacks. 'Biliary colic' is an exception (and the term colic may be a misnomer) in that pain often waxes and wanes on a plateau, and there are no pain-free intervals.

- Parietal pain such as that caused by parietal peritonitis is mediated by somatic nerves and is localized to the area of inflammation.

- Reflex guarding and rigidity of the overlying muscles is usually present, and the patient is reluctant to move for fear of exacerbating the pain.

- Some areas of the peritoneum are 'non-demonstrative' in that parietal peritonitis may be present without tenderness or guarding of overlying muscles (e.g. the pelvis, posterior abdominal wall).

---

caused by the movement of the inflamed gallbladder striking the examining hand.

- **Boas's sign** In acute cholecystitis pain radiates to the tip of the scapula and there is a tender area of skin just below the scapula, which is hyperaesthetic.
- **Grey-Turner's and Cullen's signs** In patients with severe advanced cases of acute pancreatitis, bruising and discoloration can be seen around the umbilicus (Cullen's sign) and in the left flank (Grey-Turner's sign). Cullen's sign was actually first described in relation to ruptured ectopic pregnancy, but is now often also associated with acute pancreatitis.
- **Rovsing's sign** In acute appendicitis palpation in the left iliac fossa produces pain in the right iliac fossa

Investigations

Following initial clinical assessment, and during assessment in the critically ill, measures should be taken to resuscitate the patient. During this period further investigations can be organized to help in the diagnostic process. It is important to remember that in all patients a working list of differential diagnoses must be made after clinical assessment so that only appropriate investigations are instituted. There is no point in organizing investigations the results of which will not influence the clinical management.

The most common investigations carried out on the patient with acute abdominal pain include full blood count (FBC), urea and electrolytes (U&Es), amylase, plain radiology (erect chest and supine abdominal X-rays) and an ultrasound scan.

Blood tests Blood tests, with the exception of a serum amylase level (which is the best diagnostic test for acute pancreatitis), rarely influence the clinical decision in patients with acute abdominal pain. However, FBC and U&Es are often taken as a baseline for future reference.

FBC and U&Es A single reading of a raised white cell count taken on its own is fairly non-discriminatory, but a persistent elevation or a rise suggests underlying inflammation and/or infection. Obviously U&Es are essential in patients who might be hypovolaemic in order to monitor fluid replacement, particularly if surgery is being considered. Similarly, an abnormal haemoglobin level may be significant and require correction.

Serum amylase A serum amylase >1000 IU is highly suggestive of acute pancreatitis. Lesser values are non-specific and can be the result of a wide range of conditions. However, as many as 20% of patients with acute pancreatitis may have normal amylase levels on admission. Other causes of a raised amylase are shown in Table 16.9. In patients with acute pancreatitis who present more than 48 hours after the onset of pain the serum amylase may have returned to normal. In these patients measurement of the urinary amylase may be of value.

Table 16.9	Causes of hyperamylasaemia
Pancreatic conditions	Acute pancreatitis Pancreatic cancer Pancreatic trauma
Other intra-abdominal pathology	Perforated peptic ulcer Acute appendicitis Ectopic pregnancy Intestinal infarction Acute cholecystitis
Decreased clearance of amylase	Renal failure Macroamylasaemia
Miscellaneous	Head injury Diabetic ketoacidosis Drugs (e.g. opiates)

Liver function tests Liver function tests are increasingly becoming available on an emergency rather than a routine basis in many hospitals, as clinicians have recognized their value in the assessment and subsequent management of acute hepatobiliary and pancreatic disorders.

Inflammatory markers C-reactive protein (CRP), an acute-phase protein, and the erythrocyte sedimentation rate (ESR), are both markers of acute inflammation when raised but, like the white cell count, tend to be of most value if trends are observed rather than one-off results.

Arterial blood sampling is often used to monitor the acid–base status and the efficacy of gas exchange in the seriously ill patient. Patients with sepsis and intestinal ischaemia are likely to demonstrate a metabolic acidosis.

Serum calcium Patients with hypercalcaemia may complain of abdominal pain as a result of abnormal gastro-intestinal motility, nephrolithiasis, peptic ulcer disease, pancreatitis or malignancy. A low calcium level is one of the poor prognostic factors in patients with severe acute pancreatitis.

Sickle tests Sickle cell crises are a rare cause of acute abdominal pain. Blood should be sent for testing on all at-risk patients.

Blood glucose Measurement of blood glucose is important as diabetic ketoacidosis may present with acute abdominal pain, and also because any serious illness can result in poor glycaemic control, particularly in diabetic patients.

Urinalysis

Dipstick testing Haematuria may result from a wide range of conditions but in the context of acute abdominal pain may indicate a urinary tract tumour, infection or nephrolithiasis. Glucose or ketones in the urine indicate recent starvation or possible diabetic ketoacidosis. Protein, bilirubin or casts in the urine suggest renal or liver disease. In patients with an inflamed retrocaecal appendix urine testing may demonstrate the presence of protein, and urgent microscopy (which will confirm or refute the presence of bacteria) should be arranged to determine whether there is an underlying urinary tract infection or whether another condition, such as appendicitis, might be the cause.

Bacteriology If the clinical picture is suggestive of a urinary tract infection and the urine dipstick demonstrates blood or protein, urgent microscopy and culture should be requested. Specimens from any other potential sites of infection should also be submitted for bacteriological analysis (stool, blood, pus etc).

Pregnancy test A pregnancy test should be performed in all women of childbearing age who present with acute abdominal pain in whom the chance of pregnancy cannot be excluded. Not only is this important if X-rays are to be taken, but it will also reveal the possibility of an ectopic pregnancy if positive.

Urinary porphobilinogen Quantitative assay of urinary porphobilinogen is the most important diagnostic test for porphyria, which may present with acute abdominal pain, and should be considered in difficult cases.

Radiological investigations

Plain X-rays The role of plain radiography in the investigation of the patient with acute abdominal pain has been well studied. The erect chest X-ray (CXR) is the most appropriate investigation for the detection of free intra-peritoneal gas (Fig. 16.6) and should be carried out in any patient who might have a perforation. If the condition of the patient prevents an erect film being taken then a left lateral abdominal decubitus film might be helpful. Although a visceral perforation is the commonest cause of free intra-peritoneal gas, other causes exist and should be considered where appropriate (Table 16.10).

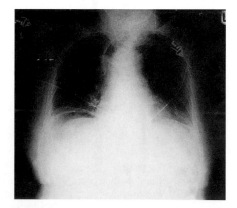

Fig. 16.6 Gas under the diaphragm in a patient with a perforated peptic ulcer seen on the erect chest X-ray.

Table 16.10 Causes of free subdiaphragmatic gas on AXR
Perforation of an intra-abdominal viscus Gas-forming infection Pleuroperitoneal fistula Iatrogenic: laparoscopy, laparotomy Gas introduced per vaginam: postpartum Interposition of bowel between liver and diaphragm

The role of plain abdominal radiographs remains controversial despite many studies which have demonstrated that, with the exception of suspected intestinal obstruction (Fig. 16.7A), they rarely help in the diagnosis and even less in altering the clinical decision. However, the supine abdominal X-ray (AXR) can be of use in patients whose diagnosis is unclear and in whom the presence of calcification (e.g. ureteric colic) and abnormal gas shadows (e.g. possible intestinal ischaemia) may be helpful.

An erect AXR is only of value in patients with intestinal obstruction, although it is well known that even then the information obtained over and above that from the supine film is small. In patients with suspected obstruction whose supine film does not show significant bowel dilatation, an erect film might reveal fluid levels (Fig. 16.7B).

Contrast radiology Contrast may be administered orally, down a nasogastric or nasojejunal tube, or per rectum to examine the bowel in patients with acute abdominal pain. In the emergency setting the contrast used is usually water soluble, as free egress of barium into the peritoneal cavity can cause inflammatory reactions and makes subsequent surgery more difficult. As water-soluble contrast does not adhere well to the bowel mucosa, the information obtained is less specific and detailed than with barium, but in the patient with acute abdominal pain the main issues that require the use of contrast X-rays are in determining the presence or absence of obstruction.

In up to 50% of patients with a perforated peptic ulcer no free gas can be identified on plain radiography. If the diagnosis remains uncertain based on clinical assessment, a

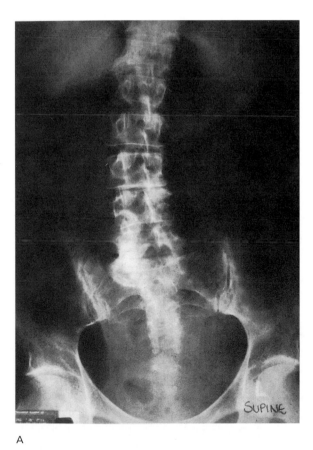

A

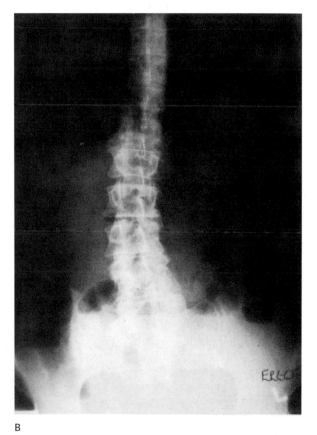

B

Fig. 16.7 **A** Supine abdominal X-ray in a patient with small bowel obstruction due to an obstructed right femoral hernia. **B** Erect abdominal X-ray in the same patient demonstrating multiple fluid levels.

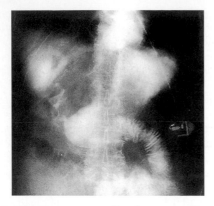

Fig. 16.8   Contrast seen exuding from a small perforated duodenal ulcer in a patient whose erect chest X-ray did not show any free gas.

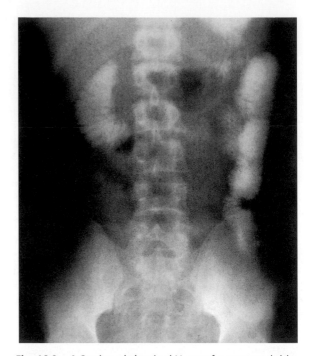

Fig. 16.9   **A** Supine abdominal X-ray of a water-soluble contrast follow-through in a patient with small bowel obstruction, taken after 90 minutes. Note the obvious distended small bowel. The contrast failed to reach the caecum after 4 hours and laparotomy confirmed complete small bowel obstruction from adhesions.

water-soluble contrast meal might be diagnostic (Fig. 16.8). In patients with small bowel obstruction a water-soluble small bowel follow-up can help, not only in confirming or refuting obstruction, but also in predicting which patient is likely to require surgery. Failure of contrast to reach the caecum by 4 hours suggests complete obstruction, and these patients will not usually settle with nonoperative management (Fig. 16.9).

A water-soluble contrast enema is now considered essential in the assessment of patients with large bowel obstruction in order to differentiate between pseudo-obstruction and an obstruction caused by a mechanical problem (Fig. 16.10). Carrying out an unnecessary operation on a patient with pseudo-obstruction is associated with a high morbidity and mortality and cannot be defended.

Intravenous pyelography confirms the diagnosis of renal obstruction by calculi and may be helpful in the diagnosis of other types of renal pain.

Ultrasonography   Ultrasound is increasingly being used in the investigation of patients with acute abdominal pain. As a general investigation it might reveal small amounts of intraperitoneal fluid in conditions such as perforation and infection, whereas in specific conditions such as acute cholecystitis, biliary obstruction, aortic aneurysms and ovarian cysts it can be diagnostic. Some studies have reported high levels of sensitivity and specificity in the diagnosis of acute appendicitis, but ultrasonography in these cases is highly operator dependent and a negative result cannot be relied upon, particularly if the clinical picture suggests otherwise.

Computerized tomography (CT)   CT is not used routinely as a first-line investigation in the acute abdomen. Its main role in the emergency situation is to evaluate traumatic injuries and intra-abdominal sepsis (such as acute

diverticular abscess), in addition to suspected leaking abdominal aortic aneurysms. Contrast-enhanced CT is used routinely to detect pancreatic necrosis in patients with severe acute pancreatitis.

Angiography   Mesenteric angiography is the investigation of choice in suspected mesenteric ischaemia, will differentiate arterial from venous causes, and distinguish occlusive from non-occlusive disease. Angiography is also of use in the diagnosis and management of lower gastrointestinal haemorrhage, although this rarely presents with acute abdominal pain.

Endoscopic investigations

Rigid sigmoidoscopy should be routine in all patients who present with an acute abdomen associated with rectal bleeding, and in those patients with large bowel obstruction to evaluate the anorectum. Additional information can be obtained from a flexible sigmoidoscopy or colonoscopy. Furthermore, a sigmoid volvulus can often be deflated by

Fig. 16.10   **A, B** Supine abdominal X-rays in patients with large bowel obstruction. **C** Contrast enema in patient A shows no mechanical cause, i.e. pseudo-obstruction. **D** An obstructing carcinoma of the sigmoid colon in patient B.   ▶

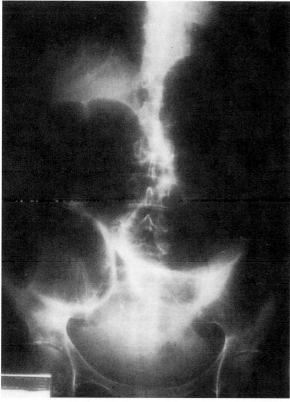

A

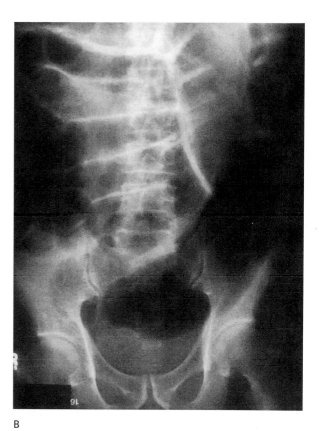

B

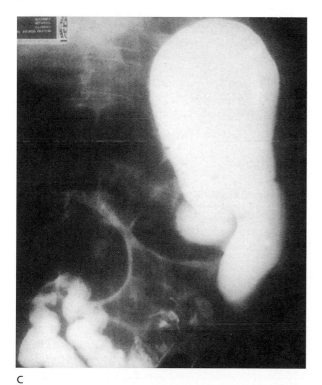

C

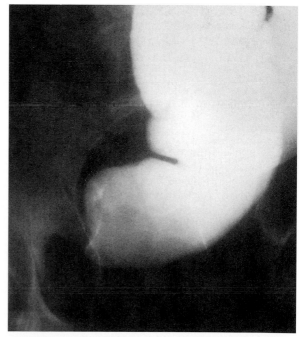

D

careful sigmoidoscopy. Upper gastrointestinal endoscopy is used to investigate patients with acute upper abdominal pain in whom a perforated peptic ulcer has been excluded, as discussed above.

Peritoneal investigations

Peritoneal lavage Peritoneal lavage has been used for many years now as one of the first-line investigations in patients suspected of having intra-abdominal haemorrhage from trauma, although its use has been increasingly overtaken by CT. It has also been used sparingly but with some success to evaluate the acute abdomen, and in those patients who present a diagnostic dilemma it can be helpful. It is carried out by inserting a dialysis catheter into the peritoneal cavity under local anaesthetic and infusing 1 L of normal saline. The effluent is removed and examined for white cell count, amylase, bacteria and bile.

Fine catheter aspiration peritoneal cytology This technique works on a similar principle to peritoneal lavage except that a much smaller catheter is inserted (4.5 Ch umbilical catheter through a 14 G venous cannula). Any fluid aspirated is deposited on to a slide and stained for white cells. A high percentage of polymorphs confirms underlying inflammation, but does not reveal the cause.

Laparoscopy Many studies have demonstrated that laparoscopy can significantly improve surgical decision making in patients with acute abdominal pain. It is particularly useful in patients for whom the decision to operate is in doubt, and in the elderly when findings from the history and examination can be misleading. Young women probably benefit the most from laparoscopy, as it is so difficult to differentiate acute appendicitis in this group from acute gynaecological conditions, many of which do not require surgery.

MANAGEMENT

General

All patients admitted with acute abdominal pain require resuscitation and close monitoring with regular re-evaluation. It is a good clinical rule that initial treatment should be based around the ABC principle (airway, breathing and circulation). Except in the management of overwhelming haemorrhage (e.g. ruptured abdominal aortic aneurysm and ruptured ectopic pregnancy), when resuscitation takes place on the way to the operating theatre, all patients with acute abdominal pain, including those requiring urgent surgery, benefit from adequate resuscitation. This will usually involve the administration of several litres of normal saline, intravenous antibiotics and oxygen by face mask. Monitoring by means of temperature, pulse, blood pressure, urine output and central venous pressure will

depend on the clinical circumstances and will not be detailed further here. Suffice to say that good preoperative assessment, resuscitation, monitoring and regular reviewing of the patient with acute abdominal pain (initially every 30 minutes to 2 hours, depending on the state of the patient) is an essential prerequisite for a satisfactory clinical outcome. Indeed, following the first assessment, close observation and regular reassessment should be carried out on **all** patients without a definitive diagnosis, as their condition may well change and the underlying cause or the correct management become more obvious. Until this time it is common practice to keep the patient fasted, and if there are signs or symptoms of obstruction, a nasogastric tube is inserted. Appropriate analgesia should be administered early to keep the patient as comfortable as possible. Deep venous thrombosis prophylaxis should also be commenced as a routine.

Specific

The management of most conditions presenting as an acute abdomen will be covered in detail in the relevant chapters. The remainder of this chapter will cover the principles that underpin the management of intestinal obstruction and acute appendicitis.

INTESTINAL OBSTRUCTION

The term intestinal obstruction refers to any form of impedance to the normal passage of bowel content through the small or large intestine. Intestinal obstruction is a common cause of acute abdominal pain, and is associated with a high morbidity and mortality if managed incorrectly. Intestinal obstruction is broadly classified as shown in Table 16.11, but the main differentiation lies between the small and the large bowel. The two entities are usually

Table 16.11 Classification of intestinal obstruction
Small bowel (high/low)
Large bowel
Mechanical   Functional
Simple   Strangulated
Partial   Complete

Acute
   Subacute
   Acute-on-chronic
   Chronic

Table 16.12 Causes of mechanical obstruction

Intrinsic
Congenital atresia
Inflammatory strictures
  Crohn's disease
  Tuberculosis
Tumours
  Benign
  Malignant
 	
Extrinsic
Adhesions
Hernias
Volvulus
Intussusception
Congenital bands
Inflammatory masses
Tumours
  Benign
  Malignant
 	
Luminal
Foreign bodies
Gallstones
Parasites
Bezoars

Table 16.13 Causes of functional obstruction

Systemic
Metabolic
  Hypokalaemia
  Hyponatraemia
  Hypothermia
  Hypoxia
  Diabetic ketoacidosis
  Uraemia
Drugs (tricyclic antidepressants)
General anaesthesia
Dehydration
Sepsis (acute pancreatitis)
Retroperitoneal malignancy (Ogilvie's syndrome)
Trauma
  Head injury
  Spinal injury
  Pelvic surgery
 	
Local
Infection
  Intra-abdominal infection/peritonitis
  Strongyloides
Trauma
Postoperative
 	
Vascular (mesenteric ischaemia)

considered separately as the aetiologies and clinical presentations differ, as does their management. However, they do share some basic principles, which will be discussed here.

Pathophysiology

Mechanical obstruction

A physical blockage causing impedance to the passage of bowel contents results in mechanical obstruction. These causes are usually divided into those that compress the bowel from the outside, those that arise from the wall of the bowel and obstruct the lumen, and those that arise within the lumen (Table 16.12). Adhesions remain the commonest cause of small bowel obstruction in the UK (60%), followed by hernias (20%) and malignancy (both primary and secondary – 10%). In the large bowel malignancy is the most common cause (65%), followed by complicated diverticular disease (10%) and volvulus (5%).

Adhesions are thought to result from a reduction in peritoneal plasminogen-activating activity (PAA), which in turn leads to a failure to break down the postoperative fibrinous adhesions that follow all intra-abdominal operations. This reduction in PAA is increased by drying and abrasion of the peritoneum during laparotomy, in addition to foreign substances such as talc (which has now been removed from surgical gloves).

Functional obstruction

This form of obstruction results from atony of the intestine with loss of normal peristalsis, in the absence of a mechanical cause. In the small bowel it is usually referred to as **paralytic ileus**, whereas in the large bowel the term **pseudo-obstruction** is used. The atony of the bowel may be localized to one segment or may be generalized. The pathophysiology is complex, but in essence results locally from an abnormality within the myenteric plexus of the bowel wall, and generally from an imbalance between sympathetic and parasympathetic nerve supply. A wide variety of underlying causal conditions is recognized (Table 16.13).

Clinical presentation and management

General

The bowel proximal to the physical obstruction dilates as a result of the accumulation of fluid and gas. The amount of fluid sequestrated in the bowel can be large, particularly in distal small bowel obstruction, and the gas that accumulates is mainly swallowed air, with luminal putrefaction making a small contribution. Absorption from the lumen is diminished and there is a net loss of water and electrolytes into the bowel lumen, some of which may then be lost in vomiting. The patient will therefore show signs of dehydration and hypovolaemia, with a decreased skin turgor, dry tongue, hypotension and tachycardia. The dilatation of the bowel activates stretch receptors in the wall, resulting in reflex contraction of smooth muscle. This produces colicky abdominal pain and abdominal distension. The bowel distal to the obstruction collapses as gas and fluid no longer pass into it, and as a result peristalsis within it eventually ceases. If the obstruction is not overcome the reflex activity proximal to the obstruction will eventually cease and the bowel becomes atonic, unless strangulation or perforation intervenes. In the absence of strangulation or perforation, hypovolaemia and ultimately starvation are the main factors that threaten life. As already discussed, fluid replacement is the mainstay of early treatment, and subsequent management will depend on other factors as detailed below.

Small bowel obstruction

Colicky pain and vomiting are early features of small bowel obstruction, with constipation appearing late and distension only really occurring if the obstruction is fairly distal. Patients usually give a short history, but the presenting event may not be the first, especially in those who have had previous abdominal surgery. Adhesions are the com-

monest cause of small bowel obstruction (60%) in the UK. In distal small bowel obstruction the onset may be more insidious and the vomiting may become faeculant (obstructed and stagnant small bowel contents, with resultant bacterial proliferation and overgrowth). Hernial orifices must be carefully examined and bowel sounds are likely to be high-pitched and tinkling. A full examination should be carried out. Rectal examination may reveal faecal impaction or the presence of a rectal tumour, diverticular masses or malignant deposits in the pouch of Douglas.

The major concern for the attending clinician is to exclude the possibility of strangulation. Although it is difficult to be certain, this is unlikely if abdominal tenderness (guarding or rebound) on palpation, tachycardia (after any associated hypovolaemia has been treated by rehydration), pyrexia or elevated white cells count are absent. If any of these signs is present then the possibility of strangulation rises accordingly, and operative treatment must be considered early. Similarly, if the colicky pain is either replaced by a continuous dull ache or is associated with a background constant pain, the possibility of strangulation increases. Strangulation is much more likely to occur if there is a closed loop obstruction (Fig. 16.2) within which the intraluminal pressure cannot be decompressed. Strangulation follows impairment of the blood supply to and from the bowel wall and leads to infarction. It is a surgical emergency and requires urgent operative intervention.

Following clinical assessment appropriate X-rays are organized. Small bowel distension (>2.5 cm in diameter) confirms the diagnosis and resuscitation is instituted. Small bowel can be differentiated from the colon by the 'valvulae conniventes', which completely cross the bowel wall (unlike the taeniae coli of the large bowel, which are incomplete), their relatively central position and their diameter (the small bowel rarely distends more than 4–5 cm in diameter, whereas the colon can distend to 10 cm and more in severe cases). If strangulation is not suspected, a period of non-operative treatment is then commenced. This will involve intestinal decompression by means of a nasogastric tube and intravenous fluid replacement. Quite marked hypokalaemia can occur in addition to the hypovolaemia, due primarily to the renal preservation of sodium, and needs to be closely monitored and corrected.

The period of non-operative treatment varies from patient to patient and can take many days. Care must be taken to ensure that strangulation or starvation does not occur, and therefore most surgeons would consider 2–3 days as the limit. A water-soluble small bowel contrast follow-through (as shown in Fig. 16.9) can be helpful in determining whether there is complete or incomplete obstruction. Failure of contrast to reach the caecum within 4 hours generally implies that surgery will be required.

Intussusception

Intussusception is a common cause of intestinal obstruction in the first year of life. The terminal ileum is peristalsed into the caecum and ascending colon thus causing intestinal obstruction (ileo-colic intussusception). This most commonly occurs after a viral illness which is thought to lead to enlargement of the Peyer's patches in the terminal small intestine. These patches become the lead point in the intussusception. In older children, small bowel polyps, tumours, intestinal wall haematomata seen in Henoch-Scholein purpura and Meckel's diverticulae can act as lead points in an intussusception (ileo-colic, ileo-ileal or ileo-ileo-colic).

Affected children present with a short history of screaming attacks, often said to be associated with attacks of pallor and drawing up of the knees. Anorexia and vomiting are common and the normal pattern of stooling can be disrupted. The abdomen becomes distended and tender and the child may pass the classic 'red-currant jelly' stool. Dehydration is common and affected infants may become drowsy and unrousable.

Initial assessment of affected infants must pay attention to rehydration. Intravenous access is essential (and often very difficult to obtain) and resuscitation with crystalloid or colloid solutions initiated. The history is often very characteristic, but differentiation from gastroenteritis can sometimes be difficult.

Abdominal examination may reveal a relatively 'empty' right iliac fossa and a sausage-shaped mass may be felt in the right upper quadrant. Abdominal x-rays may help clinch the diagnosis but may be unhelpful. Abdominal ultrasound scan has now become one of the main methods used to confirm the diagnosis. A target sign is seen when the intussusception is scanned transversely (the rings of the target represent the various layers of the bowel wall).

Treatment involves an attempt at pneumatic reduction of the intussusception using an air enema. A small tube is passed into the rectum and air pumped in using a pressure-limited valve. The reduction is monitored using x-ray screening. A second and third attempt after a delay of an hour or so between attempts may succeed where the initial attempt fails. Overall success rates for pneumatic reduction in excess of 80% have been reported. Failure to reduce the intussusception in this way requires laparotomy and reduction or resection of the affected intestine.

Large bowel obstruction

Although large bowel obstruction is three to four times less common than small bowel obstruction, it is more likely to require surgery and the associated morbidity and mortality is much higher. Malignancy is the most common cause of mechanical large bowel obstruction in the UK, but in third-world countries volvulus is more frequently encountered, and carcinoma and diverticulitis are rare. In the UK volvulus is predominantly a disease of the elderly and the mentally impaired. It is predisposed by the presence of a large redundant sigmoid loop based on a narrow mesentery. Most patients have a history of chronic constipation and laxative abuse.

Compared to small bowel obstruction, abdominal distension and constipation are common early features of large bowel obstruction, with colicky pain being less marked and vomiting only appearing very late. Although the rectum may be empty and complete obstruction results in absolute constipation (failure to pass faeces or flatus), a partial obstruction may result in the frequent passage of soft or liquid stools as a result of proximal peristaltic activity. These episodes of spurious diarrhoea often alternate with periods of constipation. Rectal examination is mandatory, although a cause for the obstruction is rarely palpable with the examining finger. However, the presence of blood and mucus on the glove is suggestive of a distal

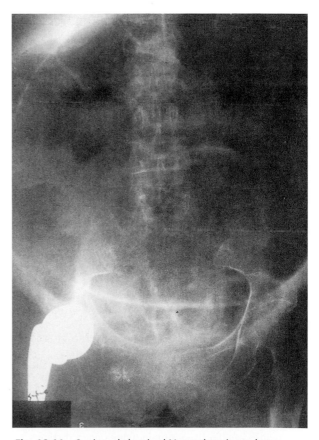

Fig. 16.11 Supine abdominal X-ray showing a huge sigmoid volvulus.

neoplasm. Sigmoidoscopy should be performed for two reasons: first, the obstructing lesion may be visible, and secondly a sigmoid volvulus (Fig. 16.11) might be decompressed.

If the ileocaecal valve is competent a closed loop obstruction exists and perforation of the caecum becomes a real possibility, particularly if its diameter measures 10 cm or more on plain X-rays. In such cases, following resuscitation and confirmation of the diagnosis with a water-soluble contrast enema, urgent laparotomy is carried out. The procedure performed varies according to the condition of the patient, the extent and site of the disease, and the experience of the operating surgeon. All these factors will be discussed in more detail in Chapter 22. If the ileocaecal valve is incompetent there is less urgency to perform surgery, but similar principles apply.

Pseudo-obstruction

This term refers to the presence of colonic obstruction for which no mechanical cause can be found. A wide variety of causes predisposes to this condition (Table 16.13), and once diagnosis has been established by water-soluble contrast enema, treatment is based on correction of the underlying disorder. Occasionally, in exceptional circumstances decompression is required, and this is carried out colonoscopically where possible. Operative decompression is rarely required.

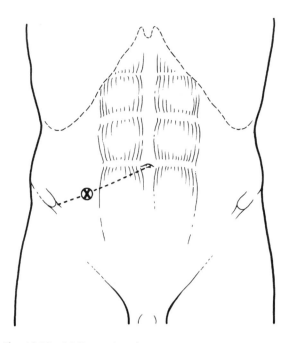

Fig. 16.12   McBurney's point.

ACUTE APPENDICITIS

Anatomy

The appendix is a worm-shaped blind-ending tube that arises from the posteromedial wall of the caecum 2 cm below the ileocaecal valve. It varies in length from 2 to 25 cm, but is most commonly 6–9 cm long. Externally the base of the appendix is found at the point of convergence of the three taeniae coli of the caecum. On the surface of the abdomen this point lies one-third of the way along a line drawn between the right anterior superior iliac spine and the umbilicus (McBurney's point; Fig. 16.12). The appendix has its own mesentery, the mesoappendix, and its blood supply comes from the appendicular artery, a branch of the ileocolic artery. The position of the appendix is variable, depending on its length and mobility. In cadaveric dissections the commonest site is retrocaecal, but data from diagnostic laparoscopy indicate that the pelvic position is probably more common (Fig. 16.13). In children there are abundant lymphoid follicles in the submucosa, but these atrophy with age.

Epidemiology

In the UK appendicitis is the most common cause of acute abdominal pain requiring surgery, and it has been estimated that 16% of the population of western countries will

---

SUMMARY BOX

Treatment of intestinal obstruction

- In paralytic ileus treatment is directed at the underlying cause (e.g. peritonitis, pancreatitis).

- In mechanical obstruction prompt diagnosis and management are normally essential to avoid the danger of strangulation. Management consists of vigorous restoration of fluid and electrolyte balance, followed by prompt surgical intervention.

- Strangulated bowel is blue or black, lacks sheen and peristaltic activity, and has no arterial pulsation in the adjacent mesentery. Strangulated bowel has to be resected with end-to-end anastomosis or exteriorization of the ends of the divided intestine.

- Situations in which conservative treatment of mechanical intestinal obstruction may sometimes be justifiable include adhesion obstruction, widespread intra-abdominal malignancy, Crohn's disease and postoperative obstruction.

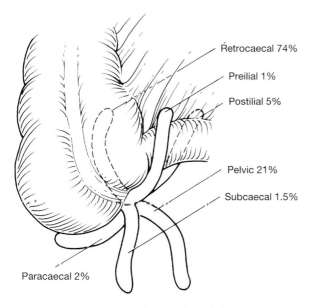

Fig. 16.13 Variations in the position of the appendix.

Retrocaecal 74%

Preilial 1%

Postilial 5%

Pelvic 21%

Subcaecal 1.5%

Paracaecal 2%

undergo appendicectomy for presumed appendicitis during their lifetime. There has been a decline in the incidence of appendicitis over the last 20 years, but the reason for this is unknown. There is an equal incidence in males and females. Appendicitis is uncommon in patients below the age of 2 and above the age of 65, and it is commonest in the under 40s, with a peak incidence between 8 and 14 years. There is a geographical variation in the incidence, being rare in Asia and Central Africa, which is thought to be due to environmental factors. In western countries it is seen more frequently in cities than in rural areas.

Aetiology

Despite its prevalence, the aetiology of acute appendicitis remains unclear. Several different mechanisms have been proposed, with a diet lacking in fibre resulting in a slow transit time and an alteration in bacterial flora being one of the more popular causes. However, this theory is challenged by the decline in incidence of appendicitis over recent years which has not been matched by an increase in dietary fibre intake. Others have suggested that viral infection may be an aetiological agent, as there is an association between appendicitis and concurrent viral illness and because there is a seasonal variation in the incidence of appendicitis.

Pathogenesis

Obstruction of the lumen of the appendix is thought to play the main role in the initiation of inflammation. Faecoliths,

lymphoid hyperplasia, foreign bodies, carcinoid tumours and strictures may all cause luminal obstruction and subsequently lead to acute appendicitis. Following obstruction, the wall of the appendix becomes inflamed, commencing in the mucosa and spreading to involve the submucosa, muscular and serosal layers. A fibrinopurulent exudate forms on the serosal surface and extends to any adjacent peritoneal surface. Inflammation of the wall of the appendix causes venous congestion, which may compromise arterial inflow, leading to ischaemia and infarction. Organisms from the lumen of the appendix enter the submucosa through an ischaemic ulcer, causing liquefaction of the wall and ultimately perforation.

As a result of the transmural inflammation small bowel and omentum adhere to the appendix, creating a localized area of sepsis. If left untreated this may progress to form an appendix mass or even an abscess. If perforation occurs early in the clinical course the inflamed area will not have had time to be walled off, and generalized peritonitis follows.

Clinical features

History

Classically the onset of acute appendicitis is associated with the gradual onset of poorly localized, central abdominal pain. After a variable amount of time the pain moves to the right iliac fossa and changes in character, to become sharper, constant and well localized. It is aggravated by movement and coughing. As described earlier, this change in the nature of the pain occurs when the parietal peritoneum overlying the appendix becomes involved in the inflammatory process. In general most patients present within 24 hours of the onset of the central abdominal pain. Many patients also admit to anorexia and occasional vomiting.

In children, the classic history and physical findings of appendicitis are often not seen. Non-specific symptoms (anorexia, nausea, vomiting, diarrhoea) and signs (fever, foetor, pallor, abdominal distension) can confuse the inexperienced clinician. The finding of tenderness and guarding in the right iliac fossa usually make the diagnosis without the need for other investigations.

Examination

The patient with established acute appendicitis looks unwell, is flushed and has a dry furred tongue with a foetor. The temperature is usually only mildly elevated (37.3–38.5°C) and there is often a tachycardia. Classically the area of maximal tenderness is over McBurney's point, with guarding and rebound (percussion) tenderness. Palpation in the left iliac fossa may reproduce the pain in the right iliac fossa (Rovsing's sign) and the patient may find it painful to extend the right hip owing to irritation of the psoas muscle (psoas stretch sign). Although rectal and vaginal examinations are frequently normal, they can be useful when the abdominal signs are vague, particularly if the acutely inflamed appendix lies within the pelvis, when tenderness may be elicited with the examining finger. In young women, either rectal or vaginal examination is extremely useful in helping to differentiate acute appendicitis from acute gynaecological disorders.

Variations in clinical features

The symptoms and signs of acute appendicitis are influenced by a variety of factors, which include age, sex, personality, and the position of the appendix. Only 50% of patients with acute appendicitis give a typical history. An inflamed retrocaecal appendix may produce poorly localized abdominal pain, and an inflamed pelvic appendix lying close to the bladder may produce symptoms of frequency and dysuria. In this scenario, as with a retrocaecal appendix which overlies the ureter, it may be quite difficult to differentiate between urinary infection and acute appendicitis. Dipstick examination of the urine may reveal microscopic haematuria and proteinuria in both cases. However, urgent microscopy and Gram stain of the urine will demonstrate bacteria in urinary tract infection. An inflamed pelvic appendix lying near the rectum causes irritation and diarrhoea, and is commonly mistaken for gastroenteritis. However, gastroenteritis is a dangerous diagnosis to make in the acute abdomen as it almost never causes abdominal tenderness (compared to abdominal pain). A very long appendix extending up to the right upper quadrant might even mimic acute cholecystitis.

Acute appendicitis is most dangerous in the very young, the very old and pregnant women.

Because it is uncommon under the age of 2 years, when it does occur it is often incorrectly diagnosed as gastroenteritis. The symptoms and signs are atypical and generalized peritonitis quickly develops. In contrast, in elderly patients the onset is more insidious. The inflamed area tends to wall off, with the development of a mass, and symptoms and signs of obstruction may be present. In the pregnant patient the appendix is displaced upwards by the enlarged uterus, and the site of the pain and tenderness is high in the abdomen. Appendicitis in pregnancy carries a high rate of morbidity and mortality for both mother and fetus.

A list of conditions that should be considered in the differential diagnosis of acute appendicitis is given in Table 16.14:

Complications

Gangrenous appendicitis and perforation tend to occur after a significantly more prolonged period of pain than uncom-

Table 16.14 Differential diagnosis of acute appendicitis
Mesenteric adenitis
Meckel's diverticulitis
Regional ileitis (Crohn's disease)
Carcinoma of the caecum
Gynaecological disorders
Ruptured ovarian follicle (Mittelschmerz)
Acute salpingitis
Ruptured ectopic pregnancy
Torsion of an ovarian cyst
Genitourinary
Pyelonephritis
Ureteric colic
Urinary tract infection
Right-sided testicular torsion

plicated appendicitis. Generalized peritonitis results if the inflamed area is not walled off by omentum and loops of bowel. If walling off does occur, either an appendix mass or an abscess will develop. A perforated pelvic appendix will lead to a pelvic abcess, and on examination there may be very little in the way of abdominal signs.

Investigations

The various investigations used in patients with suspected appendicitis have already been discussed earlier in the chapter. However, the diagnosis of acute appendicitis is based on clinical assessment and there are no specific diagnostic tests. Ultrasonography in skilled hands might demonstrate a swollen non-compressible appendix, free fluid, or even a mass in the right iliac fossa. If, after clinical assessment, the diagnosis remains in doubt, the clinician must proceed along one of two lines: either to carry out laparoscopy and undertake appendicectomy if indicated or to institute a short policy of close and repeated observation with reassessment every hour.

Management

The treatment of appendicitis is almost always surgical. However, studies have shown that in patients without overt peritonitis antibiotic treatment can be successful, and this is often used in areas of the world where ready access to surgery is impossible. In these conditions there is a high incidence of recurrent problems and as such it is not favoured. If, by the time the patient presents, a mass can be felt, non-operative treatment with intravenous fluids and antibiotics is the treatment of choice provided there are no signs of peritonitis (when an operation should be carried out). In these patients an ultrasound should be arranged to look for an underlying abscess which, if present, should be drained either under radiological guidance or surgically.

Following successful non-operative treatment of an appendix mass, it used to be traditional practice to carry out an interval appendicectomy 6–12 weeks later. This prevents further attacks, and in the elderly makes sure that there is not an underlying carcinoma of the caecum. Although this remains good practice, surgeons are increasingly finding that at the time of the appendicectomy the appendix is shrunken and fibrotic. Several studies have confirmed that after the successful non-operative treatment of either an appendix mass or an abscess only a few patients develop recurrent problems, and most of them do so within the first few months. It is therefore reasonable not to carry out an interval appendicectomy unless the patient experiences further symptoms or complications. However, especially in older patients, it is essential that a carcinoma of the caecum is first excluded by either double contrast barium enema or colonoscopy. An interval appendicectomy should be undertaken if this course is not pursued.

Prognosis

The overall mortality of appendicitis is less than 1%, rising to 5% if perforation occurs, and increases with age. The postoperative morbidity is mainly related to wound infection and late-onset intestinal obstruction from adhesions. The former can be kept to a minimum by perioperative prophylactic antibiotics (metronidazole), and the latter by careful surgery and perhaps the increasing use of laparoscopic appendicectomy. It used to be thought that fertility in female patients was adversely affected by appendicectomy, but this no longer seems to be the case and even in cases of perforated appendicitis there appears to be no increased risk of infertility.

NON-SPECIFIC ABDOMINAL PAIN (NSAP)

The term NSAP is often applied to patients in whom no cause can be found for their abdominal pain. In studies its incidence is around 40% for all patients admitted with acute abdominal pain, dropping to around 25% if investigations such as laparoscopy are used to improve diagnostic accuracy. The major concern in reaching a diagnosis of NSAP is that a serious underlying condition has been missed. It has been reported that 10% of patients over 50 years of age who are discharged with NSAP from hospital after an acute admission with abdominal pain have an underlying malignancy, of which half are colonic. Another group of patients who tend to be diagnosed with NSAP are young females who may have a gynaecological condition,

such as pelvic inflammatory disease or ovarian cyst pathology. With the more widespread use of laparoscopy in the investigation of patients with acute abdominal pain the incidence of NSAP will continue to fall.

GYNAECOLOGICAL CAUSES OF THE ACUTE ABDOMEN

Mittelschmerz and ruptured corpus luteum

The Graafian follicle normally ruptures 14 days after the start of the last menstrual period, and release of the ovum may be complicated by bleeding. The follicle normally becomes a corpus luteum, which degenerates before the start of the next period unless conception occurs. Bleeding from the corpus luteum is an occasional cause of pain in the late stages of the menstrual cycle.

Patients with these causes of pain are usually between 15 and 25 years of age, and experience sudden pain in one or other iliac fossa. Tenderness and guarding in the right iliac fossa can simulate acute appendicitis, and a few patients bleed sufficiently to suggest rupture of an ectopic pregnancy. Rectal or vaginal examination may reveal tenderness in the rectovaginal pouch.

The patient is treated conservatively unless appendicitis or ruptured ectopic pregnancy cannot be excluded. Laparoscopy may help to avoid unnecessary surgery, as ultrasonography alone will not be diagnostic.

Ruptured ectopic pregnancy

A fertilized ovum implants at an abnormal site in 1 in 200 pregnancies and the fallopian tube is by far the commonest site. The erosive trophoblast may penetrate the wall of the tube, and often ruptures after about 6 weeks. Alternatively, the conceptus may be extruded from the fimbrial end of the tube.

Bouts of cramping iliac fossa pain may be associated with fainting and vaginal bleeding. Rupture produces sudden severe pain, bleeding and circulatory collapse. The abdominal pain often becomes generalized. A missed period is reported by most patients.

Torsion of an ovarian cyst

Benign ovarian cysts are a common cause of torsion. Dermoid cysts often have a long pedicle and account for 50% of torsions in young women.

Severe cramping lower abdominal pain is often associated with a smooth round mobile mass which lies higher in the abdomen than might be expected. Tenderness and guarding may be present, particularly if there is leakage, and rupture results in diffuse peritonism. Torsion of a fallopian tube or fibroid may produce a similar picture.

At laparoscopy the twisted pedicle is transfixed and ligated and the cyst is removed. Care must be taken to avoid rupture in case the cyst is malignant. Further radical surgery may be needed if histological examination reveals malignancy.

Acute salpingitis

Acute salpingitis may be due to streptococcal infection, but gonococcal or tuberculous infection can also be responsible. Both tubes are often involved and adhesions may seal the fimbriated end, producing a pyosalpinx.

Bilateral pain is felt just above the pubis and inguinal ligaments. There may be urinary frequency, irregular menstration, pyrexia and leukocytosis. Vaginal examination reveals unusual warmth, a tender cervix and a vaginal discharge. The cervix appears red and inflamed, and a swab reveals the causative organism. Vaginal findings may be less marked when there is a closed pyosalpinx.

Treatment consists of antibiotic therapy. Laparoscopy is used increasingly to avoid unnecessary laparotomy if acute appendicitis cannot be ruled out. The tubes appear inflamed and oedematous, and 'milking' them gently produces a purulent discharge from which a bacteriological swab is taken.

SUMMARY BOX

Gynaecological causes of pain and the acute abdomen

- Non-specific abdominal pain (i.e. pain for which no cause is defined) is particularly common in female adolescents and young women, and often mimics acute appendicitis. Laparoscopy may prove increasingly valuable when the diagnosis is in doubt and the need for surgery cannot be excluded.

- Minor intraperitoneal bleeding at the time of rupture of the Graafian follicle may cause midcycle pain (Mittelschmerz) in the iliac fossa in young girls.

- Rupture of an ectopic pregnancy causes intraperitoneal bleeding and more severe abdominal pain, with circulatory collapse. Signs of pregnancy are seldom present and pregnancy testing may be unhelpful. Elevation of the foot of the bed may produce shoulder-tip pain and underline the need for laparotomy.

- Torsion of an ovarian cyst often causes cramping lower abdominal pain. Ovarian cysts can become very large and produce visible abdominal swellings which lie higher than might be expected. Some cysts prove to be malignant and care must be taken to avoid rupture at operation.

- Acute salpingitis is often due to gonococcal infection and produces bilateral suprapubic pain which is often associated with urinary frequency, a tender cervix and vaginal discharge.

17 The oesophagus

K. Munro, S. Paterson-Brown

SURGICAL ANATOMY

The oesophagus extends from the cricoid cartilage (at the level of C6 vertebra) to the gastric cardia and is 25 cm long. It has cervical, thoracic and abdominal portions. The oesophagus passes through the diaphragm at the level of the 10th thoracic vertebra and the final 2–4 cm lie within the peritoneal cavity. The relationships are shown in Figures 17.1 and 17.2.

The oesophagus has an upper sphincter, the cricopharyngeus, and a lower sphincter which cannot be defined anatomically but is a 3–5 cm high pressure area located in the region of the oesophageal hiatus of the diaphragm. The oesophagus is held loosely in the hiatus by a thickening of fascia, the phreno-oesophageal ligament.

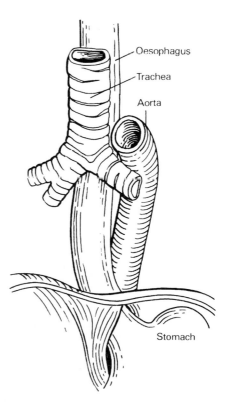

Fig. 17.1 Anatomical relationships of the oesophagus.

221

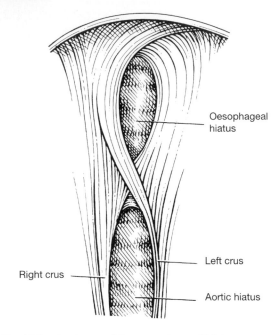

Fig. 17.2 Anatomy of the oesophageal hiatus.

The oesophageal wall can be divided into several layers:

- An outer advential connective tissue layer
- Outer longitudinal muscle layer
- Inner circular muscle layer, the upper third consisting of striated muscle and the lower part smooth muscle
- Auerbach's neural plexus lies between the two muscle layers
- The submucosa consists of mucous glands, lymphatics and Meissner's neural plexus
- The mucosa consists of stratified squamous epithelium, except for the distal 1–2 cm, which are lined by columnar epithelium.

The oesophagus receives its blood supply from the inferior thyroid artery in the cervical region, the bronchial arteries and branches from the thoracic aorta in the thorax, and the inferior phrenic and left gastric arteries in the abdomen.

Venous drainage is to the inferior thyroid veins in the neck, the hemiazygous and azygous veins (systemic circulation) in the thorax, and the left gastric (portal circulation) in the abdomen. The connection between these veins is important in the development of varices in patients with portal hypertension.

Sympathetic nerve supply is derived from preganglionic fibres from spinal cord segments T5 and T6, and postganglionic fibres from the cervical vertebral and coeliac ganglia. Parasympathetic supply comes from the glossopharyngeal, recurrent laryngeal and vagus nerves.

The lymphatics run in the submucosa and drain to the regional lymph nodes and subsequently to the posterior mediastinal, supraclavicular and coeliac lymph nodes.

SYMPTOMS OF OESOPHAGEAL DISORDERS

Dysphagia

Dysphagia is defined as difficulty in swallowing. It is a serious symptom and requires assessment. Certain points in the history are helpful in leading to a diagnosis:

- **Onset:** Sudden onset suggests a foreign body. In carcinoma the dysphagia occurs over a period of weeks, whereas in achalasia and benign strictures symptoms tend to develop over a number of years.
- **Site:** The actual site of obstruction correlates poorly in general to where the patient feels the discomfort, although some patients who feel the obstruction to be high may have a pharyngeal pouch.
- **Progression:** Dysphagia progresses rapidly in carcinoma and slowly in benign strictures and achalasia.
- **Severity:** Difficulty in swallowing solids is initially typical of carcinoma, whereas achalasia tends to be associated with dysphagia to liquids at first.
- **Causes:** A list of the common causes of dysphagia is shown in Table 17.1.

Pain

Heartburn is a retrosternal burning sensation, and is associated with reflux of acid into the mouth. It tends to occur after eating and is exacerbated by bending and lying down. It can be relieved with antacids and is associated with gastro-oesophageal reflux disease, peptic ulcer disease, benign strictures and primary motility disorders. Carcinoma of the oesophagus may progress to produce a constant central chest pain, which can be referred to the back between the shoulder blades. Retrosternal chest pain radiating to the back can also be a symptom of oesophageal perforation following recent instrumentation or vomiting. Achalasia tends to be painless. Angina is a differential diagnosis of retrosternal chest pain. Odynophagia is pain on swallowing, and may coexist with dysphagia.

Regurgitation

This is an effortless process whereby food is regurgitated into the mouth. There is no associated nausea and the patient does not vomit. It is associated with achalasia, hiatus hernia and pharyngeal pouches, in which regurgitation can lead to coughing and aspiration pneumonia.

Table 17.1 Causes of dysphagia

	Intraluminal	Intramural	Extrinsic
Pharynx/upper oesophagus	Foreign body	Pharyngitis/tonsillitis Moniliasis Sideropenic web Corrosives Carcinoma Myasthenia gravis Bulbar palsy	Thyroid enlargement Pharyngeal pouch
Body of oesophagus	Foreign body	Corrosives Peptic oesophagitis Carcinoma	Mediastinal lymph nodes Aortic aneurysm
Lower oesophagus	Foreign body	Corrosives Peptic oesophagitis Carcinoma Diffuse oesophageal spasm Scleroderma Achalasia Postvagotomy	Paraoesophageal hernia

EXAMINATION

Physical examination might reveal signs that will aid in the diagnosis of oesophageal disorders. A smooth tongue, pallor and koilonychia are signs of iron deficiency anaemia, which can be present in oesophageal carcinoma, oesophagitis and Plummer–Vinson syndrome.

Lymphadenopathy, particularly in the supraclavicular region, hepatomegaly, abdominal mass, ascites and evidence of weight loss are associated with malignancy. Crepitus in the neck is a sign of surgical emphysema which would suggest an oesophageal perforation. Neurological examination may reveal a neurological cause for the symptoms.

INVESTIGATIONS

Blood tests

A full blood count may exclude anaemia. Serum urea and electrolytes may show dehydration secondary to dysphagia. Liver function tests might show low plasma proteins, abnormal clotting and elevated enzymes in the presence of metastatic disease, and portal hypertension.

Radiology
Chest X-ray

A chest X-ray may show any of the following signs:

- Consolidation and fibrosis following aspiration in patients with oesophageal motility disorders and oesophageal carcinoma
- Air/fluid level behind the heart shadow from a hiatus hernia
- Mediastinal mass of lymph nodes and pulmonary metastases in oesophageal carcinoma
- The gastric air bubble may be indented by a carcinoma of the cardia
- Air may be seen in the mediastinum and neck after perforation of the oesophagus.

Barium swallow

A barium swallow may provide the following information:

- Reflux in the head-down position
- Smooth benign strictures
- Irregular malignant strictures
- A fusiform dilation with a tapered lower end may be evident in achalasia. The normal gas bubble in the stomach is also absent, as the oesophagus never completely empties
- Water-soluble contrast is used if perforation of the oesophagus is suspected, as barium is irritant to the mediastinum.

Endoscopy

Flexible oesophagogastroduodenoscopy (OGD) is now the first-line investigation for almost all oesophageal disorders, particularly those that present with symptoms of dyspepsia, dysphagia, haematemesis, atypical chest pain and weight loss. Flexible OGD is carried out either under light intravenous sedation or using a local anaesthetic throat spray. The patient should be fasted for 4 hours before the procedure. It is important to monitor pulse and oxygen saturation throughout the procedure to identify and rectify any possible respiratory depression that might follow the sedation.

The technique of OGD is used to inspect the oesophageal mucosa and allows biopsies to be taken. Therapeutic procedures, such as dilatation of strictures, insertion of stents, thermal ablation of tumours (using laser or Argon beam coagulation), removal of foreign bodies and control of bleeding varices and ulcers by injection of adrenaline, sclerotherapy, banding and thermocoagulation, can also be carried out.

Endoscopy can be complicated by perforation of the oesophagus, which occurs most frequently during stricture dilatation.

Computerized tomography (CT)

CT is used most commonly to investigate and stage oesophageal tumours (Fig. 17.3). In addition to the high dose of radiation required, even the most up-to-date spiral CT scanners still have a significant incidence of over- and understaging of tumours. As a result, endoscopic ultrasound is rapidly overtaking CT as the best staging modality for oesophageal tumours.

Ultrasonography

Percutaneous abdominal ultrasound is a relatively inexpensive and simple method for detecting liver metastases, which can be biopsied if required. Similarly, there have been several recent reports on the use of ultrasonography in the neck to identify metastatic lymphadenopathy from oesophageal tumours. However, endoscopic ultrasonography (EUS) is likely to revolutionize the investigation of oesophageal disorders, and particularly carcinoma (Fig. 17.4). Not only can all the layers of the oesophagus be clearly seen, with excellent assessment of any tumours, but invasion outside the lumen and adjacent lymph node enlargement can also be identified and biopsied if necessary.

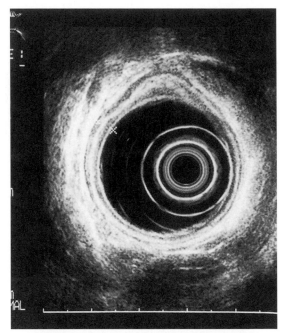

A

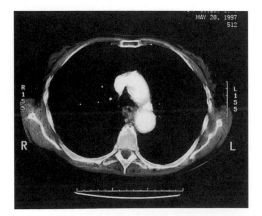

Fig. 17.3 Contrast-enhanced CT of thorax demonstrating a thickened oesophagus due to carcinoma.

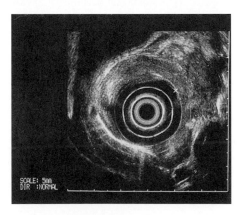

B

Fig. 17.4 EUS demonstrating **A** the normal layers of the oesophagus and a small carcinoma at 12-o-clock; **B** a large carcinoma of the oesophagus extending outside the muscle layer.

Laparoscopy

Laparoscopy which can be combined with laparoscopic ultrasound is useful to exclude liver and peritoneal metastases from lower oesophageal carcinoma before surgical resection is undertaken.

Manometry and pH studies

Measurements of lower oesophageal pH, using intraluminal electrodes, and pressure, obtained from a series of saline-perfused tubes connected to pressure transducers passed down the oesophagus, can be used to investigate various motility disorders of the oesophagus, in addition to gastro-oesophageal reflux disease (Fig. 17.5).

 The main tools for the investigation of oesophageal disease in children are contrast radiology, pH studies and upper gastrointestinal endoscopy.

IMPACTED FOREIGN BODIES

Swallowed foreign bodies are particularly common in children after accidental ingestion, and obstruction of the oropharynx and tracheal opening by a large food bolus can rapidly be fatal. The obstruction can usually be removed by coughing or a sharp blow to the back, or alternatively by the Heimlich manoeuvre (Fig. 17.6). The level at which foreign bodies tend to stick correlates with anatomical areas of narrowing, which can be found at:

● Arches of the fauces
● Vallecula
● Piriform fossae
● Cricopharyngeus
● Where the left main bronchus crosses the oesophagus
● Where the arch of the aorta crosses the oesophagus
● The diaphragm
● The gastro-oesophageal junction.

Foreign bodies can, however, become lodged at any level where there is a benign or a malignant stricture. Patients can present in severe distress, with chest pain and retching. In severe cases there may be a perforation, resulting in mediastinitis and haematemesis.

Investigation

A chest X-ray may show the foreign body if it is radio-opaque and/or there are signs of perforation. A water-soluble contrast swallow can provide confirmation. Endoscopy will allow direct visualization of the foreign body.

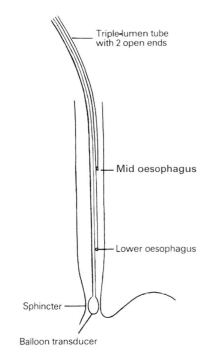

A

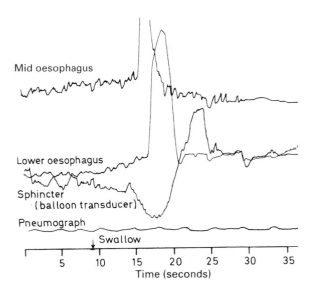

B

Fig. 17.5 Recording of the luminal pressure within the oesophagus. **A** Balloon pressure transducer and open-tipped catheter assembly in place. **B** Pressure recordings of swallowing responses in healthy subject. Note that relaxation of the lower oesophagus sphincter precedes the arrival of the peristaltic wave.

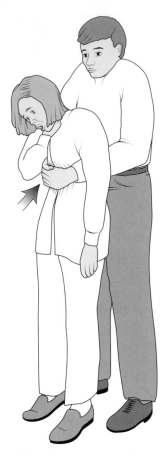

Fig. 17.6 Heimlich manoeuvre to remove an impacted foreign body in the pharynx. The patient's dentures are removed and an attempt is made to remove the bolus by hooking it out with a finger. The arms are grasped firmly over the epigastrium and lower chest from behind the patient. Following the last gasp, a firm squeeze is given to the upper abdomen. This is repeated every 10 seconds for half a minute.

Treatment

Some patients can be treated conservatively and observed until the foreign body has passed, but in the majority endoscopic removal is advisable. This can be carried out using either flexible endoscopy under sedation or rigid oesophagoscopy under general anaesthesia. The latter is particularly useful if the bolus is impacted.

CORROSIVE OESOPHAGITIS

Ingestion of strong acid or alkali occurs accidentally, especially, in children, and deliberately in attempted suicide. It results in severe chemical burns to the mouth, pharynx and oesophageal mucosa, particularly at the sites of anatomical narrowing owing to hold-up of the flow. Oedema, ulceration and inflammation follow, which in turn can lead to acute obstruction and perforation. The inflamed tissue then heals by fibrosis and stricture formation. Patients complain of severe continuous pain, which is exacerbated by swallowing. On examination the oropharynx may be inflamed, the patient may be shocked and the oesophagus may have perforated.

Alkaline solutions are the most common cause of corrosive oesophageal injuries in children, particularly in the Middle East and in developing countries. Acid ingestion causes both oesophageal and gastric injuries. Careful, early upper gastrointestinal endoscopy under general anaesthesia is essential to assess the extent and severity of the injury. Passage of a nasogastric or nasojejunal tube under the same anaesthetic will allow enteral feeding to commence and provide a passage for a guidewire should subsequent balloon dilatation for stricture formation be necessary.

Investigation

Endoscopy or barium swallow will demonstrate the extent and severity of the injury at the time of the acute event, and later to assess stricture formation.

Treatment

In the first instance an accurate history should be obtained and a detailed examination undertaken. The patient should be resuscitated and given appropriate opiate analgesia. They should also be encouraged to drink water to dilute the corrosive. Thereafter the oesophagus should be rested and the patient kept nil by mouth and commenced on intravenous fluids and antibiotics. The use of steroids to reduce the extent of the inflammation and subsequent stricture formation remains controversial. Vomiting should be actively discouraged, as this can cause further burns and risks perforation. If the patient's oropharynx is severely inflamed, an artificial airway (tracheostomy) may be required. Feeding is usually established with TPN or a feeding jejunostomy or gastrostomy. The patient is observed for perforation and later for stricture formation.

Strictures will usually require treatment with balloon dilatation. Long-term management may involve local resection of the stricture and primary anastomosis, or a more extensive resection with reconstruction using stomach, jejunum or colon. The stomach is often also damaged in the same disease process and, if so, cannot be used for reconstruction. Regular endoscopic surveillance will be required, as corrosive injury predisposes the oesophagus to malignant change.

PERFORATION

Causes

1. Intraluminal
   - swallowed foreign body or during its removal during instrumentation, with rigid endoscopy having a much greater risk than flexible. The most common sites of perforation tend to coincide with the sites of anatomical narrowing. Perforation most commonly occurs during balloon dilatation of malignant or benign strictures.
2. Outside the wall
   - caused by penetrating injuries (rare).
3. Spontaneous
   - This follows episodes of violent vomiting (Boerhaave's syndrome). The perforation is frequently on the left posterolateral aspect of the lower oesophagus. A tear to the oesophageal mucosa only, following vomiting, is known as a Mallory–Weiss tear and tends to cause haematemesis.

Clinical features

The clinical symptoms depend to some extent on the site and size of the perforation. If is in the cervical region, the patient complains of pain in the neck and local tenderness and surgical emphysema is present. Perforation of the thoracic oesophagus causes retrosternal chest pain and dysphagia. Clinically the patient may be shocked, short of breath and cyanosed owing to a pneumothorax or pleural effusion if the pleural space is involved. Perforation in this area can lead to mediastinitis and septic shock. Perforation of the abdominal oesophagus can lead to peritonitis and a rigid abdomen.

Investigations

The differential diagnosis of a perforated oesophagus includes myocardial infarction and duodenal ulceration. Investigations therefore need to exclude these two diagnoses in particular, at the same time including examination of the oesophagus for perforation.

Erect chest X-ray In addition to excluding a perforated duodenal ulcer (air under the diaphragm, see Chapter 16) an erect chest X-ray may show surgical emphysema with gas in the soft tissues of the mediastinum, often extending up to the neck. The mediastinum may also be widened, and if the pleural cavity has also been ruptured there will be a hydropneumothorax (Fig. 17.7).

Contrast swallow The diagnosis is confirmed by a water-soluble contrast swallow, which will also demonstrate whether the perforation is localized to the medi-

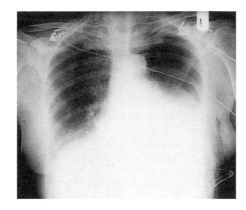

Fig. 17.7 Erect chest X-ray in a patient with Boerhaave's syndrome. Note the left-sided hydropneumothorax.

astinum or open into the pleural or peritoneal cavities. If there is any doubt on contrast swallow a contrast-enhanced CT scan should be arranged.

Treatment

Perforation of the cervical oesophagus can be treated non-operatively with intravenous fluids, withdrawal of oral fluid and diet, and the administration of antibiotics. If an abscess develops in the superior mediastinum this will require surgical drainage.

Perforation of the thoracic oesophagus has a much higher morbidity and mortality. Localized and small perforations which do not communicate with either pleural cavity can be treated non-operatively, as outlined above. However, if the perforation follows the dilatation of a carcinoma in a patient suitable for resection, emergency oesophagogastrectomy is indicated following appropriate resuscitation. In other situations perforation into either pleural cavity will usually require thoractomy, drainage and surgical repair.

MOTILITY DISORDERS

The most common motility disorders of the oesophagus are the non-specific variety commonly found in gastro-oesophageal reflux disease (which will be discussed later), achalasia, diffuse oesophageal spasm, nutcracker oesophagus, those associated with connective tissue disorders such as scleroderma, and neuromuscular diseases.

Achalasia

This disorder affects the whole oesophagus. The main feature is failure of relaxation of the lower oesophageal sphincter and, as the disease progresses, the obstructed lower oesophagus dilates and peristalsis becomes unco-ordinated.

Achalasia is thought to be due to a partial or complete degeneration of the myenteric plexus of Auerbach, and in the later stages of the disease loss of the dorsal vagal nuclei within the brain stem can be demonstrated.

Infestations with the protozoan *Trypanosoma cruzi*, which occurs in South America (Chagas' disease), also causes degeneration of the myenteric plexus, leading to a motor disorder of the oesophagus which is indistinguishable from achalasia.

Clinical features

The disease affects 1 in 100 000 of the western population. The patient is typically aged between 30 and 40 years and females are affected more often than males (3:2).

There is progressive dysphagia over several years, often for both solids and liquids. Gravity rather than peristalsis is responsible for food leaving the oesophagus and the patient finds it easier to eat when standing. There may also be retrosternal pain, which gradually decreases in severity as the oesophagus loses peristaltic activity.

Other common symptoms include weight loss, halitosis and regurgitation of undigested food, which can lead to aspiration pneumonia, particularly at night, resulting in bouts of coughing and recurrent chest infections. In the longer term achalasia can predispose to squamous cell carcinoma of the oesophagus.

Investigations

Chest X-ray An erect chest X-ray might demonstrate a widened mediastinum produced by the dilated oesophagus. A fluid level behind the heart may also be seen, sometimes with evidence of aspiration pneumonia. The gastric air bubble is usually absent as a result of incomplete emptying of the oesophagus.

Barium swallow A barium swallow will show dilatation of the oesophagus, leading to a tapered narrowing at the lower end (Fig. 17.8). As the disease progresses there will be absent peristalsis in the body of the oesophagus.

Endoscopy OGD is essential to exclude other causes of lower oesophageal narrowing, in particular carcinoma.

Oesophageal manometry The demonstration of a high-pressure non-relaxing lower oesophageal sphincter with poor or absent peristalsis of the oesophageal body is diagnostic of achalasia.

Treatment

Treatment involves either balloon dilatation of the lower oesophageal sphincter or surgical myotomy (division of the

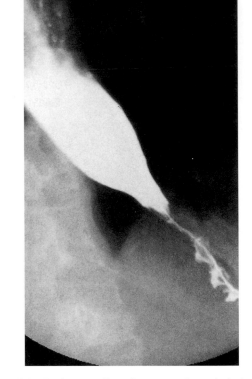

Fig. 17.8 Barium swallow demonstrating achalasia.

muscles over the lower oesophagus and proximal stomach). Endoscopic injection of the gastro-oesophageal junction with botulinum toxin has been shown to improve symptoms in a small group of patients, but recurrent problems occur. Balloon dilatation of the gastro-oesophageal junction disrupts the lower oesophageal sphincter (Fig. 17.9) and improves symptoms in 80–90% of patients, but carries with it the risk of oesophageal perforation. Patients who require more than two dilatations should be considered for surgery.

Operative treatment involves a Heller's cardiomyotomy. The lower oesophagus is exposed by either an abdominal or a left thoracic approach, and increasingly both procedures are being carried out using laparoscopy. The lower oesophageal sphincter is divided down to the mucosa for 5 cm above the oesophagogastric junction and 3 cm down the stomach. Early complications include perforation and late complications include reflux oesophagitis, stricture formation, the development of an oesophageal diverticulum and recurrent dysphagia from an inadequate myotomy. In order to reduce the risks of perforation and the development of reflux, most surgeons now prefer the abdominal route and carry out a partial anterior fundoplication at the same

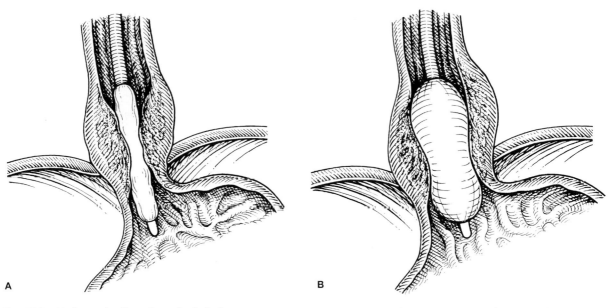

Fig. 17.9 Hydrostatic dilatation of achalasia.

time. This helps to protect the area of the mytomy if there has been a small perforation of the mucosa, keeps the edges of the muscle apart and reduces post-operative gastro-oesophageal reflux (Fig. 17.10).

Diffuse oesophageal spasm

This disorder tends to occur in middle-aged to elderly patients. Complaints are of intermittent dysphagia and retrosternal pain, which can mimic angina. The symptoms are caused by repetitive irregular peristalsis of the oesophageal body.

Investigations

Barium swallow shows a characteristic corkscrew oesophagus caused by the contracted muscle indenting the lumen (Fig. 17.11), and oesophageal manometry confirms the diagnosis.

Treatment

Medical treatment includes calcium channel blockers and proton pump inhibitors. Surgical treatment involves a long myotomy.

Nutcracker oesophagus

In this uncommon disorder the symptoms are caused by repetitive forceful peristalsis. Manometry demonstrates

normal peristalsis but with excessive amplitudes and pressures exceeding 150 mmHg. Medical treatment is similar to that of diffuse oesophageal spasm, but the results are disappointing. Dilatation and surgical myotomy also have poor results.

PLUMMER–VINSON SYNDROME

This syndrome, first described by Paterson and Brown Kelly, is characterized by a post cricoid web that results in dysphagia. The web is related to iron deficiency anaemia, but may be congenital or traumatic in origin. The squamous epithelium becomes hyperplastic and there is hyperkeratosis and desquamation, which leads to web formation.

Clinical features

Patients are commonly middle-aged women. Dysphagia is the main presenting complaint, but there may also be symptoms and signs of anaemia, including koilonychia, smooth tongue and angular stomatitis.

Investigations

A full blood count will show hypochromic microcytic anaemia and serum ferritin levels will be low. Barium swallow demonstrates a narrowing of the upper oesophagus with a web in the anterior wall, which is confirmed by

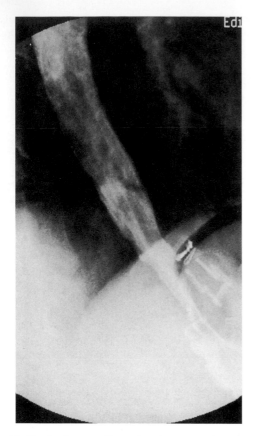

Fig. 17.10   Barium swallow after laparoscopic cardiomyotomy (Heller's procedure) with an anterior fundoplication in the same patient with achalasia as shown before surgery in Figure 17.8.

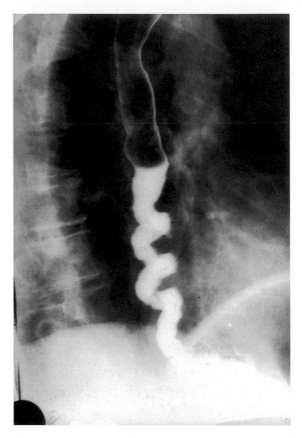

Fig. 17.11   Barium swallow showing appearances of diffuse oesophageal spasm.

endoscopy when a friable web can be seen across the lumen of the oesophagus.

Treatment

The web is dilated endoscopically and biopsies should also be taken, as there is an association with postcricoid carcinoma. The iron deficiency status is corrected by oral iron therapy.

POUCHES

Pouches are protrusions of mucosa through a weak area in the muscle wall. The best-known pouch lies in the pharynx and is associated with raised cricopharyngeal pressure, with the pouch developing through Killan's dehiscence, between the thyropharyngeus and cricopharyngeus muscles. Incoordination of swallowing and failure of relaxation of the cricopharyngeus muscle cause the hernia-

tion. The pharyngeal pouch usually develops posteriorly and is then forced by the vertebral column to deviate to the side, usually the left. Oesophageal pouches can occur around the tracheobronchial tree in relation to pressure from adjacent lymph nodes, if enlarged, and also just above the gastro-oesophageal junction in patients with raised lower oesophageal sphincter pressure.

Clinical features

Most patients are elderly and males are more commonly affected. Symptoms include regurgitation of food, halitosis, dysphagia, gurgling in the throat, aspiration and a lump in the neck (pharyngeal pouch); or the patient may be asymptomatic.

Investigation

Barium swallow demonstrates the pouch and the uncoordinated swallowing. Endoscopy also confirms the diagnosis but must be performed with care to avoid accidental perforation of the pouch.

Treatment

Surgical myotomy of the cricopharyngeus and resection of the pouch used to be the surgical treatment of choice, but endoscopic stapling is now more common.

GASTRO-OESOPHAGEAL REFLUX

Gastro-oesophageal reflux is the commonest cause of dyspepsia, affecting up to 30% of the population. It is caused by retrograde flow of gastric acid through an incompetent cardiac sphincter into the lower oesophagus. The cardiac sphincter usually prevents reflux by the following mechanisms:

- A physiological high-pressure zone (not a true sphincter) in the lower end of the oesophagus
- The mucosal rosette at the cardia acts like a plug
- The angle at which the oesophagus joins the stomach between the left border of the oesophagus and the fundus (angle of His)
- The diaphragmatic sling (crura) acts like a pinchcock at the lower end of the oesophagus
- The high-pressure area at the lower end of the oesophagus caused by the positive intra-abdominal pressure.

Clinical features

The reflux of acid causes inflammation and ulceration to the oesophageal mucosa, which manifests as:

- Heartburn: retrosternal burning pain, radiating to the epigastrium and through to the back
- Regurgitation of acid stomach contents into the mouth (acidbrash)
- Waterbrash, which is salivation due to reflex salivary gland stimulation as acid enters the gullet
- Dysphagia from benign strictures or the development of non-specific motility disorders, both of which follow chronic reflux oesophagitis.

Investigations

The differential diagnosis includes myocardial ischaemia, peptic ulcer disease, cholecystitis and carcinoma of the oesophagus, and appropriate investigations are undertaken to exclude these other disorders.

Barium swallow and meal A barium study might demonstrate a hiatus hernia, the presence of severe ulceration (if present), benign strictures and reflux of contrast from the stomach into the oesophagus in the head-down position (Fig. 17.12).

Endoscopy OGD will confirm reflux if oesophagitis is seen. Biopsies should be taken to establish the presence of inflammation and identify whether Barratt's metaplasia exists. Strictures can be dilated, but must also be biopsied to exclude malignancy.

pH monitoring and oesophageal manometry Ambulatory 24-hour pH monitoring is the gold standard in establishing the diagnosis of acid reflux, although patients must have been off all proton pump inhibitor therapy for 7 days. Manometry is carried out at the same time to exclude other motility disorders, in particular achalasia, and to ensure that there is adequate muscular contraction in the lower oesophagus to prevent postoperative dysphagia if surgery is being considered.

Treatment

General treatment includes weight loss, sleeping with additional pillows and raising the head of the bed, and the avoidance of smoking, coffee, fatty foods and alcohol.

Medical treatment

Pharmacological treatment is extremely effective and involves H_2 receptor antagonists or proton pump inhibitors to reduce gastric acid production, alginates to coat the

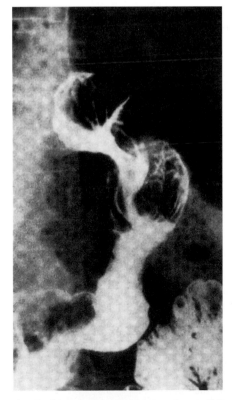

Fig. 17.12   Barium swallow demonstrating a sliding hiatus hernia and free gastro-oesophageal reflux.

oesophagus, and prokinetic agents such as metoclopramide to improve the lower oesophageal muscle tone and promote gastric emptying.

Antireflux surgery

Although surgical treatment of patients with severe antireflux disease has always been associated with good long-term outcomes, it has taken the introduction and refinements of laparoscopic techniques to bring the surgical option to more patients. The indications for surgery include those whose symptoms cannot be controlled by medical therapy, those with recurrent strictures despite treatment, and young patients who do not wish to continue taking acid suppression therapy for several decades. Symptoms that fail to be brought under control with acid suppression therapy are usually due to high-volume alkaline reflux, and surgery is an extremely effective cure. The presence of Barratt's metaplasia alone is not yet considered a suitable indication for antireflux surgery.

Surgery involves reduction of the hiatus hernia, if present, approximation of the crura around the the lower oesophagus, and some form of fundoplication. This takes the form of mobilizing the fundus of the stomach from its attachments to the undersurface of the left hemidiaphragm and the left crus, and then wrapping it around the oesophagus, either anteriorly or posteriorly. The most common procedure currently performed is the Nissen fundoplication, in which the fundoplication is taken posteriorly around the lower oesophagus and sutured to the left anterior surface of the left side of the proximal stomach as a 360° wrap (Fig. 17.13). Other procedures involving a partial (incomplete) fundoplication include the Toupet (posterior 270° wrap) and the Watson (anterior 180°) repairs. Current data do not demonstrate much difference between the various approaches, provided the surgeon is experienced in the technique. All procedures have a success rate in curing the symptoms of reflux of around 95%. Unwanted complications after surgery (compared with those occurring in the perioperative period) include gas bloat (inability to belch) and dysphagia. These usually follow the formation of a wrap that is too tight, and are more likely after a complete fundoplication. These operations are now carried out laparoscopically, with excellent results in skilled hands.

Gastro-oesophageal reflux disease is one of the commonest causes of vomiting in the first few months of life. In the majority of affected infants, simple measures including the addition of thickening agents to milk feeds, the administration of alginates (e.g. Gaviscon) with or after feeds and the use of H_2 receptor blockers, will control symptoms. Most affected children outgrow this form of reflux disease. In a small minority, surgery is required. The indications for fundoplication include failure to thrive despite optimal medical therapy, recurrent aspiration and chest infections, oesophageal stricture and haemorrhage from severe oesophagitis.

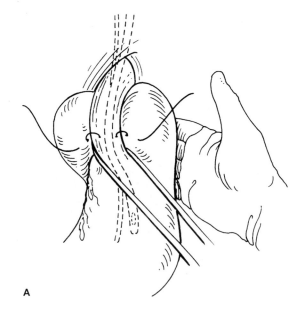
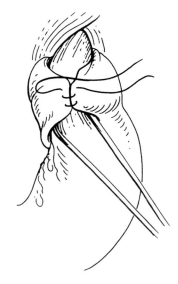

A   B

Fig. 17.13   Fundoplication for reflux oesophagitis. **A** gastric fundus wrapped around lower oesophagus. **B** Fundal wrap sutured in position.

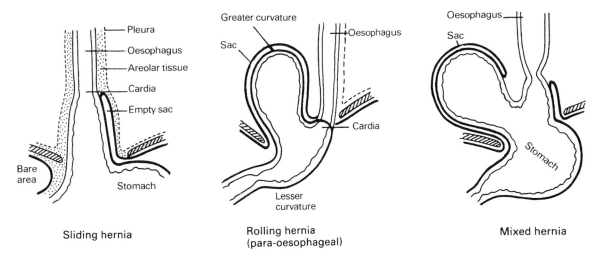

Fig. 17.14 Types of hiatus hernia.

Hiatus hernia

A hiatus hernia is an abnormal protrusion of the stomach through the oesophageal diaphragmatic hiatus into the thorax. There are two types (Fig. 17.14): sliding (90%) and rolling (10%). A sliding hernia occurs when the stomach slides through the diaphragmatic hiatus, so that the gastro-oesophageal junction lies within the chest cavity. It is covered anteriorly by peritoneum, and posteriorly is extraperitoneal.

A rolling or paraoesophageal hernia is formed when the stomach rolls up anteriorly through the hiatus (Fig. 17.15) but the cardia remains in its normal position and therefore the cardio-oesophageal sphincter remains intact.

Rolling and sliding hernias are caused by weakness of the muscles around the hiatus. They tend to occur in middle-aged and elderly patients. Women are affected more frequently than men and there is a higher incidence in the obese.

Clinical features

Hiatus hernias are often asymptomatic, but can produce some or all the following symptoms:

- Heartburn and regurgitation owing to an incompetent lower oesophageal sphincter, which is aggravated by stooping and lying flat at night, and can be relieved by antacids
- Oesophagitis results from persistent acid reflux and leads to ulceration, bleeding with anaemia, fibrosis and stricture formation
- Epigastric and lower chest pain, especially in para-oesophageal hernias as the herniated part of the stomach (usually the fundus) becomes trapped in the hiatus. This

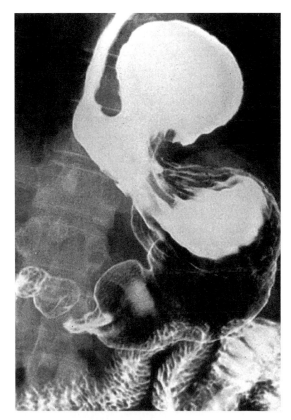

Fig. 17.15 Barium meal demonstrating a paraoesophageal hiatus hernia.

can be a surgical emergency owing to the obstruction and strangulation of the stomach

- Palpitations and hiccups are symptoms caused by the mass effect of the hernia in the thoracic cavity irritating the pericardium and the diaphragm. In patients with a large rolling hiatus hernia the whole stomach may result in a volvulus into the chest, producing symptoms of vomiting from gastric outflow obstruction.

Investigations

The diagnosis of hiatus hernia may be confirmed by performing a barium swallow and meal (Fig. 17.12 and 17.15), or by upper GI endoscopy. A chest X-ray may show a fluid level behind the heart and a widened mediastinum (Fig. 17.16).

Treatment is as for gastro-oesophageal reflux disease; however, paraoesophageal hernias should always be surgically repaired to prevent strangulation.

Barrett's oesophagus

Barrett's oesophagus is columnar metaplasia of the lower oesophagus which extends at least 3 cm above the gastro-oesophageal junction. It results from chronic damage by acid and bile reflux. The risk of adenocarcinoma is increased 40–90-fold by Barrett's oesophagus, and is particularly high in the presence of intestinal metaplasia. Patients discovered to have Barrett's oesophagus during endoscopy should be considered for endoscopic surveillance programmes. If severe

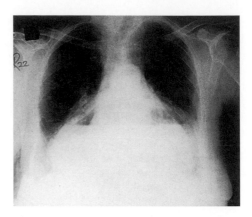

A

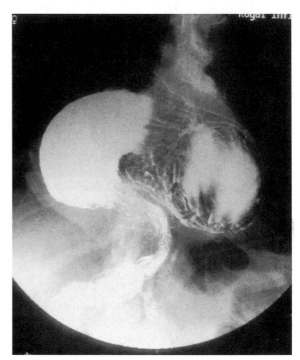

B

Fig. 17.16 **A** Erect chest X-ray in a patient with a large hiatus hernia with intrathoracic stomach. Note the air–fluid level behind the heart and the widened mediastinum. **B** Barium meal in the same patient. (Reproduced from Hamilton Bailey's emergency surgery, 13th edn, with permission from Butterworth–Heinemann.)

SUMMARY BOX

Hiatus hernia

- Almost 95% of hiatus hernias are of the sliding type. Paraoesophageal (rolling) hernias are rare and mixed hernias are exceptional.

- Sliding hernias are often associated with reflux oesophagitis and heartburn, but reflux can occur in the absence of herniation.

- Symptomatic sliding hiatus hernias can be managed non-operatively in 85% of cases; some form of fundoplication is indicated if symptoms cannot be controlled by conservative measures.

- Long-standing reflux may give rise to ulceration (with risk of bleeding, perforation and stenosis) and metaplasia may produce a Barrett's oesophagus and the risk of developing adenocarcinoma.

- Paraoesophageal hernias are not normally associated with reflux, but frequently give rise to symptoms and may strangulate, so that surgical correction is advisable.

---

dysplasia or carcinoma in situ is detected, and confirmed with repeat biopsies and by a second pathologist, subtotal oesophagectomy should be considered. Current data suggest that in this group of patients an underlying carcinoma is detected in about 50% of surgical resections.

Investigation

The diagnosis is made at endoscopy and confirmed histo-logically.

Treatment

In those in whom a new diagnosis of Barratt's oesophagus has been made, repeat biospies after a course of proton pump inhibitors is recommended as it is sometimes difficult for the pathologist to assess dysplasia in the presence of severe inflammation. There is no evidence at present that either long-term proton pump inhibitor therapy or antireflux surgery results in regression of Barratt's oesophagus, although they might prevent the subsequent development of dysplasia. This is currently an area of great interest and research.

TUMOURS OF THE OESOPHAGUS

Benign tumours

These account for less than 1% of oesophageal neoplasms. The commonest is the benign mixed stromal cell tumour (which used to be called a leiomyoma). This is usually asymptomatic, but may cause bleeding or dysphagia. It is best treated by local enucleation, with good results.

Carcinoma of the oesophagus

The incidence of carcinoma of the oesophagus has risen in western populations over the last two decades to a figure of around 15/100 000 in parts of the UK, due primarily to an increase in adenocarcinoma. The male to female ratio is 3:1 and adenocarcinoma is predominantly a disease of western white males. In the Far East and other parts of the world, particularly among some black males, there is a greater incidence of squamous cell carcinoma.

The most important risk factors for adenocarcinoma of the oesophagus are reflux and obesity, with a slightly increased risk of cardia tumours with smoking. Risk factors for squamous cell carcinoma include alcohol, smoking, leukoplakia, achalasia, and the consumption of salted fish, pickled vegetables, chewing tobacco and betel nuts.

Clinical features

Dysphagia which progresses from solids to liquids is one of the most common presentations. The average duration of symptoms at the time of presentation is between 3 and 9 months, and as a result around 70% of patients are not operable at the time of diagnosis. Retrosternal pain on swallowing (odynophagia), regurgitation and aspiration pneumonitis are other forms of presentation.

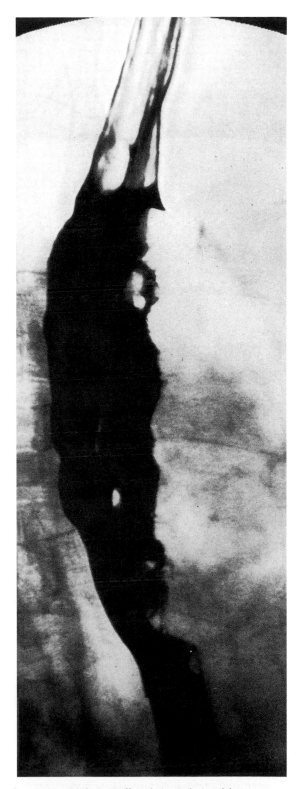

Fig. 17.17 Barium swallow in a patient with a carcinoma of the mid-oesophagus.

Occasionally patients may present with metastatic disease, including enlarged cervical lymph nodes, jaundice, hepatomegaly, hoarseness from recurrent laryngeal nerve involvement, and chest pain from mediastinal invasion. Other general features of malignancy include weight loss, anorexia, anaemia and lassitude.

Investigations

The diagnosis is often made initially by barium swallow (Fig. 17.17) but must always be confirmed by endoscopy and biopsy. Thereafter investigations are aimed at accurate staging of the disease (Table 17.2) so as to assess resectability, determine a prognosis and identify patients who might benefit from neoadjuvant therapy. Local T (tumour) stage and N (nodal) spread is best assessed by endoscopic ultrasonography (see Fig. 17.4). M (metastases) stage can be assessed with chest X-ray (lung secondaries), abdominal ultrasound (liver metastases and ascites), CT chest and abdomen (lung and liver metastases, distant lymphadenopathy) and laparoscopy (peritoneal metastases). Routine blood tests may reveal anaemia, liver disease and malnutrition, all of which require full assessment if surgery is to be considered. In those patients with proximal and middle-third tumours adjacent to the tracheobronchial tree, bronchoscopy can be a valuable investigation to assess airway invasion. If enlarged distant lymph nodes are detected these should be aspirated for cytology, as surgical resection is contraindicated if these are positive for malignancy.

Treatment

The aim of treatment is to cure those with potentially curable disease and restore swallowing in the remainder. The overall 5-year survival rate remains very low (<10%), although in patients who are suitable for resection 5-year survival figures of 20–30% have been reported.

Surgical resection

Patients with disease confined to the oesophagus and who are fit for surgery should be considered for resection. A certain proportion will be found to have more extensive disease at operation, but with better preoperative staging this figure should be small. Although surgical resection can provide reasonable palliation in some patients, setting out to perform a palliative resection has become less common because of improvements in non-surgical palliative techniques.

There are several methods currently used to resect the oesophagus:

- **Ivor Lewis two-phase oesophagectomy**. This involves a laparotomy during which the stomach is fully mobilized on its vascular pedicles along with the lower oesophagus. A right thoracotomy is then carried out to resect the oesophagus, and the mobilized stomach is brought up into the chest and anastomosed to the proximal oesophagus. This is the preferred choice for middle-third tumours (Fig. 17.18).
- **Left thoracolaparotomy** This is a good approach for lower oesophageal and cardia tumours, but experienced surgeons can also remove more proximally located tumours. If the tumour is found to extend higher than anticipated, this approach can also incorporate a cervical incision and anastomosis in the neck.
- **Transhiatal oesophagectomy** This approach involves two surgeons, one operating through the abdomen and the other in the neck. The stomach is mobilized as for the Ivor Lewis procedure and the oesophagus is mobilized through the hiatus. The surgeon operating in the neck mobilizes the upper oesophagus and extends the dissection into the chest. The stomach is brought up into the neck and anastomosed to the proximal oesophagus. This technique is best suited for elderly patients with lower oesophageal tumours, in whom a thoracotomy should be avoided if possible. Patients in whom endoscopic ultrasound has demonstrated early tumours with no obvious lymph node metastases, particularly those with severe dysplasia in Barrett's oesophagus, are also suitable for this approach. A segment of colon or small bowel can be used if it is not possible to reconstruct the oesophagus with stomach for any of these three techniques.

Postoperative care

In the early postoperative period patients are managed in a high-dependency or intensive care unit. Nutrition can be

---

Table 17.2	TNM staging of oesophageal carcinoma

T
1 Tumour confined to submucosa
2 Tumour extends into musculararis propria
3 Tumour extends outside muscle layers
4 Tumour invades adjacent structures (bronchus, aorta etc.)

N
1 Lymph node metastases to paraoesophageal, cardia or left gastric regions

M
0 No other metastatic spread
1 Lymph node metastases to all other areas
   Metastases to liver, lung, brain, bone etc.

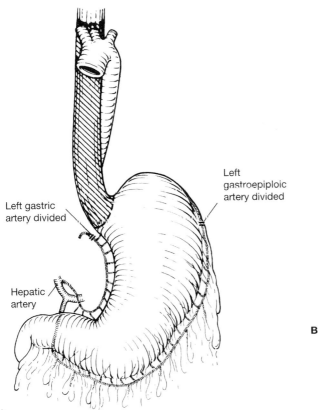

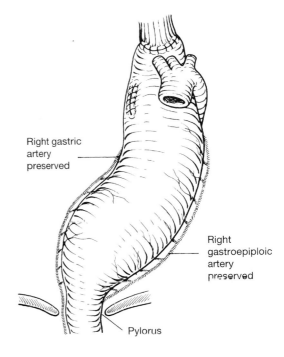

Fig. 17.18 Reconstruction after subtotal oesophagectomy.

provided by means of a feeding jejunostomy if a slow recovery is anticipated.

Complications

Chest infections are the most common complication associated with pulmonary collapse and pneumothorax after thoracotomy. Adequate chest drainage, good analgesia and chest physiotherapy are all important in reducing this complication.

Anastomotic leakage occurs in 5–10% of patients and is the single most common reason for perioperative mortality, which should be less than 10% and is approximately 5% in most specialist units. Anastomotic breakdown in the first few days after surgery represents a technical failure and usually results from ischaemia in the proximal part of the mobilized stomach. Early reoperation and revision of the anastomosis is the treatment of choice. Leaks that occur later are often well controlled by the chest drains, and provided the patient remains stable, can be managed non-operatively by nutritional support, antibiotics and naso-gastric drainage. Assessment of the anastomosis is obtained by water-soluble contrast swallow.

Radiotherapy and chemotherapy

Radical chemoradiation can be used with curative intent on both adenocarcinoma and squamous cell carcinoma in patients not suitable for surgical resection. Although postoperative radiotherapy and/or chemotherapy (adjuvant therapy) have been shown to provide no additional survival advantage in patients with resectable disease, neoadjuvant therapy (preoperative treatment) has produced encouraging results in recent randomized controlled clinical trials, and further developments can be expected in this area.

Palliation

Palliative treatment is used for patients with extensive disease and in those who are unfit for surgery. Treatment is aimed at the relief of symptoms, particularly dysphagia.

Endoscopic dilatation may provide short-term relief and must be repeated at ever-shortening intervals.

SUMMARY BOX

Carcinoma of the oesophagus

- Risk factors include chronic irritation (smoking, alcohol, betel nut, spices), obesity nutritional deficiencies and environmental carcinogens (nitrosamines, *Aspergillus flavus*).

- Premalignant conditions, including achalasia, Barrett's oesophagus, Plummer–Vinson syndrome, hiatus hernia and corrosive strictures.

- Worldwide histologically more oesophageal cancers are squamous carcinomas and fewer are adenocarcinomas which arise from columnar epithelium in the lower third (or extend upwards from the stomach). In the UK adenocarcinoma is more common.

- Late presentation with obstruction (dysphagia and regurgitation), aspiration pneumonitis, local invasion (recurrent laryngeal nerve, bronchus, mediastinum) and metastases is common.

- Approximately 30% of oesophageal cancers are resectable. Squamous carcinomas may be radiosensitive.

- Dysphagia in patients with unresectable cancers can be relieved by endoscopic or surgical intubation, laser treatment or surgical bypass (now rarely used).

- Overall 5-year survival rates are only 5%.

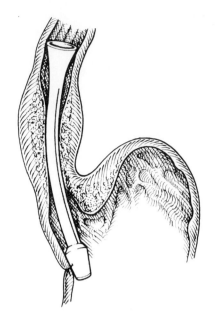

Fig. 17.19 Insertion of a Celastin tube to relieve dysphagia caused by obstructing cancer of the lower oesophagus. When the tube is inserted at laparotomy it is anchored to the stomach by a suture. This is not possible when the tube is inserted endoscopically.

Stent insertion using expandable metal or rigid plastic stents (Fig. 17.19) provides good relief of dysphagia. These can be inserted at surgery when an unresectable tumour is found, at endoscopy, or by interventional radiologists. The main problems include perforation during insertion, migration of the tube, blockage, and tumour ingrowth. The latter can be rectified by laser ablation.

Laser ablation can be carried out endoscopically and provides very good palliation of dysphagia, but does require to be repeated at regular intervals of 1–2 months. Perforation can result.

Radiotherapy and chemotherapy have been used for palliation with limited success.

Analgesia and terminal care are extremely important areas in palliation and are best provided by a multidisciplinary palliative care team.

18 Gastroduodenal disorders

S.J. Wakelin, T.J. Crofts

SURGICAL ANATOMY

Stomach

The stomach is an easily distensible viscus partly covered by the left costal margin. The diaphragm and left lobe of the liver lie on its anterior surface. Posteriorly the stomach bed is formed by the diaphragm, spleen, left adrenal, upper part of the left kidney, splenic artery and pancreas. The greater and lesser curvatures correspond to the long and short borders of the stomach respectively, and the organ can

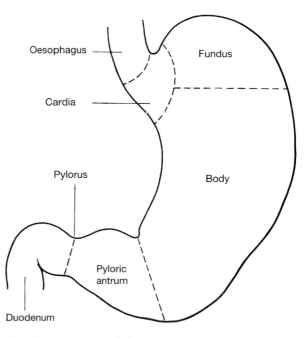

Fig. 18.1 Anatomy of the stomach.

be further divided anatomically into four distinct areas based on the mucosal appearance. The *cardia* is a very short segment proximally. The *fundus* is the area of the stomach that rises above the oesophageal opening (hiatus) in the diaphragm. The *body* extends from the level of the cardia to the incisura, a notch on the lesser curvature. The *pyloric antrum* is the area immediately proximal to the pylorus (Fig. 18.1). The stomach is limited at its proximal end by the oesophagogastric junction, a physiological sphincter that prevents stomach contents from regurgitating into the oesophagus. Distally the stomach is limited by the pylorus, a true anatomical sphincter. It is composed of greatly thickened inner circular muscle and helps to regulate the emptying of stomach contents into the duodenum.

DUODENUM

The duodenum is approximately 25 cm long and is divided into four parts, which are closely applied to the head of the pancreas. The first part is approximately 5 cm in length and its importance lies in the fact that it is the commonest site for peptic ulceration to occur. The second part has on its medial wall the ampulla of Vater, where the conjoined pancreatic duct and common bile duct deliver their contents to the upper gastrointestinal tract. The third and fourth parts pass behind the transverse mesocolon into the infracolic compartment.

BLOOD SUPPLY, LYMPHATICS AND NERVES

Blood supply

The *stomach* has an extensive blood supply (Fig. 18.2) derived from the coeliac axis, which is of great importance to the surgeon. When the stomach is used as a conduit in the chest, as in an oesophagectomy, the left gastric, left gastroepiploic and short gastric vessels are divided, and the stomach then relies on the right gastric and right gastroepiploic vessels for viability. Ischaemia does not usually result because of the free communication between the vessels supplying the stomach.

The blood supply to the *duodenum* is derived from both the coeliac axis and the superior mesenteric artery, a coeliac axis branch supplying the proximal duodenum via the gastroduodenal artery and a branch of the superior mesenteric artery supplying the distal half of the duodenum.

The veins from the stomach accompany the arteries and drain into the portal venous system. These assume greater importance in the patient with portal hypertension, giving rise to varices at the oesophagogastric junction or the

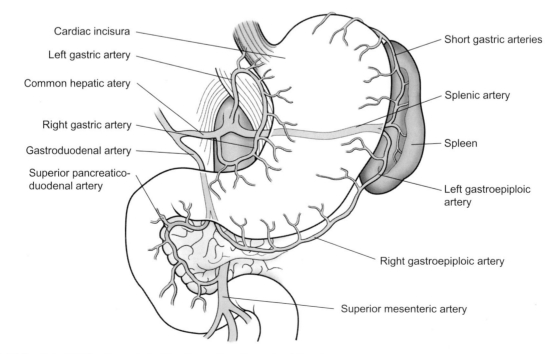

Fig. 18.2   Arterial blood supply to the stomach and proximal duodenum.

gastric fundus. The veins from the duodenum, like those of the stomach, ultimately drain into the portal circulation.

Lymphatics

The lymphatics from the *stomach* accompany the arteries and drainage is to nodes around these vessels. Thereafter drainage is to other groups around the aorta, splenic hilum and pancreas, and then to the coeliac nodes. The lymphatics of the *duodenum* drain into the nodes located at the coeliac axis and superior mesenteric vessels.

Nerve supply

The parasympathetic nerve supply to the *stomach* is derived from the anterior and posterior vagal trunks. These pass through the diaphragm with the oesophagus. The anterior trunk gives off branches to the liver and gallbladder and descends along the lesser curvature. The posterior trunk gives off a coeliac branch and descends along the lesser curvature of the stomach, going on to supply the pancreas, small intestine and large intestine as far as the distal transverse colon. The parasympathetic system supplies motor fibres to the stomach wall, inhibitory fibres to the pyloric sphincter thus effecting relaxation of the sphincter and secretomotor fibres to the glands of the stomach. Sympathetic fibres accompany the gastric arteries to reach the stomach from the coeliac ganglion. These provide motor fibres to the pyloric sphincter. The *duodenum* receives a sympathetic and parasympathetic supply from the coeliac and superior mesenteric plexuses.

SURGICAL PHYSIOLOGY

GASTRIC MOTILITY

Food is passed from the oesophagus into the stomach, where it is stored, ground and partially digested. As food enters the stomach the muscles in the stomach walls relax and intragastric pressure rises only slightly. This effect occurring in the body and fundus of the stomach is known as receptive relaxation, and is mediated by the vagus nerve. It is followed by muscular contractions that increase in amplitude and frequency, starting in the fundus and moving down towards the body and antrum. In the antrum the main role is the grinding of food and propulsion of small amounts (now called chyme) into the duodenum when the pyloric sphincter relaxes.

Gastric emptying is controlled by two mechanisms: hormonal feedback and a neural reflex called the enterogastric reflex. In the former, fat in the chyme is the main stimulus

for the production of a number of hormones, the most powerful being cholecystokinin, which exerts a negative feedback effect on the stomach, decreasing its motility. The enterogastric reflex is initiated in the duodenal wall, and this further slows stomach emptying and secretion.

GASTRIC SECRETIONS

Classically gastric secretion has been divided into three phases.

Cephalic (neural) phase Signals arise in the central cortex or appetite centres triggered by the sight, smell, taste and thought of food, and travel down the vagus nerves to the stomach. Thus acetylcholine released directly stimulates the peptic and parietal cells, causing pepsin and acid to be secreted.

Gastric phase Food (in particular protein digestion products) causes the release of acid, this release being subject to a negative feedback mechanism dependent upon the pH of the stomach. The gastric phase accounts for the greatest part of daily secretion of approximately 1.5 L.

Intestinal phase The presence of food in the duodenum triggers the release of a number of hormones, including

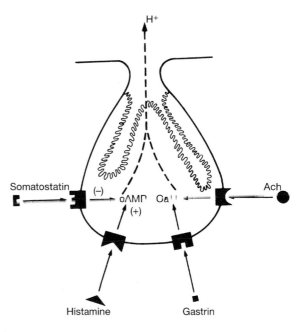

Fig. 18.3 Diagrammatic representation of the parietal cell showing receptor sites for the three major stimulants of acid secretion. Somatostatin inhibits secretion by inhibiting mucosal histamine release and by binding to somatostatin receptors. In addition to liberating acetylcholine (Ach), vagal stimulation may also increase mucosal histamine release and inhibit somatostatin release.

duodenal gastrin. These exert a positive feedback effect on the stomach, causing a small increase in gastric secretion. These hormones have a similar structure to that of gastrin.

Mucus is produced by all regions of the stomach. It is composed mainly of glycoproteins, water and electrolytes, and serves two important functions: it acts as a lubricant, and it protects the surface of the stomach against the powerful digestive properties of acid and pepsin. Bicarbonate ions are secreted into the mucus gel layer and this creates a protective buffer zone to the effects of the low pH secretions. Alkaline mucus is produced in the duodenum and small intestine, where it has a similar function of mucosal protection.

The parietal cells in the stomach are responsible for the production of *acid*. Acid secretion by these cells is stimulated by three main factors (Fig. 18.3): acetylcholine released by the vagus nerve, gastrin from the antrum, and histamine from cells neighbouring the peptic and parietal cells. The three agents act synergistically and each needs to bind to its specific receptor to exert its effect. If one of the agents is absent or decreased the result is a reduced acid

secretion. Somatostatin, gastric inhibitory peptide and vasoactive intestinal peptide inhibit acid secretion.

Pepsin is a proteolytic enzyme produced in its precursor form, pepsinogen, by the peptic cells found in the body and fundus of the stomach. Pepsinogen production is stimulated by acetylcholine from the vagus nerve. The precursor is then converted to its active form pepsin by the acid contents of the stomach.

Intrinsic factor is also produced by the parietal cells. It is a glycoprotein which binds to vitamin B_{12} present in the diet and carries it to the terminal ileum. Here specific receptors for intrinsic factor exist and the complex is taken up by the mucosa. Intrinsic factor is broken down and vitamin B_{12} is then absorbed into the bloodstream.

PEPTIC ULCERATION

Peptic ulceration affects areas of mucosa exposed to acidic gastric contents. It can only occur in the presence of acid, and the main pathology is an imbalance between the acid–pepsin system and the mucosal ability to resist digestion.

Ulceration can occur in a number of sites, including the oesophagus, stomach, duodenum, and in the jejunum following a gastrojejunostomy. Rarely ulceration may occur in the ileum close to a Meckel's diverticulum containing acid-secreting gastric mucosa.

GASTRIC AND DUODENAL ULCERATION

Peptic ulcer disease occurs more commonly in men, with a male to female ratio of 5:1 for duodenal ulcers and 2:1 for gastric ulcers. Duodenal ulcers occur four times more commonly than gastric ulcers.

Pathology

Duodenal ulcers usually occur in the first part of the duodenum and 50% occur on the anterior wall. The majority of gastric ulcers develop on the lesser curvature in the distal half of the stomach. They may coexist with duodenal ulcers in 10% of patients.

Duodenal ulcers may be acute or chronic. Ulcers with a history of less than 3 months' duration and with no evidence of fibrosis are considered to be acute. Gastric ulcers generally run a chronic course.

Gastric ulcers may be benign or malignant. Malignancy was once thought to be a complicating factor of benign gastric ulceration. It is now realized that malignant change in a benign ulcer is rare, and that such ulcers are in fact

---

SUMMARY BOX

Surgical physiology of gastric secretion

- Hydrochloric acid secreted by the parietal cells of the gastric corpus produces an environment in which the proteolytic enzyme pepsin is maximally active.

- Acid–pepsin secretion is stimulated by the vagus (acetylcholine), gastrin (hormone secreted by the gastric antrum) and histamine (paracrine regulator).

- Truncal vagotomy reduces acid–pepsin secretion by abolishing the direct vagal drive (and, to a minor degree, by reducing antral gastrin secretion).

- Truncal vagotomy impairs gastric motility by abolishing receptive relaxation of the gastric corpus (reduced reservoir) and diminishing the power of the antral contractions (antral mill) that grind, mix and expel food.

- Because of its effect on gastric motility/emptying, truncal vagotomy is usually combined with a drainage procedure (pyloroplasty or gastroenterostomy).

- Highly selective vagotomy denervates only the body of the stomach. Acid–pepsin secretion is reduced but antral motility is unaffected, so that a drainage procedure is not needed and gastric incontinence is avoided.

probably malignant from the outset. Duodenal ulcers are very rarely malignant.

Aetiology

Helicobacter pylori

H. pylori is present in around 50% of the world's population, its prevalence increasing with age. *H. pylori* is more prevalent in developing countries, where poor and crowded living conditions are commonplace, and here the infection is probably acquired in early life via the faecal–oral or oral–oral route. Once an individual is infected the *H. pylori* persists and in the majority of patients there are no symptoms.

H. pylori is detected in 95% of patients with duodenal ulceration. It infects the mucosa of the antrum of the stomach, where it causes an inflammatory response. This gastritis stimulates the gastrin-producing (G cells) of the antrum to increase gastrin production. The subsequent hypersecretion of acid provides an ideal environment for gastric metaplasia of the duodenal mucosa to occur. The colonization of the metaplastic areas by *H. pylori* further damages the mucosa, and ultimately duodenal ulceration occurs.

H. pylori is found in approximately 75% of cases of gastric ulcers, although its role here is less well defined. It

may be that the gastritis facilitates the access of acid and pepsin to the stomach mucosa. It seems that the key factor is decreased mucosal resistance, with excess acid having less of a role. Indeed, most patients with gastric ulceration have a normal or decreased secretory capacity.

The significance of *H. pylori* in the aetiology of dyspeptic symptoms in children remains the subject of much debate. In some children, the eradication of the organism using standard anti-*H. pylori* regimens can completely abolish symptoms; in others, such eradication can have no effect. True peptic ulceration is uncommon in children.

Non-steroidal anti-inflammatory drugs (NSAIDs)

This group of drugs includes aspirin, ibuprofen, piroxicam and azapropazone. Their role as anti-inflammatory agents centres on their inhibition of prostaglandin synthesis. NSAIDs inhibit the action of cyclo-oxygenase, which is involved in the production of the inflammatory mediator prostaglandin. In the stomach prostaglandins are responsible for the production of mucus and bicarbonate. These both help to protect the stomach mucosa from acid by maintaining an alkaline buffer zone. By inhibiting prostaglandin synthesis, NSAIDs damage the gastric mucosa and are implicated in 30% of gastric ulcers. They may also be responsible for the small number of *H. pylori*-negative duodenal ulcers.

Smoking

This is an aetiological factor in both duodenal and gastric ulceration, but is more important in gastric ulceration. Smoking also delays ulcer healing, and there is an increased likelihood of complications (e.g. bleeding, perforation) developing in smokers.

Genetic factors

First-degree relatives of patients with a duodenal ulcer are at increased risk of developing a duodenal ulcer themselves. This risk is further increased if ulcers develop in patients under 20 years of age. First-degree relatives of patients with gastric ulcers are also at increased risk of developing gastric ulcers.

Zollinger–Ellison syndrome

This is a rare syndrome found more commonly in men (male to female ratio 3:2), usually caused by a gastrin-secreting tumour (gastrinoma) which is normally found in the pancreas. The majority of tumours are malignant, and

---

SUMMARY BOX

Peptic ulceration

- Peptic ulceration results from an imbalance between acid–pepsin secretion and the ability of the mucosal defences (mucosa, mucus and trapped bicarbonate) of the gastrointestinal tract to withstand peptic digestion.

- Three factors known to cause peptic ulceration are infection with *Helicobacter pylori*, the use of non-steroidal anti-inflammatory drugs, and the rare Zollinger–Ellison syndrome.

- Duodenal ulceration is commoner than gastric ulceration; other sites which may be affected are the oesophagus, jejunum and Meckel's diverticulum.

- The incidence of peptic ulceration is declining and the need for gastric surgery has fallen dramatically with the availability of potent antisecretory drugs such as the H_2-receptor antagonists and the proton pump inhibitors.

- Despite the falling incidence, complications of peptic ulceration (bleeding and perforation) are still major causes of death in elderly patients.

they may occasionally be found in the duodenum or stomach. Approximately 30% of patients have features consistent with multiple endocrine neoplasia syndrome (MEN I). The hypersecretion of gastrin results in a greatly increased risk of peptic ulceration. Diarrhoea may be a prominent feature, owing to large volumes of acid being secreted into the small intestine. Inactivation of the pancreatic lipase causes steatorrhoea. Complications of ulceration (pain, bleeding and stenosis) are common.

The diagnosis of Zollinger–Ellison is problematic, but ulceration in unusual sites, at an early age, or ulcers persisting despite medical treatment should be reviewed with a high index of suspicion. A serum gastrin level of over 50 ng/L should warrant further investigation. Ultrasound, CT scanning and selective angiography may be used to localize the tumour and its metastases, if present.

Cure is effected by removal of the tumour wherever possible, although this may be made more difficult by the presence of metastatic disease, a very small tumour or multifocal disease. Removal is often supplemented with control of acid secretion, using, in most instances, proton pump inhibitors.

Other factors

Other patients at risk of peptic ulceration include those with *blood group O*, elevated levels of *pepsinogen I* and those with *hyperparathyroidism*. Hyperparathyroidism causes elevated calcium levels, thus stimulating acid secretion. With resolution of the condition, spontaneous ulcer healing usually occurs.

Symptomatology

Recurrent well localized epigastric pain is typical of peptic ulcer disease. Classically the pain of a gastric ulcer occurs during eating and is relieved by vomiting. Patients with duodenal ulceration characteristically describe pain when they are hungry. This pain is relieved by food, antacids, milk and vomiting. Often, however, these well defined features are not present, and it is usually impossible to differentiate between the pain of gastric and that of duodenal ulceration.

Other symptoms associated with peptic ulcer disease include heartburn, anorexia, waterbrash (sudden flow of saliva into the mouth) and intolerance of certain foods. Intermittent vomiting may occur. Where persistent vomiting is troublesome the possibility of gastric outlet obstruction should be considered. Such vomiting tends to be projectile and may contain recognizable food eaten many hours previously.

Differential diagnosis

Epigastric pain with or without the other symptoms described above may present in a variety of other conditions, both surgical and medical (Table 18.1).

The diagnosis of peptic ulcer disease may not be straightforward. This is particularly true in the elderly patient on NSAIDs. In such patients pain may be absent and they may present for the first time with complications of ulceration, such as bleeding or perforation.

Diagnosis

Blood tests The full blood count may indicate iron-deficiency anaemia in the patient with a chronically bleeding ulcer. The biochemical screen may reveal dehydration and hypokalaemia from vomiting. Where hypergastrinaemia is suspected (e.g. Zollinger–Ellison syndrome) serum gastrin may be estimated, levels over 50 ng/L being suggestive of the condition. Calcium may be elevated in patients with hyperparathyroidism.

Endoscopy Endoscopy is now preferred to contrast studies in the investigation of peptic ulcer disease. It allows good visualization and biopsy of lesions and the detection of *H. pylori* using the CLO test. In the latter a biopsy specimen taken from the antrum is placed in a gel containing urea. Ammonia released by the action of the *H. pylori*-derived urease is detected and causes a colour change – in most kits from yellow to pink/red. Biopsy of gastric ulcers is particularly important as malignancy needs to be excluded.

Contrast studies These are still used where endoscopy is contraindicated, e.g. the use of Gastrografin studies in suspected perforation. Contrast studies are not commonly used as a first-line investigation for uncomplicated disease.

Ultrasound Ultrasound may be useful to exclude coexistent pathology. Cholelithiasis and peptic ulcer disease share similar symptoms and often coexist. Ultrasound is useful to determine whether gallstones are present. It is also useful to assess the pancreas, and provides information regarding the

Table 18.1 Causes of epigastric pain	
Surgical	**Medical**
Biliary colic or acute cholecystitis	Gastro-oesophageal reflux disease
Pancreatitis	Myocardial infarction
Mesenteric ischaemia	Pulmonary embolism
Perforation of a viscus	Lower lobe pneumonia
Acute appendicitis	Irritable bowel syndrome
Gastro-oesophageal malignancy	

texture of the liver and the presence of intraperitoneal fluid or gas in the acute setting.

SPECIAL FORMS OF ULCERATION

Stress ulceration refers to erosions or ulceration of the stomach or duodenum occurring in certain circumstances. These include severe illness, trauma, prolonged mechanical ventilation, multiple organ failure, sepsis and major surgery. The aetiology is not fully defined, although acid and mucosal ischaemia appear to be key elements. Such ulcers may be commonly found among patients in intensive care units. Medical prophylaxis using proton pump inhibitors may be used in such circumstances.

Cushing's and *Curling's* ulcers are special forms of stress ulceration that occur following central nervous injury and burns, respectively. Hypersecretion of acid is not always essential for stress ulceration to occur, but does appear to be important in both of these conditions. In neurosurgical injury raised intracranial pressure may be responsible for an increase in vagal activity and hence the increase in gastric secretion. The ulcers resulting from hypersecretion are usually single and, in common with other forms of peptic ulceration, may be complicated by perforation and bleeding.

TREATMENT OF UNCOMPLICATED PEPTIC ULCER DISEASE

Since the discovery of the link between *Helicobacter pylori* and peptic ulceration the management of uncomplicated ulcer disease has changed greatly. Surgery has become outdated, its use now being limited to patients in whom malignancy has been proven or is suspected, and those in whom complications, e.g. bleeding, perforation or stenosis, have developed.

The aims of medical treatment are symptomatic relief, accelerated ulcer healing and the prevention of ulcer relapse.

Medical treatment

General measures

General measures helpful in the management of peptic ulcers include the avoidance of NSAIDs, smoking and excessive alcohol. In *H. pylori*-negative patients on NSAIDs where the use of these drugs cannot be avoided altogether, the least damaging agents should be used, e.g. ibuprofen or diclofenac. These should be prescribed with an antisecretory agent. Antisecretory agents include selec-

tive histamine receptor antagonists and proton pump inhibitors. H_2 antagonists competitively inhibit histamine at the parietal cell receptor and can decrease acid secretion by up to 80%. These have been largely replaced by the proton pump inhibitors (e.g. omeprazole or lansoprazole). These agents act by irreversibly inhibiting H^+/K^+ ATPase and thus are powerful inhibitors of acid secretion.

Other agents that may be used to supplement antisecretory agents include bismuth compounds, sucralfate, prostaglandin analogues and antacids.

Eradication of H. pylori

Duodenal ulcers Ninety-five per cent of duodenal ulcers are associated with *H. pylori* infection, and eradication of the bacterium has become the mainstay of management in those diagnosed with a duodenal ulcer at endoscopy. Eradication therapies now commonly use three agents: an antisecretory agent, typically omeprazole, together with one or more antibiotics. The course is usually given for 1–2 weeks. Commonly used regimens are shown in Table 18.2. These triple therapies have been associated with eradication rates of greater than 90%. Reinfection following successful eradication is rare. Without eradication therapy it has been shown that approximately 80% of ulcers will recur within 1 year.

Complete resolution of symptoms is a good indicator of successful eradication. However, where symptoms persist it is advisable to recheck the *H. pylori* status. This may be done using the *H. pylori* breath test. Like the CLO test, this relies on the hydrolysis of urea by *H. pylori*. Urea is labelled with ^{13}C which, when hydrolysed is expired as $^{13}CO_2$. The test should be undertaken at least 4 weeks after finishing the course of eradication therapy. Earlier testing may give rise to false negative results owing to suppression of the bacterium rather than true eradication. True persist-

Table 18.2 *Helicobacter pylori* eradication regimens

Regimen 1
Proton pump inhibitor
  Omeprazole 20 mg b.d. or
  Lansoprazole 30 mg o.d.
Metronidazole 400 mg t.d.s.
Amoxycillin 500 mg t.d.s.

Regimen 2
Proton pump inhibitor (as above)
Clarithromycin 250 mg t.d.s.
Amoxycillin 500 mg t.d.s.

Regimen 3 (if allergic to amoxycillin)
Proton pump inhibitor (as above)
Metronidazole 400 mg t.d.s.
Clarithromycin 250 mg b.d.

ing infection should be treated with an alternative eradication course (Table 18.2).

Gastric ulcers Malignancy should be excluded by endoscopic biopsy before a diagnosis of benign gastric ulcer is made. Where a patient is found to be *H. pylori* positive at endoscopy, eradication therapy should be instituted. Without eradication the relapse rate is in the region of 50%, but this falls to less than 10% with successful eradication therapy. Endoscopic surveillance of a treated ulcer should continue until healing is complete. Failure to heal warrants further biopsies.

Surgical treatment

Duodenal ulceration

Surgery for uncomplicated duodenal ulceration is extremely rare and is aimed at the reduction of acid and pepsin. This may be achieved by undertaking a vagotomy procedure, whereby the acetylcholine component of the secretion pathway is interrupted. A drawback of this procedure, however, is that stomach motility is also decreased and the pyloric sphincter fails to relax. A drainage procedure (pyloroplasty or gastrojejunostomy) is therefore needed (Fig. 18.4).

Highly selective vagotomy avoids the need for a drainage procedure, as only vagal fibres passing to the stomach body are divided, thereby preserving innervation to the antrum and pylorus (Fig. 18.5). This procedure, however, carries with it an increased ulcer recurrence rate.

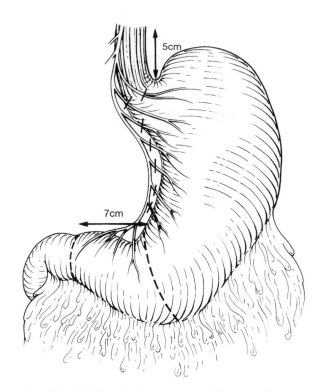

Fig. 18.5 Highly selective vagotomy. The operation divides vagal fibres to the gastric corpus and 5 cm of oesophagus should be cleared.

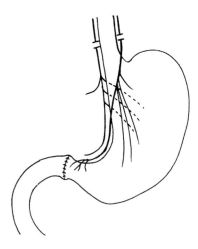

Pyloroplasty

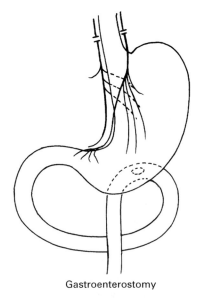

Gastroenterostomy

Fig. 18.4 Truncal vagotomy and drainage.

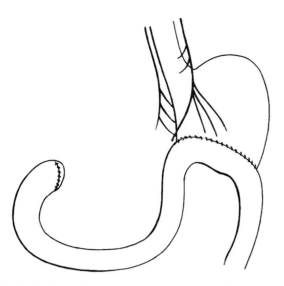

Fig. 18.6 Partial gastrectomy for duodenal ulcer (Polya or Billroth II).

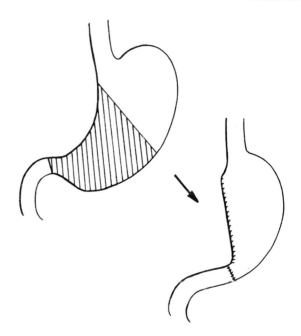

Fig. 18.7 Partial gastrectomy for gastric ulcer (Billroth I).

Prior to the use of vagotomy procedures, gastric resection was used to decrease acid and pepsin secretion, the more extensive procedures being associated with lower recurrence rates. The Billroth II or Polya partial gastrectomy (Fig. 18.6) was used for duodenal ulceration, whereby the proximal gastric remnant is anastomosed to the jejunum.

Gastric ulcers

Failure of conservative therapy to heal a gastric ulcer is an indication for surgical intervention. Where malignancy cannot be excluded or is suspected, resection of the ulcer is the treatment of choice. The extent and type of resection will be determined by the position of the ulcer within the stomach and its suspected malignant potential. Benign distal ulcers may be treated by a Billroth I gastrectomy, whereby the distal part of the stomach is removed and the proximal stump anastomosed to the duodenum (Fig. 18.7). More proximal ulcers usually necessitate a Polya-type reconstruction involving anastomosis of the gastric remnant to the jejunum.

Complications after surgery

In most patients the side-effects of surgery are minor, but in up to 10% significant morbidity may result.

Early

Haemorrhage This complication presents on the first postoperative day in the form of fresh blood in the naso-gastric aspirate. It usually settles spontaneously and further surgery is rarely indicated. Occasionally careful endoscopy and injection of adrenaline to the bleeding point may be indicated.

Stomal hold-up The commonest cause of stomal hold-up is oedema around the anastomosis following resectional surgery, and it should be suspected if large volumes of nasogastric aspirate are produced for several days after the operation. This complication usually settles spontaneously and is reflected in decreasing volumes of nasogastric aspirate, but may require surgery if it fails to settle.

Suture line leakage Anastomotic leakage is a rare but important early complication. Following a Polya partial gastrectomy duodenal stump leakage is a significant cause of death. It may present as localized peritonitis during the first week following surgery. This complication can be treated conservatively with nasogastric aspiration and intravenous feeding if the patient is stable and there is good drainage from the area. A controlled fistula develops and will close spontaneously as long as there is no distal obstruction in the intestine. Should generalized peritonitis develop there may be a place for peritoneal toilet and formal drainage of the area concerned.

Intermediate

Vomiting This complication is relatively common following gastric surgery, occurring in up to 30% of patients.

It is usually quite mild and settles spontaneously. Troublesome vomiting may result from delayed gastric emptying, biliary reflux associated with gastritis, and mechanical obstruction at the anastomosis (e.g. stenosis secondary to recurrent ulceration or oedema).

Dumping This arises in up to 20% of patients following gastric resection and encompasses a range of vasomotor symptoms, including light-headedness, tachycardia, flushing, sweats and palpitations. Occasionally these are accompanied by diarrhoea and vomiting.

Early dumping (or *dumping syndrome* proper) occurs 15–30 minutes after eating. The rapid emptying of hyperosmolar (mainly carbohydrates) gastric contents into the small intestine is responsible. This leads to the influx of fluid down an osmotic gradient into the bowel lumen. The symptoms associated with the syndrome are due to both the sudden contraction of the extracellular fluid compartment and intestinal distension causing increased peristalsis. The patient often needs to lie down until the symptoms pass. In the majority of patients symptoms improve spontaneously with conservative measures, which include taking smaller, dry and frequent meals, avoiding excessive carbohydrate intake, and avoiding liquids at mealtimes.

Late dumping is much less common than early dumping. It is a reactive hypoglycaemia caused by more rapid absorption of glucose from the upper small intestine. This causes hyperglycaemia, which in turn leads to increased insulin production a rebound hypoglycaemia. The symptoms are of a similar nature to those of the dumping syndrome proper (or early dumping), but may include hunger and confusion and occur 1–3 hours after eating. Late dumping is symptomatically controlled with sugar.

Diarrhoea This is frequently found after resectional surgery and pyloroplasty but is very uncommon following highly selective vagotomy. Rapid influx of gastric contents into the small intestine and an interruption of vagal fibres to abdominal viscera other than stomach are thought to be responsible. The diarrhoea may be associated with mild steatorrhoea. Codeine-related compounds or loperamide may be used to treat the diarrhoea, although they are not always helpful. Eating small, dry meals lacking in refined carbohydrates can help. Surgical methods to slow bowel transit have not proved to be successful.

General nutritional effects Up to 40% of patients lose weight following surgery for peptic ulcers. In the most part decreased oral intake is responsible, and this may be due to vomiting or dumping. In the dumping syndromes patients take small carbohydrate-poor meals in order to control their symptoms, and so overall intake is reduced. Early satiety following surgery (e.g. due to a small gastric remnant) may also contribute.

Malabsorption may also play a role, as there is generally accelerated emptying of gastric contents into the small intestine following surgery. Bacterial overgrowth may also contribute to malabsorption.

Anaemia Anaemia may occur some time after any form of gastric surgery and is particularly common following complete gastrectomy. The picture may be one of iron, B_{12} or folate deficiency, or a mixture of the three. Iron deficiency is the most common and may be part of a generalized poor intake, as described above. It may also result from depressed acid-dependent reduction of iron salts, this process being necessary for the body's utilization of iron. B_{12} deficiency occurs when insufficient intrinsic factor is available for its absorption. This usually only occurs after extensive gastric resection, as the stomach generally produces far more intrinsic factor than is actually needed for B_{12} absorption. Folate deficiency may result from poor oral intake.

Late

Osteoporosis and osteomalacia These conditions are associated with partial gastrectomy owing to decreased absorption of calcium and vitamin D. Such bone disease may manifest itself many years postoperatively as pathological fractures. Vitamin D and calcium supplementation on a long-term basis is indicated, especially in women.

Carcinoma Following partial gastric resection there is an increased risk of the long-term development of gastric cancer. The aetiology is not clear, but the reflux of bile into the stomach, relative hypochlorhydia and *H. pylori* infection are likely to play a role.

Cholelithiasis Current evidence suggests that there is an increased risk of developing gallstones following surgery for peptic ulcers. The mechanisms involved have not been fully established.

Tuberculosis There is an established association of tuberculosis following partial gastric resection. Careful follow-up for those with a history of tuberculosis is mandatory.

COMPLICATIONS OF PEPTIC ULCERATION REQUIRING OPERATIVE INTERVENTION

PERFORATION

Duodenal ulcers Perforation occurs in 2–4% of patients with duodenal ulcers, and of these 5–10% will have had no previous ulcer symptoms. It has a peak incidence in the fourth and fifth decades of life and its incidence is decreasing. This is probably due in part to improvements in the medical management of duodenal ulcers. Perforation usually occurs in acute ulcers on the anterior wall of the duodenum.

Gastric ulcers Gastric ulcer perforation is less common than duodenal ulcer perforation. It has a peak incidence in the elderly, and consequently the associated morbidity and mortality are higher. Gastric perforation has a strong association with NSAID use.

Symptomatology

The acute onset of severe unremitting epigastric pain is strongly suggestive that perforation may have occurred. Thereafter, the range of symptoms depends on the intra-abdominal course. The patient may be pale, shocked and peripherally shut down secondary to generalized peritonitis. Irritant stomach contents in the peritoneal cavity may give rise to shoulder-tip pain resulting from irritation of the diaphragm. Vomiting may occur. The abdomen does not move freely with respiration, and marked tenderness, guarding, fear of movement and board-like rigidity may be found on examination. Respiration is shallow and bowel sounds are usually absent. There may also be loss of liver dullness as free air escapes from the alimentary tract into the peritoneal cavity. In some patients the symptoms may appear to lessen after a few hours. This results from the dilution of the irritant fluid by peritoneal exudates. In some patients bacterial peritonitis may supersede.

Generalized peritonitis does not occur in some patients because the perforation seals over with omentum. In others the fluid tracks down the paracolic gutters, simulating acute appendicitis. Silent perforations may also occur, and are only found incidentally on a chest X-ray.

Diagnosis

In 60% cases of perforation, an erect chest X-ray will demonstrate free air under the diaphragm, although the absence of free air does not exclude a perforation (Fig. 18.8). A lateral decubitus film can be useful where an erect chest X-ray is not feasible, e.g. because of shock or disability.

A moderate hyperamylasaemia may be found with a perforated duodenal ulcer. High amylase levels are more suggestive of pancreatitis. Where there is still doubt over the diagnosis an emergency water-soluble contrast meal may be indicated.

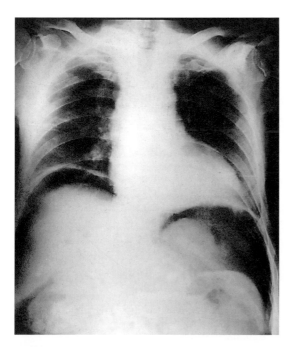

Fig. 18.8 Chest X-ray showing air under the diaphragm.

SUMMARY BOX

Perforated peptic ulcer

- Perforated duodenal ulcer is commoner than perforated gastric ulcer.
- Ulcer perforation still carries a significant mortality (10%), particularly in the elderly and those with intercurrent disease.
- Free gas beneath the diaphragm on an erect abdominal or chest film confirms the diagnosis in two-thirds of cases; a Gastrografin meal may be helpful if free gas is not present.
- Perforated duodenal ulcers can be dealt with by simple closure and the application of nearby omentum. If the ulcer is chronic (i.e. a history of more than 3 months and scarring at operation) definitive surgery in the form of truncal vagotomy and pyloroplasty can be considered.
- Patients who present late or who are deemed too ill for operation can be managed by conservative means (nasogastric aspiration and intravenous fluids, antibiotics and antisecretory drugs).
- Perforated 'gastric ulcers' frequently prove to be perforated gastric tumours (15% of cases) and may best be treated by partial gastrectomy. Lesser procedures (e.g. simple closure or ulcer excision, vagotomy and drainage) may be advisable in elderly poor-risk patients.

Management

The initial management, as for other causes of peritonitis, consists of resuscitation, intravenous antibiotics (e.g. cefuroxime and metronidazole) and the passage of a naso-gastric tube. Adequate analgesia is provided and blood is withdrawn for haematology and the measurement of urea and electrolytes. A urinary catheter enables close monitoring of urine output.

Operative management is indicated in most patients, but rapid operative intervention should not be substituted for thorough resuscitation. Although a laparoscopic approach to treatment is favoured by some, its superiority over open surgery is yet to be established.

Duodenal ulcers Surgery may involve simple closure, whereby the ulcer is underrun with sutures or plugged using an omental patch (Fig. 18.9). This approach is most appropriate for patients with acute ulcers, i.e. those with a history of less than 3 months' duration and no chronic scarring at operation, and is coupled with a thorough peritoneal lavage. Those patients found to be *H. pylori* positive are commenced on eradication therapy. Long-term proton pump inhibitors are indicated in *H. pylori*-negative patients.

In some cases there may be a place for the non-operative management of perforated ulcers. It may be appropriate in patients with silent perforations and those too ill to undergo laparotomy (e.g. due to severe cardiorespiratory disease). Where the decision has been made not to operate, management consists of supportive treatment with nasogastric suction, *H. pylori* eradication therapy, intravenous fluids and antisecretory agents.

Gastric ulcers Approximately 15% of perforated gastric ulcers prove ultimately to be malignant, and therefore, where possible, definitive surgery is preferred in these patients. Where the situation is less clear, e.g. in poor-risk patients, simple closure coupled with biopsy or local excision may still be the safest option. Regular endoscopy for the detection of ulcer recurrence is appropriate.

ACUTE HAEMORRHAGE

The differential diagnosis of upper GI bleeding is summarized in Table 18.3.

The most common causes of upper gastrointestinal bleeding in children are oesophagitis, Mallory–Weiss tear, gastritis, duodenitis and oesophageal varices. Rarely, benign tumours of the stomach including haemangiomata, islands of aberrant pancreatic tissue or hamartomata can be the source of upper gastrointestinal bleeding. Endoscopy allows for an accurate diagnosis to be made, and, in the majority, conservative management of the underlying disorder will allow the bleeding to settle. Rarely, segmental excision of a bleeding haemangioma or similar lesion may be necessary.

The rate of blood loss from a peptic ulcer determines the signs and symptoms the patient experiences. The vomiting of blood (haematemesis) may be bright red, suggestive of an acute brisk bleed, or it may have the appearance of coffee grounds. This is more suggestive of a less severe bleed and the appearance results from the partial digestion of blood in the stomach. Upper GI bleeding may present as malaena – the

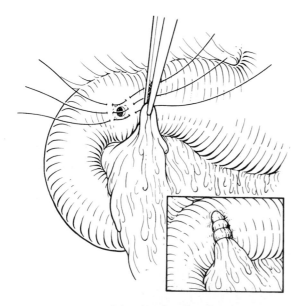

Fig. 18.9 Closure of duodenal perforation.

Table 18.3 Causes of upper GI bleeding	
Peptic ulceration	50%
Mucosal lesions including gastritis Duodenitis and erosions	30%
Mallory–Weiss tear	5–10%
Varices	5–10%
Reflux oesophagitis	5%
Angiodysphasia	2%
Carcinoma	Uncommon
Aortoduodenal fistual	Uncommon
Dieulafoy syndrome (rupture of a large tortuous submucosal artery normally found in the body of the stomach)	Rare
Coagulopathies	Uncommon

passage of black tarry stool that has a very characteristic smell. It results from the digestion of blood by enzymes and bacteria. Less commonly malaena may be the result of a bleed from the right colon. Very rarely, if bleeding is very brisk, upper GI bleeding may present as fresh rectal bleeding, in which case signs of cardiovascular instability are usually present. Slow chronic blood loss may be asymptomatic and detected on rectal examination by a positive faecal occult blood test.

Diagnosis

History and examination

A full history and examination are essential in determining the cause of the bleeding. Pointers to the diagnosis include the past medical history (peptic ulcer disease, previous bleeding, liver disease, previous surgery, coagulopathies), drug history (most importantly NSAIDs, anticoagulants) and social history (alcohol abuse).

Specific features to be looked for include those suggestive of acute substantial blood loss and shock (hypotension, tachycardia and pallor), and signs of liver disease and portal hypertension (spider naevi, portosystemic shunting and bruising). The latter are particularly important, as variceal haemorrhage necessitates specific treatment.

Blood tests

Blood tests are useful in the assessment of gastrointestinal bleeding. The full blood count may be normal immediately after an acute bleed but will fall once haemodilution has occurred. The test may also reflect anaemia, suggestive of more chronic blood loss. Urea is often high following a gastrointestinal bleed, reflecting the absorption of blood and its subsequent metabolism by the liver. Coagulation derangement occurs in the presence of significant hepatic disease.

Management

Resuscitation

Bleeding is now the commonest cause of death from peptic ulcer disease and resuscitation is vital in the management of all patients with this presentation. Intravenous access is obtained and at the same time blood taken for the investigations noted above. A sample is also taken for cross-matching, as often these patients will require a blood transfusion.

A nasogastric tube is passed to monitor the bleeding and prevent aspiration. A urinary catheter is inserted. A central line is often used to help monitor central venous pressure. The circulating blood volume should be replaced as quickly as possible. Type-specific blood is used as soon as this becomes available from the Blood Transfusion Service. Volume replacement is gauged against pulse, blood pressure, urine output and central venous pressure. Overtransfusion or rapid transfusion in those with compromised cardiac function can lead to pulmonary oedema. Oxygen is administered to all shocked patients.

Detection and endoscopic treatment

The aims of management of bleeding peptic ulcers are to identify the bleeding point, arrest the bleeding (bleeding ceases spontaneously in 90% of patients) and prevent recurrence.

Once resuscitation has stabilized the patient endoscopy can be used to detect the site of bleeding, and does so successfully in 80–90% of cases. Endoscopy may also be used in a therapeutic capacity. This is appropriate when stigmata of recent haemorrhage are present. These include active bleeding from the ulcer base, the presence of a visible vessel, and adherent clot overlying the ulcer. These features are associated with a significantly increased risk of further bleeding from the ulcer. Injection sclerotherapy (e.g. using adrenaline 1:10 000 or sclerosants) is used commonly, but other methods include the use of heat probes and lasers. Therapeutic endoscopy can also be used in the management of oesophageal and gastric varices and vascular malformations.

In patients in whom endoscopy does not identify the bleeding point angiography may be used, but the limitation of this investigation is that it can only detect active bleeding of greater than 1 mL/min. In these patients selective embolization can be used to stop the bleeding and thus avoid the need for surgery. The main drawback of this is that in some cases it may lead to mesenteric ischaemia. A technetium scan is sometimes used when a Meckel's diverticulum is suspected.

Surgical treatment

Emergency surgery may be indicated if endoscopy reveals bleeding from a major artery and where attempted injection sclerotherapy is unable to control the bleeding directly: 60% of patients with active arterial bleeding and 40% with a visible vessel at the ulcer base are ultimately likely to require surgery. Surgery is also indicated when cardiovascular stability is compromised or where bleeding recurs. Recurrent bleeding is associated with significant morbidity and mortality, particularly in the elderly. Continuing bleeding is particularly common in those with a chronic ulcer and is more common in gastric ulceration. The type of operation used depends on the site of the bleeding ulcer and the comorbidity of the patient.

Duodenal ulcers A bleeding duodenal ulcer may simply be underrun with non-absorbable sutures once it has been identified, using a pyloromyotomy (opening of the anterior wall of the pylorus) to gain access to the duodenum. The pyloromyotomy may be then closed transversely as a pyloroplasty. A biopsy of the antrum is usually taken to

Table 18.4 Causes of gastric outlet obstruction

Peptic ulcer disease
Malignancy
Stomach antrum
Pancreas
Lymphomas
Crohn's disease of duodenum
Adult hypertrophic pyloric stenosis
Inflammation of adjacent organs
Gastroparesis

establish *H. pylori* status. Alternatively, the patient may be started on *H. pylori* eradication therapy empirically.

Gastric ulcers In a bleeding gastric ulcer the possibility of malignancy must not be overlooked. The ulcer must be biopsied in all cases to determine its nature. In young fit patients the ulcer should be excised completely by undertaking a partial gastric resection. If feasible, a smaller wedge resection may be undertaken instead. In elderly patients or those with significant comorbidity, underrunning of the ulcer may be preferable, at least in the first instance. If the pathology result confirms malignancy partial gastric resection may be indicated as soon as the patient is fit enough. If the ulcer proves to be benign *H. pylori* eradication is indicated if infection is present. NSAIDs should be avoided.

PYLORIC STENOSIS

Pyloric stenosis consists of narrowing of the pyloric channel, leading to gastric outlet obstruction. The obstruc-

tion may be anywhere in the region of the pylorus, but most commonly occurs in the first part of the duodenum. The commonest cause in adults is peptic ulceration but other causes are shown in Table 18.4.

Symptoms and signs

Gastric outlet obstruction presents with symptoms of fullness and often a constant dull pain in the epigastrium. Projectile vomiting of large volumes of undigested and partially digested food matter is characteristic. This is more common later in the day and when lying down, and usually relieves the sensation of fullness. There may be associated weight loss.

On examination there is commonly epigastric fullness associated with signs of dehydration and weight loss. Visible gastric peristalsis may be seen and is diagnostic of gastric outlet obstruction. A succussion splash (i.e. an audible splashing noise when the patient is gently rocked from side to side) is often elicited.

Management

When gastric outlet obstruction is suspected a large-bore nasogastric tube is passed. Often large volumes of non-bilious gastric contents can be aspirated, and undigested food may be recognized. Intravenous access is obtained and bloods sent for full blood count, urea and electrolytes. Biochemical analysis usually reflects dehydration, with a low sodium, potassium and chloride and a high urea and bicarbonate. The further obligatory loss of potassium by the kidneys results in a hypokalaemic metabolic alkalosis. As the alkalosis worsens, potassium stores become so depleted that hydrogen ions are excreted instead of potassium by the kidney, and the result is aciduria – the so-called *paradoxical aciduria of gastric outlet obstruction*. If the history of outlet obstruction is chronic, biochemistry may also reflect a degree of starvation (i.e. hypoalbuminaemia).

Gastric outlet obstruction is further investigated using radiological contrast studies (e.g. barium meal) or endoscopy. Endoscopy is the investigation of choice, as biopsies can establish the nature of the obstruction. It is essential, however, that the stomach is empty before either investigation is attempted.

In most patients there is no indication for urgent laparotomy and their fluid and electrolyte balance should be corrected prior to any surgery. In long-standing cases there may also be some benefit from intravenous feeding prior to surgery to improve the patient's overall nutritional status. Surgery is not always necessary and, assuming the pathology is benign, a course of proton pump inhibitors may be sufficient to heal the ulceration and relieve the obstruction. In most cases surgery is necessary, and where the pathology is benign a pyloroplasty or gastrojejunostomy is used, which may be coupled with a vagotomy procedure to avoid ulcer recurrence. Where malignancy is identified clearly more radical surgery is necessary.

INFANTILE HYPERTROPHIC PYLORIC STENOSIS

Infantile hypertrophic pyloric stenosis is a common cause of vomiting in the first eight weeks of life. Male, first-born infants are most frequently affected and there is a higher incidence in the presence of an affected male relative. The infant presents with vomiting of increasing amounts of milk feed, until the child vomits after every meal. The vomiting is classically described as 'projectile', but the fact that the vomiting occurs after every feed is a much more important observation. The child will cry with hunger after vomiting the feed but further attempt to satisfy this hunger will result in further vomiting.

Continuing vomiting will result in dehydration, loss of gastric acid, and the classic picture of a hypokalaemic, hypochloraemic, metabolic alkalosis. The child may have paradoxical aciduria.

The diagnosis can be made clinically. Visible gastric peristalsis and the palpation of the hypertrophied pyloris during feeding clinches the diagnosis. This is possible in 60–75% of cases. In the remainder, ultrasound scan will reveal thickening and lengthening of the pyloric canal.

After a period of careful rehydration using half-strength (0.45%) saline containing potassium to correct the biochemical imbalances, the child is taken to the operating theatre. A pyloromyotomy is performed using an open, or in a few centres, a laparoscopic technique. The serosa of the pyloris is cut with a scapel and the thick, hypertrophied muscle tumour is split down to the mucosa using an artery forceps.

Complications following this operation are rare, but include haemorrhage, inadequate myotomy, wound infection and wound dehiscence.

GASTRIC NEOPLASIA

BENIGN GASTRIC NEOPLASMS

Benign tumours of the stomach may arise from epithelial or mesenchymal tissue. Adenomatous polyps may be single or multiple and are the commonest benign epithelial neoplasm. Leiomyoma is the commonest of the stromal tumours, and neurogenic tumours, fibromata and lipoma are rare. Such benign lesions may be an incidental finding during investigation, but can give rise to bleeding or intermittent pyloric obstruction with vomiting. The benign nature of these lesions is confirmed by endoscopic biopsy. Small lesions may be removed at endoscopy by diathermy wire, but large polyps should be resected surgically in view of the risk of malignancy.

MALIGNANT GASTRIC NEOPLASMS

Gastric carcinoma

Epidemiology

Gastric adenocarcinoma is the most common of the malignancies affecting the stomach. It accounts for 90% of malignant tumours found within the stomach, lymphomas and smooth muscle tumours comprising the remaining 10%. Gastric cancer is responsible for 7500 deaths per year in the UK. Its incidence has decreased substantially throughout the latter part of the 20th century. Gastric cancer principally affects those in the 60–80-year age group, but is not infrequently seen in younger patients. Where once the tumour was more commonly noted in the gastric antrum, its incidence in this region has diminished and a corresponding increase in incidence in the proximal stomach has occurred. The male:female ratio is 2:1. Gastric cancer has the fifth poorest 5-year survival rate after cancer of the pancreas, liver, oesophagus and lung.

Aetiological factors

No definitive aetiological agents have been recognized but the environment is thought to have considerable influence. Environmental factors include diet and socioeconomic status. In addition several conditions have been described which are associated with the development of malignant change within the stomach.

Diet Gastric cancer is noted more commonly where malnutrition is prevalent. It has also been associated with the use of certain preservatives in food: nitrates, nitrites and nitrosamines have been implicated. Where soils are rich in nitrates or dietary intake is high, gastric carcinoma is more common. A high vitamin intake is thought to be protective against the development of cancer of the stomach. Diets rich in carotene and vitamins C and E have been shown to reduce the incidence of intestinal metaplasia in the stomach, a condition thought to be associated with malignant change.

Helicobacter pylori infection Recent epidemiological studies have suggested that *H. pylori* may be associated with an increased incidence of malignant change within the stomach. At the present time it is thought that its ability to produce ammonia as well as other mutagenic chemicals may play a part in neoplastic transformation of the gastric mucosa. Such changes are thought to be enhanced by lack of vitamin C.

Gastric polyps Hyperplastic and adenomatous polyps are the most frequently found but only the latter have significant malignant potential. Studies have shown that over a quarter of adenomatous polyps may show malignant changes within them. Furthermore, gastric carcinoma is frequently encountered in stomachs affected by polyps. This suggests that conditions necessary for the development of polyps may also enhance the development of malignancy.

Gastroenterostomy Where there has been a previous gastric resection or duodenal bypass for benign disease and the remaining stomach has been anastomosed to the bile-containing upper gastrointestinal tract, the stomach remnant is more vulnerable to malignant change than the intact stomach. The risk of malignant change increases with the time elapsed since surgery. Patients having had gastric resections with gastroenterostomy may be four to five times more liable to develop gastric carcinoma in the stomach remnant than the normal population.

Chronic gastric ulcer disease It is thought that chronic peptic ulceration in the stomach increases the risk of malignant change within the ulcer. It has been extremely difficult to assess the true level of risk with such ulcers, but it is thought to be low. Such chronic ulcers, however, deserve close observation by endoscopy and biopsy at frequent intervals until they have healed.

Chronic atrophic gastritis This condition is associated with a loss of the gastric glands from the stomach mucosa. It has been noted to be more frequent in patients at increased risk of developing stomach cancer. Chronic atrophic gastritis is associated with pernicious anaemia, which is linked to an increased risk of gastric cancer. Such patients have a fourfold increased risk compared to the normal population.

Intestinal metaplasia This condition arises when the gastric mucosa is replaced by mucosa-containing glands which have features more in common with those found in the small intestine. Such changes are usually found in the distal part of the stomach and are associated with an increased risk of development of gastric carcinoma.

Gastric dysplasia When the gastric mucosal cells become less uniform in size, shape and organization, dysplastic changes may result and may be mild, moderate or severe. Only in the most severe cases is there concern regarding associated malignant change.

Host factors Blood group A is associated with an increased risk of developing gastric cancer. Oncogenes have recently been discovered which have been found to be activated in patients with stomach cancer.

Early gastric cancer

Early gastric cancer (Fig. 18.10) results when neoplastic cells are limited to the mucosa or submucosal layers of the stomach wall. By definition, this type of cancer is confined to the most superficial layers of the stomach wall but it can be associated in a small minority of patients with lymph node metastases. Such tumours, if adequately treated surgically, are associated with 5-year survival rates in excess of 90%. The survival rate will depend upon the depth of invasion of the tumour and the presence or absence of lymph node metastases at the time of surgical excision. Early gastric cancer in Britain accounts for approximately 10% of all resected cases of gastric adenocarcinoma.

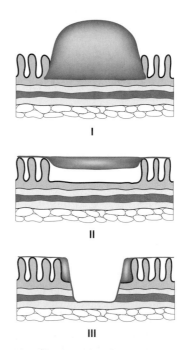

Fig. 18.10 Classification of early gastric cancer.
   Type I (protruded): protrusion into the gastric lumen.
   Type II (flat): hardly any noticeable elevation from or depression in the surrounding mucosa.
   Type III (excavated): marked excavation in the gastric wall.

Advanced gastric cancer

The vast majority of malignant tumours found in the stomach are of the advanced gastric adenocarcinoma type (Fig. 18.11). These tumours have penetrated more deeply into the stomach wall than those of early gastric cancers, and many will have transgressed the stomach wall to invade adjacent structures. Lymphatics are more frequently involved than in early gastric cancer. Should the entire thickness of the stomach wall have been penetrated, transperitoneal spread and invasion of surrounding structures by tumour is frequent. Haematogenous spread also occurs via the portal system and may lead to metastases in the liver. Advanced gastric cancer is therefore frequently associated with a variety of distant manifestations that preclude surgical resection for cure.

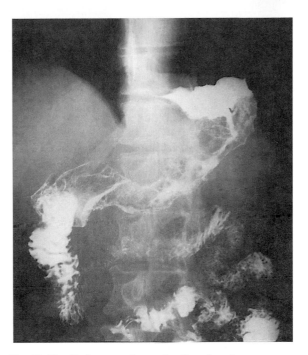

Fig. 18.12 Barium meal examination showing extensive gastric carcinoma causing narrowing of the gastric lumen.

Advanced gastric adenocarcinomas are classically described as four morphological types: polypoid and fungating; excavated crater cancer; ulcer cancer with infiltrative margins; and a diffuse cancer with thickening of the stomach wall, making it diffusely rigid and known as linitis plastica (Fig. 18.12).

Factors affecting survival in advanced gastric cancer

The survival of the patient with advanced gastric cancer depends upon their state of fitness at the time of diagnosis and the stage of the cancer when it is discovered and treated. Treatment usually implies surgical resection, as this is the only effective means of possible cure available at present. For surgery to be curative excision must be adequate, with margins clear of the tumour and with satisfactory en-bloc resection of all possible involved lymph nodes. Such surgery will offer the best chance of cure or a prolonged disease-free interval before recurrence. Only half of patients diagnosed with gastric cancer will be suitable for gastric resection.

Poor survival has been correlated with depth of invasion of the tumour through the stomach wall, involvement of tumour resection margins and the presence of lymph node metastases. Transgression of the tumour through the stomach wall is associated with very poor survival, as the

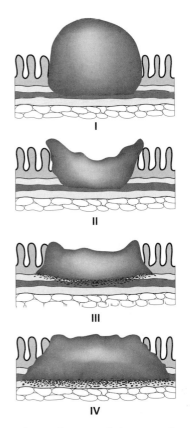

I

II

III

IV

Fig. 18.11 Advanced cancer of the stomach may be classified according to Borrmann's morphologic descriptions of the gastric lesions. (1) Borrmann I: fungating type of carcinoma. (2) Borrmann II: carcinomatous ulcer without infiltration of surrounding mucosa. (3) Borrmann III: carcinomatous ulcer with infiltration of surrounding mucosa. (4) Borrmann IV: diffuse infiltrative carcinoma.

Table 18.5 TNM Classification of gastric carcinoma. From Sobin L. H., Whittekind C. 1997 UICC: TNM classification of malignant tumours, 4th edn. Springer, New York	
T1	Tumour extends to lamina propria or submucosa
T2	Tumour extends into muscle
T3	Tumour extends to serosa
T4	Tumour invades adjacent structures
N0	No lymph node involvement
N1	Fewer than 7 lymph nodes involved by tumour
N2	7–15 lymph nodes involved by tumour
N3	More than 15 lymph nodes involved by tumour
M0	No metastases
M1	Metastases present

tumour is able to spread transperitoneally and therefore seed the peritoneum with malignant cells, making complete surgical excision impossible.

A comprehensive pathological classification of tumours has enabled the prognosis of a particular stage of cancer to be estimated. Such staging is usually classified according to the tumour size (T), the node status (N) and the presence or absence of distant metastases (M) (Table 18.5).

Clinical features of gastric malignancy

The symptomatology of gastric carcinoma may be subtle and mild symptoms of indigestion, flatulence or dyspepsia may be the early signs of malignancy. Such symptoms should not be overlooked and should not be treated without further investigation, particularly in patients in a vulnerable age group (> 40 years).

The severity of symptoms is not invariably associated with the stage of disease. More advanced gastric cancer tends to be associated with weight loss, anaemia, dysphagia, vomiting, epigastric or back pain, or the presence of an epigastric mass. The patient may also manifest signs of more widespread distant metastases, such as jaundice (liver secondaries or compression of the biliary tree by enlarged lymph nodes), ascites, spurious diarrhoea (secondary to pelvic infiltration), and signs and symptoms of intestinal obstruction secondary to malignant deposits on the bowel.

Diagnosis

Diagnosis is made on the basis of a thorough medical history and clinical examination. By the time of referral weight loss may be evident. An epigastric mass may be pal-

pable and ascites may be present. The liver and supraclavicular lymph nodes should be palpated for mesenteric disease. A digital rectal examination may detect transcolonic spread to the pelvis. Thereafter general tests assessing the patient's nutritional status, renal and hepatic function, as well as a full blood count, should be carried out. Specific tests to confirm and further elucidate the nature of the disease should include upper gastrointestinal endoscopy and biopsy of any suspicious lesions. Following histological diagnosis care should be taken to evaluate accurately the level of fitness of the patient to ascertain the likelihood of their being amenable to radical treatment should staging of the disease be favourable.

Staging of gastric carcinoma

Having confirmed the nature of the malignancy within the stomach further assessment is required to stage the degree of advancement of the disease and allow a rational approach to treatment. Investigations will include ultrasound scanning of the liver in order to exclude liver metastases, CT scanning to visualize the retroperitoneal lymph nodes that may be affected by gastric carcinoma, and endoscopic ultrasound to assess the degree of penetration through the gastric wall, as well as spread to associated lymphatics. Laparoscopy and laparoscopic ultrasound may help to detect small metastases within the liver, and laparoscopy alone may detect small amounts of ascites and very small tumour nodules within the peritoneum.

Where the disease is thought to be resectable and the patient sufficiently fit, aggressive surgical resection with the associated lymphatic drainage can take place. For this to be considered the tumour has to be confined to the stomach wall (T1–T3) and there must be no evidence of distant metastases. Occasionally, when there has been direct invasion of other structures from the stomach tumour (T4), wide resection for cure involving the resection of adjacent organs can be considered.

Treatment

Prior to treatment the patient's preoperative condition should be optimized by improving nutritional status and anaemia, as well as the state of hydration if appropriate. Attention should be paid to physiotherapy and ensuring the cessation of smoking.

With advanced disease, or if the patient is unfit, palliative measures such as more conservative resection, bypass, or lesser measures such as intubation or laser therapy, may be required to control the worst symptoms of the tumour. Chemotherapy and radiotherapy have only a limited role in the palliation of disease in a small proportion of patients. Recent trials have suggested that combinations of drugs, including epirubicin, cisplatin and 5-fluorouracil, may cause shrinkage of some gastric carcinomas and may in some circumstances render previously inoperable tumours operable.

Resection with curative intent – radical total gastrectomy

This procedure involves the removal of the entire stomach together with the distal part of the abdominal oesophagus and the proximal part of the duodenum. In such a radical procedure attention is also paid to the removal of surrounding structures in which metastases may occur. These include the greater and lesser omenta and related lymph nodes.

Reconstruction involves refashioning the small bowel, allowing bile to enter lower down the gastrointestinal tract, thereby preventing regurgitation of corrosive bile into the lower oesophagus. The most common form of reconstruction is Roux-en-Y (Fig. 18.13).

On occasion it may be possible to carry out radical subtotal gastrectomy, where 90–95% of the stomach is removed and a small proximal cuff is left close to the cardia, thereby allowing a small gastric reservoir to remain. This is thought to allow better digestive functioning post operatively, but such gastric preservation can only take place if appropriate clearance of the tumour has been achieved.

Such radical procedures should carry a mortality of less than 5%.

Palliative resection

In such operations attention is aimed primarily at reducing symptomatic tumour bulk and reconstituting gastrointestinal continuity, avoiding tumour-bearing areas. Palliative resection is preferred primarily for bleeding or obstruction, but only in patients deemed surgically fit and properly appraised of their tumours. Such tumours are usually distal, as proximal tumours are not generally amenable to palliative resection.

Palliative bypass

These operations are designed principally for advanced distal gastric tumours that are unresectable for cure and fixed to vital structures such as the common bile duct or major vessels or pancreas. Bypass is achieved by anastomosing the small bowel (jejunum) to the stomach proximal to the obstructing lesion (Fig. 18.14).

Prognosis

When the tumour is confined to the mucosa or submucosa without lymph node or distant metastases a 5-year survival of the order of 95–100% can be achieved. With increasing penetration of the tumour through the stomach wall and increasing numbers of nodes involved, the 5-year survival decreases. A further deterioration occurs when distant metastases are present, when 5-year survival is unusual (Table 18.6).

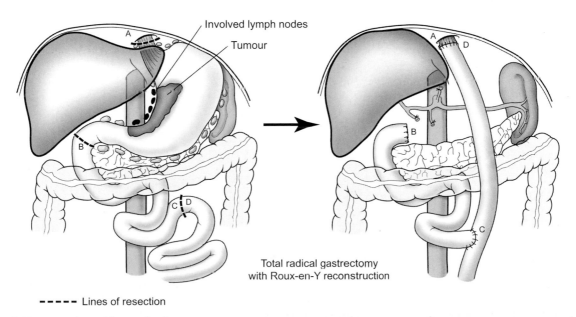

Total radical gastrectomy with Roux-en-Y reconstruction

– – – – – Lines of resection

Fig. 18.13 Resection with curative intent.

Table 18.6 Examples of stages of gastric cancer and their prognosis

Stage	5-yr survival (%)
$T_1N_0M_0$	95+
$T_1N_1M_0$	70–80
$T_2N_1M_0$	45–50
$T_3N_2M_0$	15–25
M_1	0–10

OTHER GASTRIC TUMOURS

Gastrointestinal stromal tumours

These were previously described as leiomyomas or leiomyosarcomas, according to their malignant potential as judged by the pathologist, and account for less than 1% of all gastric malignancies. Such tumours are more commonly found in resected or postmortem specimens as incidental findings. Only infrequently do they contribute to clinical problems such as bleeding or obstruction. These tumours are now considered to be stromal tumours, as it is believed that they may arise from stromal fibroblasts, whereas previously they were thought to have arisen from smooth muscle cells. It is difficult to ascertain the malignant potential of these tumours, but histological features (mitotic figure counts) as well as size are significant indicators.

Lymphomas

The stomach represents the commonest site for gastrointestinal lymphomas, which are malignant aggregations of

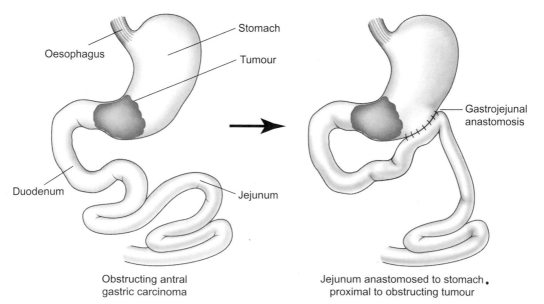

Fig. 18.14 Palliative bypass procedure for gastric carcinoma.

lymphatic tissue. Many lymphomas are thought to arise from mucosa-associated lymphoid tissue and are therefore frequently referred to as MALT lymphomas. In such cases there is a frequent association with the presence of *H. pylori* infection, which it is thought may bring about a lymphomatous change. Such lymphomas are usually low grade and may respond to treatment of the underlying *H. pylori* infection with antibiotics. Occasionally such lymphomas may transform to a high-grade type tumour which carries a poorer prognosis. Such tumours are more likely to require more aggressive treatment, such as surgery and/or chemotherapy.

Carcinoid tumours

These are tumours of neuroendocrine origin and vary enormously in their malignant potential. The vast majority encountered are benign, but occasionally malignant carcinoids can be extremely aggressive. When associated with liver secondary spread they may result in carcinoid syndrome related to the overproduction of 5-hydroxytrytamine.

MISCELLANEOUS DISORDERS OF THE STOMACH

Ménétrier's disease A condition of gastric mucosal hypertrophy on which the mucosal rugal folds are grossly enlarged in the fundus and body of the stomach; the antrum is usually spared.

Mucosal hypertrophy may lead to abnormally large secretions of mucus or acid. Oversecretion of acid and protein-rich mucus may contribute to symptoms of epigastric pain and hypoproteinaemia.

Ménétrier's disease is associated with a high incidence of malignancy in the stomach and, once diagnosed, total gastrectomy is indicated in the otherwise fit patient.

Gastritis This common condition is due to inflammation of the gastric mucosal lining. It may be caused by a variety of injurious agents, both chemical and bacteriological. It is frequently associated with overindulgence of alcohol. Biliary gastritis is seen in the presence of bile in the stomach (frequently seen after Polya-type partial gastrectomy).

Gastritis may arise as a consequence of extreme stress resulting from shock, and this form is therefore more frequently encountered in the intensive care situation. Such gastritis is thought to be a consequence of mucosal hypoperfusion and acidosis secondary to a shock-like state. This combination leads to mucosal ischaemia and resulting stress gastritis, which can cause loss of mucosa resulting in erosions which may on occasion bleed profusely.

Gastritis may be lessened or prevented by rapid treatment of the shock-like state, administering mucosal protective agents, and neutralizing or minimizing gastric acid

secretion. Surgery is undertaken rarely to control massive haemorrhage resulting from gastritis.

Dieulafoy's lesion A condition of profuse bleeding from an abnormal vessel situated in the gastric mucosa and not associated with ulceration. Usually found in the upper stomach. Such bleeding is usually treated initially by injection sclerotherapy, but may require open gastrotomy and oversewing of the bleeding point.

Gastric volvulus Volvulus results from twisting of the stomach about its long axis between the two relative fixed points of the oesophageal hiatus and the duodenum. It is usually associated with paraoesophageal hiatus hernia and, if complete, can give rise to complete obstruction to the upper gastrointestinal tract, with compromise to the blood supply to the stomach leading to infarction.

The diagnosis is confirmed by chest X-ray and contrast studies. Immediate laparotomy is advised to reduce the hernia, repair the diaphragmatic defect and anchor the stomach in the abdomen to prevent recurrence.

Bezoars Accumulations of hair (trichobezoars) or vegetable matter (phytobezoars) or combinations of the two (trichophytobezoar). They may on occasion form a complete cast of the stomach, and the ensuing reduced nutritional intake contributes to malnourishment. The diagnosis is made by barium examination and surgical removal is advisable.

MISCELLANEOUS DISORDERS OF THE DUODENUM

DUODENAL OBSTRUCTION

Common causes of duodenal obstruction are pyloric stenosis and carcinoma of the pancreas. Rarer causes include blockage by mesenteric lymph nodes, duodenal diverticulum, duodenal atresia, annular pancreas and chronic duodenal ileus (Fig. 18.15). If surgical treatment is required, bypass by duodenojejunal or gastrojejunal anastomosis is often appropriate. Symptomatic diverticula may have to be excised. Chronic duodenal ileus is an ill-defined entity which may affect visceroptotic females and rapidly-growing, thin children. It has been suggested that the duodenum is obstructed by the superior mesenteric vessels as they cross its third part, but most surgeons are sceptical about this explanation. The condition is usually self-limiting in children, but in adults surgical bypass may have to be considered.

DUODENAL DIVERTICULA

The duodenum is the second commonest site for diverticulum formation in the gastrointestinal tract. The diverticula rarely develop before the age of 40 years, and are often

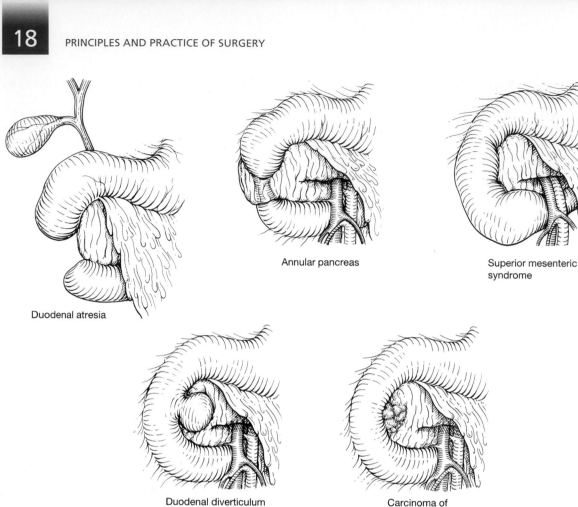

Duodenal atresia

Annular pancreas

Superior mesenteric syndrome

Duodenal diverticulum

Carcinoma of head of pancreas

Fig. 18.15 Causes of duodenal obstruction.

found at the point of entry of the common bile duct. They are frequently discovered incidentally at endoscopy or on barium meal examination, but can cause obstruction, bleeding and inflammation (diverticulitis). Symptomatic diverticula should be excised if it is certain that they are the cause of problems.

Duodenal trauma

Duodenal damage may follow severe crush injury of the upper abdomen (see Chapter 9).

SECTION 4
HEPATOBILIARY SURGERY

19 The liver and biliary tract
O.J. Garden

THE LIVER

ANATOMY

The liver is the largest abdominal organ, weighing approximately 1500 g. It extends from the fifth intercostal space to the right costal margin. It is triangular in shape, its apex reaching the left midclavicular line in the fifth intercostal space. In the recumbent position the liver is impalpable under cover of the ribs. The liver is attached to the undersurface of the diaphragm by suspensory ligaments which enclose a 'bare area', the only part of its surface without a peritoneal covering. Its inferior or visceral surface lies on the right kidney, duodenum, colon and stomach.

Topographically the liver is divided by the attachment of the falciform ligament into right and left lobes; fissures on its visceral surface demarcate two further lobes, the quadrate and caudate (Fig. 19.1). From a practical standpoint it is the segmental anatomy of the liver, as defined by the distribution of its blood supply, that is important to the surgeon.

Segmental anatomy

The portal vein and hepatic artery divide into right and left branches in the porta hepatis. Occluding either branch at

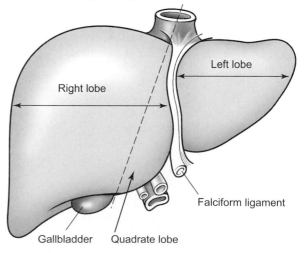

Fig. 19.1   Surgical anatomy of the liver.

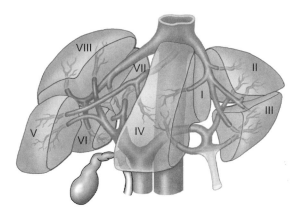

Fig. 19.2 Segmental anatomy and venous drainage.

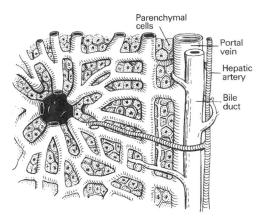

Fig. 19.3 The hepatic lobule: sinusoids drain into the central hepatic vein.

surgery produces an easily visible line of demarcation which runs from the gallbladder bed behind and to the left of the inferior vena cava, thus separating the two hemilivers. Each hemiliver is further divided into four segments corresponding to the main branches of the hepatic artery and portal vein. In the left hemiliver, segment I corresponds to the caudate lobe, segments II and III to the left lobe and segment IV to the quadrate lobe. The remaining segments (V–VIII) comprise the right hemiliver (Fig. 19.2).

Blood supply

The liver normally receives 1500 mL of blood per minute and has a dual blood supply: 65% comes from the portal vein and 35% from the hepatic artery. Because of its better oxygenation the hepatic artery supplies 50% of the oxygen requirements.

The principal venous drainage of the liver is by the right, middle and left hepatic veins, which leave the back of the liver to enter the vena cava (Fig. 19.2). In 25% of individuals there is an inferior right hepatic vein and numerous small veins drain direct into the vena cava from the caudate lobe (segment I). The functional unit of the liver is the hepatic acinus. Sheets of liver cells (hepatocytes) one cell thick are separated by interlacing sinusoids through which blood flows from the peripheral portal tract into the hepatic acinus to the central branch of the hepatic venous system. Bile is secreted by the liver cells and passes in the opposite direction along the small canaliculi into interlobular bile ducts located in the portal tracts (Fig. 19.3).

The liver is responsible for storing glucose in the form of glycogen, or converts it to lactate for release into the systemic circulation. Amino acids are utilized for hepatic and plasma protein synthesis or catabolized to urea. The liver has a central role in the metabolism of bilirubin and bile salts, drugs and alcohol. In addition to acting as a store for a number of vitamins, it is responsible for the production of the vitamin K-dependent factors II, VII, IX and X.

The liver is also the largest reticuloendothelial organ in the body and its Kupffer cells play a role in the removal of damaged red blood cells, bacteria, viruses and endotoxin, much of which enter the body from the gut.

JAUNDICE

Jaundice is a yellowish discoloration most obvious in the skin, sclera and mucous membranes. It is caused by an increase in the level of circulating bilirubin and becomes obvious clinically when levels exceed 50 μmol/L. Jaundice may result from excessive destruction of red cells (haemo-

---

SURGICAL ANATOMY

- The liver is divisible into right and left hemilivers (each having four segments) by a line running from the gallbladder fossa to the inferior vena cava.

- Each hemiliver receives a branch of the hepatic artery and portal vein; 65% of liver blood flow and 50% of its oxygen supply are provided by the portal vein.

- The hepatocytes are arranged in lobules, each of which has a central branch of the hepatic vein and peripheral portal tracts (containing a branch of the hepatic artery, portal vein and bile duct).

- Liver anatomy allows the surgeon to perform right hepatectomy, left hepatectomy and extended right hepatectomy (i.e. resecting all of the liver to the right of the falciform ligament). Resection of individual segments is also possible.

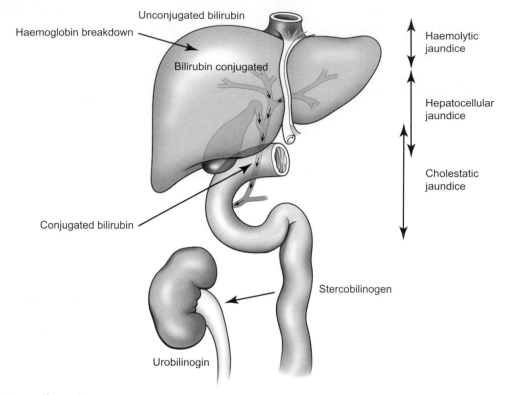

Haemoglobin breakdown

Unconjugated bilirubin

Bilirubin conjugated

Haemolytic jaundice

Hepatocellular jaundice

Cholestatic jaundice

Conjugated bilirubin

Stercobilinogen

Urobilinogin

Fig. 19.4   Types of jaundice.

lytic jaundice), from failure to remove bilirubin from the bloodstream (hepatocellular jaundice), or from obstruction to the flow of bile from the liver (cholestatic jaundice) (Fig. 19.4). Congenital non-haemolytic hyperbilirubinaemia (Gilbert's syndrome) is a relatively rare cause of jaundice due to defective bilirubin transport; the jaundice is usually mild and transient, the prognosis is excellent, and the condition must not be confused with more serious causes of jaundice.

To the surgeon the most important type of haemolytic jaundice is that caused by hereditary spherocytosis, in which splenectomy may be necessary (see Ch. 21). Haemolytic jaundice may also occur after blood transfusion and after operative or accidental trauma, where haematoma formation produces a pigment load that exceeds hepatic excretory capacity.

Hepatocellular jaundice is usually a medical rather than a surgical condition, although its recognition in patients presenting with abdominal pain is important, as surgical intervention may aggravate the hepatocellular injury.

Cholestatic jaundice due to intrahepatic obstruction of bile canaliculi may be a feature of acute and chronic liver disease and can be caused by drugs (e.g. chlorpromazine). This form of jaundice must be differentiated from that due to extrahepatic obstruction, the cause of which has most

surgical relevance. Extrahepatic obstruction most commonly results from gallstones or cancer of the head of the pancreas. Other causes include cancer of the periampullary region or major bile ducts, extrinsic compression of the bile ducts by metastatic tumour, iatrogenic biliary stricture and choledochal cyst.

Diagnosis

History and clinical examination

An accurate diagnosis of the cause of jaundice must be made as quickly as possible to allow prompt institution of appropriate treatment. The age, sex, occupation, social habits, drug and alcohol intake, history of injections or infusions, and general demeanour of the patient must be considered. A history of intermittent pain, fluctuant jaundice and dyspepsia suggests calculous obstruction of the common bile duct, whereas a history of weight loss and relentless progressive jaundice favours a diagnosis of neoplasia. Obstructive jaundice is likely if there is a history of passage of dark urine and pale stools, and if the patient complains of pruritus (owing to an inability to secrete bile salts into the obstructed biliary system). Hepatocellular jaundice is likely if there are stigmata of chronic liver disease, such as liver palms, spider naevi, testicular atrophy and gynaecomastia. The abdomen must be examined for evidence of hepatomegaly or gallbladder distension, and for signs of portal hypertension such as splenomegaly, ascites and large collateral veins (caput Medusae) in the abdominal wall.

Biochemical and haematological investigations

Haemolytic jaundice is suggested if there are high circulating levels of unconjugated bilirubin but no bilirubin in the urine. Serum concentrations of liver enzymes are normal in these circumstances and the appropriate haematological investigations should be set in train.

In jaundice due to biliary obstruction the circulating bilirubin is conjugated by the liver and rendered water soluble; it can then be excreted in the urine and gives it a dark colour. As bile cannot pass into the gastrointestinal tract, the stool becomes pale and urobilinogen is absent from the urine. Obstruction increases the formation of alkaline phosphatase from the cells lining the biliary canaliculi and produces raised serum levels. In biliary obstruction the rise in serum alkaline phosphatase precedes that of bilirubin and its fall is more gradual once obstruction is relieved. Serum transaminase and lactic dehydrogenase levels also often rise in obstruction. Conversely, swelling of the parenchyma in hepatocellular jaundice frequently produces an element of intrahepatic biliary obstruction and a modest rise in serum alkaline phosphatase concentration.

Serum hepatitis B surface antigen status should be determined in all jaundiced patients. A full blood count and coagulation screen should be undertaken as a matter of routine. The presence of anaemia may signify occult blood loss, and a low white cell or platelet count may indicate hypersplenism due to portal hypertension. Prolongation of the prothrombin time may be present in both hepatocellular and cholestatic jaundice, but should readily correct within 36 hours with the administration of parenteral vitamin K when jaundice is cholestatic.

Radiological investigations

If the clinical picture and biochemical investigations suggest that jaundice is obstructive, radiological techniques can be used to define the site and nature of the obstruction.

Ultrasonography In skilled hands this key investigation is safe, non-invasive and reliable. In the present context it is used to define whether the patient has duct dilatation or gallbladder distension due to obstruction, and to confirm the need for more invasive investigations. Ultrasonography will also detect gallstones and space-occupying lesions in the liver and pancreas, although overlying bowel gas may prevent a clear view of the pancreas.

Magnetic resonance cholangiopancreatography (MRCP) This non-invasive investigation is likely to replace other forms of invasive radiological imaging of the bile duct and pancreas. Magnetic resonance imaging (MRI) has the advantage that it does not introduce infection into an obstructed biliary system or the pancreatic duct; it also enables assessment of the vascular anatomy and the parenchyma of the liver and pancreas. This is important in patients presenting with symptoms suggestive of malignant obstructive jaundice.

Endoscopic retrograde cholangiopancreatography (ERCP) This examination outlines the biliary and pancreatic systems by injecting dye through a cannula inserted into the papilla of Vater by means of an endoscope passed into the duodenum. It gives more detailed information than ultrasonography and, as will be discussed later, also allows endoscopic treatment of gallstones, biopsy of periampullary tumours, and relief of obstructive jaundice by the insertion of stents. The investigation may be complicated by acute pancreatitis and prophylactic antibiotics should be administered to reduce the risk of cholangitis. Haemorrhage and perforation are less frequent complications.

Percutaneous transhepatic cholangiography (PTC) Used less often than formerly, this is useful in assessing obstruction of the upper biliary tree. It provides a clear outline of the biliary system by the injection of dye through a slim flexible needle passed percutaneously into the liver. Although diagnostic cholangiograms can be obtained in virtually all patients with ductal obstruction, the technique may cause bleeding or bile leakage and can be complicated by bacteraemia and septicaemia. Coagulation status must be checked prior to PTC and the procedure should be covered by antibiotics. Facilities for emergency surgery should be available, although they are seldom needed.

Computerized tomography (CT) This can be used to identify hepatic, bile duct and pancreatic tumours in jaundiced patients. It often demonstrates the dilated biliary tree to the level of the obstruction, and may show dissemination to adjacent lymph nodes.

Other radiological investigations These are seldom needed. Isotopic liver scanning has been superseded by ultrasonography and CT scanning. Selective angiography is not used to diagnose the cause of jaundice, but is used by some to assess resectability if there is neoplastic obstruction: it also identifies vascular anomalies. Barium meal examination and hypotonic duodenography are now obsolete investigations in jaundiced patients given the ready availability of ERCP.

Liver biopsy

Liver biopsy is valuable in patients with unexplained jaundice in whom an obstructing lesion has been excluded by ultrasonography. It may be preceded by a CT scan to determine whether metastatic disease is present. If lesions have been identified, a 'targeted' liver biopsy can be conducted under ultrasound or CT control. It may be preferable and safer to undertake biopsy at laparoscopy. Prothrombin time, platelet count and hepatitis B surface antigen (HBsAg) status must always be determined and clotting abnormalities corrected before biopsy is undertaken. In patients with a persistent bleeding disorder liver biopsy can be undertaken through the hepatic veins, employing a transjugular approach.

Laparoscopy

Laparoscopy is used increasingly in the evaluation of liver disease and obstructive jaundice. It is best undertaken under general anaesthesia. In patients with malignant obstruction of the biliary tree it may have a vital role in the staging of the tumour, as peritoneal dissemination and small hepatic metastases may be apparent.

Laparotomy

Laparotomy is no longer necessary to establish the cause of jaundice and is only undertaken to remove the causal lesion or relieve biliary obstruction. Intraoperative ultrasonography and operative cholangiography may give useful additional information in patients with neoplasia and biliary obstruction. Appropriate preoperative preparation is particularly important in jaundiced patients (see Ch. 2).

CONGENITAL ABNORMALITIES

Simple cysts within the liver are common. They are often referred to as biliary cysts, as they are lined by biliary epithelium. They contain serous fluid, are usually solitary, but never communicate with the biliary tree. They rarely produce symptoms, are associated with normal liver function, and on ultrasound or CT scan have no discernible wall (Fig. 19.5). In the few patients who develop symptoms it is evident that all cysts tend to recur following aspiration, and sclerosis by alcohol injection is of little value for large symptomatic cysts. Surgical management consists of deroofing and may be undertaken by laparoscopic means. Polycystic disease is a rare cause of liver enlargement and may be associated with polycystic kidneys as an autosomal dominant trait. In symptomatic patients it may be necessary to combine a deroofing procedure with hepatic resection.

Cavernous haemangiomas are one of the commonest benign tumours of the liver and may be congenital. Women are six times more commonly affected than men. Most haemangiomas are small solitary subcapsular growths found incidentally at laparotomy or autopsy, but they are sometimes detected on ultrasound examination as densely hyperechoic lesions that mimic hepatic tumours. These lesions rarely give rise to pain. Resection may be considered for symptomatic lesions exceeding 5 cm in diameter.

Anatomical abnormalities of the extrahepatic bile ducts are common.

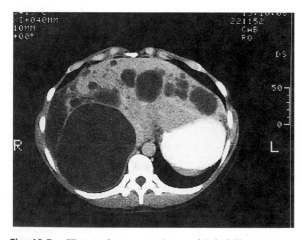

Fig. 19.5 CT scan demonstrating multiple biliary cysts appearing as hypodense areas within both lobes of the liver.

> **SUMMARY BOX**
>
> **Jaundice**
>
> - Jaundice is a yellowish discoloration of the tissues which becomes apparent clinically when serum bilirubin levels exceed 50 μmol/L (normal <20 μmol/L).
>
> - It may be due to excessive haemolysis, hepatic insufficiency or cholestasis; cholestatic (obstructive) jaundice is the type encountered in surgical practice.
>
> - The two commonest causes of surgical obstructive jaundice are cancer of the head of the pancreas and stones in the common bile duct (choledocholithiasis).
>
> - In cholestatic jaundice the bilirubin has been conjugated by the hepatocytes and is therefore soluble in water and can be excreted in the urine; patients with obstructive jaundice typically have dark urine and pale stools and may have pruritus (thought to be due to the accumulation of bile salts).
>
> - Obstructive jaundice is characterized by elevated serum alkaline phosphatase levels in addition to hyperbilirubinameia, and may be accompanied by modest elevations in transaminase (aminotransferase) levels, reflecting liver damage.

LIVER TRAUMA

After the spleen, the liver is the solid organ most commonly damaged in abdominal trauma, particularly following road traffic accidents. Stab injuries and gunshot wounds of the liver are also increasing in incidence. These are considered in Chapter 9.

HEPATIC INFECTIONS AND INFESTATIONS

Liver abscesses can be classified as bacterial, parasitic or fungal. Bacterial abscess is the commonest type in western medicine, but parasitic infestation is an important cause worldwide. Fungal abscesses are found in patients receiving long-term broad-spectrum antibiotic treatment or immuno-suppressive therapy, and may complicate actinomycosis.

Pyogenic liver abscess

Bacteria may gain access through a number of routes. Infection from the *biliary system* is now more common with the increasing use of radiological and endoscopic intervention. Infection may spread through the *portal vein* from abdominal sepsis (e.g. appendicitis, diverticulitis), via the *hepatic artery* from a septic focus anywhere in the body, or by direct spread from a *contiguous organ* (e.g. empyema of the gallbladder). Abscess formation may follow *blunt or penetrating injury*, and in one-third of patients the source of infection is *indeterminate* (cryptogenic). Anaerobic organisms such as *Streptococcus milleri* are common in cryptogenic infections and those arising from the portal system. Gram-negative bacteria, notably *Escherichia coli*, are present in most cases and are particularly frequent in infections arising from the biliary tree. *Staphylococcus aureus* is invariably the causal organism in abscesses arising from haematogenous spread.

Clinical features

The onset of symptoms is often insidious and the patient may present with a pyrexia of unknown origin. There is sometimes a history of sepsis elsewhere, particularly within the abdomen, and pain in the right hypochondrium. Other patients present with swinging pyrexia, rigors, marked toxicity and jaundice.

Investigation

The liver is often enlarged and tender. Plain radiographs may show elevation of the diaphragm, pleural effusion and basal lobe collapse. Leukocytosis is usually present and liver function tests (LFTs) are deranged. Ultrasonography or CT scanning is used to define the abscess (which is often irregular and thick walled) and to facilitate percutaneous aspiration for culture. ERCP may be useful if biliary obstruction is thought to be responsible.

Treatment

Untreated abscesses often prove fatal because of spread within the liver to multiple sites, septicaemia and debility. The principles of treatment are percutaneous drainage of accessible abscesses under ultrasound guidance, and antibiotic therapy selected on the basis of culture of blood or pus. It is unusual to have to resort to formal surgical drainage. Percutaneously or surgically placed drainage tubes are left in place and the size of the cavity is monitored by serial X-rays following the injection of contrast material. Multiple small abscesses may require prolonged treatment with antibiotics for up to 8 weeks.

Amoebic liver abscess

Entamoeba histolytica is a protozoal parasite that infests the large intestine and is endemic in many tropical regions. Trophozoites released by the cyst in the intestine may penetrate the mucosa to gain access to the portal venous system and so spread to the liver. The abscess is large and thin-walled, is usually solitary and in the right lobe, and contains brown sterile pus resembling anchovy sauce.

Clinical features

The onset of symptoms may be sudden or insidious. Right upper quadrant pain is the most striking symptom and this may be accompanied by anorexia, nausea, weight loss and night sweats. Tender enlargement of the liver is invariable, although jaundice is uncommon. Other signs include basal pulmonary collapse, pleural effusion and leukocytosis.

Investigation

Ultrasound and CT liver scans are used to demonstrate the site and size of the abscess, which often has poorly defined margins. The stools should be examined for amoebae or cysts. Direct and indirect serological tests to detect amoebic protein are available.

Treatment:

Early diagnosis and prompt treatment are important, and treatment may be commenced empirically in areas where the problem is endemic. If untreated, an amoebic abscess may rupture into the peritoneal cavity or into a bronchus. Treatment consists of the administration of metronidazole (800 mg 8-hourly for 5 days) and usually results in rapid resolution. If there is no clinical response within 72 hours the abscess should be aspirated by needle puncture, although this is rarely necessary. Drainage by open operation is rarely required, and even for the few cases of secondary bacterial infection not responding to therapy, percutaneous aspiration should be adequate.

Hydatid disease

This less common infestation is caused in humans by one of two forms of tapeworm, *Echinococcus granulosus* and *E. multilocularis*. The adult tapeworm lives in the intestine of the dog, from which ova are passed in the stool; sheep or humans serve as the intermediate host by ingesting the ova (Fig. 19.6). The condition is most common in sheep-rearing areas. Ingested ova hatch in the duodenum and the embryos pass to the liver through the portal venous system. The wall of the resulting hydatid cyst is surrounded by an adventitial layer of fibrous tissue and consists of a laminated membrane lined by germinal epithelium on which brood capsules containing scolices develop.

Clinical features

The disease may be symptomless, but chronic right upper quadrant pain with enlargement of the liver is the common presentation. The cyst may rupture into the biliary tree or peritoneal cavity, the latter sometimes causing an acute anaphylactic reaction due to absorption of foreign hydatid

protein. Other complications include secondary infection and biliary obstruction with jaundice.

Investigation

Eosinophilia is common and serological tests, such as the complement-fixation test, are available to detect the foreign protein. Hydatid cysts commonly calcify and may be seen on a plain film of the abdomen. Alternatively, they can be detected by ultrasound or CT scan of the liver and are recognizable by their thick wall, which may contain multiple daughter cysts.

Treatment

In asymptomatic patients small calcified cysts may require no treatment. Large symptomatic cysts are best treated by complete excision of the cyst, together with its contained parasites. At surgery, the liver is isolated by carefully positioned packs to avoid spillage of the cyst contents, which are aspirated via a cannula. Scolicidal agents should never be injected into the cyst as there is invariably a communication with the biliary tree, which is at risk of secondary sclerosing cholangitis as a consequence. The cyst and its contents are shelled out from the liver, taking care to remove the laminated membrane completely. In longstanding cysts it may be preferable to remove the fibrous ectocyst and minimize the risk of subsequent bile leakage, subphrenic collection and recurrence from contained daughter cysts. Some surgeons advocate packing the residual cavity with the greater omentum.

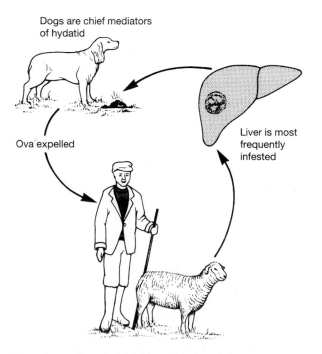

Fig. 19.6   Lifecycle of *Echinococcus granulosus*.

Dogs are chief mediators of hydatid

Ova expelled

Liver is most frequently infested

Table 19.1	Causes of portal hypertension
Obstruction to portal flow	
Prehepatic	Congenital atresia of the portal vein
	Portal vein thrombosis
	Neonatal sepsis
	Pyelophlebitis
	Trauma
	Tumour
	Extrinsic compression of the portal vein
	Pancreatic disease
	Lymphadenopathy
	Biliary tract tumours
Intrahepatic	Cirrhosis
	Schistosomiasis
Posthepatic	Budd–Chiari syndrome
	Constrictive pericarditis
Increased blood flow (rare)	
	Arteriovenous fistula
	Increased splenic blood flow in hypersplenism

Mebendazole has been used as an alternative to surgical treatment but its value remains uncertain.

PORTAL HYPERTENSION

Portal hypertension is usually caused by increased resistance to portal venous blood flow, the obstruction being prehepatic, hepatic or posthepatic. Rarely it results primarily from an increase in portal blood flow. The normal pressure in the portal vein varies from 5 to 15 cmH_2O. When the portal venous pressure is consistently raised above 25 cmH_2O there may be serious clinical consequences. The causes of portal hypertension are shown in Table 19.1.

Portal vein thrombosis is a rare cause. It is most commonly due to neonatal umbilical sepsis, though the effects may not be manifest for many years.

By far the commonest cause of portal hypertension is cirrhosis of the liver. This results from chronic liver disease and is characterized by liver cell damage, fibrosis and nodular regeneration. In micronodular cirrhosis there is an even distribution of nodules a few millimetres in diameter; in macronodular cirrhosis the nodules vary in size and are sometimes very large. Macronodules are usual in end-stage cirrhosis, irrespective of the aetiology. The fibrosis obstructs portal venous return and portal hypertension develops. Arteriovenous shunts within the liver also contribute to the hypertension.

Alcohol is the commonest aetiological factor in western countries, whereas in North Africa, the Middle East and China schistosomiasis due to *Bilharzia mansonii* is a common cause. In alcoholic cirrhosis the abnormal resistance is predominantly postsinusoidal, as shown by an increase in wedge hepatic venous pressure. The hepatic veins become distorted by regenerative nodules, there is narrowing of the central veins by centrilobular collagen deposition, and swelling of the hepatocytes encroaches on the sinusoidal lumen. In schistosomiasis, granulomas from parasitic involvement are seen in the portal triads and the hypertension is presinusoidal. Ultimately, as macronodules appear the obstruction becomes postsinusoidal. Chronic active hepatitis and primary and secondary biliary cirrhosis may result in portal hypertension, but in a large number of patients the cause remains obscure (cryptogenic cirrhosis).

Posthepatic portal hypertension is rare. It is most frequently due to spontaneous thrombosis of the hepatic veins and this has been associated with neoplasia, oral contraceptive agents, polycythaemia and the presence of abnormal coagulants in the blood. The resulting Budd–Chiari syndrome is characterized by portal hypertension, liver failure and gross ascites.

Effects of portal hypertension

As a result of gradual chronic occlusion of the portal venous system, collateral pathways develop between the portal and systemic venous circulations. Portosystemic shunting occurs at three principal sites (Fig. 19.7).

The most important consequence of shunting is the development of varices in the submucosal plexus of veins in the lower oesophagus and gastric fundus. The oesophageal varices may then rupture, to cause acute massive gastrointestinal bleeding. Such bleeding occurs in about 40% of patients with cirrhosis. The initial episode of variceal haemorrhage is fatal in about one-third of patients, and the great majority of those who survive the initial haemorrhage bleed again. Bleeding from retroperitoneal and periumbilical collaterals is troublesome during abdominal surgery, and collaterals may develop and cause bleeding at the site of stomas. Anorectal varices are not uncommonly found at proctoscopy but rarely cause bleeding.

Progressive enlargement of the spleen occurs as a result of vascular engorgement and associated hypertrophy. Haematological consequences are anaemia, thrombocytopenia and leukopenia. (The resulting syndrome of hypersplenism is discussed in more detail in Ch. 2.) *Ascites* may develop and is due to an increased formation of hepatic and splanchnic lymph, hypoalbuminaemia, and retention of salt and water. Increased aldosterone and antidiuretic hormone levels may contribute.

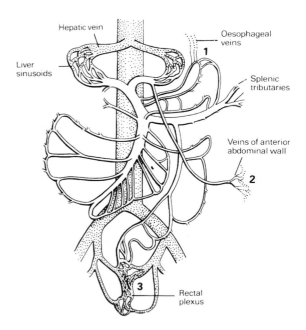

Fig. 19.7 The portal venous system. Sites of portosystemic shunting are marked 1–3. Retroperitoneal communications also exist.

Portosystemic *encephalopathy* is due to an increased level of toxins such as ammonia in the systemic circulation. This is particularly likely to develop where there are large spontaneous or surgically created portosystemic shunts. Gastrointestinal haemorrhage increases the absorption of nitrogenous products and may precipitate encephalopathy.

Clinical presentation

Patients with cirrhosis frequently develop anorexia, generalized malaise and weight loss. Clinical manifestations of liver disease may be present, such as hepatosplenomegaly, ascites, jaundice and spider naevi. The serum bilirubin may be elevated and the serum albumin depressed. Anaemia may be present and the leukocyte count can be raised (or depressed if there is hypersplenism). The prothrombin time and other indices of clotting may be abnormal. Clinical and biochemical parameters are used as the basis of the Child's classification (Table 19.2). Patients allocated to grade A have a good prognosis, whereas those in grade C have the worst prognosis.

Patients with portal hypertension usually present to a surgeon because of active uncontrolled bleeding from oesophageal varices, or for consideration of elective surgery for varices which have been resistant to non-surgical management.

Acute variceal bleeding

Patients presenting with acute upper gastrointestinal bleeding are carefully examined for evidence of chronic liver disease. Distended collateral veins may be visible, particularly around the umbilicus, where they give rise to a 'caput medusae'. Slurring of speech, a flapping tremor or dysarthria may point to encephalopathy, and this may be precipitated or intensified by the accumulation of blood in the gastrointestinal tract.

The key investigation during an episode of active bleeding is endoscopy. This allows the detection of varices and defines whether they are or have been the site of bleeding. It is important to remember that peptic ulcer and gastritis are common complaints that occur in 20% of patients with varices. Even though a patient is known to have chronic liver disease and varices, bleeding cannot be assumed to be due to the varices.

Management

The priorities in the management of bleeding oesophageal varices are summarized in Table 19.3.

Active resuscitation Blood is withdrawn for grouping, cross-matching and a clotting screen; a free-flowing intravenous line is established, a urinary catheter is inserted to measure hourly urine output, pulse rate and blood pressure are monitored, and a central venous line is inserted to monitor central venous pressure. Large volumes of blood may be lost rapidly and the aim is to replace blood loss quickly with a view to urgent endoscopy. Many patients bleeding from varices have coagulation defects from the outset, and thrombocytopenia is a common manifestation of hypersplenism. Fresh blood is preferred for transfusion purposes and the advice of the haematologist is sought regarding the use of fresh-frozen plasma (FFP) or platelet transfusion.

Table 19.2 Assessment of patients with portal hypertension by a modification of Child's grading system

Criterion	Points scored		
	1	2	3
Encephalopathy	None	Minimal	Marked
Ascites	None	Slight	Moderate
Bilirubin (μmol/L)	<35	35–50	>50
Albumin (g/L)	>35	28–35	<28
Prothrombin ratio	<1.4	1.4–2.0	>2.0

Grade A = 5–6 points; grade B = 7–8 points; grade C = 10–15 points.

Table 19.3 Priorities in the management of bleeding oesophageal varices

- Active resuscitation
  Group and cross-match blood
  Establish i.v. infusion line(s)
  Monitor: pulse
            blood pressure
            hourly urine output
            central venous pressure
- Assessment of coagulation status
  Prothrombin time
  Platelet count
- Urgent endoscopy
- Control of bleeding
  Tamponade (Minnesota tube) or injection sclerotherapy
  Pharmacological measures (e.g. vasopressin/somatostatin)
- Treatment of hepatocellular decompensation
- Treatment/prevention of portosystemic encephalopathy
- Prevention of further bleeding from varices
  Injection sclerotherapy
  Stapled oesophagogastric junction
  Portosystemic shunting/TIPSS
  Liver transplantation

Endoscopy This is performed at the earliest opportunity, and in patients threatened by massive bleeding, active resuscitation is instituted and continued in the endoscopy suite. The tortuous varices are usually in three columns and most prominent in the lower third of the oesophagus. If varices are the source of blood loss, this usually occurs from the lowest few centimetres of the oesophagus. Rarely, bleeding occurs from varices in the gastric fundus.

Control of bleeding Of the medical agents used to lower portal venous pressure and arrest bleeding, the synthetic form of somatostatin, octreotide, is most commonly employed. If variceal haemorrhage is apparent at the initial endoscopy the injection of a sclerosant such as ethanolamine, or the application of bands, is now used to arrest the bleeding. If haemorrhage is torrential and prevents direct injection, balloon tamponade may be used to stop the bleeding.

The four-lumen Minnesota tube (Fig. 19.8) has largely replaced the three-lumen Sengstaken–Blakemore tube. The four lumina allow:

- Aspiration of gastric contents
- Inflation of a gastric balloon with 150 mL of water to which a radio-opaque dye (Hypaque) has been added so that balloon position can be checked radiologically (this balloon compresses the gastric fundus and oesophago-gastric junction, thereby reducing the flow of blood into the oesophageal varices)
- Inflation of an oesophageal balloon with air to a pressure of 40 mmHg using a sphygmomanometer (this balloon applies direct pressure to the oesophageal varices)
- Aspiration of the oesophagus and pharynx above the oesophageal balloon, so reducing the risk of aspiration pneumonitis and pneumonia.

Traction is applied to the Minnesota tube by pulling the gastric balloon up against the oesophagogastric junction and taping a spatula to the tube as it emerges from the angle of the mouth. A trained nurse should be in constant attendance, and the pharynx and stomach are aspirated at 15–30 minute intervals. Balloon tamponade arrests bleeding from varices in over 90% of patients, but the tube is not left in place for more than 24–36 hours for fear of causing oesophageal necrosis. Tamponade should be regarded as a holding measure which allows further resuscitation and treatment of hepatic decompensation. Unless more definitive measures are used to prevent further variceal bleeding (see below), two-thirds of individuals rebled while still in hospital and 90% rebled within a year.

Further resuscitation and treatment of hepatocellular decompensation Control of variceal bleeding allows blood loss to be made good and permits a full assessment of coagulopathy. Blood may be evacuated from the gut by a bowel washout to reduce the risk of portosystemic encephalopathy. Lactulose (15–30 mL 8-hourly) is prescribed to reduce bacterial degradation of blood in the gut

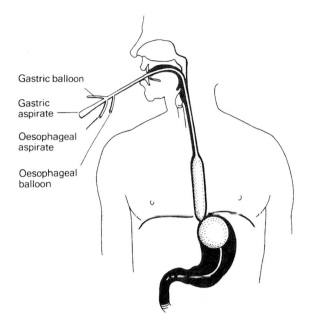

Gastric balloon

Gastric aspirate

Oesophageal aspirate

Oesophageal balloon

Fig. 19.8   Oesophageal tamponade using a Minnesota tube.

lumen and further reduce the risk of encephalopathy. Patients with oesophageal varices due to liver disease frequently have major defects in both the intrinsic and extrinsic clotting systems, which may prove refractory to therapy. Vitamin K_1 is prescribed to aid restoration of the extrinsic system, but FFP, factor concentrates and platelet transfusion may all be required to cover specific procedures such as sclerotherapy. It should be stressed that these transfusion measures have transient effects on blood coagulation, and that the ultimate coagulation status depends upon restoration of hepatic function.

Prevention of further bleeding

A number of methods are now available to reduce the risk of further variceal bleeding.

Injection sclerotherapy Although originally undertaken by means of a rigid oesophagoscope under general anaesthesia, this is now carried out routinely by fibreoptic endoscopy. Injection is repeated at weekly or fortnightly intervals until the varices are completely sclerosed. Following complete ablation, fibreoptic examination is repeated periodically and any recurrent varices are injected. Excessive or too frequent injection may be complicated by ulceration and necrosis, sometimes with a fatal result. Controversy exists as to whether the sclerosant should be injected directly into the varix or into the surrounding mucosa. The increased use of injection sclerotherapy has substantially reduced the number of patients undergoing surgery, and it is most successful in patients with well-preserved liver function. Although sclerotherapy reduces the risk of further variceal bleeding, it is still uncertain whether it improves long-term survival.

Endoscopic banding Just as haemorrhoids can be managed by the application of elastic bands, endoscopic applicators are now available which can be used to occlude varices at the oesophagogastric junction. The reduced risk of oesophageal ulceration and perforation has resulted in this technique being favoured in many centres.

Surgical disconnection This is rarely used in the management of variceal haemorrhage. The gastric vein and short gastric veins are ligated and the distal oesophagus is transected and reanastomosed just above the cardia using a stapling gun (Fig. 19.9). Stapled oesophageal transection occludes flow into the varices, but the procedure is technically difficult in patients who have been submitted to repeated injection sclerotherapy and carries considerable morbidity and mortality when employed as a last resort in the emergency situation.

Emergency portosystemic shunting This has a high mortality and has been abandoned in most centres. Elective portosystemic shunting is still used occasionally to decompress the portal system and reduce the risk of further variceal haemorrhage, but portosystemic encephalopathy can be troublesome and it is uncertain whether shunting prolongs life in patients with parenchymal liver disease. Operation is rarely considered in patients whose condition is complicated by jaundice, ascites or encephalopathy, and where there is a clear indication for liver transplantation.

Types of shunt procedure There are several anatomical sites at which portosystemic shunts can be performed (Fig. 19.10). The distal splenorenal (Warren) shunt selectively decompresses the lower oesophagus and upper stomach and maintains liver blood flow, and is preferred by many surgeons. The incidence of encephalopathy is lower than after other shunt procedures.

Transjugular intrahepatic portosystemic stent shunting (TIPSS) In this procedure a metal stent is inserted via the transjugular route using a guidewire passed through the hepatic vein to the intrahepatic branches of the portal vein. The technique is a relatively safe means of decompressing the portal system as general anaesthesia and laparotomy are avoided. The risk of encephalopathy is similar to that of a surgical portosystemic shunt, but is now considered routinely before surgical intervention in both the acute and the elective setting.

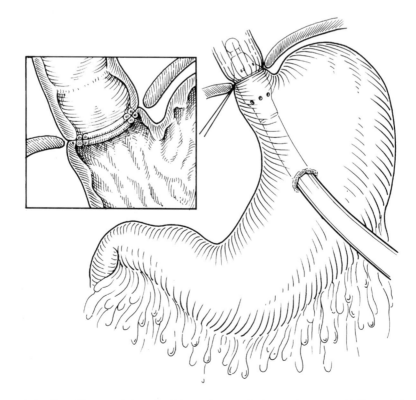

Fig. 19.9 Oesophageal stapling. The gun is inserted through an anterior gastrostomy. A ligature is tied just above the cardia, invaginating a flange of oesophageal wall between the two parts of the gun. Inset: the gun has been fired, simultaneously resecting a full-thickness ring of oesophageal wall and anastomosing the cut ends with staples.

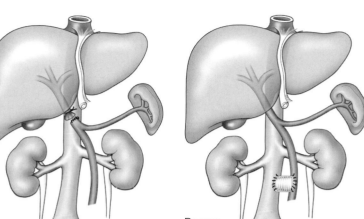

Splenic vein

Portal
vein

IVC

Superior
mesenteric
vein

Normal

End-to-side
portocaval shunt

Dacron
graft

Mesocaval shunt
(Dacron graft interposition)

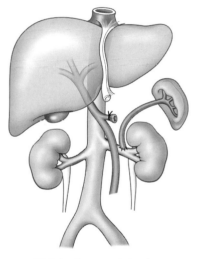

Distal splenorenal shunt

TIPSS

Fig. 19.10 Types of portosystemic shunt.

Ascites

Ascites can be controlled by bed rest, salt and water restriction and a diuretic such as the aldosterone-inhibitor spironolactone. If refractory, ascites can be treated by inserting a peritoneojugular (LeVeen) shunt, which allows one-way flow between the peritoneum and the jugular vein (Fig. 19.11). It is unusual for the shunt to remain patent for more than 12 months, but this may suffice for patients with refractory ascites and advanced liver disease who are not candidates for liver transplantation.

TUMOURS OF THE LIVER

Hepatic tumours can be benign or malignant, primary or secondary. Primary tumours may arise from the parenchymal

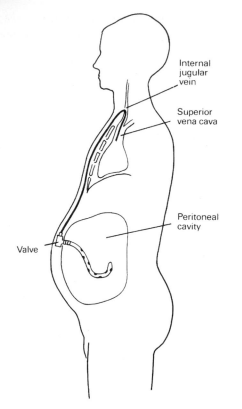

Internal jugular vein

Superior vena cava

Peritoneal cavity

Valve

Fig. 19.11 Peritoneovenous (Le Veen) shunt to relieve ascites.

SUMMARY BOX

Portal hypertension

- Portal hypertension is almost always due to obstruction to portal flow (rather than increased inflow) and may be prehepatic, hepatic or posthepatic.

- Cirrhosis of the liver is the commonest cause of portal hypertension in western countries, and alcoholic cirrhosis is most often responsible.

- Portosystemic shunts develop between gastric and oesophageal veins, in the retroperitoneum and periumbilical area, and occasionally in the anorectum. Varices in the submucosa of the lower oesophagus are a common source of major bleeding, but gastritis (portal gastropathy) can be responsible.

- Child's grading (A, B or C) is based on encephalopathy, ascites, bilirubin and albumin levels, and porthrombin time, and is a valuable prognostic index.

- Variceal bleeding may be controlled by injection sclerotherapy or endoscopic banding, although balloon tamponade (four-lumen Minnesota tube) may sometimes be needed.

- Surgical portosystemic shunts effectively decompress oesophageal varices and reduce rebleeding, but can cause encephalopathy and have been largely replaced by TIPSS.

- Although injection sclerotherapy (or banding) reduces the risk of rebleeding and may improve survival rates, long-term outcome is determined by the nature and severity of the underlying liver disease.

cells, the epithelium of the bile ducts, or the supporting tissues.

Benign hepatic tumours

Cavernous haemangioma is the commonest benign liver tumour. Most are asymptomatic and are detected on ultrasonography as a dense hyperechoic lesion, or are found incidentally at laparotomy. These lesions rarely reach a sufficient size to produce pain, abdominal swelling or haemorrhage. Heart failure occasionally develops if there is a large arteriovenous communication. Lesions discovered incidentally at laparotomy should be left alone and needle biopsy can be hazardous. Large symptomatic lesions should normally be resected by an experienced surgeon.

Biliary hamartomas are small fibrous lesions which are often situated beneath the capsule of the liver. They can be mistaken for a small metastatic tumour unless a biopsy is obtained.

Liver cell adenomas are relatively uncommon and are found almost exclusively in women. They may be associated with the use of high oestrogen-containing contraceptives. The majority present as solitary, well encapsulated lesions, but malignant transformation has been reported. They may be asymptomatic but generally present with right hypochondrial pain as a result of haemorrhage within the tumour. Superficial tumours may bleed spontaneously and present with symptoms of haemoperitoneum.

The adenomas may be detected by ultrasonography or CT scanning. LFTs and serum α-fetoprotein levels are usually normal. Percutaneous biopsy should be avoided because of the risk of haemorrhage.

Treatment consists of formal hepatic resection because of the difficulties of differentiating adenoma from a well-differentiated hepatoma, concerns that lesions may undergo malignant transformation, and the known risk of spontaneous haemorrhage.

Focal nodular hyperplasia of the liver is more common in females. The lesion is generally asymptomatic and may regress with time or on withdrawal of the contraceptive pill.

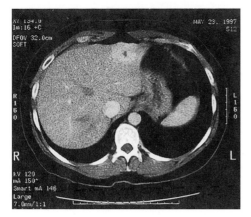

Fig. 19.12 Intravenous enhanced CT scan demonstrating a hypervascular lesion in the left lobe of the liver. This symptomatic focal nodular hyperplastic lesion was removed by left lobectomy.

Hyperplasia does not undergo malignant transformation and does not require excision unless symptomatic.

Hyperplasia can be differentiated from adenoma by the central fibrous scar, which is often visible on ultrasound or CT (Fig. 19.12). Whereas other hepatic lesions produce a filling defect on isotope scan, hyperplastic nodules often produce no filling defect because the isotope is taken up by Kupffer cells within the lesion. Such lesions should only be resected if there is doubt about the diagnosis, or if the lesion is symptomatic.

Primary malignant tumours of the liver

Hepatocellular carcinoma (hepatoma)

Hepatocellular carcinoma (hepatoma) is relatively uncommon in the western world but is common in Africa and the Far East. Environmental factors are probably important, and in American blacks the incidence is the same as that found in white Americans. In the west, about two-thirds of patients have pre-existing cirrhosis and many others have evidence of hepatitis B infection. In Africa and the east, 'aflatoxin' (derived from the fungus *Aspergillus flavus*, which contaminates maize and nuts) is an important hepatocarcinogen. In recent years, hepatitis C virus infection has become increasingly important as an aetiological factor.

Clinical features The diagnosis is usually made late in the course of the disease. In non-cirrhotic patients the tumour may have grown to a considerable size before giving rise to abdominal pain or swelling.

In cirrhotic patients hepatoma may become manifest as sudden deterioration in liver function, often associated with extension of the tumour into the portal venous system.

Common presenting features include abdominal pain, weight loss, abdominal distension, fever, and spontaneous intraperitoneal haemorrhage. Jaundice is uncommon unless there is advanced cirrhosis. Examination may reveal features of established liver disease and hepatomegaly is invariable.

Investigation Liver function tests are generally deranged. Although early detection of hepatocellular carcinoma in susceptible individuals can be pursued by a policy of serial measurement of α-fetoprotein (an oncofetal antigen) and ultrasound scanning, this tumour marker is present in only one-third of the white population with hepatocellular carcinoma, compared to 80% of African patients with this disease.

The diagnosis is made on the history and the radiological features of a solid mass in the liver in the absence of primary tumour elsewhere. The lesion may be detected and characterized by abnormal ultrasound scanning. Percutaneous needle aspiration cytology and needle biopsy for histological confirmation should be reserved for patients who are not being considered for hepatic resection, as these investigations carry a small but significant risk of tumour dissemination and haemorrhage.

Abdominal CT scanning or MRI is valuable in planning resection and excluding the presence of nodal involvement. Pulmonary metastases may not be evident on chest X-ray and their presence should be excluded by a CT scan of the thorax if resection is contemplated. Peritoneal dissemination of the tumour may only be excluded by laparoscopy. Hepatocellular carcinoma is seen as an extremely vascular lesion on arteriography, and propagation of tumour thrombus along the portal vein or its branches may be demonstrated.

Treatment In non-cirrhotic patients large tumours (particularly those of the fibrolamellar type) may be amenable to extensive liver resection. Cirrhotic patients have less hepatic functional reserve, and even those with well-preserved liver function may only tolerate limited segmental or subsegmental resection of the liver. The only prospect of cure lies in complete surgical resection of the tumour. In cirrhotic patients multicentricity is common and satellite lesions often surround the primary tumour, so that cure is uncommon.

For advanced tumours, hepatic arterial ligation and local infusion of chemotherapeutic agents through a surgically implanted catheter in the hepatic artery have been used in the past. Systemic chemotherapy with doxorubicin (Adriamycin), methotrexate or 5-fluorouracil may have palliative value, although response rates of less than 20% are the norm. More encouraging results have been reported following local embolization of these agents plus lipiodol by selective arteriography (chemoembolization).

The disease is usually advanced at presentation and the 5-year survival rate is less than 10%. Liver transplantation has been used in the treatment of this tumour, but recurrence in the transplanted liver and elsewhere is common in immunosuppressed patients. The best results following transplantation are reported in cirrhotic patients undergoing transplantation and in whom an incidental hepatoma has been found on examination of the resected specimen.

Cholangiocarcinoma

This adenocarcinoma may arise anywhere in the biliary tree, including its intrahepatic radicles. It accounts for less than 10% of malignant primary neoplasms of the liver in western medicine, although its incidence is said to be rising. Risk factors include chronic parasitic infestation of the biliary tree in the Orient, and choledochal cysts (see below).

Jaundice, pain and an enlarged liver are the common presenting features, although there may be coexisting biliary infection causing the tumour to masquerade as a hepatic abscess. Resection offers the only prospect of cure but is seldom feasible when cholangiocarcinoma arises in the liver substance. Cholangiocarcinoma arising from the extrahepatic bile ducts is considered later.

Other primary malignant tumours

Angiosarcoma (Fig. 19.13). This rare tumour of the liver may arise after industrial exposure to vinyl chloride or exposure to the previously used radiological contrast medium Thorotrast.

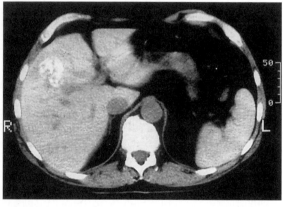

A

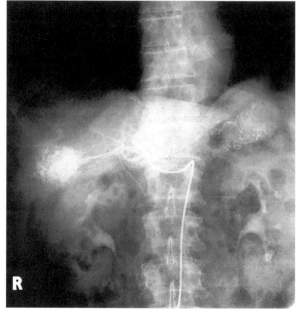

C

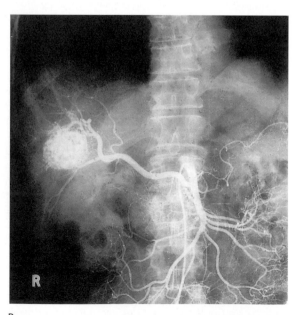

B

Fig. 19.13 **A** CT scan demonstrating a lesion in segment V. Previous ultrasound-guided biopsy had suggested an angiosarcoma. **B** Angiography shows an extremely vascular lesion taking its blood supply mainly from an aberrant right hepatic artery arising from the superior mesenteric artery. **C** The lesion derives some of its blood supply from the left hepatic artery. The patient underwent a curative resection of the lesion by extended right hepatectomy (segments IV–VIII).

Haemangioendothelioma This presents as a diffuse multifocal tumour and is rarely resectable at presentation.

Biliary cystadenoma This rare condition of the liver, with a marked female predominance, has a 1:4 risk of malignant transformation and should be resected.

All of these rare tumours generally present late and resection is seldom feasible. The prognosis is generally poor.

Metastatic tumours

The liver is a common site for metastatic disease: secondary liver tumours are 20 times more common than primary ones. In 50% of cases the primary tumour is in the gastrointestinal tract; other common sites are the breast, ovaries, bronchus and kidney. Almost 90% of patients with hepatic metastases have tumour deposits in other sites.

Hepatomegaly and tenderness are distinctive features, and individual deposits may be palpable. The patient is often cachectic, and ascites or jaundice may be present. Pyrexia occurs in up to 10% of patients. LFTs are abnormal, notably the alkaline phosphatase and γ-glutamyl transpeptidase, which are often raised. Ultrasound and CT scans may demonstrate multiple filling defects. The diagnosis can be confirmed by aspiration cytology or needle biopsy undertaken under ultrasound control. Such invasive investigation may be unnecessary when resection is being considered.

There is no effective treatment for most patients with hepatic metastases. Both lobes of the liver are usually involved, making surgical resection impossible. Hepatic artery ligation, local and systemic chemotherapy, and chemoembolization have given disappointing results.

In some tumours, notably those arising from the colon and rectum, apparently solitary metastases or metastases confined to one or other lobe may be resected. A careful search for other metastases is required, including a search for local recurrence of the original primary tumour (e.g. colonoscopy) and dissemination elsewhere (e.g. CT of the thorax). In well selected patients 5 year survival rates of 30–40% have been reported following resection. Non-curative resection may be considered as a means of palliation in patients with symptomatic hepatic metastases from a carcinoid tumour.

LIVER RESECTION

Resection involves mobilization of the liver from its peritoneal attachments. Following isolation, ligature and division of the appropriate vessels, the devascularized lobe or segment is separated by careful dissection, which may be facilitated by the use of an ultrasonic dissector. Intervening biliary and vascular channels can be defined and divided between ligatures. The hepatic veins or tributaries are con-trolled by suture ligation following removal of the resected specimen.

Modern techniques of hepatic resection have greatly reduced operative blood loss, with a subsequent reduction in morbidity and mortality. Adequate drainage of the operating field following resection may minimize the consequences of postoperative bile leakage or bleeding. Postoperative monitoring should include blood gas, glucose and lactate measurement. Hepatic dysfunction may be evident from prolongation of the prothrombin time in major liver resectional surgery.

LIVER TRANSPLANTATION

This is considered in Chapter 31.

THE GALLBLADDER AND BILE DUCTS

ANATOMY OF THE BILIARY SYSTEM

The biliary tree consists of fine intrahepatic biliary radicles which drain individual liver segments before forming the right and left hepatic ducts. The left hepatic duct runs a mainly extrahepatic course and joins the right hepatic duct

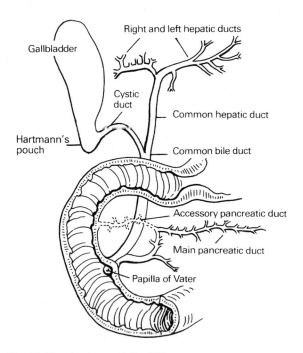

Fig. 19.14   Anatomy of the biliary tree.

to form the common hepatic duct. This is joined at a variable position by the cystic duct to form the common bile duct, which ends at the papilla of Vater, usually in the second part of the duodenum (Fig. 19.14).

The common bile duct is approximately 8 cm long and up to 10 mm in diameter. It lies in the free edge of the lesser omentum before passing behind the first part of the duodenum and through the head of the pancreas. It is usually joined by the pancreatic duct just before entering the duodenum.

The gallbladder lies in a bed on the undersurface of the liver between its right and left halves. It is a muscular structure with a fundus, body and neck. Hartmann's pouch is a dilatation of the gallbladder outlet adjacent to the origin of the cystic duct, in which gallstones frequently become impacted. The gallbladder is supplied by the cystic artery, a branch of the right hepatic artery.

PHYSIOLOGY

Bile salts and the enterohepatic circulation

Bile acids are sterols synthesized by the liver from cholesterol. The primary bile acids, chenodeoxycholic and cholic acid, are conjugated with glycine or taurine to increase their solubility in water, and the conjugates (e.g. glycocholic and taurocholic acid) form sodium and potassium bile salts. In the intestine, bacterial action produces the secondary bile salts deoxycholic and lithocholic acid.

Bile salts can combine with lipids to form water-soluble complexes called micelles (Fig. 19.15), within which lecithin and cholesterol can be transported from the liver. Bile salts are also detergents and a reduction in surface tension allows fat to be emulsified in the intestine, thus facilitating its digestion and absorption. On reaching the distal ileum, 95% of the bile salts are reabsorbed, transported back to the liver and passed once again into the biliary system. This enterohepatic circulation (Fig. 19.16) allows a relatively small bile salt pool (2–4 g) to circulate through the intestine some 6–12 times a day. The daily faecal loss equals that of hepatic synthesis (0.2–0.6 g/24 h). When bile is excluded from the intestine, 25% of ingested fat may appear in the faeces and there is a marked malabsorption of fat-soluble vitamins, including vitamin K.

The gallbladder has a capacity of 50 mL and can concentrate bile by a factor of 10. It contracts in response to cholecystokinin (CCK), which is released from the duodenal mucosa by the presence of food, notably fatty acids. Gallbladder contraction is accompanied by reciprocal relaxation of the sphincter of Oddi. The secretion of bile is promoted by the hormone secretion. The vagus nerve also stimulates bile secretin and gallbladder contraction. Some 1–2 L of bile are produced by the liver.

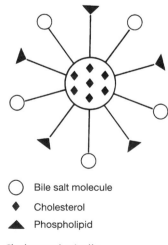

○ Bile salt molecule
◆ Cholesterol
▲ Phospholipid

Fig. 19.15 Cholesterol micelle.

> **SUMMARY BOX**
>
> **Bile salts**
>
> - The primary bile acids chenodeoxycholic and cholic acid are conjugated with glycine or taurine and form sodium or potassium bile salts (e.g. sodium taurocholate).
>
> - The bile salts are vital for the excretion of cholesterol in bile; cholesterol is insoluble in water and must be transported in water-soluble complexes (micelles) with bile salts and lecithin.
>
> - Bile salts are detergents, and on reaching the intestine they emulsify fat and facilitate the digestion and absorption of fat and fat-soluble vitamins.
>
> - Bile salts must not be confused with bile pigments (e.g. bilirubin), which are waste products and excreted in bile. The small bile salt pool (2–4 g) is conserved by reabsorption of bile salts from the terminal ileum.
>
> - Disease or resection of the terminal ileum prevents the enterohepatic circulation of bile salts and is associated with a high incidence of cholesterol gallstones and diarrhoea (owing to the cathartic action of bile salts on the colon).

CONGENITAL ABNORMALITIES

Congenital abnormalities of the gallbladder and bile ducts are common. The gallbladder may be absent (agenesis),

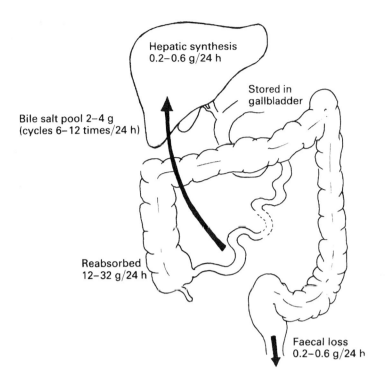

Hepatic synthesis
0.2–0.6 g/24 h

Stored in
gallbladder

Bile salt pool 2–4 g
(cycles 6–12 times/24 h)

Reabsorbed
12–32 g/24 h

Faecal loss
0.2–0.6 g/24 h

Fig. 19.16 The enterohepatic circulation.

double, intrahepatic, partitioned with a fold in the fundus (Phrygian cap), or multiseptate. The cystic duct may be absent or join the right hepatic duct rather than the common hepatic duct, and accessory ducts may be present. The cystic artery may be duplicated or may arise from the common hepatic or left hepatic artery. These anomalies are important in that great care must be taken to avoid the inappropriate division of major ducts and arteries in the course of cholecystectomy.

Biliary atresia

Failure of development of the duct system occurs once in every 20 000–30 000 births and is the commonest cause of prolonged jaundice in infancy. The condition may be acquired after birth, rather than truly congenital, in that it has not been described in autopsies of newborn infants. The site and extent of the atresia are variable and the duct system may be entirely replaced by solid fibrous strands. Fortunately, intrahepatic atresia is rare and the extrahepatic system is usually most affected.

Jaundice usually becomes apparent in the first 2–3 weeks of life and the liver and spleen usually enlarge. LFTs show an obstructive pattern, although the serum transaminase levels are often elevated. Liver biopsy reveals cholestatic jaundice, but differentiation from neonatal hepatitis is often surprisingly difficult.

In extrahepatic biliary atresia, a Roux loop of jejunum is anastomosed to the intrahepatic duct system in the hilus of the liver (Kasai operation). A delay in treatment may allow cirrhosis to develop, with portal hypertension and ascites. The prognosis for infants with extrahepatic biliary atresia has improved, although recurrent fibrosis and stricture may lead to troublesome cholangitis and abscess formation. Intrahepatic atresia is rarely correctable and liver transplantation may be needed.

Choledochal cysts

Cystic transformation of the biliary tree (choledochal cyst) is rare. The most common type results in a saccular dilatation of the common bile duct, which often has an abnormal termination that enters the pancreatic duct within the head of the pancreas. This may allow reflux into the biliary system, resulting in pain, inflammation, calculus formation and malignant transformation. The abnormalities are probably congenital, although diagnosis may be delayed until adult life.

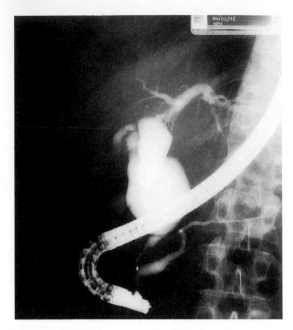

Fig. 19.17 ERCP demonstrating the common type of choledochal cyst involving the common bile duct.

In the neonate the cyst may present with jaundice or spontaneous perforation. The adult patient usually presents with intermittent pain and jaundice and may have attacks of pancreatitis. Localized abdominal tenderness and a mass may be present in the right hypochondrium. LETs show a cholestatic pattern, and ultrasonography and cholangiography (MRCP or ERCP) establish the diagnosis (Fig. 19.17). In view of the significant risk of malignant transformation, excision of the cyst is indicated. However, the risk of developing intrahepatic cholangiocarcinoma is not completely removed by excision of the extrahepatic biliary tree.

Caroli's disease consists of cystic biliary dilatation which is more marked in the peripheral intrahepatic ducts. Recurring infection may progress to cirrhosis and liver failure. When Caroli's disease is found in association with congenital hepatic fibrosis, portal hypertension is often present. Endoscopic, percutaneous and surgical manipulation of the biliary tree is best avoided, and liver transplantation may have a valuable role in management.

GALLSTONES

Pathogenesis

Gallstones are common in Europe and North America and less so in Asia and Africa. Their incidence increases with age. In 'developed' countries they occur in at least 20% of women over the age of 40; the incidence in males is about one-third of that in females. The disease has increased markedly in frequency and cholecystectomy is the commonest elective abdominal operation in many western countries.

Gallstones are formed from the constituents of bile. The great majority result from failure to keep cholesterol in micellar form in the gallbladder, and pigment stones are less common. Most cholesterol stones become mixed with bile pigments as they increase in size; such 'mixed' stones are much more common than pure cholesterol stones.

Cholesterol stones

Cholesterol stones are particularly common in middle-aged obese multiparous women. Stone formation is encouraged if bile becomes supersaturated with cholesterol (i.e. lithogenic), either by excessive cholesterol excretion or by a reduction in the amount of bile salt and lecithin available for micelle formation. Supersaturation is most likely to occur while the bile is concentrated in the gallbladder, and is favoured by stasis or decreased gallbladder contractility. The formation of cholesterol crystals is the key event, and this 'nucleation' may be due to coalescence of cholesterol molecules or their precipitation around particles of mucus, bacteria, calcium bilirubinate or mucosal cells. Pure cholesterol stones are yellowish-green with a regular shape but rough surface. They are usually solitary, whereas mixed stones are darker and are usually multiple.

Cholesterol stones are particularly common in some tribes of North American Indians, where more than 75% of women over 40 are affected. Such individuals have a small bile salt pool. Conversely, the high incidence of stones in Chilean women reflects high levels of cholesterol excretion. Obesity and high-calorie or high-cholesterol diets favour cholesterol stone formation by producing highly supersaturated gallbladder bile. Drastic weight reduction and diets designed to lower serum cholesterol levels may also promote stone formation by mobilizing cholesterol and increasing its excretion.

Disease or resection of the terminal ileum and drugs such as cholestyramine favour cholesterol nucleation by reducing the bile salt pool. Hormonal influences are reflected in an increased incidence of stone formation in women taking oral contraceptives or postmenopausal oestrogen replacement. Pregnancy may also have an effect by increasing stasis within the gallbladder.

Pigment stones

Pigment stones consist of calcium bilirubinate and are usually multiple and small. Stones found in Occidental patients are usually composed of black pigment, whereas brown pigment stones are common in Orientals. Pigment stones account for 25% of all gallstones in western patients, but for 60% of those in some Oriental countries such as Japan.

Chronic haemolysis favours pigment stone formation by increasing pigment excretion, and stone formation is common in congenital spherocytosis, haemoglobinopathy and malaria. Cirrhosis and biliary stasis are also important associations. Some patients with brown pigment stones have increased amounts of unconjugated bilirubin in the bile. In Oriental patients this may be due to the action of β-glucuronidase produced by *E. coli*, an organism that invades duct systems infested with *Clonorchis sinensis* or *Ascaris lumbricoides*.

Pathological effects of gallstones
Acute cholecystitis and its complications

This is usually produced by obstruction of the neck of the gallbladder or cystic duct by a stone. Bacteria are cultured from the bile in approximately one-half of patients with gallstones, and unrelieved obstruction in the presence of this infected bile may produce an **empyema**. The thickened gallbladder becomes intensely inflamed, oedematous and occasionally gangrenous. The fundus of the distended, inflamed gallbladder may perforate, giving rise to localized abscess formation and occasionally to biliary peritonitis. The common organisms implicated in inflammation of the gallbladder are *E. coli*, *Klebsiella aerogenes* and *Streptococcus faecalis*. Staphylococci, clostridia and salmonella are occasionally present. These organisms may be cultured from the blood if there is bacteraemia.

Chronic cholecystitis

Repeated bouts of biliary colic or acute cholecystitis culminate in fibrosis, contraction of the gallbladder and chronic inflammatory change with marked thickening of the wall. The gallbladder ceases to function. Chronic inflammatory change may be present in the absence of gallstones, as is the case in the gallbladders of typhoid carriers.

Mucocele

A mucocele develops when the outlet of the gallbladder becomes obstructed in the absence of infection. The imprisoned bile is absorbed, but clear mucus continues to be secreted into the distended gallbladder.

Choledocholithiasis

When gallstones enter the common bile duct they may pass spontaneously or give rise to obstructive jaundice, cholangitis or acute pancreatitis. Gallstone pancreatitis most commonly occurs when a small stone becomes temporarily arrested at the ampulla of Vater.

Gallstone ileus

This uncommon form of intestinal obstruction occurs when a large gallstone becomes impacted in the intestine. Stones large enough to block the gut generally gain access by eroding through the wall of the gallbladder into the duodenum.

Carcinoma

The incidence of carcinoma of the gallbladder is increased in patients with long-standing gallstones.

Common clinical syndromes associated with gallstones

The majority of individuals with gallstones are asymptomatic or have only vague symptoms of distension and flatu-

---

SUMMARY BOX

Gallstones

- Most gallstones form because of failure to keep cholesterol in solution. This can result in pure cholesterol stones, but more commonly the stones also acquire a content of bile pigment as they enlarge, forming 'mixed' stones.

- Pigment stones are the commonest type of stone in some Oriental countries, but are less common in western society, where they are associated with chronic haemolysis, biliary stasis and cirrhosis.

- Only 15% of stones contain enough calcium to be seen on a plain film.

- The majority of individuals with gallstones are asymptomatic and remain so; the presence of gallstones is not in itself an indication for cholecystectomy.

- Gallbladder stones may cause flatulent dyspepsia, biliary colic, acute cholecystitis and gallbladder cancer (although this is so rare that this consideration does not affect the decision not to treat asymptomatic stones).

- Gallstones that migrate into the bile duct can cause obstructive jaundice, cholangitis and acute pancreatitis, although they often remain asymptomatic.

- Gallstone ileus is a rare form of intestinal obstruction: stones large enough to obstruct the gut are usually too large to pass through the ampulla of Vater and have gained access to the gut by an internal fistula involving the gallbladder.

lence. Fewer than half of such patients develop symptoms or complications from their gallstones within 10 years.

Biliary colic

Biliary colic is due to transient obstruction of the gallbladder from an impacted stone. There is severe gripping pain, often developing after meals or in the evening, which is maximal in the epigastrium and right hypochondrium with radiation to the back. Despite being continuous, the pain may wax and wane in intensity over several hours, and vomiting and retching are common. Resolution occurs when the stone falls back into the gallbladder lumen or passes onward into the common bile duct. The patient then recovers rapidly, but repeated bouts of colic are common. In some cases, the obstruction does not resolve and the patient develops acute cholecystitis.

Acute cholecystitis

Acute cholecystitis is a more prolonged and severe illness. It usually begins with an attack of biliary colic, though its onset may be more gradual. There is severe right hypochondrial pain radiating to the right subscapular region, and occasionally to the right shoulder, together with tachycardia, pyrexia, nausea, vomiting and leukocytosis. Abdominal tenderness and rigidity may be generalized but are most marked over the gallbladder. Murphy's sign (a catching of the breath at the height of inspiration while the gallbladder area is palpated) is usually present. A right hypochondrial mass may be felt. This is due to omentum 'wrapped' around the inflamed gallbladder.

In 85–90% of cases the attack settles within 4–5 days. In the remainder, tenderness may spread and pyrexia and tachycardia persist or worsen. The development of a tender mass associated with rigors and marked pyrexia signals empyema formation. The gallbladder may become gangrenous and perforate, giving rise to biliary peritonitis.

Jaundice can develop during the acute attack. Usually this is associated with stones in the common bile duct, but compression of the bile ducts by the gallbladder may be responsible.

Acute cholecystitis must be differentiated from perforated peptic ulcer, high retrocaecal appendicitis, acute pancreatitis, myocardial infarction and basal pneumonia. Acute cholecystitis can develop in the absence of gallstones (acalculous cholecystitis), although this is rare.

Chronic cholecystitis

Chronic cholecystitis is the most common cause of symptomatic gallbladder disease. The patient gives a history of recurrent flatulence, fatty food intolerance and right upper quadrant pain. The pain is worse after meals and is often associated with a feeling of distension and heartburn.

SUMMARY BOX

Acute cholecystitis

- In the great majority of cases acute cholecystitis is associated with gallstones and results from obstruction of gallbladder outflow.

- In contrast to biliary colic, which results from obstruction alone, acute cholecystitis is associated with infection and is a systemic illness.

- The patient appears unwell, has pyrexia and tachycardia, and is tender in the right hypochondrium: Murphy's sign is almost always positive.

- In 90% of cases acute cholecystitis will settle with conservative treatment (nil by mouth, i.v. fluids, antibiotics, nasogastric suction if appropriate).

- In 10% of cases disease progression leads to life-threatening complications, notably empyema, gangrene and perforation.

- Given that the gallbladder is permanently diseased and that complications may supervene, most surgeons now advocate early cholecystectomy (i.e. within 5 days) for acute cholecystitis.

The differential diagnosis includes duodenal ulcer, hiatus hernia, myocardial ischaemia, chronic pancreatitis and gastrointestinal neoplasia.

Mucocele

In this condition the patient often presents with a history of biliary colic and a non-tender piriform swelling in the right hypochondrium. There is little systemic upset and no pyrexia.

Choledocholithiasis

Stones may be present in the common bile duct of some 5–10% of patients with gallstones. There is little muscle in the wall of the bile duct, and pain is not a symptom unless the stone impedes flow through the sphincter of Oddi. The vast majority of stones in the common bile duct originate in the gallbladder. 'Primary' duct stones are extremely rare.

Impaction of a stone at the sphincter obstructs the flow of bile, producing jaundice, pale stools and dark urine. Obstruction commonly persists for several days but may clear spontaneously, as a result of either passage of the stone or of its disimpaction. Small stones may pass through the common bile duct without causing symptoms.

In long-standing obstruction the bile ducts become markedly dilated and the diameter of the common bile duct may exceed its upper limit of 10 mm. A totally obstructed duct system becomes filled with clear 'white bile', as back pressure on the hepatocytes prevents clearance of bilirubin and mucus secretion is increased.

Infection of an obstructed biliary tract causes cholangitis, which is characterized by attacks of pain, pyrexia and jaundice (the so-called triad of Charcot), frequently in association with rigors. Long-standing intermittent biliary obstruction may lead to secondary biliary cirrhosis.

Acute pancreatitis may be associated with a stone in the common bile duct (see Ch. 20).

Obstructive jaundice due to stones in the common bile duct has to be distinguished from other causes of obstructive jaundice, notably malignant obstruction and cholestatic jaundice. Acute viral or alcoholic hepatitis may occasionally be confused with obstructive jaundice.

Courvoisier's law Fibrosed gallbladders that contain stones cannot distend when pressure increases in the obstructed biliary tree. Courvoisier's law states that if the gallbladder is palpable in the presence of jaundice, the jaundice is unlikely to be due to stone. This law is not inviolate.

Distended gallbladders are not always easy to feel but can be detected readily by ultrasound.

Other benign conditions of the gallbladder

Cholesterosis

Cholesterosis or 'strawberry gallbladder' is a condition in which the mucous membrane of the gallbladder is infiltrated with lipid and cholesterol. It affects middle-aged and elderly patients of either sex.

Cholesterol stones are found in the gallbladders of half of these patients. Macroscopically the mucosa is brick-red and speckled with bright yellow nodules. Symptoms of acute and chronic cholecystitis may be produced, and cholecystectomy is required in the symptomatic patient.

Adenomyomatosis

This rare condition is characterized by mucosal diverticula (Rokitansky–Aschoff sinuses) which affect particularly the fundus and penetrate the muscular layers to the serosa. Muscular hypertrophy and inflammatory cell infiltrates are present. The diagnosis is often only made following cholecystectomy, as the gallbladder often contains stones or biliary gravel.

Acute acalculous cholecystitis

About 5% patients with acute cholecystitis have acalculous inflammation. The condition may be precipitated by major surgery, bacteraemia, trauma, pancreatitis or other serious illness, and may complicate parenteral nutrition. The inflammatory reaction in the gallbladder wall may be intense and severe, leading to gangrene and perforation. In ill patients percutaneous drainage (cholecystostomy) under ultrasound guidance may be considered, but urgent cholecystectomy is often advisable.

Investigation of patients with suspected gallstones

Blood tests

A full blood count may reveal a neutrophilia in acute cholecystitis or its complications. An elevated serum bilirubin or alkaline phosphatase may signify the presence of common duct stones.

Plain abdominal X-ray

As only 15% of gallstones contain enough calcium to be seen on a plain radiograph, this investigation is seldom used in diagnosis. Gas is occasionally seen outlining the biliary tree if there is a fistula between the biliary tract and the gut, as in gallstone ileus or following choledochoduodenostomy. Previous endoscopic sphincterotomy also allows gas to enter the biliary tree.

Ultrasonography

Ultrasonography using a real-time scanner has become the mainstay of investigation of suspected gallstone disease. It permits inspection of the gallbladder, its wall and its contents, and demonstrates dilatation of the intrahepatic and extrahepatic biliary tree. Stones reflect the ultrasonic wave and are thrown into prominence by the acoustic shadow they produce (Fig. 19.18). The technique is extremely accurate in skilled hands. As it does not depend on hepatic excretion of contrast, it can be used both in jaundiced and non-jaundiced patients.

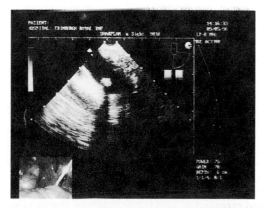

Fig. 19.18 Ultrasound scan of the gallbladder demonstrating the hyperechoic features of a solitary gallstone along with the typical acoustic shadow.

Oral cholecystography and intravenous cholangiography

These investigations are rarely used in the assessment of the gallbladder or common bile duct. Neither will visualize these structures adequately if the liver function tests are abnormal.

Although intravenous cholangiography has been more frequently used by some surgeons in the laparoscopic cholecystectomy era, intravenous injection of an iodine-containing compound carries a small but definite risk of severe (and even fatal) anaphylactoid reaction.

Magnetic resonance cholangiopancreatography (MRCP)

This non-invasive investigation is finding increasing use in the assessment of the biliary tree. Recent improvements in image quality have resulted in a technique that can be used to assess accurately the biliary and pancreatic ducts.

Endoscopic retrograde cholangiopancreatography (ERCP)

Using a side-viewing fibreoptic endoscope, the papilla of Vater may be seen and cannulated. Contrast is injected to outline the biliary and pancreatic duct systems. If stones are detected in the common bile duct they can be removed at the same time, following endoscopic sphincterotomy. Complications include cholangitis and pancreatitis.

Percutaneous transhepatic cholangiography (PTC)

In patients with obstructive jaundice the intrahepatic biliary system can be entered percutaneously using a slim flexible needle through which a radio-opaque dye is injected. The site and nature of any obstruction can than be defined. Ultra-sonography is usually performed first to confirm that there is duct dilatation. PTC is less successful in patients who do not have a dilated duct system. Leakage of bile or bleeding from the puncture site are now rare complications, but antibiotic cover is required and coagulation status must be checked before the procedure is undertaken. This investigation is more likely to be used in the evaluation of biliary malignancy.

Surgical treatment of gallstones

Patients with symptomatic gallstones are usually advised to undergo cholecystectomy to relieve symptoms and avoid complications. Patients with asymptomatic gallstones are treated expectantly, particularly if they are elderly or suffering from medical conditions likely to increase the risk of surgery. In younger patients there may be a stronger case for surgery despite the absence of symptoms, particularly if the stones are multiple and likely to cause complications, such as acute pancreatitis.

Irrespective of whether open or laparoscopic cholecystectomy is undertaken, the principles of surgical technique remain the same. The gallbladder and its contained stones are removed, while ensuring that no stones remain within the ductal system. 'Open' cholecystectomy may be required if the equipment and expertise for laparoscopic cholecystectomy are not available, but is now undertaken in less than 10% of patients with symptomatic gallstones. A laparoscopic procedure may not be possible in the patient who has previously undergone multiple abdominal operations or who is grossly obese. Pregnancy is considered a relative contraindication to laparoscopy because of the risk of anaesthetic agents to the developing fetus in the first trimester, and because of the risk of spontaneous abortion. There is continuing debate as to whether laparoscopic cholecystectomy should be used in patients with acute complications of biliary disease, as the risk of complications is said to be greater than for open cholecystectomy.

Conversion from a laparoscopic procedure to open cholecystectomy should be seen as a limitation of the minimally invasive technique and not as a failure of the surgeon. Laparotomy is mandatory when the anatomy in the area of the cystic duct and artery cannot be defined readily, if uncontrolled bleeding occurs, or if the bile duct is injured.

Open cholecystectomy

The gallbladder is usually approached through a right subcostal incision. Following careful inspection and palpation of the abdominal contents to exclude other pathology, the cystic duct and artery are identified. Intraoperative cholangiography is performed by cannulating the cystic duct and taking serial radiographs after the injection of contrast. The cholangiogram displays the anatomy of the duct system, identifies ductal stones, and confirms that dye passes freely into the duodenum (Fig. 19.19). Once the films have been inspected the cystic duct and artery are ligated and divided and the gallbladder is removed. A retrograde approach in which the gallbladder is mobilized 'fundus first' can be used when inflammation makes visualization of the biliary anatomy difficult.

Some surgeons pursue a policy of selective cholangiography, obtaining a cholangiogram only in patients at high risk of having ductal stones. The presence of such stones may be suspected if there is a history of jaundice or pancreatitis, preoperative LFTs are abnormal, or dilatation of the common bile duct or multiple gallbladder stones has been detected on ultrasound. At surgery, a stone may be palpable in the duct system.

Following removal of the gallbladder, haemostasis is secured and the wound is closed. Many surgeons leave a or postoperative period to exclude the presence of common bile duct stones.

The cystic duct and artery are divided between metal clips and the gallbladder is dissected from the liver using diathermy. Extraction of the gallbladder through a cannula site may require extension of the incision or the tedious removal of individual stones from the gallbladder. Care must be taken to secure haemostasis, and many surgeons leave a drain in the subhepatic space.

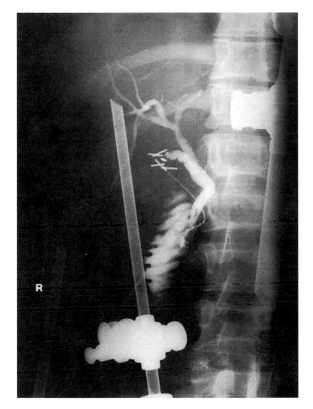

Fig. 19.19 Operative cholangiogram undertaken at laparoscopic cholecystectomy (note the radio-opaque ports). The extrahepatic ducts are not particularly dilated and there is flow of contrast into the duodenum, but there is a small solitary radiolucent calculus at the lower end of the common bile duct.

drain in the subhepatic space to prevent the development of a collection and to identify leakage of bile, although the value of this approach has been questioned.

Laparoscopic cholecystectomy

Access to the peritoneal cavity is obtained through three or four cannula inserted through the anterior abdominal wall and following insufflation of the peritoneal cavity with CO_2. The gallbladder is retracted by grasping forceps inserted through the most lateral cannula in order to display the structures at the porta hepatis. An excellent view of the operating field is obtained with the laparoscope, and the cystic duct and artery are isolated by dissection with instruments passed through the remaining cannulae. Some surgeons have found it difficult to undertake operative cholangiography routinely with this approach, and have either abandoned its use or relied upon intravenous cholangiography, MRCP or ERCP in the pre-

> **SUMMARY BOX**
>
> **Cholecystectomy**
>
> - Cholecystectomy is the standard treatment for symptomatic gallbladder stones; alternatives (stone dissolution, extracorporeal lithotripsy) are now seldom used.
>
> - Open cholecystectomy has been largely superseded by laparoscopic cholecystectomy, but conversion to open operation is still sometimes needed.
>
> - Cholecystectomy now has a low operative mortality (0.2%); inadvertent injury to the bile duct (0.2% incidence) remains the main source of major morbidity.
>
> - Some 5–10% of patients coming to cholecystectomy have ductal stones, many of which are unsuspected. Opinions vary as to whether intraoperative cholangiography should be undertaken routinely to detect such stones.
>
> - In the era of laparoscopic cholecystectomy there is a growing tendency not to perform routine operative cholangiography, and to extract symptomatic duct stones by non-operative means (i.e. at endoscopic papillotomy).
>
> - If ductal stones cause symptoms they frequently give rise to cholangitis and Charcot's triad of pain, jaundice and fever (often with rigors).

Exploration of the common bile duct

This is undertaken much less often with the free availability of ERCP and sphincterotomy. At open surgery, if stones are present in the duct system the common bile duct is opened longitudinally between stay sutures (choledochotomy) and the stones are extracted with forceps (Desjardin forceps) or a Fogarty balloon catheter. Following exploration, further check cholangiogram films are obtained, or the interior of the duct can be inspected with a rigid or fibreoptic choledochoscope.

The opening in the common bile duct is closed around a T-tube, the long limb of which is brought out through a stab incision in the abdominal wall (Fig. 19.20). This

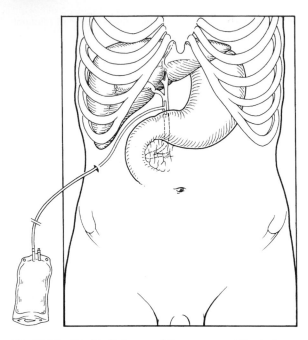

Fig. 19.20   T-tube drainage of the common bile duct.

serves as a safety valve to allow the escape of bile if there is a temporary obstruction to flow into the duodenum following duct exploration. It also facilitates the installation of iodine-containing dye to obtain a T-tube cholangiogram some 7–10 days following surgery. If this shows free flow of dye into the duodenum and no residual duct stones, the T-tube can be clamped before removal. If at operation there is gross duct dilatation and the bile duct contains multiple stones and debris, some surgeons follow duct exploration by anastomosing the common bile duct to the adjacent duodenum (choledochoduodenostomy), but this is rarely necessary.

If at operation a stone is firmly impacted at the lower end of the common bile duct, it may have to be removed through the duodenum. Transduodenal sphincterotomy and sphincteroplasty increase the risk of postoperative morbidity and mortality, and are rarely undertaken.

With the reluctance of some surgeons to perform operative cholangiography during laparoscopic cholecystectomy, increasing reliance has been placed on removing common bile duct stones at ERCP. Other surgeons continue to adhere to the principles employed at open cholecystectomy and explore the common bile duct by means of a choledochotomy or through the dilated cystic duct. Retained stones can be removed with the aid of a small-diameter fibreoptic choledochoscope under direct vision, or by means of a wire basket or an inflatable balloon catheter. The surgeon can suture or leave a drain in the cystic duct, or can oversew the choledochotomy over a T-tube or stent.

Complications of cholecystectomy

The postoperative stay of patients undergoing open cholecystectomy may exceed 7 days. Respiratory complications are not uncommon and there is a significant risk of wound infection (see below). Operative mortality following elective open cholecystectomy is low (0.2%), but is increased tenfold if there is obstructive jaundice or if the common bile duct has to be explored.

Postoperative stay is reduced greatly with laparoscopic cholecystectomy, which in some centres is undertaken as a day-case procedure. Complications resulting from a major abdominal wound are undoubtedly avoided, but there is concern regarding the apparent increased incidence of injury to the bile duct. The development of abdominal pain or the need for additional analgesia in the immediate postoperative period should cause the surgeon to consider the complications of haemorrhage or bile leakage. Mortality and morbidity related to the laparoscopic procedure have also been reported. None the less, the advantages to the patient of this minimally invasive technique has led to its widespread adoption by surgeons.

Haemorrhage

This may originate from the cystic artery or the gallbladder bed. Significant intra-abdominal bleeding may not be readily apparent, but should be suspected from the development of pain or if the patient exhibits early features of hypovolaemic shock. Blood may issue from the drain, if this is present, and re-exploration is mandatory.

Infective complications

Wound infection from organisms present in the bile (notably *E. coli*, *Klebsiella aerogenes* and *Strep. faecalis*) can be reduced following cholecystectomy by the intravenous administration of a cephalosporin at the time of induction of anaesthesia although their routine use at laparoscopic cholecystectomy has been questioned recently. A longer course of antibiotics may be prescribed when operating on patients with obstructive jaundice, cholangitis, or complications such as acute cholecystitis or empyema when significant bile contamination of the peritoneal cavity has occurred. Collections of bile and/or blood readily become infected after cholecystectomy. Formal drainage may be needed if this progresses to the formation of a subhepatic or subphrenic abscess.

Bile leakage

This may be due to a ligature or clip slipping off the cystic duct, the accidental division of an unrecognized accessory duct, damage to the common bile duct, or retention of a duct stone after exploration. This may be evidenced by the development of localized or generalized abdominal pain. Bile leakage may be contained if a drain is in place. In the absence of biliary peritonitis, a persistent leak requires investigation by means of endoscopic cholangiography. Surgery may be needed if biliary peritonitis develops.

Retained stones

Following bile duct exploration, the postoperative T-tube cholangiogram (see above) may reveal a retained stone in the bile duct. Small stones can sometimes be flushed into the duodenum by irrigating the T-tube with saline, and their passage may be facilitated if glucagon is given to relax the sphincter of Oddi. If the duct cannot be cleared by irrigation, delayed extraction of the stones may be undertaken under radiological control. The patient is discharged with the T-tube in place. This is removed 4–6 weeks later and a steerable catheter passed along its track into the bile duct. A wire basket (Dormia basket) can be passed along the catheter to catch and withdraw the retained calculus (Fig. 19.21).

In some patients unsuspected stones may be left in the bile duct at cholecystectomy. Such stones may remain asymptomatic, but usually give rise to complications such as jaundice, cholangitis and pancreatitis in the months and years following cholecystectomy. ERCP can be used to

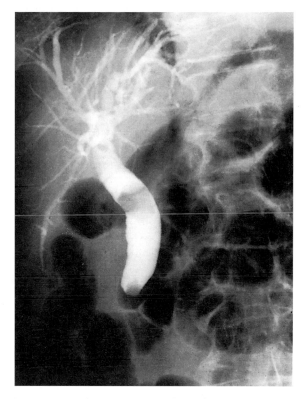

Fig. 19.22 Endoscopic retrograde cholangiography demonstrating multiple stones within the biliary tree. The endoscope has been withdrawn to enable clear visualization of the lower end of the bile duct, which is markedly dilated. These calculi were removed successfully by balloon extraction following sphincterotomy.

confirm the presence of such retained stones (Fig. 19.22) and endoscopic papillotomy is performed to recover them (Fig. 19.23). In this technique a diathermy wire attached to a cannula is passed through the duodenoscope and used to divide the sphincter of Oddi. The stones can then be extracted with a Dormia basket or balloon catheter. The same method can be used to extract stones detected in the immediate postoperative period. If the stones are too large to be withdrawn or the patient is unwell, a stent or a catheter can be left in the biliary system (nasobiliary catheter). The stones can be crushed (lithotripsy) and removed at a later date by means of a repeat endoscopic examination. It is uncommon to have to operate to retrieve retained bile duct stones.

Bile duct stricture

About 90% of benign duct strictures result from damage during cholecystectomy, in which the duct is divided, ligated or devascularized. This last mechanism appears to

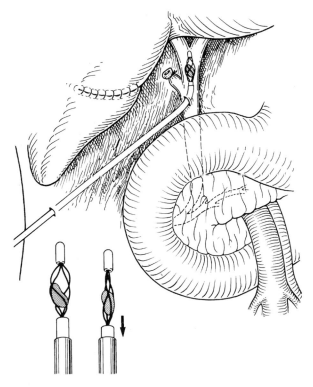

Fig. 19.21 Removal of a retained common bile duct stone.

abdominal trauma or erosion of the bile duct by a gallstone (Mirizzi syndrome).

If the common bile duct is completely occluded, progressive obstructive jaundice develops in the postoperative period. If there is a partial stricture, attacks of pain, fever and obstructive jaundice signal the development of cholangitis. The serum alkaline phosphatase and transaminase concentrations are usually elevated, and blood cultures may be positive during attacks of fever. If left untreated, persistent cholangitis and obstruction progress to secondary biliary cirrhosis, hepatic abscess formation, portal hypertension and liver failure.

The site and extent of the stricture must be defined radiologically. After ultrasonography has been performed, MRCP, ERCP and/or PTC are undertaken. Reconstructive surgery is undertaken in a specialist centre and usually necessitates bringing up a Roux loop of jejunum and anastomosing this to the distended biliary system above the stricture (Fig. 19.24).

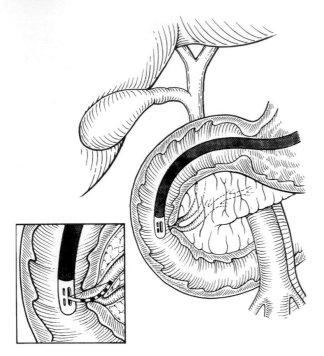

Fig. 19.23 Endoscopic papillotomy to remove retained stones.

be a common cause of injury at laparoscopic cholecystectomy. Other causes of injury include division of a ligated common bile duct which has been mistaken for the cystic duct, division of the right hepatic duct below the point of anomalous insertion of the cystic duct, and encirclement of the common bile duct by the ligature or clip used to close off the cystic duct. Strictures only occasionally result from

Post-cholecystectomy syndrome

This term is used to embrace a group of complaints such as postprandial flatulence, fat intolerance, epigastric and right hypochondrial discomfort, and heartburn which may follow cholecystectomy. The complaints tend to be more troublesome when cholecystectomy has been performed in the absence of gallstones. Investigations are usually negative, but some patients prove to have retained stones or other alimentary disorders such as peptic ulceration, gastritis and chronic pancreatitis. It is possible that some patients develop pain because of functional abnormalities of the sphincter of Oddi (see below).

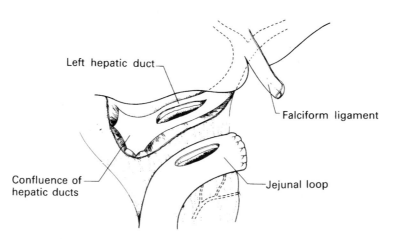

Left hepatic duct

Falciform ligament

Confluence of hepatic ducts

Jejunal loop

Fig. 19.24 Relief of bile duct stricture by anastomosis of a loop of jejunum to the distended biliary tree above the stricture (hepaticojejunostomy Roux en Y).

Management of acute cholecystitis

Patients with acute cholecystitis are admitted to hospital. The pulse, blood pressure and temperature are monitored, and analgesics, intravenous fluid and a broad-spectrum antibiotic such as a cephalosporin are prescribed. The patient is given nothing by mouth and a nasogastric tube is passed if they are vomiting. The majority of patients settle within a few days on this regimen. Failure to settle suggests the presence of an empyema.

Some surgeons delay operation for 2–3 months after the attack in the expectation that the acute inflammatory reaction will have resolved by then, but most now prefer to perform cholecystectomy during the same admission and within 72 hours of the onset of the attack. Provided the operation is carried out by an experienced surgeon and under antibiotic cover, 'early' cholecystectomy is not associated with an increased incidence of complications. The duration of the illness and hospitalization is reduced, and further attacks of acute cholecystitis during the waiting period for elective surgery are averted. It should be noted that this is a planned procedure carried out after appropriate investigation (ultrasonography) and with all facilities, on a routine elective list. 'Emergency' cholecystectomy at the time of admission is not advised, except for empyema of the gallbladder or when there is a suspicion of biliary peritonitis. Laparoscopic cholecystectomy is more difficult to perform in the acute setting, but is the method preferred by most surgeons.

If surrounding inflammation makes identification of the relevant anatomical structures difficult, drainage of the gallbladder with removal of stones (cholecystostomy) may be performed as an interim measure. Elective cholecystectomy is usually performed approximately 2 months later.

Atypical 'biliary' pain

More difficulty arises with patients who have attacks of pain consistent with biliary colic but in whom investigations such as ultrasonography, oral cholecystography and ERCP reveal no abnormality. Some of these patients with 'acalculous biliary pain' may eventually prove to have non-biliary disease, such as peptic ulceration, chronic pancreatitis or 'irritable' colon. In the majority no explanation for the symptoms can be found, although recent evidence suggests that some may be suffering from a functional disorder of the sphincter of Oddi (Fig. 19.25). Endoscopic manometry may be useful in identifying patients who may benefit from endoscopic sphincterotomy.

Laparoscopy or laparotomy is sometimes needed to exclude other pathology, to confirm that there are no stones in the biliary tree, and to remove the gallbladder as the potential source of symptoms. The results of cholecystec-

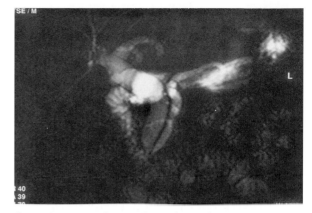

Fig. 19.25 MRCP in a patient who underwent laparoscopic cholecystectomy 5 years before the development of recurrent right upper quadrant pain. The bile and pancreatic ducts are dilated secondary to biliary dyskinesia.

tomy in these patients are extremely variable, and many continue to have symptoms.

Non-surgical treatment of gallstones

Dissolution therapy with bile salts is no longer popular in the management of gallstone disease.

Percutaneous extraction or dissolution of gallstones is possible, but the efficacy and complications of this approach have been questioned. Destruction of stones by extracorporeal shock-wave lithotripsy has been used in selected patients but, like the previous treatments, has largely been made redundant with the advent of laparoscopic cholecystectomy.

Management of acute cholangitis

This condition is caused by incomplete obstruction of the biliary tree and is more commonly due to common bile duct stones. It is not often observed as a presenting feature of malignancy, but may result from instrumentation of the biliary tree during the investigation or treatment of malignant obstructive jaundice.

The patient is often extremely unwell, with evidence of septic shock. The principles of treatment are resuscitation, the administration of appropriate antibiotics, and decompression of the biliary tree. Given the high associated morbidity and mortality of surgical intervention, this is normally achieved by endoscopic means. When common bile duct stones are responsible it may be necessary to drain the biliary tree temporarily by means of a stent, even if sphincterotomy and stone extraction have been apparently successful.

OTHER BENIGN BILIARY DISORDERS

Asiatic cholangiohepatitis

There has been a decline in the incidence of this condition, which occurs in the Far East and is particularly common in coastal Chinese communities. Suppurative cholangitis develops and pigment stones form in the intrahepatic and extrahepatic biliary tree. Deconjugation of bilirubin glucuronide by bacteria may be implicated in stone formation, and *E. coli* and *Strep. faecalis* can often be isolated from the bile and portal blood.

The clinical features are those of obstructive jaundice, pain and fever, and liver abscesses may form. Cholangitis is treated with antibiotics, and stones in the duct can be removed by percutaneous, endoscopic and operative means. Ductal obstruction may be treated by choledochoduodenostomy or hepaticojejunostomy. A limb of the Roux loop of jejunum may be left in a subcutaneous position to facilitate subsequent percutaneous manoeuvres to treat residual or recurrent calculi. Hepatic resection may be indicated if suppuration and obstruction have led to regional destruction of liver tissue.

Primary sclerosing cholangitis

In this condition both intrahepatic and extrahepatic bile ducts may become indurated and irregularly thickened. There is a marked chronic inflammatory cell infiltrate and fibrous narrowing of the biliary tree. The aetiology of the condition is unknown, but it may have an immunological basis. Over three-quarters of patients also suffer from ulcerative colitis; other associated conditions include retroperitoneal fibrosis, immunodeficiency syndromes, and pancreatitis. Bile duct carcinoma can develop, and obstruction can give rise to bacterial cholangitis and secondary biliary cirrhosis.

The condition frequently affects young adults and gives rise to intermittent attacks of obstructive jaundice, pruritus and pain. ERCP and liver biopsy are the mainstays of diagnosis. Medical treatment is generally unsatisfactory, and the outlook is extremely variable. Duct strictures can sometimes by treated by surgical bypass or the insertion of stents, but such manoeuvres may compromise the ability to undertake successful liver transplantation, which offers the only prospect of cure.

TUMOURS OF THE BILIARY TRACT

Carcinoma of the gallbladder

Carcinoma of the gallbladder is rare and almost invariably associated with the presence of gallstones. The condition is four times as common in females as in males. About 90% of lesions are adenocarcinomas, the remainder are squamous carcinomas.

Direct invasion commonly obstructs the bile duct or porta hepatis and early lymphatic and haematogenous dissemination is common. Initial symptoms are indistinguishable from those of gallstones, but jaundice is unremitting. A mass is frequently palpable. Many tumours are detected incidentally at cholecystectomy for the treatment of gallstones. Some surgeons recommend an aggressive approach of segmental resection, involving segments IV, V and VI of the liver and dissection of the regional lymph nodes. Tumours presenting with jaundice cannot be cured by resection, and palliation by endoscopic or percutaneous insertion of a stent or surgical bypass is required. The 5-year survival rate is less than 5%.

Carcinoma of the bile ducts

Cholangiocarcinoma is a relatively uncommon cancer that affects the elderly and which may be increasing in fre-

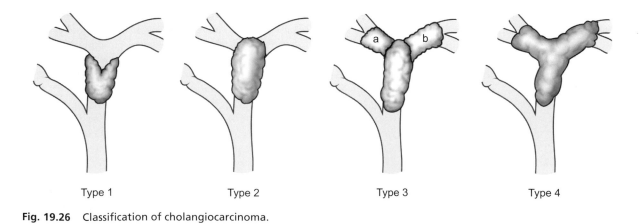

Type 1   Type 2   Type 3   Type 4

Fig. 19.26   Classification of cholangiocarcinoma.

quency. The tumour may arise at any site within the biliary tree and can be multifocal. Tumours can be classified based on the level of involvement of the biliary tree (Fig. 19.26). Polypoidal tumours are uncommon but carry a more favourable outlook. Sclerotic lesions involving the confluence of the hepatic ducts (Klatskin tumour) pose considerable problems in management. The lesions are said to be slow-growing, but this has been overemphasized. Cholangiocarcinoma may develop in patients with underlying primary sclerosing cholangitis or choledochal cyst.

Clinical features

Progressive obstructive jaundice, often preceded by vague dyspeptic pain, is the usual presenting feature. The gallbladder may become obstructed because of cystic duct involvement and mucocele or empyema can develop, but generally it is impalpable. Anorexia and weight loss are common. Pruritus is often particularly distressing.

Management

The diagnosis of malignant obstruction may be made on the history and clinical findings. The presence of intrahepatic duct dilatation and a collapsed gallbladder on ultrasound scan are highly suggestive of a tumour involving the common hepatic duct. Resectability is best assessed by CT scanning (to exclude the presence of hepatic metastases and nodal involvement) and angiography (to assess vascular invasion). PTC may assist the surgeon in planning resection, although MRCP offers a useful non-invasive means of assessing resectability.

Carcinoma of the common bile duct is treated by the Whipple operation (p. 306) if the tumour is localized and the patient is fit for radical resection. Long-term survival following this procedure is better in patients with cholangiocarcinoma than in those with carcinoma of the head of the pancreas.

Carcinoma of the upper biliary tract is resectable in only 10% of patients, some of whom may require hepatic resection to achieve satisfactory clearance of the tumour. Following resection, the remaining biliary tree is anastomosed to a Roux loop of jejunum. In the majority of

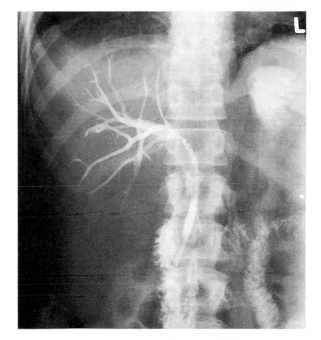

Fig. 19.27 Percutaneous transhepatic cholangiogram demonstrating a stricture at the confluence of the hepatic ducts. This lesion has the typical appearance of a cholangiocarcinoma and has been managed by percutaneous insertion of a stent.

patients not submitted to resection, palliation can be achieved by insertion of a stent by endoscopic or percutaneous transhepatic techniques (Fig. 19.27). Most stents are liable to occlusion, exposing the patient to repeated attacks of cholangitis and/or jaundice. Some surgeons prefer surgical palliation, which can be effected by intrahepatic anastomosis of a Roux loop of jejunum to the segment III duct in the left lobe of the liver. Although decompression of only one half of the biliary tree is achieved, this operation provides effective palliation in the short term. Few patients with cholangiocarcinoma survive for more than 18 months. The role of systemic chemotherapy and/or radiotherapy has yet to be established.

20 The pancreas
O.J. Garden

SURGICAL ANATOMY

The pancreas develops from separate ventral and dorsal buds of endoderm which appear during the fourth week of fetal life. The ventral pancreas develops in association with the biliary tree, and its duct joins the common bile duct before emptying into the duodenum through the papilla of Vater (Fig. 20.1). During gestation the duodenum rotates clockwise on its long axis, and the bile duct and ventral pancreas pass round behind it to fuse with the dorsal pancreas. Most of the duct that drains the dorsal pancreas joins the duct draining the ventral pancreas to form the main pancreatic duct (of Wirsung); the rest of the dorsal duct becomes the accessory pancreatic duct (of Santorini) and enters the duodenum 2.5 cm proximal to the main duct. In fetal life the common bile duct and main pancreatic duct are dilated at their junction to form the ampulla of Vater. In extrauterine life only 10% of individuals retain this ampulla, although the great majority still have a short common channel between the two duct systems.

The pancreas is deep-seated and inaccessible. It lies retroperitoneally, behind the lesser sac and stomach. The head of the gland lies within the C-loop of the duodenum, with which it shares a blood supply from the coeliac and superior mesenteric arteries (Fig. 20.2). The superior mesenteric vein runs upwards to the left of the uncinate process, and joins the splenic vein behind the neck of the pancreas to form the portal vein. The body and tail of the pancreas lie in front of the splenic vein as far as the splenic hilum, and receive arterial blood from the splenic artery as it runs along the upper border of the gland. The intimate relationship of the friable pancreas to these major blood vessels explains why bleeding is so problematic after pancreatic trauma. The close association between the common bile duct and the head of pancreas explains why obstructive jaundice is so common in cancer of the head of the pancreas, and why gallstones frequently give rise to acute pancreatitis.

SURGICAL PHYSIOLOGY

Exocrine function

The exocrine pancreas is essential for the digestion of fat, protein and carbohydrate. The pancreas secretes 1–2 L of

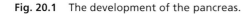

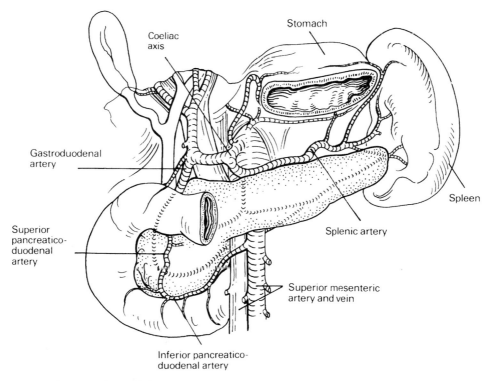

Fig. 20.1 The development of the pancreas.

Fig. 20.2 Anatomical relationships of the pancreas.

alkaline (pH 7.5–8.8) enzyme-rich juice each day. The enzymes are synthesized by the acinar cells and stored there as zymogen granules. Trypsin is the key proteolytic enzyme; it is released in an inactive form (trypsinogen) and is normally only activated within the duodenum by the brush border enzyme enterokinase. Once trypsin has been activated, a cascade is established whereby the other proteolytic enzymes become activated in turn. Lipase and amylase are secreted as active enzymes. The alkaline medium required for the activity of pancreatic enzymes is provided by the bicarbonate secreted by the ductal epithelium.

Pancreatic secretion is stimulated by eating. Hormonal and neural (vagal) mechanisms are involved. Food entering the duodenum (notably fat and protein digestion products) releases cholecystokinin (CCK), which stimulates pancreatic enzyme secretion while at the same time causing the gallbladder to contract and increase bile flow into the intestine. Acid in the duodenum releases the hormone secretion, which stimulates the pancreas to secrete watery alkaline juice.

Endocrine function

The islets of Langerhans are distributed throughout the pancreas. Although they account for only 2% of the weight of the gland, they receive 10% of its blood supply. Interaction between the endocrine and the exocrine pancreas is facilitated by the close proximity of islets and acini, and by a local 'portal' system in which blood draining from the islets enters a capillary network around neighbouring acinar cells before entering the tributaries of the portal vein. Four types of islet cells are recognized: A cells produce glucagon, B cells insulin, D cells somatostatin, and PP cells pancreatic polypeptide. Glucagon and insulin have well established physiological roles; the function of the other islet products is uncertain, but somatostatin and pancreatic polypeptide may serve as local (paracrine) regulators, rather than as circulating (endocrine) messengers. Gastrin producing (G) cells are not normally found in the pancreas except in the rare Zollinger–Ellison syndrome (Ch. 18).

Pancreatic pain

The parasympathetic nervous system has no role in the perception of pancreatic pain. Painful stimuli from the pancreas are transmitted by sympathetic fibres which travel along the arteries of supply to the coeliac ganglion, and from there to segments 5–10 of the thoracic spinal cord via the greater (and lesser) splanchnic nerves.

CONGENITAL DISORDERS OF THE PANCREAS

Annular pancreas

This rare cause of duodenal obstruction results from failure of rotation of the ventral pancreas.

Pancreas divisum

In approximately 5% of individuals the ducts draining the dorsal and ventral pancreas fail to fuse, giving rise to pancreas divisum. This means that the secretions of the larger dorsal pancreas have to drain to the duodenum through the smaller accessory duct. There is no evidence to suggest a strong association between pancreas divisum and acute or chronic pancreatitis.

Heterotopic pancreatic tissue

Rests of pancreatic tissue may be found at a variety of sites within the gut wall, but are commonest in the duodenum, stomach and proximal small bowel. Most remain asymptomatic, but they can cause ulceration, bleeding and obstruction.

Cystic fibrosis (mucoviscidosis)

Cystic fibrosis affects the sweat glands, pancreas and bronchial mucous glands. Meconium ileus can produce surgical problems by giving rise to intestinal obstruction in neonates.

PANCREATITIS

Pancreatitis may be acute or chronic. After an attack of acute pancreatitis the gland usually returns to anatomical and functional normality, whereas chronic pancreatitis is associated with a permanent derangement of structure and function. Some patients suffer from recurrent acute pancreatitis but enjoy relatively normal health between attacks.

ACUTE PANCREATITIS

Acute pancreatitis is a common cause of emergency admission to hospital. Britain has 100–200 new cases per million of the population each year and the incidence continues to rise, possibly as a result of increasing alcohol consumption. The disease is relatively rare in children, but all adult age groups may be affected. Roughly one in four patients proves to have severe disease, and of these one in four will die.

Aetiology

Conditions associated with the development of acute pancreatitis are listed in Table 20.1; gallstones and alcohol are of overriding importance.

Gallstone pancreatitis

Gallstones are present in some 50% of patients in Britain who develop acute pancreatitis. Most of these have many small stones in the gallbladder, a wide cystic duct, and a

Table 20.1	Causes of acute pancreatitis
Non-traumatic (75%)	
Major factors	Biliary tract disease (50%)
	Alcohol (20–30%)
Minor factors	Viral infection (mumps, Coxsackie)
	Drugs (e.g. steroids)
	Hyperparathyroidism
	Hyperlipidaemia
	Scorpion bites (Trinidad)
	Hypothermia
	Pancreatic cancer
	Polyarteritis nodosa
	Previous Polya gastrectomy
Traumatic (5%)	Operative trauma
	Blunt or penetrating injury
	Investigation (ERCP or angiography)
Idiopathic (20%)	

Alcohol-associated pancreatitis

The proportion of cases of acute pancreatitis linked to alcohol varies in different parts of the world. In Scotland the figure is around 30%, whereas in some parts of France and North America it may be as high as 50–90%. The mechanism responsible is uncertain. Alcohol consumption normally exceeds 80 g day immediately prior to an attack, but genetic vulnerability to the mechanism is likely. Alcohol may cause the secretion of unduly viscid juice, with the formation of protein plugs and impairment of flow, and may also generate toxic free radicals that directly damage the gland. Alcohol-associated pancreatitis frequently causes permanent damage to the gland, with progression to chronic pancreatitis.

Other causes

A proportion of patients labelled as having idiopathic pancreatitis will eventually be diagnosed as having gallstone disease. Of the other rarer causes, pancreatitis following ERCP has assumed a greater importance because of the increasing number of such diagnostic procedures being undertaken, and owing to the particularly severe form of disease following over injection of contrast into the pancreatic duct. A small number of patients may have a family history of acute pancreatitis. There is a high incidence of pancreatic cancer when familial pancreatitis proceeds to its chronic form.

Acute pancreatitis in children is rare. The symptoms are often non-specific and back pain, in particular, is a very inconsistent complaint. The most common causes are the mumps virus, trauma (particularly from the ends of bicycle handlebars impacting on the epigastrium) and multi-organ failure. In most cases the disease is benign and self-limiting and can be managed conservatively in the

common channel between the common bile duct and the main pancreatic duct (Fig. 20.3). It is now believed that stones or biliary sand may impact transiently in the common channel and so promote the reflux of bile into the pancreatic duct and/or impair the normal flow of pancreatic juice. Stones ranging in diameter from 1 to 12 mm have been recovered from the faeces in the days following an attack of acute pancreatitis, supporting the concept of transient impaction. It has also become apparent that many patients with 'idiopathic acute pancreatitis' are actually suffering from pancreatitis caused not by stones per se, but by debris containing microcrystals of cholesterol and calcium bilirubinate granules (so-called biliary sludge). The causal significance of gallstones and biliary sludge in acute pancreatitis is underlined by the fact that further attacks are exceptional once biliary tract disease has been eradicated.

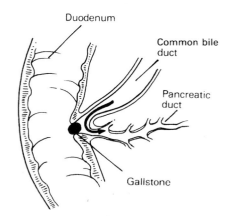

Fig. 20.3 A common channel shared by the bile duct and the pancreatic duct may allow gallstone pancreatitis.

same way that adult disease is managed. Almost 50% of affected children will develop a pancreatic pseudocyst, but only a small minority of these require surgical drainage.

Pathophysiology

Pancreatic inflammation ranges in severity from mild oedema to severe necrosis and haemorrhage. In general, *oedematous* pancreatitis is usually mild and settles on conservative treatment, whereas *necrotizing* pancreatitis is frequently severe, often leading to complications, the need for operation and death.

Local effects

The exact mechanism responsible for acute pancreatitis remains uncertain. Reflux of duodenal juice and/or bile into the pancreatic duct, and obstruction to the flow of pancreatic juice, may trigger premature activation of pancreatic enzymes within the duct system. Intraduct activation of trypsin, chymotrypsin, phospholipase, catalase and elastase may then unleash a chain reaction of cell necrosis, further enzyme release, and changes in the microcirculation. Rupture of the duct system permits autodigestion of the gland. The continued release of activated proteolytic enzymes is responsible for increased capillary permeability, protein exudation, retroperitoneal oedema and peritoneal exudation. Vasoactive kinins such as kallikrein are also released, and activated macrophages may release cytokines such as tumour necrosis factor (TNF) and interleukins 1 and 6 (IL-1, IL-6). Alcohol induces spasm of the sphincter of Oddi and increases the sensitivity of acinar cells to cholecystokinin hyperstimulation, resulting in enhanced intracellular protease activation.

General effects

The majority of patients who develop severe pancreatitis have evidence of early organ dysfunction at the time of admission or soon thereafter. Worsening organ failure is associated with a poor outcome. Profound hypovolaemic shock may follow the fluid, protein and electrolyte loss that results from altered capillary permeability, and metabolic upsets result from cytokine release. Endotoxin can be detected in the systemic circulation in many patients, indicating that bacteria and their products may also be implicated in the circulatory upset. Other factors that contribute to the systemic upset include acute renal failure (possibly due to a combination of hypovolaemia, endotoxaemia and local intravascular coagulation), adult respiratory distress syndrome (ARDS) (due to altered permeability in pulmonary capillaries), consumptive coagulopathy, and altered liver function (due to hepatocyte depression and/or obstruction of the common bile duct by a gallstone or pancreatic oedema).

Clinical features

Severe or agonizing constant pain in the epigastrium, with radiation through to the back, is usually prominent. Pain can also be experienced in either hypochondrium. Nausea, vomiting and retching are often marked.

Clinical examination often reveals much less tenderness, guarding and rigidity than might have been expected from the patient's history. Shock is often present in severe pancreatitis. Bruising around the umbilicus (Cullen's sign) or brawny discoloration of the flanks (Grey-Turner's sign) are uncommon, relatively late signs of severe pancreatitis but are indicative of a poor prognosis. Obstructive jaundice may be apparent in patients with pancreatitis due to an impacted gallstone, but is usually transient. A pleural effusion may be detected in about 20% of cases, and is almost always left-sided; it probably represents the effect of inflammation tracking retroperitoneally to involve the pleura.

Diagnosis

The key to the diagnosis of acute pancreatitis is a high index of suspicion and measurement of the serum amylase concentration. Previous attacks of flatulent dyspepsia, biliary colic or jaundice may suggest biliary pancreatitis. Alcohol intake should be carefully documented.

Biochemistry

The diagnosis is usually supported by a raised total serum amylase of at least three times the upper limit of normal (generally > 1000 iu/L). Hyperamylasaemia reflects the rupture of acinar cells and parts of the ductal system, with the release of amylase into the circulation. The serum amylase levels usually rise rapidly (within 6 hours) but are often raised only transiently, returning to normal within 48 hours. Serum lipase levels also rise in acute pancreatitis, the rise being slower but more sustained, although this test is not generally undertaken routinely by most laboratories.

As shown in Table 20.2, a number of other conditions can produce hyperamylasaemia, although the rise is seldom as high as 1000 iu/L. Most conditions causing such 'false positive' rises in serum amylase demand prompt surgical intervention, whereas surgery is usually avoided whenever possible in the early stages of acute pancreatitis. Approximately 30% of fatal attacks of pancreatitis are diagnosed at postmortem. If there is significant diagnostic doubt, urgent ultrasonography or CT scanning may reveal the true diagnosis; some surgeons occasionally use diagnostic peritoneal lavage in this situation, the diagnosis of pancreatitis being confirmed by the return of amylase-rich fluid and the absence of bile, blood or intestinal content. False negative results occur in 5–10% of cases of acute pancreatitis, in that the patient is seen before (exceptional) or after the hyper-

Table 20.2 Non-pancreatic disorders capable of causing hyperamylasaemia

Acute cholecystitis
Perforated duodenal ulcer
High intestinal obstruction
Mesenteric vascular occlusion
Bowel strangulation
Dissecting aortic aneurysm
Ruptured aortic aneurysm
Ruptured ectopic pregnancy

Table 20.3 Diagnosis of alcohol- or gallstone-associated pancreatitis

	Alcohol	Gallstones
Female patient	+/–	+
History of alcohol abuse	+++	+/–
History of gallstone disease	+/–	+++
Family history of gallstones	+/–	++
High serum amylase level	+	++
Abnormal liver function tests	+	+++
Radiological evidence of gallstones	+/–	+++

amylasaemia has occurred. There is no correlation between the height of the serum amylase level and the severity of the attack. Some of the most severe attacks are accompanied by relatively modest hyperamylasaemia. Macroamylasaemia is a rare cause of confusion in which persistent hyper-amylasaemia results from amylase being bound to globulin and forming a complex too large to be excreted by the kidney. It is found in 1–2% of the normal population and in a similar proportion of patients with acute pancreatitis.

Radiology

There are no pathognomic radiological signs of acute pancreatitis on plain films of the chest or abdomen. A left-sided pleural effusion is seen in 20% of cases and pulmonary oedema may be present in patients with ARDS. A bowel empty of gas except for a 'sentinel loop' of jejunum may reflect local ileus, and in some cases gas is seen in the hepatic and splenic flexures but not the transverse colon – the 'colon cut-off' sign. Radio-opaque gallstones may be seen in some patients with gallstone pancreatitis.

Ultrasonography may reveal swelling of the pancreas with peripancreatic fluid collections and oedema, and may detect gallstones. CT scanning is not usually performed as part of the initial diagnostic assessment but may also reveal pancreatic and peripancreatic swelling, the development of necrosis (see below) and the presence of gallstones. Although there is considerable interest in MRI it is not suitable for patients requiring significant intensive care support. Gastrografin studies are not normally indicated unless ulcer perforation cannot be excluded; the examination often shows widening of the duodenal C-loop by an inflamed head of pancreas, oedematous and coarse duodenal folds, and the 'reversed 3 sign' in which duodenal oedema produces the appearance of retraction of the papilla of Vater.

Differentiation between gallstone- and alcohol-associated pancreatitis

It may not be evident from the history and presentation whether the attack of pancreatitis is due to gallstone disease or to alcohol. On the one hand there may be a history of alcohol abuse in a patient with known gallstone disease, whereas on the other, it should be remembered that some patients with no obvious predisposing factors may be shown to have gallstones during a subsequent readmission for an attack of idiopathic pancreatitis. Table 20.3 lists some of the ways in which alcohol and gallstones can be differentiated as potential causes of an attack of acute pancreatitis.

Assessment of severity

The severity of an attack of pancreatitis can be assessed at the time of admission in a number of ways. Most patients with severe attacks have some evidence of systemic organ dysfunction at presentation. This may be obvious clinically from the shocked state of the patient, or formal 'prognostic

Table 20.4 Glasgow system used to predict severity of acute pancreatitis. Factors are assessed within 48 hours of admission and three or more positive criteria indicate the presence of severe disease

Age	> 55 years
White cell count	$> 15 \times 10^9/L$
Blood glucose (no diabetic history)	> 10 mmol/L
Serum urea (no response to i.v. fluids)	> 16 mmol/L
PaO_2	< 60 mmHg (8-kPa)
Serum calcium	< 2.0 mmol/L
Serum albumin	< 32 g/L
Serum lactate dehydrogenase	> 600 iu/L
Serum asparate aminotransferase	> 100 u/L

factor scores', such as the Glasgow system, can be used (Table 20.4). Urea and electrolyte measurements reflect the state of hydration and are helpful in managing fluid and electrolyte balance. Liver function tests (LFTs) may show hyperbilirubinaemia and elevation of liver enzymes, particularly in patients with gallstone pancreatitis. Hyperglycaemia and glycosuria can occur transiently in severe disease. Arterial blood gas analysis may reveal severe hypoxia. Moderate polymorphonuclear leukocytosis is common. Serum calcium levels may fall in severe disease. At one time it was believed that this reflected the formation of calcium soaps following fat necrosis within the abdomen, but it is now recognized that much of the fall reflects the drop in serum albumin levels caused by protein exudation. A marked reduction in the level of ionized calcium is unusual and frank tetany is exceptional.

It should be appreciated that predictive systems require 48 hours for full evaluation, by which time clinical assessment is almost as accurate. Progress can be monitored by regular clinical evaluation, and a rising APACHE II score or a rising level of C-reactive protein (see below) may help to identify patients in need of urgent investigation and surgical intervention. Serum IL-6 level has been shown to be an excellent marker of disease severity but is not generally available. Trypsinogen activation peptide and leukocyte elastase share similar disadvantages. If deterioration occurs, endoscopic retrograde cholangiopancreatography (ERCP) and endoscopic papillotomy may be considered in patients

thought to have gallstone pancreatitis, or CT scanning may be indicated to detect pancreatic necrosis.

Treatment

There is no specific treatment for acute pancreatitis and most attacks settle with conservative management. All patients with suspected severe disease should be managed in a high-dependency or intensive care environment.

Conservative treatment

Pain relief Severe pain requires the administration of opiates; pethidine is frequently prescribed.

Treatment of shock Large volumes of crystalloid solution, plasma or dextran may be needed to maintain circulating blood volume and to correct intravascular hypovolaemia. Oxygen is essential in shocked patients, in whom pulse, blood pressure, urine output and central venous pressure should be monitored (see Ch. 3).

Suppression of pancreatic function Oral fluids and diet are withheld. A nasogastric tube may relieve vomiting but there is no evidence that routine nasogastric intubation is beneficial.

Inhibition of pancreatic secretion or enzymes There is no evidence to support the use of the somatostatin analogue octreotide. Similarly, several trials have shown no advantage to support the use of the antiprotease aprotonin (Trasylol) and gabexate mesilate in the treatment of pancreatitis.

Prevention of infection Antibiotic prophylaxis has been advocated by some as a means of reducing the risk of secondary infection. Others have been concerned that the more widespread use of antibiotics will result in an increased incidence of severe fungal infection. Consensus supports the use of a prophylactic antibiotic such as an intravenous cephalosporin for predicted severe disease.

Inhibition of inflammatory response There is currently no evidence to support the use of agents such as the platelet-activating factor (PAF) antagonist lexipafant as a means of reducing the inflammatory response in acute pancreatitis.

Nutritional support A reduction in acute-phase response and septic complications may result from enteral support rather than intravenous nutrition, although this requires the passage of a nasojejunal tube. There remains doubt as to whether outcome is affected, but enteral nutrition should be favoured where possible in patients with severe pancreatitis and its complications.

Other measures Peritoneal lavage with isotonic crystalloid solutions was once advocated as a means of removing enzymes and vasoactive substances from the peritoneal cavity and so preventing their absorption. However, recent trials have shown no reduction in mortality or morbidity in patients with severe acute pancreatitis.

SUMMARY BOX

Acute pancreatitis

- Acute pancreatitis is defined as an attack of pancreatic inflammation after which the gland returns to anatomical and functional normality.

- Gallstones (50% of cases) and alcohol (30% of cases) are the outstanding causes of acute pancreatitis.

- In one in four cases the attack is severe, as assessed by prognostic factor scoring; in one in four patients with severe pancreatitis the attack proves fatal.

- In most cases the pancreatic inflammation is mild and oedematous, and settles on conservative management. Necrotizing pancreatitis is frequently severe, and often leads to complications, the need for surgery and death.

- Severe attacks of gallstone pancreatitis can often be aborted if a stone occluding the lower end of the biliary tree can be removed by endoscopic papillotomy. Once gallstones have been eradicated, recurrent attacks of gallstone pancreatitis are exceptional.

Endoscopic treatment

When gallstones are suspected to be the cause of acute pancreatitis, consideration may be given to the endoscopic retrieval of such stones from the biliary tree by a basket or balloon following endoscopic sphincterotomy. When patients are admitted with a mild attack of pancreatitis there is no need to institute such active therapy, as in most cases the offending gallstone will pass on into the duodenum spontaneously. In patients with severe disease which does not settle promptly on conservative management, endoscopic stone retrieval may abort the attack and reduce morbidity and mortality. All patients with predicted severe disease and any patient with suspected cholangitis should therefore undergo urgent ERCP and sphincterotomy.

Surgical treatment

Acute pancreatitis is managed conservatively whenever possible, but surgery is indicated under the following circumstances:

1. *When the diagnosis is uncertain.* If alternative causes of hyperamylasaemia are suspected laparotomy is occasionally needed to confirm the diagnosis. It is accepted, however, that unnecessary laparotomy increases morbidity in patients with acute pancreatitis. If acute pancreatitis is present no further action is usually needed, although when gallstones are found, consideration should be given to cholecystectomy.

2. *When the patient fails to improve on conservative management or deteriorates.* If the general condition and other indices (e.g. APACHE II score or C-reactive protein level) are deteriorating, the presence of pancreatic and peripancreatic necrosis must be suspected. A dynamic CT scan is obtained urgently, the term dynamic reflecting the fact that contrast is injected into the circulation so that it can be seen whether all of the pancreas enhances (and therefore

has a blood supply and is not necrotic). If there is extensive necrosis, and particularly when there is evidence of infected necrosis (gas visible radiologically or a positive culture on needle aspiration), urgent laparotomy is usually needed (Fig. 20.4). Necrotic pancreatic and peripancreatic tissue is removed from the lesser sac by blunt dissection with a finger, and after thorough debridement drains are inserted so that lavage can continue in the postoperative period to wash out any further necrotic material. Alternatively the wound can be left open so that repeated debridement can be carried out more easily. A gastrostomy is usually inserted at the time of necrosectomy so that the patient does not have to suffer the discomfort of prolonged nasogastric intubation in the days or weeks that may elapse before duodenal ileus resolves. A feeding jejunostomy may also be inserted so that feeding can continue without reliance on total parenteral nutrition. As might be expected, the mortality of necrotizing pancreatitis is higher (10% or more) than that of oedematous pancreatitis (2% or less).

3. *When gallstones are present.* In the past, patients thought to have gallstone pancreatitis were allowed to settle on conservative management before being investigated radiologically, and were then admitted for elective biliary surgery some 6–8 weeks later. Modern practice favours the 'early' eradication of gallstones in the course of the first admission with pancreatitis. Ultrasonography is used to confirm the presence of stones and surgery is undertaken once the attack of acute pancreatitis has settled. In patients with severe disease who fail to settle promptly, ERCP may both confirm the presence of stones and allow their removal following endoscopic sphincterotomy, thus permitting resolution of the attack. It cannot be overemphasized that patients who have had an attack of gallstone pancreatitis should not be allowed to have another because of failure to eradicate gallstones. When biliary surgery is undertaken it consists of cholecystectomy with operative cholangiography to ensure that there are no stones in the duct system that also require removal. A laparoscopic approach is normally possible in patients with mild disease during the same admission.

4. *When complications develop* (see below).

Complications

Pancreatic pseudocyst

A pancreatic pseudocyst is a collection of pancreatic secretions and inflammatory exudate enclosed in a wall of fibrous or granulation tissue. It differs from a true cyst in that the collection has no epithelial lining and is surrounded by inflammatory tissue. Pseudocysts form most commonly in the lesser sac or in the adjacent retroperitoneum, and differ from acute collections in that they persist for 4 or more weeks from the onset of acute pancreatitis. Small

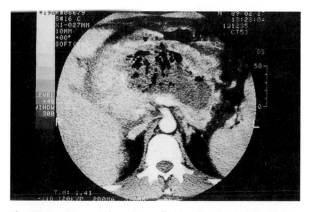

Fig. 20.4 CT scan showing a fluid collection with gas in an area of infected necrosis.

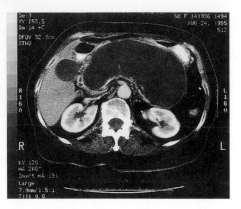

Fig. 20.5 CT scan showing a massive pseudocyst displacing the stomach and duodenum.

pseudocysts are usually asymptomatic and resolve spontaneously. In about 10% of patients larger collections persist and can pose problems.

Clinical features Pseudocysts typically do not declare themselves for some weeks after the episode of pancreatitis. Persistent or intermittent abdominal discomfort and mild to moderate hyperamylasaemia usually signal their presence, and larger collections may compress neighbouring structures to cause vomiting and obstructive jaundice. Ultrasonography is of great value in monitoring the progress of inflammation and in detecting pseudocyst formation, although a CT scan may assist better in determining the appropriate approach to treatment (Fig. 20.5). Some cysts become so large that they are palpable and, in some cases, visible.

Treatment The presence of a pseudocyst is not in itself an indication for surgical treatment. Approximately 50% of asymptomatic pseudocysts will resolve up to 12 weeks following the onset of acute pancreatitis. Treatment is indicated only if the pseudocyst is enlarging, and aims to avoid infection of the contents, haemorrhage or rupture. It normally consists of drainage of the pseudocyst into a Roux loop of jejunum (pseudocyst-jejunostomy), the stomach (pseudocyst-gastrostomy) or duodenum (pseudocyst-duodenostomy), whichever appears most appropriate (Fig. 20.6). As the tissues holding the sutures must be firm, it is desirable to avoid surgery within 6 weeks of the onset of the acute attack to allow the pseudocyst to 'mature' if possible. Ultrasound-guided puncture of the pseudocyst and the insertion of a

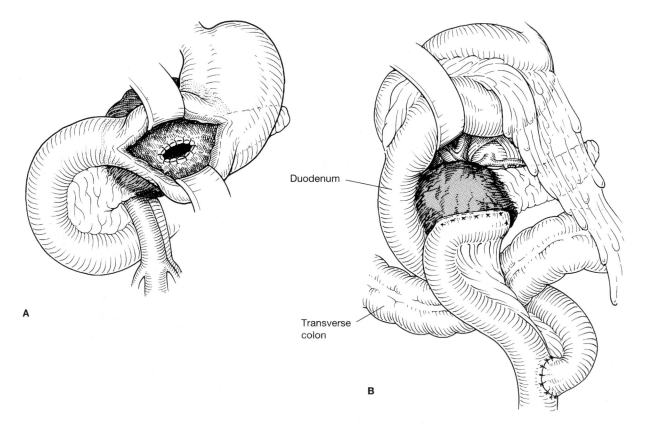

A

Duodenum

Transverse
colon

B

Fig. 20.6 Treatment of pancreatic pseudocyst. **A** Transgastric cystogastrostomy. **B** Cystojejunostomy Roux-en-Y (note that the loop is usually brought retrocolic and not antecolic as shown here).

catheter for external drainage offers an alternative to surgical drainage, particularly in ill patients. However, this approach may allow infection to supervene and is sometimes followed by the development of an external pancreatic fistula. In the absence of necrosis endoscopic cystogastrostomy may be successful, but the relative roles of surgical and endoscopic drainage are yet to be determined.

Pancreatic abscess

A pancreatic abscess is a circumscribed intra-abdominal collection of pus, usually in proximity to the pancreas, containing little or no pancreatic necrosis. The presentation often resembles that of pancreatic pseudocyst, but the patient is usually more ill, and has pyrexia and leukocytosis. The presence of an abscess is confirmed by ultrasonography or CT (Fig. 20.4). Treatment consists of adequate external drainage under antibiotic cover and is achieved by laparotomy, which allows the debridement of any associated necrosis. In the absence of necrosis, percutaneous or endoscopic drainage combined with lavage may be successful.

Pancreatic necrosis

The development of retroperitoneal necrosis is not in itself an indication for surgery. In patients with a secondary deterioration in organ failure scores or systemic signs of infection, a CT or ultrasound-guided fine-needle aspiration of the pancreatic or peripancreatic tissue is required. If the presence of infection is confirmed, surgery is required. Blunt finger debridement is undertaken and multiple retroperitoneal drains are placed before abdominal closure and postoperative lavage. Open packing of the debrided abdomen has been described; others have favoured a minimally invasive technique employing a rigid endoscope.

Progressive jaundice

Persistent or progressively deepening jaundice suggests that a gallstone is impacted at the lower end of the biliary tree, or that the bile duct is compressed by pancreatic inflammation or pseudocyst formation. ERCP can be used to define the problem and remove any impacted stones following endoscopic sphincterotomy. When this approach fails, calculous obstruction can be dealt with by cholecystectomy, operative cholangiography and the extraction of any duct stones.

Persistent duodenal ileus

Protracted ileus usually reflects continuing pancreatic inflammation. In the absence of an indication for operation (e.g. pancreatic necrosis, pseudocyst formation), conservative management is instituted and nutritional status main-

tained by tube feeding (nasoenteric fine-bore tube) or parenteral nutrition while the pancreatitis is resolving.

Gastrointestinal bleeding

Severe acute pancreatitis may be complicated by bleeding from gastritis, erosions or duodenal ulceration, and prophylactic H_2-receptor antagonists are advisable in all such cases. Splenic vein thrombosis is evident in up to 15% of patients dying from acute pancreatitis, and may contribute to blood loss as a result of gastropathy in the early stages and rarely gastric varices in the late stages. If bleeding develops, the guidelines for investigation and management are as outlined in Chapter 19. On rare occasions, laparotomy (preceded if possible by angiography) is required urgently for massive intraperitoneal bleeding due to erosion of blood vessels by the inflammatory process (Fig. 20.7).

Pancreatic ascites

Rarely amylase-rich fluid accumulates within the abdomen. This complication is increasingly associated with an alcohol-related attack in a malnourished patient. This may result from rupture of an immature pseudocyst, or of the pancreatic duct or one of its tributaries. A pleural effusion may be evident. Treatment consists of gut rest and intravenous nutritional support. An ERCP may demonstrate the leak and/or distal obstruction of the pancreatic duct. A pancreatic stent may avoid the need for pancreatic surgery.

Prognosis

Following resolution of the acute attack the prognosis depends on the aetiological factor involved. The biliary tree must be fully investigated in all cases, as gallstone pancre-

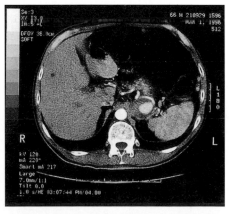

Fig. 20.7 Intravenous contrast-enhanced CT scan showing a splenic artery aneurysm secondary to pancreatic necrosis.

atitis has an excellent long-term outlook once cholecystectomy has been carried out and gallstones have been cleared from the biliary tree.

The prognosis in alcohol-associated pancreatitis is less favourable. Many patients are unwilling or unable to abstain from drinking, and suffer further attacks of acute pancreatitis with progression to chronic pancreatitis.

CHRONIC PANCREATITIS

Chronic pancreatitis is a chronic inflammatory condition characterized by fibrosis and the destruction of exocrine pancreatic tissue.

Aetiology

Chronic pancreatitis is a relatively rare disease but its incidence may be increasing with the growing problem of alcoholism. Although alcohol is much the most common aetiological factor, being implicated in some 70–80% of cases, the factors that predispose some patients to develop chronic pancreatitis are poorly understood. Smoking appears to be an important co-factor. In parts of equatorial Africa, the Middle East and India, adolescents and young adults may suffer from so-called tropical pancreatitis. This was once thought to be a consequence of malnutrition, but it is now thought that toxins in dietary staples such as cassava are responsible and that malnutrition is a result rather than a cause of the condition. Rare causes of chronic pancreatitis include hyperparathyroidism, traumatic duct strictures, gallstones and pancreas divisum, although the significance of the last is still uncertain.

Pathophysiology

The secretion of an unduly viscid pancreatic juice may allow protein plugs to form in the duct system, and these plugs calcify subsequently to form duct stones. Impaired flow of pancreatic juice then leads to inflammation, stricture formation in the duct system, and progressive replacement of the gland by fibrous tissue. Loss of acinar tissue is reflected eventually by steatorrhoea and, in time, loss of islet tissue may lead to diabetes mellitus.

Clinical features

Pain is the outstanding feature in most cases. It is characteristically epigastric with marked radiation through to the back, and is often eased by leaning forward or getting down on all fours. Some patients experience marked pain in one or both loins and gain relief by lying on one side. In some cases the pain is precipitated by eating, or the patient learns to avoid certain foods, notably fatty foods. The application of heat sometimes brings relief, and permanent discoloration of the skin may reflect the continued use of heat pads or hot water bottles. The progressive use of powerful opioid analgesics can result in drug dependency.

Weight loss is usual and reflects a combination of inadequate intake, a poor diet and malabsorption. Steatorrhoea is common, the bowel motion being pale, bulky, offensive, floating on water, and difficult to flush. Diabetes mellitus develops in about one-third of patients, but islet function is often preserved for some years following the onset of exocrine insufficiency.

Other less common manifestations of chronic pancreatitis include transient or intermittent obstructive jaundice, duodenal obstruction and splenic vein thrombosis (leading to splenomegaly, hypersplenism and gastric and oesophageal varices).

Investigation and diagnosis

Abdominal plain films and CT scans may reveal the speckled calcification typical of chronic pancreatitis. Ultrasonography and CT can be used to detect pancreatic enlargement, and may also reveal pseudocysts, dilatation of the pancreatic duct and splenomegaly. MRCP or ERCP is of great value and must always be performed if surgery is contemplated. The architecture of the pancreatic duct is revealed and any compression of the biliary tree can be evaluated. When investigating these patients it must be borne in mind that cancer of the pancreas may block the duct system and cause pancreatitis, and that the two conditions can coexist.

Pancreatic endocrine function is assessed by measurement of random blood glucose levels, supplemented if necessary by a glucose tolerance test.

Exocrine function can be measured in a multitude of ways, but insufficiency may not be detectable until 90% of the pancreatic parenchyma is destroyed. Furthermore, function tests do not differentiate between chronic pancreatitis and pancreatic cancer. If necessary, faecal fat excretion can be measured over 3–5 days while the patient's fat intake is controlled at 100 g/day (normal individuals excrete less than 5 g/day), or fat absorption can be measured by isotopic labelling of dietary fat. In practice, the key question is: does the patient have clinically obvious steatorrhoea? Duodenal intubation studies aimed at measuring pancreatic secretion after food or hormonal stimulation are now seldom employed. More often, a trial of oral pancreatic supplements is attempted.

Management

The diagnosis of chronic pancreatitis is not in itself an indication for surgery. Considerable clinical judgement is needed to determine the need for, and timing of, operation. In most cases intractable pain is the cardinal indication for surgery; operation does not restore pancreatic endocrine and exocrine function and at best merely slows their decline.

Conservative management

This consists of encouraging abstinence from alcohol, relief of pain, treatment of exocrine and endocrine insufficiency, and attempts to improve nutritional status. Relief of pain is notoriously difficult; opiates are avoided if possible, but their use may prove essential. Coeliac plexus block is rarely of value and at best provides relief for a few weeks or months. Diabetes mellitus is treated by appropriate means (diet, oral hypoglycaemic agents or insulin). Steatorrhoea is treated by pancreatic exocrine supplements, and modern position-release preparations (e.g. Creon) minimize the enzymic degradation of the supplements by acid and pepsin during their passage through the stomach. Oral pancreatic enzyme supplements in the absence of exocrine insufficiency have not been shown conclusively to reduce analgesia consumption.

Surgical treatment

This is indicated if pain is intractable; when neighbouring structures such as the common bile duct, duodenum, portal or splenic vein are compressed sufficiently to produce symptoms; when pseudocysts or abscesses develop; or when cancer cannot be excluded.

In general, the objective is to relieve pain or compression while at the same time conserving as much pancreatic tissue and function as possible. In about one-third of cases the pancreatic duct system is sufficiently dilated to allow these objectives to be achieved by a drainage operation. Demonstration of ductal anatomy is essential in determining the most appropriate option, and operative pancreatography or ultrasonography is mandatory if ERCP has not been successful. The method of drainage used depends on the extent of the obstruction. There is rarely a single area of narrowing close to the sphincter of Oddi, so that sphincteroplasty rarely suffices. More frequently there are multiple strictures throughout the length of the duct, which must be slit open so that a Roux loop of jejunum can be brought up and anastomosed to the entire length of the pancreatic duct as a longitudinal pancreaticojejunostomy (Fig. 20.8). Approximately 70% of patients remain pain free or substantially improved when assessed 5 years after this operation, and the avoid-

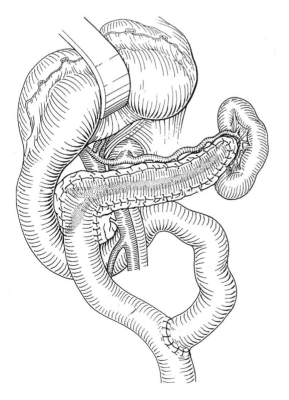

Fig. 20.8 Pancreatic duct decompression by longitudinal pancreaticojejunostomy.

SUMMARY BOX

Chronic pancreatitis

- Chronic pancreatitis is defined as pancreatic inflammation in which the pancreas does not return to anatomical and/or functional normality.

- The disease is frequently (but by no means invariably) associated with alcohol abuse, and is characterized by blockage of the pancreatic duct system by protein plugs, in which calcification occurs.

- Other causes of chronic pancreatitis include hyperparathyroidism, cholelithiasis, duct obstruction due to trauma, mucoviscidosis, haemochromatosis, pancreas divisum and nutritional disorders.

- Pain is the cardinal symptom in chronic pancreatitis; other symptoms include weight loss, steatorrhoea, obstructive jaundice and diabetes mellitus.

- Surgery is indicated if pain cannot be controlled by conservative means or if complications ensue. If the pancreatic duct system is distended, pancreaticojejunostomy is the operation of choice; if the duct system is not distended, partial or even total pancreatectomy may be necessary.

ance of resection often means that pancreatic function does not worsen appreciably. As with all aspects of chronic pancreatitis, the results of pancreaticojejunostomy are better in patients who continue to abstain from alcohol. There is little strong evidence to support a less invasive approach of ERCP, pancreatic stent placement with or without the extraction of pancreatic duct calculi.

If drainage is not feasible, part or all of the pancreas will have to be resected. This is a more difficult undertaking and may precipitate endocrine and exocrine insufficiency or compound existing insufficiency. In a few patients chronic pancreatitis is confined to the distal part of the gland, so that distal pancreatectomy is appropriate. In many patients, the disease is more severe in the head of the gland, and the Whipple operation (pancreaticoduodenectomy, see p. 311) is indicated. This approach has recently been avoided in favour of a procedure that combines a 'coring out' of the pancreatic head with pancreaticojejunostomy. In some patients the entire pancreas appears to be so diseased that total pancreatectomy is undertaken. This must be regarded as a last resort, given the permanent brittle diabetes and exocrine insufficiency that follow, and careful patient selection is vital. As with drainage operations, approximately 70% of patients are pain free or substantially improved when assessed 5 years following resection.

NEOPLASMS OF THE PANCREAS

Neoplasms of the exocrine pancreas are common and are almost always malignant, whereas neoplasms of the endocrine pancreas are rare and may be benign.

NEOPLASMS OF THE EXOCRINE PANCREAS

Benign pancreatic neoplasms such as cystadenomas frequently remain asymptomatic until their size causes pressure on surrounding structures. Such lesions are more common in females and, unlike pseudocysts, they are not associated with a preceding history of pancreatitis or alcohol abuse. The serum amylase is usually normal. Imaging techniques may not reliably differentiate such lesions from a pseudocyst (Fig. 20.9). Resection of the affected part of the pancreas is usually needed, but the prognosis thereafter is excellent.

Malignant neoplasms of the pancreas are almost invariably ductal adenocarcinomas. Acinar cell carcinomas, cystadenocarcinomas and sarcomas are all rare.

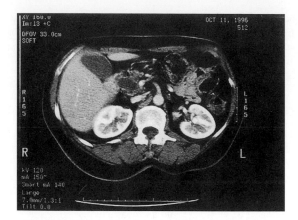

Fig. 20.9 CT scan showing a mucinous cystadenoma in the head of the pancreas.

ADENOCARCINOMA OF THE PANCREAS

Aetiology

The cause of pancreatic cancer is unknown. It is increasing in frequency and is now the fourth commonest cause of cancer death in males and the sixth commonest in females in many western countries. It affects approximately 100 per million of the population in the UK and USA, and accounts for about 10% of all cancers of the alimentary system. It carries a dismal prognosis.

Men are more commonly affected than women and the peak incidence lies between 55 and 70 years of age. Factors thought to increase the risk of pancreatic cancer include tobacco smoking and a high-fat high-protein diet. The disease may occur in family clusters.

Pathology

The great majority of adenocarcinomas arise from ductal rather than acinar tissue. The head of the gland is at least two thirds more commonly affected than the body or tail. The cancer spreads locally and disseminates to nerve bundles, local lymphatics, and to lymph nodes around the gland. Regardless of the site of origin, spread outside the reach of surgical cure is usual by the time the disease is diagnosed. It is hardly surprising that 90% of patients are dead within a year of the diagnosis being made, and that survival beyond 5 years is truly exceptional.

Cancer arising from the ampullary region, distal common bile duct and duodenum has a much better outlook than cancer of the pancreas. It may be that biliary obstruction occurs so early that the tumour is discovered at a stage where resection is still curative.

Clinical features

Obstructive jaundice, with the passage of dark urine and pale stools, is the common presenting feature of cancer of the head of the pancreas. It is usually progressive, in contrast to the intermittent jaundice of calculous obstruction. Pruritus is frequently troublesome. In keeping with Courvoisier's law, the gallbladder is frequently palpable in patients with obstructive jaundice due to pancreatic cancer, but is often felt more laterally than might be expected from its usual surface markings. When cancer arises in the body and tail of the pancreas, jaundice is more likely to be due to liver metastases or the involvement of nodes in the porta hepatis.

Weight loss is invariable and may be the first symptom, reflecting a combination of inadequate intake, malabsorption and depressed liver function. Cancer of the pancreas was once said to cause painless obstructive jaundice, but pain is present in about 70% of patients at the time of diagnosis. Most patients have ill-defined upper abdominal pain or discomfort and neoplastic infiltration can cause severe back pain, which is an ominous symptom signalling unresectability.

Pancreatic insufficiency is common in that diabetes mellitus or impaired glucose tolerance is present in one-third of patients. Steatorrhoea due to impaired digestion and absorption of fat is common, and the associated failure to absorb the fat-soluble vitamin K may cause coagulopathy.

Trousseau's sign of thrombophlebitis migrans is a late manifestation in some patients but is not specific for this form of cancer.

Investigation and diagnosis

Many patients with pancreatic cancer are anaemic at the time of diagnosis. A stool examination revealing occult blood loss should, however, raise the possible diagnosis of an ampullary tumour. In patients with jaundice, its obstructive nature is confirmed by examination of the urine, stool and blood (see Ch. 19). Ultrasonography will detect dilatation of the biliary tree, exclude gallstones, and may show the mass lesion in the pancreas or reveal liver metastases. CT may be used for the same purposes, but is no more accurate than ultrasonography in assessing the pancreatic tumour. The more recent introduction of high-quality spiral (helical) CT with thin-cut examination of the pancreas has improved the staging of pancreatic malignancy (Fig. 20.10). However, neither CT nor ultrasonography can differentiate between neoplasia and chronic pancreatitis with absolute accuracy. If biliary obstruction is present, cholangiography is used to define the site and nature of the obstruction; in the past ERCP was preferred to percutaneous transhepatic cholangiography as it causes less discomfort, displays both pancreatic and biliary duct

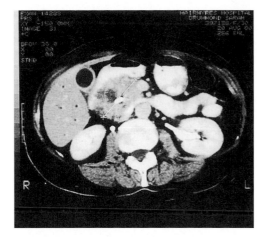

Fig. 20.10 CT scan showing a 6 cm adenocarcinoma in the head of the pancreas. A stent is evident within the invaded bile duct and the tumour comes into contact with the superior mesenteric vein.

systems, and readily allows therapeutic intervention such as stent insertion (see below; Fig. 20.11). A common finding in pancreatic cancer is the 'double duct sign', in which both the pancreatic duct and the common bile duct are narrowed as they pass through the neoplasm. Endoscopy

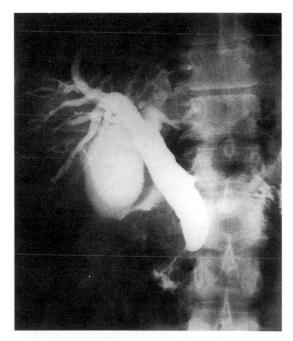

Fig. 20.11 A cholangiogram obtained at ERCP demonstrates a dilated gallbladder and biliary tree above a pancreatic cancer obstructing the intrapancreatic portion of the common bile duct.

also allows lesions in the gastroduodenal lumen to be biopsied, and pancreatic juice and bile can be sampled for cytological examination. MRCP offers a non-invasive and more accurate means of assessing potential malignant biliary obstruction, and may in the future allow better assessment of tumour resectability.

Pancreatic function tests are of no value in diagnosis. A number of circulating tumour markers (e.g. CA 19–9) have been described in pancreatic cancer, but their lack of sensitivity and specificity has prevented their use in screening and diagnosis. They may, however, be useful in the follow-up of treated patients and in the detection of recurrence following resection.

Every effort should be made to obtain cytological or histological confirmation of the malignant nature of any mass lesions revealed radiologically. This is particularly important if surgery is not contemplated, as a number of benign lesions (e.g. chronic pancreatitis) can masquerade as malignancy, whereas a number of malignancies (e.g. lymphoma) that can mimic pancreatic cancer have a far better prognosis if recognized and treated appropriately. Pancreatic tissue can be obtained safely by percutaneous fine-needle aspiration or Tru-cut needle biopsy under ultrasound or CT scan guidance, although this is not generally undertaken if resection is being considered.

If radical surgery is contemplated, selective angiography is occasionally used in some centres to display the vascular anatomy and detect invasion of major vessels, such as the portal vein, that would preclude resection. CT scanning of the abdomen should be undertaken to assess local invasion of the tumour and to exclude distant metastases. The use of laparoscopy has been promoted to exclude dissemination of disease (peritoneal seedlings or liver metastases) that might not be easily detected by conventional radiological imaging and that would preclude radical surgery.

Management

Surgical resection offers the only prospect of cure, but only about 10% of patients are candidates for radical surgery. In most cases the presence of advanced disease, advanced age or intercurrent disease means that palliation is the objective of management. In jaundiced patients, coagulopathy should be corrected by the parenteral administration of vitamin K. Patients should be well hydrated to avoid postoperative renal failure, and prophylactic antibiotics should be given.

Curative treatment

The standard operation of radical pancreaticoduodenectomy (Whipple's procedure) entails block resection of the head of the pancreas, the distal half of the stomach, the duodenum, gallbladder and common bile duct. Reconstruction is achieved by anastomoses between the jejunum and the pancreatic remnant, common hepatic duct and gastric remnant, respectively (Fig. 20.12). The operation aims to eradicate the cancer and yet retain enough pancreas to sustain endocrine and exocrine function. The procedure used to carry a prohibitively high operative mortality, but in specialist hands this should now be less than 1–2%. It has been suggested that prior drainage of the biliary tree by endoscopic or percutaneous means may introduce infection and thereby increase the risk of postoperative infection. In practice, the majority of patients have already undergone stent placement at the time of diagnostic ERCP. Although 5-year survival rates following resection of 20% have been reported in a series of selected patients, overall survival rates are little better than those obtained by palliative surgery and cure remains exceptional. Attempts to improve the radicality of resection by removing all of the pancreas have proved disappointing: total pancreatectomy offers no advantage in terms of operative mortality or long-term survival, and also confers permanent diabetes and exocrine insufficiency. Although adjuvant chemoradiation therapy is favoured in the USA following pancreatic resection, there is no strong evidence to support its routine use.

The prospects for patients with cancer of the periampullary region, distal common bile duct or duodenum are less gloomy, with 5-year survival rates ranging from 20 to 40%.

Palliative treatment

The relief of jaundice, pruritus, pain and duodenal obstruction is the objective of palliative treatment. In the past, operation was usually undertaken to bypass the obstructed biliary system (cholecyst-jejunostomy or choledocho-jejunostomy) and gastrojejunostomy was carried out to treat or prevent blockage of the duodenum by continued tumour growth. In many cases operation can now be avoided by the insertion of a prosthetic stent following endoscopic papillotomy. If this fails it may still be possible to avoid surgery by inserting the stent via the percutaneous transhepatic route. Stenting suffers from the disadvantages that it cannot deal with or prevent duodenal obstruction, and that the stents frequently encrust and block after about 3 months, so that their replacement becomes necessary. Some surgeons have therefore promoted a policy of surgical bypass in selected patients with unresectable malignancy.

Mean survival following palliative intervention is only about 4 months and few patients live for more than a year. Prolonged survival raises doubt about the diagnosis of cancer, underlining the need to have cytological or histological confirmation of the diagnosis in all cases.

Although there is evidence that survival rates can be improved by radiotherapy and/or chemotherapy, the benefits obtainable with currently available regimens do not

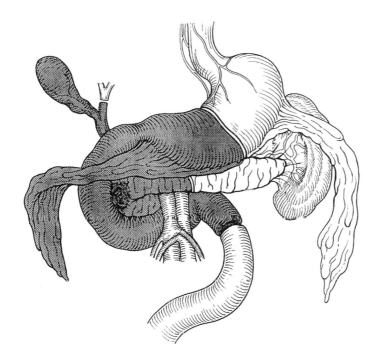

A

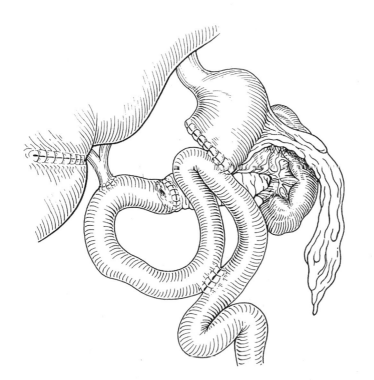

B

Fig. 20.12 Whipple procedure
showing A the area resected and
B the anastomoses performed. (The
gallbladder is usually removed.)

justify their use outside the context of controlled clinical trials. Pain relief is a vital part of the management of advanced pancreatic cancer, and coeliac plexus block should be considered if pain cannot be controlled by appropriate analgesic therapy. In some patients with intractable pain, thoracoscopic splanchnicectomy has been advocated.

NEOPLASMS OF THE ENDOCRINE PANCREAS

These rare neoplasms may give rise to defined syndromes as a result of the oversecretion of peptide products, but some tumours that appear histologically to be of neuro-endocrine origin neither contain identifiable products on immunohistochemistry nor give rise to circulating products. The commonest islet cell tumour is the insulinoma, which has an annual incidence of 1 per million of the population. It arises from B cells and results in the oversecretion of insulin, with episodes of hypoglycaemia. Gastrinomas arise from G cells and give rise to the Zollinger–Ellison syndrome (see Ch. 18). Tumours of the A cells producing glucagon are known as glucagonomas, and excessive secretion of vasoactive intestinal peptide (VIP) from vipomas produces pancreatic cholera (see below). Some tumours

> **SUMMARY BOX**
>
> **Pancreatic cancer**
>
> - Ductal adenocarcinoma of the pancreas is predominantly a disease of the ageing population and has shown a threefold increase in incidence during this century.
> - Aetiological factors include a high-fat high-protein diet and smoking, and one-third of patients have abnormal glucose tolerance.
> - As the head of the pancreas is the commonest site for tumour formation, obstructive jaundice is commonly the presenting complaint. Other features include weight loss, steatorrhoea and diabetes mellitus.
> - Late presentation is the rule and 90% of patients are dead within a year of diagnosis.
> - Only 10% of patients are potential candidates for curative resection (Whipple's operation) and overall 5-year survival rates are close to zero.
> - Endoscopic stenting now offers an alternative to palliative surgical bypass of the obstructed biliary system, but duodenal obstruction by tumour is also a problem in up to 10% of patients.

may produce more than one peptide, or the pattern of secretion may vary with time. A proportion of patients have tumours and/or hyperplasia of the parathyroid glands or anterior pituitary gland and are regarded as suffering from multiple endocrine neoplasia type I (MEN I; see Ch. 26).

INSULINOMA

Insulinomas are usually single, small (< 2 cm in diameter) benign tumours which may affect any part of the pancreas. Multiple insulinomas are usually associated with MEN I. Less than 10% of insulinomas are malignant, but such tumours are often larger than 2 cm in diameter.

Clinical features

Unlike normal islet cells, which secrete appropriate amounts of insulin in response to changing glucose concentrations, insulinomas secrete insulin autonomously and inappropriately. The resulting hypoglycaemia may give rise to mild symptoms, but over the years there is gradual intellectual and motor impairment with insidious personality changes. More severe attacks of hypoglycaemia can produce sweating, palpitations, tremulousness, and a wide variety of transient psychoneurological symptoms with episodes of bizarre behaviour. Because of memory lapses the patient may not recall these events, and the diagnosis only comes to light when they are found in a hypoglycaemic coma. Attacks are typically precipitated by fasting and relieved by taking glucose. Many patients become obese because of the associated hunger. Some patients are misdiagnosed as suffering from psychiatric illness, epilepsy, alcoholism or brain tumours, and it is not unusual for 2–3 years to elapse between the first symptom and establishment of the correct diagnosis.

Diagnosis

The diagnosis of insulinoma demands a high index of suspicion and rests on:

1. The demonstration of hypoglycaemia after fasting (blood glucose concentration of less than 2.2 mmol/L after an overnight 12–14-hour fast)
2. The confirmation that hypoglycaemia is due to inappropriate insulin secretion.

Insulin is not normally detectable when glucose levels are subnormal, but in patients with insulinoma serial plasma insulin levels remain inappropriately high in the face of falling glucose levels.

Factitious hypoglycaemia caused by insulin injection is a rare problem occasionally encountered in members of medical and nursing staff. It can be excluded by measuring C-peptide levels at the same time as insulin levels are determined. One molecule of C-peptide is normally produced for every molecule of endogenous insulin. If exogenous insulin is being administered, there is no corresponding C-peptide production.

Once the presence of an insulinoma has been confirmed, a variety of methods can be used to localize the tumour(s). Ultrasonography, CT and selective angiography are successful in less than 50% of cases owing to the small size of the tumour. Selective venous sampling from a catheter inserted into the portal and splenic veins through the liver allows plotting of the concentration of insulin at various sites, and may define the point at which excess secretion is entering the venous system. Although successful in some 90% of cases, the method is invasive and in some centres is not used routinely. Endoscopic ultrasonography has been introduced recently and appears to offer a safe, accurate method of localization. In many centres experienced in the management of such lesions, preoperative assessment is limited to confirmation of the inappropriate secretion of insulin.

Treatment

Surgical removal of the tumour is the treatment of choice, although patients can be controlled temporarily by diazoxide (a diabetogenic antihypertensive drug; 5 mg/kg daily in three divided doses, given orally). At laparotomy the pancreas is fully exposed and carefully palpated. All but a

few lesions will be evident to the surgeon's palpating hand or on intraoperative ultrasound. Most insulinomas can be enucleated, but resection of the affected part of the pancreas is occasionally necessary. If the tumour cannot be found, distal pancreatectomy used to be recommended in the mistaken belief that insulinomas were more common in the body and tail of the gland. If no tumour is found it is better to close the abdomen, control hypoglycaemia with diazoxide, and carry out interval selective venous sampling or endoscopic ultrasonography in order to localize the lesion for reoperation.

If a malignant insulinoma is found confined to the pancreas, resection is indicated. Chemotherapy using streptozotocin may prove useful if there is unresectable or metastatic disease, although this is often poorly tolerated because of its toxic side-effects. Symptoms of hyperinsulinism can be controlled by diazoxide if necessary.

GLUCAGONOMA

Excessive glucagon production may give rise to a syndrome of necrotizing dermatitis, painful glossitis, stomatitis, bowel upset, weight loss, diabetes mellitus and anaemia. Plasma levels of glucagon are raised and the tumour may be defined by CT scanning or angiography.

Resection of the tumour (which is sometimes benign) often reverses these effects. Streptozotocin may be beneficial in patients with non-resectable tumours and the somatostatin analogue octreotide (initially 50 μg twice daily by subcutaneous injection) may help to control symptoms of this rare tumour.

VIPOMA

Vipomas may be solitary and benign but half are malignant. Oversecretion of VIP (vasoactive intestinal peptide) causes a syndrome of profuse watery diarrhoea, hypokalaemia and achlorhydria also known as 'pancreatic cholera'. The systemic upset may be profound, with daily loss of 5 L or more of potassium-rich stool and the production of marked metabolic alkalosis. The patient may be confused, and ileus and abdominal distension may lead to intestinal obstruction being suspected. Alternatively, symptoms may be intermittent and the diagnosis so delayed that malignant tumours have metastasized by the time they are discovered.

Diagnosis rests on a high index of suspicion, recognition of the typical syndrome and the detection of increased levels of VIP in the circulating blood. The tumours are often large and demonstrable on CT and angiography.

SUMMARY BOX

Insulinoma

- Insulinoma is the commonest endocrine tumour of the pancreas (but is still rare, having an annual incidence of 1 per million of the population)
- The diagnosis of insulinoma is often delayed as the episodes of hypoglycaemia (usually precipitated by fasting and relieved by food) are often misinterpreted (e.g. as being due to brain tumour, psychiatric upset, epilepsy).
- The diagnosis is confirmed by demonstrating that fasting produces hypoglycaemia in association with inappropriately *high* insulin levels.
- Measurement of C-peptide levels (one molecule of C-peptide is released for every molecule of insulin) excludes factitious hypoglycaemia.
- Most insulinomas are small benign tumours which may be difficult to locate; they are usually treated by enucleation.

Adequate fluid and electrolyte replacement is essential before surgery. The aim is to remove the tumour, although this may necessitate total or subtotal pancreatectomy. In the case of solitary tumours, surgery may be curative. In unresectable cases and those with metastases, streptozotocin or octreotide may be useful in controlling symptoms.

21 The spleen

O.J. Garden

ANATOMY

The spleen is a friable blood-filled organ lying in the left upper quadrant of the abdomen behind the ninth, 10th and 11th ribs. It weighs about 150 g, is ellipsoid in shape and lies with its long axis along the line of the 10th rib. The convex outer surface of the spleen lies against the diaphragm and its lower pole rests on the splenic flexure of the colon below. Its concave inner surface is related to the fundus of the stomach, the tail of the pancreas and the upper pole of the right kidney. It has a fibrous capsule and, except at its hilus, is covered by peritoneum, which is reflected as ligaments running to adjacent organs. These are the lienorenal, lienogastric and lienocolic ligaments. The phrenicocolic ligament, which runs between the splenic flexure of the colon and the undersurface of the diaphragm, provides additional support.

The tortuous splenic artery arises from the coeliac axis (Fig. 21.1), which carries 40% of the splanchnic blood flow into the spleen. Venous blood drains into the portal venous system via the splenic vein. The splenic vessels are closely related to the pancreas; the artery runs within the lienorenal ligament and branches reach the splenic hilus, the only part of the spleen without a peritoneal covering. Further branches continue as the short gastric vessels that run within the lienogastric ligament to the upper part of the greater curvature of the stomach. Both the lienogastric and

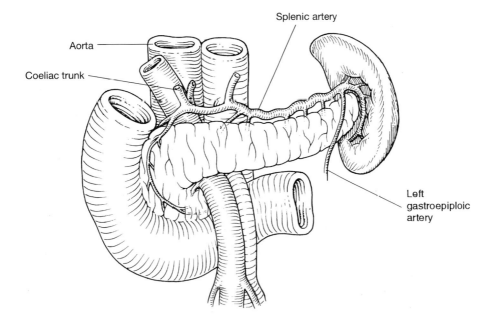

Fig. 21.1   Arterial blood supply of the spleen.

lienorenal ligaments and their contained vessels must be divided during splenectomy.

Some 25% of the lymphoid tissue of the body is contained within the spleen and forms its **white pulp**, which consists of lymphoid follicles (Malpighian bodies) and lymphatic tissue, containing lymphocytes, macrophages and plasma cells. These cells migrate to the spleen from the bone marrow and 30–50% of them are thymus dependent. The **red pulp** is a loose honeycomb of reticular tissue that contains the splenic sinusoids. The blood vessels are carried into the pulp along fibrous trabeculae, which are continuous with the capsule. Erythrocytes move in and out of the pulp tissue, so that 1% of the body's red cells and 20–30% of its platelets are sequestrated at any given moment.

The pulp of the spleen is not provided with lymphatic vessels and those present are confined to the capsule and trabeculae. Lymph nodes close to the hilus thus receive more lymph from the stomach than from the spleen, and drain to nodes along the splenic artery.

Normally the spleen is impalpable and cannot be percussed. When enlarged, it extends downwards and medially below the costal margin. It is then best palpated bimanually, with the patient lying on their right side with the left side turned slightly forward. The distinctive notch on its antero-inferior border may then be felt. On percussion an enlarged spleen causes dullness over the ninth rib in the midaxillary line. Splenomegaly is normally confirmed by abdominal ultrasound or CT scan.

FUNCTION

Haemopoiesis

In fetal life the spleen is a source of red blood cells and granulocytes. Extramedullary haemopoiesis occurs only in the myeloproliferative syndromes. In humans the spleen does not act as a reservoir for blood.

Filtration of blood cells

Normal blood cells pass through the spleen unchanged, but abnormal and ageing cells are trapped. It has been estimated that 20 ml of red cells are phagocytosed daily. White cells and platelets, particularly when coated with antibodies, are also removed. Following splenectomy there is an increased number of misshapen red cells in the peripheral blood, some containing nuclear remnants (Howell–Jolly bodies) and others containing clumps of iron (siderocytes).

Immunological function

The spleen is an important site for effecting both cell-mediated and humoral immunity. Following splenectomy, immunological responses are impaired.

INDICATIONS FOR SPLENECTOMY

Although the recommendation to remove the spleen often comes from the haematologist, the surgeon must be aware of the indications for splenectomy and the criteria that should be fulfilled before accepting a patient for operation. The common indications are outlined below.

Trauma

In recent years there has been an increasing tendency to avoid unnecessary laparotomy in trauma patients thought to have minor splenic injury. In those patients submitted to laparotomy, splenectomy is indicated only if the organ cannot be conserved by the use of haemostatic agents, local suturing or partial splenectomy. Spleens involved by pathological conditions, such as portal hypertension, polycythaemia and infective mononucleosis, are prone to rupture with minor trauma. A temporary improvement in the clinical state may precede a sudden deterioration following splenic rupture. Awareness and careful observation are critical, particularly in patients with suspected or known splenic trauma, such as subcapsular haematoma, which can lead to 'delayed rupture'. Splenic injuries are considered in more detail in Chapter 21.

In children, the conservative, non-operative approach to the management of splenic injury is now standard practice. Patients require to be closely monitored in a paediatric intensive care unit with appropriately trained paediatric surgeons close at hand. The need to replace more than half of a child's circulating blood volume (80 mL/kg) would be an indication to intervene surgically.

Haemolytic anaemias

Hereditary spherocytosis

In this autosomal dominant disorder the red blood cells are spherical rather than biconcave, are unduly fragile, and are destroyed almost exclusively in the spleen. Excess haemolysis results in anaemia, jaundice and splenic enlargement. It is a disease of remissions and relapses, with 'haemolytic crises' requiring transfusion. Pigment gallstones occur in 30–60% of cases.

Splenectomy is indicated in all cases when health is impaired, when severe haemolytic crises have occurred and when gallbladder disease is present. However, it should be avoided before the age of 3–4 years. If gallstones are present, cholecystectomy is carried out simultaneously. Both procedures can be performed by laparoscopic means.

Acquired haemolytic anaemias

Excess haemolysis may occur following exposure to agents such as chemicals, drugs or infection, with extensive burns, or it may be an immune phenomenon. In the latter the red cells are coated with an autoantibody, which can be detected by agglutination when antihuman globulin is added to a suspension of the patient's erythrocytes (positive Coombs' test).

Autoimmune haemolytic anaemia affects predominantly middle-aged women and causes severe haemolytic crises superimposed on a background of mild anaemia. Treatment consists of steroid therapy. Splenectomy is indicated if treatment fails from the outset or if there is a fall in the haemoglobin following the reduction or cessation of steroids.

The purpuras

Idiopathic thrombocytopenic purpura (ITP)

In this disease, the presence of autoantibodies causes the premature removal of platelets. The low platelet count is associated with plentiful megakaryocytes in the bone marrow. Cyclical bleeding from the gastrointestinal tract and other sites is associated with petechiae and ecchymoses. Platelet counts are below 50×10^9/L, bleeding time is prolonged but clotting time is normal. The spleen is palpably enlarged in only 2–3% of patients, and dense adhesions may form around it.

Clinical course The disease may be chronic or acute. The *acute* form often presents in children and there is usually a short history of a preceding viral illness. Spontaneous remission is common and the response to steroids or splenectomy is excellent. The *chronic* form is characterized by a course of remissions and relapses which may last several years. Its response to steroids is poor and the outcome after splenectomy less satisfactory.

Choice of treatment The acute form of the disease is treated initially with steroids. A rapid increase in the platelet count is associated with a good prospect of complete and lasting remission when therapy is stopped. If steroid therapy does not result in rapid remission splenectomy is advised, except for acute ITP in children, as spontaneous remission is likely. Splenectomy is curative in about 70% of patients with the chronic form of the disease, and is usually recommended if a patient has two relapses on steroid therapy. Patients may remain asymptomatic despite a low platelet count of $20–30 \times 10^9$/L following splenectomy.

Secondary thrombocytopenia

Splenectomy is contraindicated in secondary haemorrhagic purpuras, although it may be advised if hypersplenism is associated with symptomatic secondary thrombocytopenia.

Hypersplenism

This syndrome consists of splenomegaly and pancytopenia in the presence of an apparently normal bone marrow and the absence of an autoimmune disorder. There is sequestration and destruction of blood cells in the spleen, affecting predominantly white cells and platelets.

Hypersplenism may complicate a number of inflammatory conditions (e.g. rheumatoid arthritis), infections (e.g. malaria), and myeloproliferative and lymphoproliferative disorders. In portal hypertension splenic congestion frequently leads to splenomegaly and hypersplenism.

The effects of hypersplenism include expansion of the total blood volume to fill the increased vascular spaces of the enlarged spleen and splanchnic bed. There is increased pooling of cells within the enlarged spleen, and excess destruction. In the peripheral blood there is anaemia, leukopenia and thrombocytopenia, but marrow turnover is increased, with reticulocytosis and leukoerythroblastosis. Increased amounts of urobilinogen are present in the urine.

The removal of a grossly enlarged spleen carries appreciable morbidity and mortality and puts the patient at long-term risk from serious bacterial infection. Splenectomy must not be undertaken lightly, and the haematologist and surgeon should take into account the degree of cytopenia, the extent of splenic enlargement, the amount of discomfort caused, and the incidence of recurrent infections from leukopenia. The prognosis of the underlying cause of the hypersplenism and the potential difficulty of the surgical procedure should be taken into account.

Segmental portal hypertension

A localized form of portal hypertension associated with hypersplenism and oesophagogastric varices may follow occlusion of the splenic vein. Thrombosis may result from acute or chronic pancreatitis (Fig. 21.2), or the vessel may become compromised by direct invasion from a carcinoma

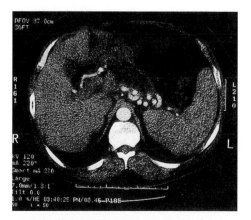

Fig. 21.2 Moderate enlargement of the spleen in a patient with segmental portal hypertension following an episode of acute pancreatitis. Contrast is seen in a tortuous splenic artery. The splenic vein did not visualize on this examination.

of the pancreas. Gastric varices are particularly prominent in this condition and often communicate directly with short gastric veins. Acute variceal haemorrhage in this situation is best managed by splenectomy with ligation of the vessels on the greater curvature of the stomach, as endoscopic sclerotherapy or banding of gastric varices is difficult. Recurrent haemorrhage is unusual following surgery and the prognosis is favourable, given that there is often no associated liver disease.

Proliferative disorders

Myelofibrosis

It is recognized that this condition is due to an abnormal pro-liferation of mesenchymal elements in the bone marrow, spleen, liver and lymph nodes, and that extramedullary haemopoiesis occurs at many sites. Most patients present over the age of 50 years. The spleen may be grossly enlarged and splenic infarcts may occur. Splenectomy decreases transfu-sion requirements and, by relieving the discomfort of a grossly enlarged spleen, also improves symptoms.

Lymphomas

In non-Hodgkin's lymphoma splenectomy is now only indi-cated in the rare event that a primary neoplasm is confined to the spleen. However, in both myelo- and lymphoprolifer-ative conditions splenectomy may be indicated to reduce transfusion requirements when hypersplenism is a problem.

Other tumours

Apart from lymphomas and leukaemias, tumours of the spleen are rare. Haemangiomas (capillary or cavernous) may reach sufficient size to cause splenic enlargement with a consumptive coagulopathy and haemorrhagic tendency. Most haemangiomas are recognized at operation, when the spleen should be removed.

Miscellaneous conditions

Cysts of the spleen

Cysts of the spleen are rare. They are usually single (Fig. 21.3) but occasionally multiple. Single cysts may be congenital, degenerative or parasitic.

Congenital cysts are due to an embryonic defect and result in a dermoid-like lesion. They are lined by flattened epithelium and contain thin bloodstained fluid or thick creamy material, sometimes with hair and teeth.

Degenerative cysts result from liquefaction of an infarct or haematoma. There may be a past history of minor trauma. The wall is fibrous and often calcified, and the cyst is filled with brownish fluid or paste-like material.

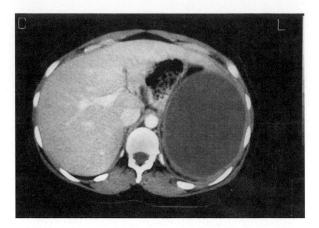

Fig. 21.3 On this CT scan the upper pole of the spleen has been completely replaced by a relatively thick-walled cyst. There was a past history of minor abnormal trauma 5 years earlier.

Parasitic cysts are usually acquired through contact with dogs and are due to infection with *Echinococcus granulosus* (hydatid disease).

Splenic cysts normally cause no symptoms and are often discovered fortuitously when splenic enlargement is found on clinical examination, abnormal calcification is shown on abdominal X-ray, or abdominal scanning is being under-taken to investigate other intraabdominal pathology. Symptomatic cysts may present with left upper quadrant pain radiating to the back or left shoulder. The lesion may be recognized by CT or ultrasound scan, investigations which are usually sufficient to characterize the nature of the cyst. Intervention is not indicated for small congenital or degenerative cysts and needle aspiration is not advised, as the cyst may be parasitic. Large symptomatic cysts are treated by partial or complete splenectomy.

Abscess of the spleen

A splenic abscess is rare. It should be suspected when pro-gressive splenic enlargement is associated with bacteraemia and abscess formation at other sites. Splenectomy, although desirable, may not prove feasible. Drainage of the abscess may be the only possible method of treatment.

Splenic infarct

Splenic infarct may present with acute onset of left upper quadrant pain in a patient with known hypersplenism. Asymptomatic infarcts may be observed in patients follow-ing a severe attack of pancreatitis (Fig. 21.4). These may resolve with the formation of a splenic cyst, but do not require surgical intervention.

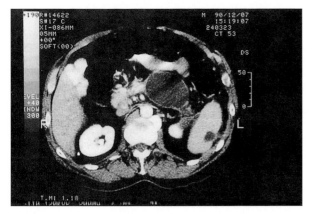

Fig. 21.4 A splenic infarct is seen on this CT scan in a patient who has developed a pseudocyst following a severe attack of pancreatitis.

Splenic artery aneurysm

This is a relatively common complication of atherosclerosis in elderly patients. The calcified wall of the aneurysm is visible on X-ray and there is obvious calcification of the tortuous splenic artery. The presence of a small uncomplicated atherosclerotic aneurysm is not necessarily an indication for surgical treatment. The natural history of these lesions is not well known, particularly as they often affect elderly, frail patients. Bleeding can occur, however, and operation is then mandatory. A splenic aneurysm may rarely arise from a peripancreatic abscess following an attack of acute pancreatitis. Haemorrhage in this setting is associated with a high mortality rate.

Rarely, a congenital aneurysm affects the splenic artery. Such aneurysms are more common in women and may rupture during pregnancy. An asymptomatic congenital aneurysm may be discovered on abdominal X-ray as a thin calcified ring shadow. Because of the risk of rupture, it should be treated electively. As most congenital aneurysms lie close to the splenic hilus splenectomy is usually required, although it may occasionally be possible to conserve the spleen by relying on the collateral arterial blood supply from the short gastric arteries.

Other indications for splenectomy

Removal of the spleen may be required as part of other surgical procedures, such as radical gastrectomy for carcinoma and, less frequently, for certain types of splenorenal shunt.

SPLENECTOMY

Preoperative preparation

In the preoperative period particular attention must be paid to the full blood count and coagulation status. In the presence of any bleeding tendency, transfusion of blood, fresh frozen plasma, cryoprecipitate or platelets may be required to bring the coagulation profiles to as near normal as possible before surgery. For thrombocytopenia, platelets should be available to cover the operation and the postoperative phase.

Accessory spleens in the splenic hilus, splenic pedicle or omentum may account for relapse of the condition for which the splenectomy was performed. Scintiscanning after the administration of ^{51}Cr-labelled red cells may be used to detect functioning accessory splenic tissue, although a careful search at operation should identify these.

The degree of splenic enlargement will have been established by CT scan before operation. A massively enlarged spleen, particularly if due to tropical disease, may give a spurious impression of mobility despite gross adhesion formation. This results from movement of the attenuated diaphragm. Where there is reason to suspect that blood loss during surgery may be considerable, preoperative selective embolization of the splenic artery may minimize intraoperative haemorrhage.

Prophylactic antibiotics should be administered with the premedication because of the increased risk of infection. As the stomach is handled during splenectomy, a nasogastric tube should be inserted.

In children, the administration of antipneumococcal vaccine some weeks prior to elective splenectomy, has been shown to offer some protection against infection by this organism. Children under two years of age do not seem to benefit from vaccine administration. Long-term prophylactic antibiotic administration is recommended for all splenectomized children.

In cases of suspected splenic trauma laparotomy is normally undertaken through a long vertical incision. For an elective splenectomy, access is usually gained via a left subcostal incision. Rarely a thoracoabdominal incision is necessary to remove a large spleen. Laparoscopic splenectomy is now favoured by some surgeons, although delivery of an enlarged spleen from the abdomen may pose difficulties.

Technique

A normal-sized non-adherent spleen is removed after first mobilizing it medially by dividing its lateral peritoneal attachments. The splenic artery and vein are doubly ligated and divided. Finally, the lienogastric ligament with its contained short gastric vessels is divided between ligatures.

When the spleen is enlarged or adherent to surrounding organs or the diaphragm, preliminary mobilization may not be possible and the vascular pedicle is dissected first. The lienogastric ligament is divided between ligatures, before the splenic artery is identified at the upper border of the pancreas and doubly ligated and divided. Alternatively, the splenic artery may first be ligated in continuity so that the spleen shrinks in size, allowing it to be mobilized and the vessels to be ligated close to the splenic hilus.

Drainage of the abdomen is not normally required after the removal of a normal-sized spleen. After removal of an enlarged organ, bleeding from the pedicle should not occur if the splenic vessels have been doubly ligated, but oozing from adhesions and the cut edge of the peritoneum is common. This should be controlled by electrocautery or, if large collateral vessels are present, by oversewing of the peritoneal edge.

Drains are not used (as they may actually increase the incidence of subphrenic sepsis) unless there is a possibility that the tail of the pancreas has been injured or there is persistent oozing due to a coagulation defect.

Postoperative course and complications

Any bleeding tendency increases the likelihood of postoperative haemorrhage. Hypotension and circulatory collapse within 48 hours of surgery indicate the need to re-explore the abdomen.

Pancreatitis occasionally follows splenectomy owing to handling and bruising of the tail of the pancreas during mobilization of the spleen. Serum amylase levels should be monitored in the immediate postoperative period. Pancreatic fistula formation is uncommon, although gastric fistula (involving the greater curvature of the stomach) can follow injury to the greater curvature of the stomach when the short gastric vessels are ligated in the lienogastric ligament.

Left lower lobe collapse or atelectasis is the most frequent complication of splenectomy but usually responds to conservative measures. The later development of atelectasis and pleural effusion may also signal the development of a subphrenic abscess. Subphrenic abscess may arise from pancreatic or gastric injury, inadequate haemostasis or inappropriate use of drains. Pancreatic and gastric fistulae are rare complications of splenectomy.

Following splenectomy there is a transient increase in the platelet and white cell count. This may predispose to venous thrombosis. In patients with portal hypertension splenectomy may be complicated by splenic vein thrombosis, with propagation of clot into the portal vein. Low-dose heparin is advised in all patients undergoing splenectomy.

Loss of lymphoid tissue reduces immune activity and impairs the response to bacteraemia. The risk of overwhelming postsplenectomy sepsis is greatest when splenectomy is performed in childhood, but a slightly increased incidence of death from pneumonia, complicated by disseminated intravascular coagulation and adrenal failure, has also been reported in adults. As most infections occur within 3 years of splenectomy, some surgeons advise prophylactic penicillin for this period. Although this is mandatory in young children, there remains some debate regarding its benefit in adults.

Elective splenectomy should be preceded by the administration of pneumococcal, meningococcal and *Haemophilus influenzae* vaccine. These are best administered 2–3 weeks prior to surgery, but are still effective if given postoperatively.

SUMMARY BOX

Splenectomy

- The spleen is the intra-abdominal organ most frequently ruptured during blunt abdominal trauma. Rupture is particularly liable to occur if the spleen is pathologically enlarged.

- Other indications for splenectomy include hereditary spherocytosis, acquired haemolytic anaemia, idiopathic thrombocytopenic purpura, hypersplenism, and myeloproliferative disorders such as myelofibrosis.

- Following traumatic rupture or laceration of the spleen there is now increased emphasis on conservation rather than splenectomy, whenever this is safe and feasible.

- Splenectomy in childhood (and to a lesser extent in adult life) carries an appreciable risk of overwhelming postsplenectomy sepsis, and pneumococcal infection is frequently responsible.

- If splenectomy is unavoidable, the patient should receive pneumococcal, meningococcal and *Haemophilus influenzae* vaccine (before splenectomy if possible), and may benefit from prophylactic penicillin. The duration of penicillin therapy is uncertain but the risk of sepsis is greatest in the first few years after splenectomy.

SECTION 5
LOWER GASTROINTESTINAL TRACT

22 Intestine and appendix

M.G. Dunlop

Conditions affecting the intestine are a common source of admission to the surgical ward. Symptoms attributable to intestinal disease can develop at any time in life, with causes ranging from episodes of infective diarrhoea in childhood to diverticular disease in later years (Table 22.1). It is important to differentiate chronic conditions that need timely diagnosis and active intervention from those where conservative management is appropriate (Table 22.2). Hence there is conflict between the need for prompt diagnosis of conditions such as colonic cancer, where intervention at an early stage in the natural history of the disease has been shown to be beneficial, and the need to differentiate cancer from other common conditions, such as diverticular disease, where surgery can be avoided in most cases.

APPLIED SURGICAL ANATOMY

Anatomy and function of the small intestine

The small bowel extends from the pylorus to the ileocaecal valve and ranges in length from 3 to 9 metres. The jejunum, which comprises two-fifths of the small intestine, is of wider calibre than the ileum and the diameter of the gut lumen narrows progressively from the duodenojejunal flexure to the ileocaecal valve. The small bowel mucosa comprises a single layer of columnar cells interspersed with mucus-secreting cells, Paneth cells and APUD (amine precursor uptake and decarboxylation) cells. The epithelium is

Table 22.1 Principal symptoms associated with disorders of appendix and intestine	
Appendix	**Intestine**
Abdominal pain	Change in bowel habit
Mid-gut or RIF (parietal) pain	Rectal bleeding (fresh or melaena)
Abdominal mass (RIF)	Passage of mucus or pus per rectum
Systemic toxicity	Abdominal pain (midgut, hindgut or parietal)
	Abdominal distension
	Abdominal mass
	Anorexia and weight loss
RIF = right iliac fossa.	

Table 22.2   Principal disorders of appendix and intestine relevant to surgical practice

Appendix	Small intestine	Colon and rectum

Appendicitis
Tumours, benign
or malignant
	Crohn's disease
	Tumours, benign and malignant
	Mesenteric ischaemia
	Jejunal diverticulosis
	Paralytic ileus
	Mechanical obstruction
	Meckel's diverticulum
	Radiation damage
		Diverticular disease
		Tumours, benign and malignant
		Mesenteric ischaemia
		Colitis
		   Crohn's disease
		   Ulcerative colitis
		   Pseudomembranous colitis
		   Infective
		Irritable bowel syndrome
		Volvulus
		Angiodysplasia
		Pseudo-obstruction
		Megacolon – Hirschsprung's disease or acquired

supported on a strong submucosa. Between the inner layer of circular muscle and the outer longitudinal layer runs Auerbach's myenteric plexus, which comprises vagus parasympathetic fibres and sympathetic fibres from the lesser and greater splanchnic nerves. This plexus controls orderly, propulsive contractions of the muscular layers of the gut wall. The sympathetic nervous system mediates the sensation of visceral pain and a submucosal plexus (Meissner's plexus) of autonomic nerves innervates the glandular cells in the epithelium.

The small intestine is suspended by a mesentery, the root of which runs from the left of L2 to the right sacroiliac joint. The superior mesenteric artery runs in the root of the mesentery and supplies the small bowel by a series of straight vessels originating from arterial arcades (Fig. 22.1). These midgut vessels communicate through the pancreaticoduodenal arcade with the coeliac axis. Venous blood drains via the superior mesenteric vein to the portal vein. Lymphoid aggregates in the submucosa (Peyer's patches) are more numerous in the ileum and lymph drains to regional nodes in the root of the mesentery before passing to the cisterna chyli.

The principal function of the small bowel is absorption, but its secretory and digestive functions supplement those of the upper digestive tract. The mucosa is thrown into circular folds (plicae semilunares) and is carpeted by finger-like villi, giving an absorptive area of 200–500 m². Vitamin B_{12} and iron are specifically absorbed in the small intestine. Some 5–8 L of fluid enter the jejunum each day, of which only 1–2 L normally pass to the colon.

Anatomy and function of the large intestine

The large bowel actively absorbs sodium and water, particularly on the right side, whereas the left colon and rectum act as a reservoir until defecation is appropriate. Mucus is secreted as a lubricant, and when there is inflammation may become visible as a covering layer or discharge. The large bowel extends from the ileocaecal valve, which has relevance in the presence of colonic obstruction, because if it remains competent increasing pressure within the colon may result in perforation. The caecum is a blind pouch in the right iliac fossa and the appendix opens from its base at the point where the taeniae coli converge. The ascending colon passes to the hepatic flexure, which overlies the lower pole of the right kidney. The transverse colon runs to the

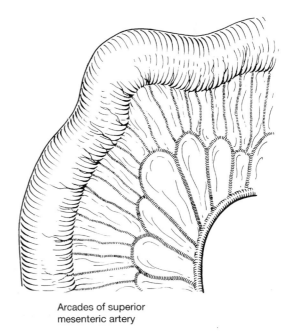

Arcades of superior
mesenteric artery

Fig. 22.1   Blood supply of small intestine showing arterial arcades.

splenic flexure, suspended by the transverse mesocolon. At the brim of the pelvis the descending colon becomes the sigmoid colon. The sigmoid colon is suspended by a sigmoid mesocolon, which forms an inverted V at the point where the left ureter crosses the bifurcation of the left common iliac artery. The transverse and sigmoid colons have mobility by virtue of their mesenteries. In most people the immobile ascending and descending colons are peritonealized on only their fronts and sides.

The large bowel mucosa consists of columnar epithelium interspersed with mucus-secreting goblet cells. Crypts pass down to the muscularis mucosa, which is supported by a strong submucosa. The true rectum is demarcated by coalescence of the taenia coli of the sigmoid colon to form a continuous outer muscular tube. The upper third of the rectum has peritoneal cover on its front and sides, but the middle third is peritonealized only anteriorly as it passes downwards in the hollow of the sacrum to the anorectal junction. The lower third of rectum lies beneath the peritoneal floor of the pelvis.

The inferior and superior mesenteric arteries supply the colon and anastomose via a marginal artery (Fig. 22.2) which allows collateral supply in the event of arterial occlusion, but at the splenic flexure this arterial communication is tenuous. The superior rectal artery is the continuation of the inferior mesenteric artery and supplies the rectum and anastomoses with the middle and inferior rectal arteries (branches of the internal iliac arteries).

Blood from the inferior mesenteric vein drains into the splenic vein. Lymph drains from the colon to epicolic and paracolic nodes close to the bowel wall, and to regional nodes at the origin of the superior and inferior mesenteric vessels (Fig. 22.3). Lymph from the rectum drains upwards to superior rectal and inferior mesenteric nodes, whereas anal canal lymph drains to inguinal nodes.

Anatomy of the appendix

The appendiceal lumen is lined by colonic epithelium and the submucosa contains lymphoid follicles, which are prominent in childhood but regress in adolescence. In older patients the lumen may eventually be obliterated by fibrosis. It develops as a conical diverticulum, which projects from the medial wall of the caecum some 2 cm below the ileocaecal junction as the taeniae coli converge on the root of the appendix. The appendix lies generally behind the caecum or hangs down over the pelvic brim (Fig. 22.4).

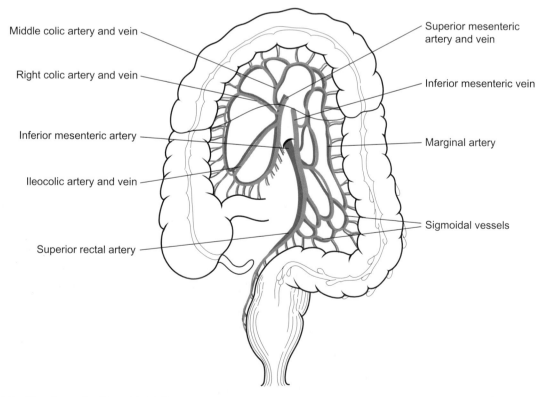

Middle colic artery and vein

Right colic artery and vein

Inferior mesenteric artery

Ileocolic artery and vein

Superior rectal artery

Superior mesenteric artery and vein

Inferior mesenteric vein

Marginal artery

Sigmoidal vessels

Fig. 22.2   Blood supply of large intestine.

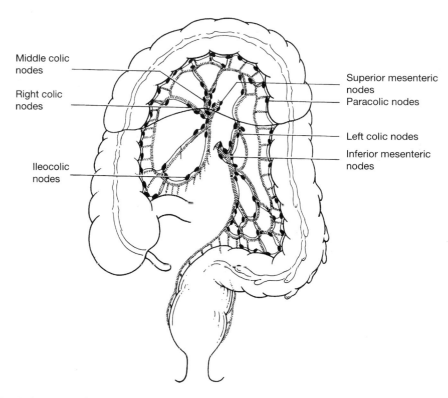

Fig. 22.3 Lymphatic drainage of the colon.

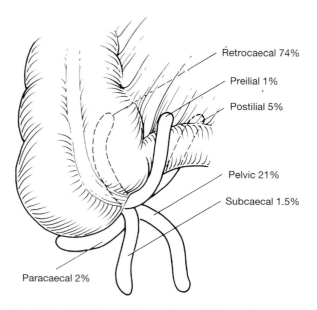

Fig. 22.4 Variations in the position of the appendix.

DISORDERS OF THE APPENDIX

Appendicitis

Acute appendicitis is predominantly a disease of western civilization, although its incidence (which is currently 1.5/1000 population) in the UK has fallen over the past 30 years. In developing countries its incidence may be increasing with the adoption of low-residue western-style diets. Acute appendicitis remains the commonest acute abdominal emergency in childhood, adolescence and early adult life. It is uncommon before the age of 2, and less than 5% of cases occur in patients aged over 60 years.

Aetiology and pathophysiology

The accumulation of secretions in the obstructed appendix may lead to distension, necrosis of the mucosa, and translocation of gut bacteria across the wall. The peak age of incidence of appendicitis overlaps the period of maximal development of lymphoid tissue, suggesting that lymphoid hyperplasia within the wall predisposes to obstruction. In older patients, inspissated faeces (faecoliths), fibrosis, adhesions and neoplasia are all potential causes of obstruction. Threadworms can cause signs and symptoms resembling mild acute appendicitis but are incriminated in only a few cases.

Although acute inflammation of the appendix may resolve spontaneously, symptomatic patients may progress to gangrene and perforation if the appendix is not removed, as continuing obstruction may impair the blood supply. Before frank perforation occurs, bacteria migrate through the damaged wall to infect the peritoneal cavity and inflame the parietal peritoneum. If the infection remains contained following perforation, an appendix abscess or mass will result, but generalized peritonitis is more common. The omentum is not fully developed in infants and localization of the infection is less effective.

Clinical features

'Typical' signs and symptoms of acute appendicitis are not always present or may appear late. Pain normally begins as periumbilical colic, which ranges in severity from mild discomfort to severe pain. The colic represents visceral pain due to appendiceal obstruction and its periumbilical location reflects the embryonic origin of the appendix as a midline midgut structure. Classically, the pain remains periumbilical for several hours before shifting to the right iliac fossa as parietal peritonitis ensues. Whereas periumbilical colic is ill localized, the somatic pain is sharply localized and is exacerbated by moving or coughing. In one-third of cases the pain commences and remains in the right iliac fossa. When the appendix is retrocaecal, somatic pain is perceived in the flank and loin. Pelvic appendicitis may be associated with bladder irritation. Anorexia is almost invariable and nausea is common, but vomiting is rarely a prominent feature. Some patients experience fullness and may misguidedly take aperients to gain relief. Diarrhoea may occur when pelvic appendicitis irritates the neighbouring rectum.

Tenderness and muscle guarding are the cardinal signs of acute appendicitis. Tenderness is often maximal over McBurney's point, which is located one-third of the way along a line from the right anterior iliac spine to the umbilicus. There is often associated rebound tenderness and hyperaesthesia of the skin. Fever and tachycardia are *not* early signs of appendicitis, and may not develop until perforation has occurred. Fetor oris is a non-specific sign. Less reliable signs include Rovsing's sign (pressure on the left iliac fossa producing pain in the right iliac fossa) and the psoas sign (pain during passive extension of the right hip). Bowel sounds may be normal or reduced in frequency. There may be no signs in the right iliac fossa in retrocaecal appendicitis. Tenderness, if present, is maximal in the right flank or loin. Pelvic appendicitis often produces little tenderness or guarding on abdominal examination, but tenderness is usually present on digital rectal examination, which is a valuable means of excluding gynaecological and other causes of pain.

Perforation of the appendix with diffuse peritonitis leads to generalized tenderness, guarding and rigidity, although even at this stage tenderness is often still maximal in the right iliac fossa. If infection remains localized, a mass of omentum and neighbouring viscera may become palpable on abdominal or rectal examination.

Diagnosis

The diagnosis of acute appendicitis is primarily a clinical one. Repeated clinical assessment over a period of a few hours will usually exclude other diagnoses. Abdominal ultrasonography may be used in the early assessment of female patients to exclude gynaecological conditions. A urinary immunological pregnancy test may be performed to exclude ruptured ectopic pregnancy. Polymorphonuclear leukocytosis is not specific for appendicitis, and the urine may contain a few pus or red cells if the inflamed appendix lies near to the urinary tract.

Abdominal radiography may show distended small intestinal loops due to a localized ileus. Obliteration of the psoas border and free gas in the right iliac fossa are occasional signs of *late* appendicitis. The diagnosis can be secured by laparoscopy, but this requires general anaesthetic and so the patient must consent and be prepared to proceed with appendicectomy if required. Other imaging techniques to diagnose appendicitis include CT and MRI, although these are not used routinely in the UK.

Differential diagnosis of acute appendicitis

Acute appendicitis should be considered in the differential diagnosis of all acute abdominal pain, unless the appendix has already been removed. Non-surgical causes of abdominal pain, such as basal pneumonia and diabetic ketoacidosis, should be considered. Gastroenteritis, intestinal obstruction, and rare infections such as *Yersinia enterocolitica*, tuberculosis and actinomycosis, should be excluded. Acute mesenteric adenitis, acute terminal ileitis and inflammation of Meckel's diverticulum may present with right iliac fossa pain. Acute salpingitis, rupture of an ectopic pregnancy and mittelschmertz may present in females. Ureteric colic, perinephric abscess or acute pyelonephritis may mimic retrocaecal appendicitis. Acute cholecystitis and perforated duodenal ulcer may produce right-sided abdominal pain. Diverticular disease or perforation of a colonic carcinoma can occasionally produce symptoms suggestive of acute appendicitis. A mass in the right iliac fossa raises the suspicion of intussusception (in young children), Crohn's disease, ovarian cyst and bowel neoplasia.

Appendicitis in special situations

Pregnancy Early diagnosis in the pregnant woman is vital but may be confounded by the gravid uterus. By the third trimester the appendix is displaced upwards, and so pain and tenderness are more superior than would be expected. Rectal and vaginal examination may be unhelpful, the white cell count is normally elevated in pregnancy, and the use of X-rays is contraindicated. Delay is harmful to both mother and unborn child, and the threshold for diagnosis and surgery must be no different from that applied in non-pregnant women. Fetal mortality in uncomplicated appendicitis is 3%; that following perforated appendicitis is 30%.

The elderly Gangrene and perforation are five times commoner in patients over the age of 60, possibly because of the earlier loss of appendiceal blood supply. Awareness of the diagnosis, despite atypical presentation, and prompt surgery are the keys to successful management.

Appendix abscess and appendix mass

When an appendix abscess or mass is present the differential diagnosis of Crohn's disease should always be borne in mind. Increasing pyrexia, pain and tenderness is likely to be due to loculated pus, and a diagnosis of appendix abscess is probable. Abscesses behind the caecum or terminal ileum may produce psoas spasm, such that the patient prefers to lie with the right hip flexed. Ultrasound or CT are helpful in identifying loculated pus or matted loops of terminal ileum without abscess formation.

Appendix abscess is best treated by surgical drainage and appendicectomy, avoiding the dissemination of infection throughout the peritoneal cavity. An appendix mass can be treated with parenteral antibiotics, intravenous fluids and nil by mouth, with an interval appendicectomy performed some weeks later. Immediate surgery is made difficult by the inflammatory mass but has the benefit of a shorter overall hospital stay, and is now the approach preferred by most surgeons. There is a high risk of relapse when an initial conservative approach is undertaken.

Treatment of appendicitis

Treatment comprises surgical removal of the appendix before gangrene and perforation occur. Preoperative resuscitation is only required in the presence of generalized peritonitis. Metronidazole and a broad-spectrum cephalosporin are normally administered. The operation can be performed open through a small incision in the right iliac fossa or by laparoscopic means, which is dependent on the equipment and expertise available. The appendix should always be sent for histological examination to confirm the diagnosis and exclude malignancy, and a swab is taken for bacteriological culture. In the rare instance where there is gross purulent or faecal peritonitis it may be prudent to close only the deeper layers of the wound, leaving the skin and subcutaneous tissues open for some 4–5 days. The clean wound can be sutured by delayed primary closure, although in most instances the skin will heal without the need for suture.

The normal appendix found at operation in a patient with suspected appendicitis In 10–20% of emergency appendicectomies a normal appendix is removed. Although every effort should be made to avoid unnecessary laparotomy, delaying operation until the diagnosis is certain can lead to an unacceptable incidence of gangrene and perforation, resulting in increased morbidity as well as mortality.

If a normal appendix is found at operation, other pathologies should be excluded. Mesenteric adenitis may be associated with clear yellow peritoneal fluid, perforated peptic ulcer with bile-stained fluid, colonic perforation with faecal fluid, and gut infarction with bloodstained fluid. Free blood suggests rupture of a vessel or ectopic pregnancy. Faecoliths are the commonest cause of a palpable mass within the appendix and, although mobile, may be mistaken for neoplasms in obstructed appendicitis. The distal ileum should be examined to exclude Meckel's diverticulum, terminal ileitis or Crohn's disease. Both ovaries and Fallopian tubes should be inspected and an attempt made to visualize the sigmoid colon. Even if other pathology is present, a normal appendix should be removed when operating through an incision, as this avoids confusion if appendicitis develops in a patient bearing an appendicectomy scar.

Complications of appendicitis

Although most patients recover well thanks to modern diagnostic approaches and safe surgery, an appreciable number of deaths occur in the UK every year, some even in children. Uncomplicated appendicitis has an overall mortality of less than 0.1%, whereas following perforation in the elderly mortality rates may be as high as 5%.

Perforated appendicitis may be associated with temporary easing of pain, but the onset of diffuse abdominal pain and tenderness, fever and tachycardia indicate the onset of generalized peritonitis. Prompt appendicectomy following vigorous resuscitation with intravenous fluids and systemic broad-spectrum antibiotics is essential. A limited right hemicolectomy may be necessary if the appendiceal base has ruptured.

Gangrenous perforated appendicitis is more likely to result in wound infection and intra-abdominal abscess formation. Pelvic abscesses are palpable on digital rectal examination and may produce few abdominal signs. Subphrenic abscess should be suspected where there is a swinging pyrexia and respiratory signs or symptoms. The complication may be suggested by chest X-ray but the

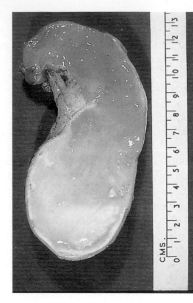

Fig. 22.5 Mucocele of the appendix.

diagnosis is secured by ultrasound scan. Portal vein thrombophlebitis with hepatic abscess formation is a rare complication and may be suspected by a swinging pyrexia and icterus. Gas may be seen radiologically in the portal system. Vigorous antibiotic treatment offers the only hope of survival, and surviving patients often develop portal hypertension owing to portal vein occlusion.

Chronic appendicitis

It is debatable whether recurring bouts of low-grade appendicitis can give rise to intermittent right iliac fossa pain. The 'grumbling' appendix is something of a diagnostic scapegoat and appendicectomy should be advised only when all other investigations have proved negative.

Mucocele of the appendix and pseudomyxoma peritonei

This rare condition results from chronic obstruction of the appendix, with the resulting accumulation of mucin (Fig. 22.5). Obstruction of the appendix lumen is usually due to fibrosis, but sometimes a malignant mucus-secreting papillary adenocarcinoma is responsible. Such simple mucoceles are cured by appendicectomy, but pseudomyxoma peritonei is a rare complication of rupture of a mucocele. The resultant seeding of the peritoneal cavity with mucus-secreting cells that have a low mitotic rate can cause pressure symptoms owing to the amount of mucin produced. In a substantial proportion of cases death results

from the need for repeated excisions. The underlying basis of the condition may be a true malignant mucus-secreting adenocarcinoma of the appendix. Treatment requires surgical debulking, as these lesions respond poorly to chemotherapy and radiotherapy, although encouraging results have been obtained recently by combined surgery and topical mitomycin C.

Yersinia ileitis

This is a self-limiting infection caused by the Gram-negative bacteria *Yersinia enterocolitica* or, rarely, *Yersinia pseudotuberbulosis*. It may mimic acute appendicitis clinically, and at operation the terminal ileum is red and thickened but the caecum and appendix are normal. Mesenteric adenitis is a dramatic feature, but histological examination of the lymph nodes reveals non-specific changes and the diagnosis is best confirmed serologically or by node culture. When acute terminal ileitis was confused with Crohn's disease, it was thought that appendicectomy was contraindicated because of the risk of fistula formation. However, modern practice has shown that appendicectomy in the presence of Crohn's disease or *Yersinia* is safe if the appendix is not involved.

Meckel's diverticulitis

Symptoms minicking acute appendicitis may arise from a Meckel's diverticulum if there is ectopic acid-secreting gastric mucosa causing peptic ulceration. Diverticular inflammation is rare but cannot be distinguished clinically from acute appendicitis. An inflamed diverticulum should be resected if found at laparotomy, but there is no need to look for an incidental Meckel's diverticulum if an inflamed appendix is found.

Tumours of the appendix
Carcinoid tumour

The appendix is the commonest site for carcinoid tumours, which arise from argentaffin cells of the APUD system and are usually distinct yellow submucosal lesions located near the tip of the appendix. They account for 85% of all appendiceal tumours and are found in 0.5% of all appendices removed surgically. The vast majority are benign, but tumours larger than 2 cm can infiltrate the wall of the appendix and spread to the mesenteric and regional lymph glands. It is exceptional for appendiceal carcinoids to give rise to liver metastases and the carcinoid syndrome.

Appendicectomy is sufficient treatment for most appendiceal carcinoid tumours, but right hemicolectomy is necessary if the tumour is larger than 2 cm, involves the caecum, or if the lymph nodes are affected.

Adenocarcinoma

Adenocarcinoma of the appendix is an uncommon but highly malignant neoplasm which frequently presents with involved regional lymph nodes at diagnosis. The clinical presentation may mimic acute appendicitis or appendix mass. Right hemicolectomy is the treatment of choice, even in cases where the diagnosis is only apparent at histological assessment of an appendicectomy specimen. In cases with involved lymph nodes consideration should be given to the place of adjuvant chemotherapy with 5-fluorouracil. Appendix adenocarcinoma often affects younger patients, and may arise in association with the autosomal syndrome of hereditary non-polyposis colorectal cancer (HNPCC).

> **SUMMARY BOX**
>
> **The appendix**
>
> - The common positions for the appendix are pelvic and rectrocaecal.
>
> - The incidence of acute appendicitis has declined, but it is still the commonest acute abdominal condition in childhood, adolescence and early adulthood.
>
> - The typical history of periumbilical colic (visceral midgut pain), followed within several hours by right iliac fossa pain (somatic pain from parietal peritonitis), is not always present.
>
> - Tenderness and muscle guarding in the right iliac fossa are the most reliable signs of acute appendicitis. Leukocytosis, high temperature and radiological signs are manifestations which may denote gangrene and perforation.
>
> - The objective is to carry out appendicectomy before gangrene and perforation supervene (with an associated increase in morbidity and mortality).
>
> - Gangrene and perforation are common and/or particularly dangerous in infants (diagnosis not considered in children under 2 years), pregnant women (desire to avoid negative laparotomy) and the elderly (more rapid progression of disease).

> **SUMMARY BOX**
>
> **Tumours of the appendix**
>
> - The appendix is the commonest site of carcinoid tumour in the gastrointestinal tract, and 85% of all appendiceal tumours are carcinoids.
>
> - Carcinoid tumours are found in 0.5% of all appendices removed surgically.
>
> - The tumour usually takes the form of a small firm yellowish nodule near the tip of the appendix.
>
> - Although carcinoid tumours frequently show spread to the serosa, lymph node involvement is rare and distant metastases are extremely rare.
>
> - Appendicectomy is usually adequate treatment, although subsequent right hemicolectomy may be considered in patients who prove to have involved lymph nodes.

SMALL AND LARGE INTESTINE – CLINICAL ASSESSMENT

History and clinical examination

Obstruction of the small bowel (midgut) produces periumbilical colic, whereas obstruction of the distal large bowel (hindgut) produces colic in the lower abdomen. Nausea and vomiting are early and predominant features of small bowel obstruction, particularly high small bowel obstruction. In contrast, large bowel conditions present with the predominant feature of constipation, diarrhoea, or alternating bouts of each. Large bowel obstruction presents with abdominal distension and absolute constipation, whereas vomiting is a late feature.

Normal bowel habit may range from the passage of one motion every 3 days to three per day. The passage of blood or mucus per rectum is a common feature of large bowel disease. It is essential to differentiate 'outlet-type' bleeding from sinister blood loss, where the blood is mixed with the stool and there may be associated altered bowel habit or tenesmus. Outlet bleeding is typically bright red and may be present only on the paper or spattered in the pan separate from the stool. There may be associated perianal pain, due to fissure or prolapsed piles. Blood originating from the distal bowel is usually bright red, whereas blood coming from the upper gastrointestinal tract is often so altered by gut bacteria that it is black (melaena). In some cases blood is not obvious on inspection of the stool, but the faecal occult blood (FOB) test is positive. Weight loss, malaise and anaemia are common non-specific features of intestinal disease.

The oral mucous membrane, hands and fingernails should be inspected. Examination of the abdomen may reveal distension, a mass or visible peristalsis. In thin subjects the caecum is often palpable, and the descending and sigmoid colon may be palpable when loaded with faeces. Hepatomegaly due to metastatic disease should be excluded. Abdominal auscultation determines the presence and pitch of bowel sounds and occasionally reveals an arterial bruit. Digital rectal examination is essential to detect for blood and mucus. Three-quarters of rectal cancers and up to one-third of all colorectal cancers can be felt rectally. In patients with lower gastrointestinal symptoms there is no rationale for checking the faeces for occult blood, as the sensitivity of the Guiac FOB test is only 55%.

Investigation of surgical disease

The standard small bowel investigation is the barium follow-through or the small bowel enema, where barium is instilled directly through a tube placed in the duodenum. Long fibreoptic enteroscopes are available to inspect and biopsy at least a proportion of the small intestine. The terminal ileum can be inspected at colonoscopy, where the ileocaecal valve can be cannulated. Radiolabelled red cell scans may reveal occult bleeding in the small bowel if a lesion such as a Meckel's diverticulum is the suspected cause of persistent blood loss. CT and MRI are useful in identifying mass lesions and in diagnosing Crohn's disease, especially in the acute phase.

Direct inspection of the large bowel includes proctoscopy, rigid sigmoidoscopy, flexible sigmoidoscopy and colonoscopy. These techniques allow biopsy and facilitate snare removal of colorectal polyps using cauterizing diathermy. Contrast radiography of the colon is undertaken routinely using double contrast (air and barium) to allow detailed inspection of the mucosa. Cross-sectional imaging using CT and MRI is also widely used in the staging of colorectal cancer. Other investigations available include tests of colonic transit using ingested radio-opaque markers. This investigation is not used routinely but is relevant to the assessment of megacolon and slow-transit constipation.

PRINCIPLES OF OPERATIVE INTESTINAL SURGERY

The crucial role of the small bowel in maintaining nutrition requires that resectional surgery should aim to retain the maximum possible length of bowel. Consideration must be given to the absorptive function of specific regions of the small intestine. Ileocaecal resection for Crohn's disease may result in gallstone formation and megaloblastic anaemia owing to poor absorption of bile salts and vitamin B_{12}. The main function of the large intestine is the reabsorption of water and to act as a reservoir for faecal material. Consequently, loss of the large bowel can be tolerated with little impact on nutritional status.

Small intestinal anastomoses heal well owing to their excellent blood supply and to a rich submucosal arteriolar plexus. Small bowel content clears after 12 hours of fasting, and so apart from fasting the patient no specific bowel preparation is required for planned small bowel resection. The large intestine microcirculation consists of a series of small end-arteries which, combined with the presence of faeces with a high density of bacterial colonization, results in poor anastomotic healing compared to those of the small intestine. This results in a higher anastomotic leak rate for colocolic or colorectal anastomoses.

In view of the risk of anastomotic leakage there is a lower threshold for the formation of a stoma in patients who require large bowel anastomosis, particularly in the emergency setting when the bowel lumen contains liquid faeces, which increases the risk of peritoneal contamination. In specialist centres every effort is made to reconstitute large bowel continuity in both elective and emergency resectional surgery. The faecal content of the bowel is reduced by ensuring a low-residue diet for 2 days preoperatively and a liquid diet for the day before surgery. The bowel is cleared using mechanical bowel preparations comprising cathartic laxatives, such as Picolax, or osmotic laxatives such as polyethylene glycol (KleanPrep). Prophylactic antibiotic therapy usually comprises a single dose of a broad-spectrum cephalosporin such as Cefotaxime, to cover coliforms, in combination with metronidazole to cover anaerobic bacteria.

In emergency surgery for left-sided colonic obstruction or perforation, a total colectomy with anastomosis of the ileum to the rectum may be considered to avoid a colorectal anastomosis in the presence of faecal loading. Segmental left-sided resection and the formation of a colostomy (Hartmann's operation) avoids an anastomosis, but many specialist colorectal surgeons prefer left-sided resection with on-table colonic lavage and primary anastomosis.

INTESTINAL STOMA AND FISTULA

Stoma

Intestinal stomas have an important place in the management of small and large intestinal disease. An ileostomy is formed by bringing out the ileum through the abdominal wall, usually the right rectus muscle in the right iliac fossa. Ileal bowel content is irritant to skin and a spout is fashioned to allow appliances to be fitted and prevent skin contact with bowel content. Ileostomy comprises either an 'end' stoma or a 'loop' or 'defunctioning' stoma. It may be employed as an adjunct to resectional surgery where the disease process prevents reanastomosis, or as a temporary stoma to allow a distal anastomosis to heal, such as for a low colorectal or ileoanal anastomosis. End-ileostomy is used when the colon has been removed, and occasionally where small intestine distal to the stoma has been removed, as in extensive Crohn's disease.

The colon can be brought out as an end or a loop colostomy (Fig. 22.6), usually in the left iliac fossa, although a transverse colostomy is brought out in the right

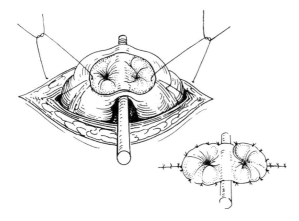

Fig. 22.6 Loop colostomy (the rod is kept in place for approximately 7 days).

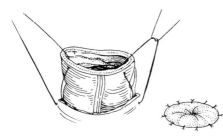

Fig. 22.7 End-colostomy.

upper quadrant. A colostomy does not require a spout as faeces are not usually irritant to the skin. End-colostomy (Fig. 22.7) is used as part of a Hartmann's procedure and is an integral part of an abdominoperineal resection for rectal cancer (see below). A loop colostomy of the sigmoid colon is used to divert faeces from a diseased anorectum, such as during the management of complex perianal fistula or faecal incontinence surgery. It may also be used as palliation for pelvic cancer or during radical radiotherapy for rectal cancer. A transverse colostomy is very seldom used in modern colorectal surgical practice.

Intestinal fistula

A fistula is an abnormal communication between two epithelialized surfaces, and can manifest as a communication between intestine and other parts of the GI tract, skin, urinary tract or vagina. Intestinal fistulae may arise as part of a disease process or as an iatrogenic complication, such as leak from a surgical anastomosis or after radiotherapy. Anastomotic leak usually results in a cutaneous fistula, with bowel content appearing through the wound several days after intestinal surgery. The overall leak rate from colorectal surgery is around 5%, but 10% for rectal anastomoses. Occasionally post-surgical leak can present as a rectovaginal fistula and management is usually conservative. Peritonitis requires laparotomy and the anastomosis may have to be taken down, with the formation of a stoma. Radiation fistula typically presents several months or years after the primary treatment owing to the late development of endarteritis obliterans and chronic microvascular ischaemia. Radiation-induced rectovaginal fistula in patients cured of the original malignancy is best treated by rectal excision and coloanal anastomosis, to allow healing to occur in healthy non-irradiated bowel.

Disease processes resulting in fistula formation include Crohn's disease. Although complicated diverticular disease usually manifests as diverticulitis and rarely causes a fistula, it is none the less the commonest cause of colovesical fistula, owing to the close proximity of the sigmoid colon and the dome of the bladder. Malignant tumours of the upper and lower intestine can result in any combination of fistulation. Actinomycosis and tuberculosis are rare

---

SUMMARY BOX

Intestinal fistula

- A fistula is an abnormal communication between two surfaces lined by epithelium (commonly an intestinal fistula involves other loops of bowel, bladder, vagina or skin).

- Gastrointestinal fistulae may be a complication of surgery (90%) or intestinal disease (Crohn's disease, diverticular disease, carcinoma).

- Small bowel fistulae frequently have a high output (e.g. several litres per day) and irritate the skin (the fluid contains activated pancreatic enzymes).

- Large bowel fistulae are usually low output and do not irritate the skin.

- The principles of management are:
  - ensure adequate external drainage
  - maintain fluid and electrolyte balance
  - provide nutritional support (usually by parenteral nutrition)
  - protect the skin
  - ensure that there is no distal obstruction by contrast studies.

- In the absence of distal obstruction or intrinsic bowel disease (Crohn's disease or carcinoma) the great majority of fistulae will close with conservative management.

causes of cutaneous fistula. Treatment of disease-related fistula usually requires management of the primary problem.

INFLAMMATORY BOWEL DISEASE

In view of the similarities in clinical presentation and in aspects of the management of both conditions, it is useful to discuss Crohn's disease and ulcerative colitis together (Table 22.3). The key difference between the two conditions is that ulcerative colitis affects the colon and rectum exclusively, whereas Crohn's disease can affect the whole GI tract. There are also important implications for prognosis, as surgery for ulcerative colitis is curative, whereas Crohn's disease usually follows a relapsing course, despite medical or surgical intervention.

Crohn's disease

Although this was originally described as a disease affecting the terminal ileum, it is now clear that any part of the gastrointestinal tract can be involved, from mouth to anus. In 50% of cases both small and large bowel are involved, whereas in 25% of cases large bowel alone is affected. The incidence is increasing in developed countries and the annual rate is currently 5–7 cases per 100 000 population in the UK. The underlying aetiology remains enigmatic, although nutritional deficits, increased intestinal permeability and immunological factors have been postulated. At the time of initial clinical presentation the features of Crohn's disease may be indistinguishable from those of ulcerative colitis. Indeed, in cases of colonic Crohn's disease it may be difficult to differentiate the two conditions, even after resection and histological assessment.

Pathological features

Macroscopically, Crohn's disease produces a cobblestone appearance in which oedematous islands of mucosa are separated by crevices or fissures, which can extend through all coats of the bowel wall. Serpiginous ulceration is common, and fibrosis produces strictures of varying number and length. Multiple areas of inflammation are common but intervening bowel appears normal (i.e. skip lesions). Full-thickness involvement of the bowel wall leads to serosal inflammation, adhesion to neighbouring structures, and sinus or fistula formation. Microscopically, these are deep fissuring ulcers, oedema and inflammatory cell infiltrates with foci of lymphocytes. In 50% of cases there are non-caseating granulomas similar to those found in sarcoid.

Clinical features

Crohn's disease is a chronic disorder with exacerbations, remissions and a varied clinical presentation. Continuous or episodic diarrhoea is associated with recurring abdominal pain and tenderness, lassitude and fever. Declining general health, malabsorption, weight loss with failure to thrive and to reach developmental milestones is common in affected children.

Examination may reveal malnutrition and there may be a palpable abdominal mass. There may be features of subacute intestinal obstruction and this may be due to active disease, stricturing of 'burnt-out' disease, or adhesions from previous surgical intervention. Fistula formation occurs in 20% of patients with small and large bowel disease and in 10% of those with large bowel disease only. The fistula may communicate with other loops of bowel, other viscera (e.g. bladder, vagina) or the skin. External fistulae most often result from surgical intervention and commonly involve the anterior

Table 22.3   Comparison of clinical features of ulcerative colitis and Crohn's disease

	Crohn's disease	Ulcerative colitis
Incidence	5–7 per 100 000 and rising	10 per 100 000 and static
Extent	May involve entire gastrointestinal tract	Limited to large bowel
Rectal involvement	Variable	Almost invariable
Disease continuity	Discontinuous (skip lesions)	Continuous
Depth of inflammation	Transmural	Mucosal
Macroscopic appearance of mucosa	Cobblestone, discrete deep ulcers and fissures	Multiple small ulcers, pseudopolyps
Histological features	Transmural inflammation, granulomas (50%)	Crypt abscesses, no granulomas
Presence of perianal disease	75% of cases with large bowel disease 25% of cases with small bowel disease	25% of cases
Frequency of fistula	10–20% of cases	Uncommon
Colorectal cancer risk	Elevated risk (RR = 2.5) in colonic disease	25% risk over 30 yrs for pancolitis

abdominal wall or perineum. Abscesses can result from sub-clinical bowel perforation. Free perforation is uncommon because the inflamed segment usually adheres to surrounding structures. Although less common than in ulcerative colitis, toxic dilatation can complicate colonic disease.

Crohn's disease is associated with an elevated (2.5 times increased) risk of carcinoma of the colon. It is important to consider the possibility of malignancy in patients with relapsing symptoms from long-standing disease which has been relatively quiescent. There is no evidence that surveillance is beneficial, and many patients with colonic Crohn's eventually require to have the colon removed.

One-quarter of patients with small bowel Crohn's disease and three-quarters of those with large bowel disease have troublesome anal lesions, including ulceration, abscess, oedematous skin tags, fissure and fistula. Anal fissures are often multiple and indolent and extend to involve any part of the perineum, including the vagina or scrotum.

Systemic manifestations include anterior uveitis, iritis, polyarthropathy, ankylosing spondylitis, liver disease (e.g. sclerosing cholangitis) and erythema nodosum. Disease of the terminal ileum or its resection increases the incidence of gallstones.

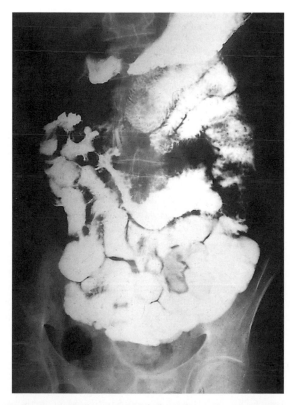

Fig. 22.8 Barium meal and follow-through examination in Crohn's disease, showing strictures in the distal ileum.

Investigation

In the non-emergency situation general assessment includes evaluation of nutritional status and the detection of anaemia, which may be due to iron deficiency from chronic blood loss. Normocytic anaemia of chronic disease or macrocytic anaemia due to vitamin B_{12} or folate malabsorption may result. Elevated ESR and acute-phase proteins such as C-reactive protein are useful in monitoring disease, but are not specific for diagnostic purposes. The standard diagnostic investigation is barium follow-through (or small bowel enema). Active disease produces radiological evidence of thickening, luminal narrowing and separation of loops, and is often associated with ulceration, spike-like fissures and a cobblestone appearance (Fig. 22.8). Skip lesions and fistula formation may be apparent. Enteroscopy is being used increasingly to assess the extent and activity of the disease. Proctoscopy, sigmoidoscopy and colonoscopy are used to determine the presence and extent of large bowel disease. Biopsy of macroscopically normal rectum at sigmoidoscopy or colonoscopy may reveal occult large bowel involvement, particularly where there has been troublesome perianal involvement. Double-contrast barium enema may be useful in assessing the extent of disease and may delineate fistula formation.

Treatment

Medical management Attention to nutritional state is essential and anaemia should be corrected by iron or vitamin supplements. Malnourishment should be managed by a high-protein, low-residue or elemental diet. Hydrophilic colloid preparations and codeine phosphate may help diarrhoea, and cholestyramine can be used to bind bile salts and prevent their cathartic effects on the colon in patients with small bowel disease.

Steroids can be used in the acute phase (prednisolone 30–60 mg daily by mouth), but every attempt should be made to avoid long-term steroid therapy in view of the risk of complications. There are no drugs that can guarantee freedom from relapse, but large bowel Crohn's disease may respond to sulfasalazine (3–4 g daily by mouth). Small bowel disease does not respond to sulfasalazine because colonic bacteria are required to metabolize the compound to its active principles, sulfapyridine and 5-aminosalicylate. Aminosalicylates, such as mesalazine and olsalazine, may be useful in some relapsing cases, but there is no clear evidence that maintenance therapy prevents relapse in the long term. Azathioprine (3 mg/kg daily) can be used in resistant cases. Monoclonal antibodies to tumour necrosis factor-α (TNF-α) have reached clinical use and may have a place in patients with fistulating Crohn's disease where steroid therapy has failed.

Surgical management Almost 90% of patients with Crohn's disease require surgery at some stage. Surgery may have a role in the acute management of abscess or perforation, and in the chronic situation where there are frequent relapses on maximum medical management or failure to respond in subacute disease. Perianal and chronic burnt-out disease with fibrosis and stricturing may necessitate intervention for intermittent bowel obstruction. Operation is reserved for patients who are not thriving on medical management or who have complications (notably obstruction, abscess, perforation and fistula). Uninvolved bowel should be preserved and the residual small bowel length documented. Strictureplasty is a useful technique which involves longitudinal division of the strictured small bowel with closure of the defect transversely to widen the intestinal lumen. Radical surgery is contraindicated, as the risk of recurrence is determined by the natural history of the disease rather than the extent of surgery. The recurrence rate following small bowel resection is around 30%, as opposed to less than 20% in colonic disease. In the initial phases of colonic Crohn's disease segmental resection is preferred to bypass of affected segments. However, many patients eventually undergo proctocolectomy and ileostomy. Surgery carries an operative mortality of up to 5% due to sepsis, but late deaths bring overall mortality to around 10%.

In perianal Crohn's disease loculated pus can be drained and radical surgery should be avoided, as the disease tends to recur. Fistulae should be laid open and complex reconstructions avoided.

Ulcerative colitis

In western countries the annual incidence is approximately 10 new cases per 100 000 population. The cause is unknown, but most interest centres on an immunological basis for the disease. Ulcerative colitis affects all age groups but the peak incidence occurs in young adults. Unlike Crohn's disease, the incidence of ulcerative colitis is static.

Although ulcerative colitis is primarily a disease of the large bowel, systemic manifestations (iritis, polyarthritis, sacroiliitis, hepatitis, erythema nodosum, pyoderma gangrenosum) can occur. In 95% of cases the disease is contiguous, affecting the rectum and extending proximally (Table 22.3). In 5% of cases it is segmental and the rectum is occasionally spared. There is substantial risk of colorectal adenocarcinoma in cases with pancolitis (Table 22.3).

Pathological features

The characteristic feature of ulcerative colitis is that it involves only the mucosal lining of the large bowel. However, when severe there may be full-thickness involvement, with inflammatory infiltrate. Abscesses form at the base of the colonic crypts, which may burst horizontally or

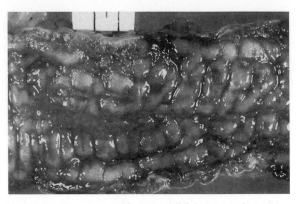

Fig. 22.9   Macroscopic features of fulminant ulcerative colitis.

occasionally radially to involve deeper layers of the bowel wall. The abscesses have a surrounding inflammatory infiltrate and coalesce to form ulcers which undermine the mucosa (Fig. 22.9). The intervening mucosa becomes oedematous and may form inflammatory pseudopolyps. The bowel loses its haustrations and becomes thick and rigid, although strictures are uncommon.

Clinical features

Ulcerative colitis characteristically runs an intermittent course of relapse and remission, although some patients may have a chronic continuous variant. In some cases the initial attack is fulminant, and toxic dilatation with exacerbation of abdominal and systemic symptoms may occur at any time. Diarrhoea with the passage of mucus and blood is typical of relapse. Passage of 10 or more stools each day is not unusual and there is often incapacitating faecal urgency. Abdominal pain and tenderness may be present and intermittent pyrexia is common.

Careful rectal examination should detect anal complications such as fissure, fistula and haemorrhoids, which are present in 25% of cases. The rectal mucosa often feels thick and boggy. Sigmoidoscopy (with biopsy) is the key investigation and reveals a red, matt granular mucosa with contact bleeding. In the early stages of disease the only sign on sigmoidoscopy may be loss of the rectal mucosal vessels. As the disease progresses severe ulceration leads to fulminant colitis, the complications of which include toxic dilatation and severe bleeding. During an exacerbation the dilated colon may become paper-thin.

Investigations

A barium enema is valuable to assess the extent of the disease (Fig. 22.10) but is contraindicated in the acute phase for fear of precipitating perforation. Typical changes

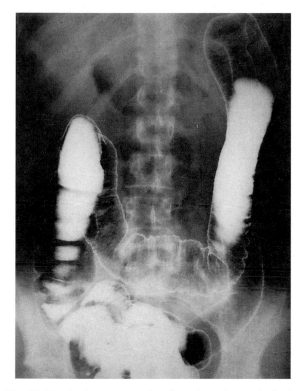

Fig. 22.10 Barium enema showing ulceration typical of pan-ulcerative colitis.

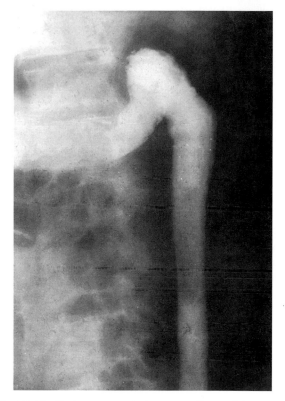

Fig. 22.11 Barium enema in long-standing colitis, showing a featureless colon with loss of haustrations.

include loss of haustrations, fluffy granularity of the mucosa, and pseudopolyps. Ultimately the bowel may become short and featureless, resembling a smooth tube (Fig. 22.11). Undermining ulcers may create a double contour to the edge of the colon (Fig. 22.12). Widening of the retrorectal space, due to perirectal inflammation and reduced distensibility of the rectum, is common. So-called 'backwash ileitis' may produce a dilated and featureless terminal ileum in which the mucosa appears granular. Colonoscopy has an important place in the diagnosis and surveillance of colitis by detecting evidence of dysplasia.

In an acute attack plain films of the abdomen may reveal a dilated gas-filled colon in which pseudopolyps are evident. When toxic dilatation is suspected, daily plain X-rays are essential to monitor progress.

Cancer surveillance in ulcerative colitis

Cancer surveillance is important in the long-term management of patients with chronic ulcerative colitis and is a major factor in the decision to operate. There is clear evidence of a substantial elevation in cancer risk, most likely owing to the presence of chronic inflammation and increased mucosal cell proliferation. Early age at onset and total involvement (pancolitis) are strong predictors of cancer risk. In pancolitis the overall risk appears to be around 25% after 30 years. Carcinoma is often difficult to detect in colitis, is usually poorly differentiated and has a poor prognosis. Random biopsies should be taken at surveillance colonoscopies, as dysplasia indicates a high risk of cancer occurrence. There is no direct evidence that screening such patients provides benefit in early detection, but it is important to discuss the cancer risk with patients. Restorative proctocolectomy in patients with pancolitis may be considered, especially when ulcerative colitis was diagnosed before the age of 15 years, rather than accepting the uncertainties of a prolonged surveillance programme without proven benefit.

Treatment

Medical management

With fluid and electrolyte replacement, correction of anaemia, adequate nutrition and steroid therapy, and timely surgical intervention when appropriate, 97% of patients survive their first attack. However, 70% are destined to have recurrent episodes. High-dose systemic steroids

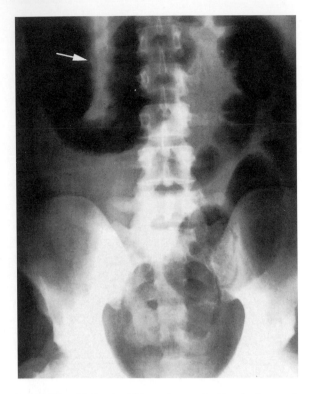

Fig. 22.12   Abdominal X-ray demonstrating features of toxic megacolon due to inflammatory bowel disease. Grossly thickened bowel wall is apparent (arrowed) and the patient required total colectomy.

(prednisolone, methylprednisolone or hydrocortisone) are needed during an acute relapse. Immunosuppression with either azothioprine or cyclosporine may be helpful for those who do not respond. Topical steroids delivered by enema or suppository usually control mild attacks of proctocolitis. Long-term aminosalicylates such as mesalazine or olsalazine are now preferred to sulfasalazine and have been shown to reduce the risk of relapse when a patient is in remission. Around 15% of patients eventually require surgery. The risk varies from 1 in 50 for those with mild proctitis, to 1 in 20 for those with moderately severe colitis, to 1 in 3 for those with extensive disease.

Elective surgery

Surgery is indicated for failure of medical management or repeated relapses on medical treatment. Failure to thrive, as reflected in retardation of growth and sexual development in children, or malnourishment and anaemia in adults, is a common indication for operation. Local complications that influence the decision to operate include those affecting the perineum and the rare instance when a stricture has formed.

The onset of biopsy-proven dysplasia or early carcinoma in chronic disease and the onset of fulminant colitis unresponsive to maximal medical management necessitate surgical intervention. Toxic megacolon or perforation and severe extracolonic manifestations may occasionally require colonic resectional surgery, although both ankylosing spondylitis and liver disease are unaffected.

Operative options

In the acute setting bowel reconstruction is inadvisable and an ileostomy is required. In the elective situation panprotocolectomy involves excision of the colon, rectum and anus, with a permanent ileostomy. This remains a valuable option and is useful when there is an associated low rectal cancer involving the sphincter muscles. Another historical option involved colectomy and ileorectal anastomosis, but such patients suffered continuing proctitis and diarrhoea and also required regular surveillance for rectal cancer.

Modern surgical practice aims to preserve continence following removal of the diseased bowel. The Koch's pouch involves a stoma following panproctocolectomy but the patient does not require a stoma bag as the pouch is emptied by cannulating the spout. The more common approach involves proctocolectomy with retention of the anal sphincters and reconstruction by formation of a terminal ileal pouch, which is anastomosed to the upper anal canal. This approach has the benefits of removing all but a tiny cuff of rectal mucosa in the upper anal canal, and also maintaining the ability of the patient's bowel to move normally. The operation is complex and may require a temporary ileostomy to protect the ileoanal anastomosis. The overall quality of life is excellent, despite the passage of four to six liquid motions per day.

Emergency surgery

Perforation, toxic dilatation and massive bleeding are all indications for emergency surgery. Acute fulminant colitis which fails to respond promptly to aggressive medical therapy may also mandate urgent operation. Modern management comprises a 'first aid' operation of colectomy and ileostomy to allow the patient to recover from the associated sepsis and nutritional depletion. The rectum is closed over as a stump in the pelvis, or by bringing out the distal end as a mucous fistula, but is subsequently removed as there can be persistent active disease in addition to a substantial cancer risk. Completion proctectomy and the formation of an ileoanal pouch is undertaken following recovery from the emergency operation.

as a result of intussusception or bleeding, particularly in the case of leiomyoma.

Malignant tumours

The diagnosis of a malignant tumour of the small intestine is notoriously difficult as symptoms are ill defined and intermittent. Small bowel imaging, such as a follow-through contrast study, may not reveal a lesion because of overlying loops of unaffected small bowel. Abdominal CT or MRI may be useful.

Adenocarcinoma The duodenum and upper jejunum are the most common sites of these rare tumours. The tumours, which are usually poorly differentiated and are mucin secreting, may be associated with hereditary non-polyposis colorectal cancer. Resection of the affected segment is carried out, but palliative bypass may be all that is possible as the disease often presents late.

Lymphoma Coeliac disease is a predisposing factor in small bowel T-cell lymphoma which, along with B-cell lymphoma, can cause intermittent obstruction, bleeding or perforation. The disease should be staged preoperatively to allow further systemic or local treatment to be planned. Antigliadin and antiendomysial antibodies should be determined and a biopsy of adjacent normal small intestine or duodenal biopsy should be assessed for villous atrophy.

Carcinoid tumour The small bowel is the second most common site for carcinoid tumour after the appendix. Metastasis to lymph nodes is common at presentation, and obstruction and bleeding are the usual mode of presentation. There may be features of the carcinoid syndrome in the presence of liver metastasis, but blood 5-HT levels are determined in the absence of liver metastasis. The primary tumour should be resected where possible.

Peutz–Jeghers syndrome

Peutz–Jeghers syndrome is an autosomal dominant inherited disorder with high penetrance. The gene, *LKB1/STK11*, is located on the short arm of chromosome 19 and mutations are causative in most families, although some cases are due to as yet unmapped genes. The clinical manifestations include gastrointestinal polyps and melanin pigmentation at mucocutaneous junctions, and occasionally on the dorsum of the hands and feet. Small intestinal and gastric cancers occur in around 7% of patients and the lifetime risk of colorectal cancer is 10%.

Pathology Polyps occur most commonly in the jejunum and have a short pedicle with a lobulated surface resembling that of an adenomatous polyp, or sometimes a villous tumour. On microscopy the hamartomas consist of branches of muscularis mucosae covered by epithelium and lamina propria. Adenocarcinomatous change may occur but it is

DISORDERS OF THE SMALL INTESTINE

Small bowel neoplasms

Small bowel tumours account for less than 5% of all gastrointestinal neoplasms.

Benign tumours

Solitary neoplasms include adenomatous or villous polyps, hamartomas, lipomas, haemangiomas and leiomyomas. Multiple hamartomas are found in the Peutz–Jeghers syndrome (see below). Benign tumours are rarely symptomatic and so the true incidence is unknown. Symptoms may arise not clear whether this arises in a hamartoma or in an area of normal epithelium.

Clinical features Most cases present in childhood or adolescence. There are usually dark brown or bluish spots on the lips and inside the mouth. The face, palms, soles, arms and perianal region can also be affected, but patients without pigmentation have been described. The usual presentation is with abdominal pain or obstruction due to intussusception of a polyp, but rectal bleeding and iron deficiency anaemia are also common.

Treatment Treatment is conservative wherever possible, but enterotomy and polypectomy is recommended as polyps tend to develop at the anastomosis. Upper and lower GI surveillance endoscopy is recommended to exclude cancer.

Diverticula of the small intestine

Meckel's diverticulum This is the commonest congenital abnormality of the gastrointestinal tract and comprises persistence of part of the vitellointestinal duct. The diverticulum arises from the antimesenteric border of the ileum some 2 feet from the ileocaecal valve in 2% of people, and is on average 2 inches long. It is a true diverticulum and in 10% of cases its tip is connected to the umbilicus by a fibrous cord. Heterotopic mucosa is found in 50% of symptomatic diverticula and is most often acid-secreting gastric mucosa.

Only 5% of Meckel's diverticula ever cause symptoms, most frequently in childhood or early adult life. Bleeding from peptic ulceration is the commonest cause of severe gastrointestinal bleeding in childhood. Intestinal obstruction may occur due to intussusception of the diverticulum, or to a loop of bowel becoming trapped beneath or twisted around (volvulus) a band extending to the umbilicus. Acute diverticulitis produces abdominal pain and tenderness, pyrexia and leukocytosis, and may mimic acute appendicitis.

Symptomatic Meckel's diverticula should be excised. Asymptomatic diverticula found incidentally at laparotomy should be left alone unless the neck is narrow or nodularity suggests that the diverticulum contains abnormal mucosa. In patients with unexplained gastrointestinal bleeding, heterotopic mucosa within a Meckel's diverticulum can be detected by scintiscanning after injection of ^{99m}Tc-labelled sodium pertechnetate.

Jejunal diverticulosis Jejunal diverticula are acquired during adult life. Only one or two diverticula may be present, but often diverticulosis is very extensive, with multiple wide-mouthed sacs caused by herniation of mucosa into the mesentery at the site of vessel penetration of the gut wall. Jejunal diverticulosis may first be diagnosed at laparotomy for complicated disease, or incidentally by barium studies or at operation. The diverticula may cause bleeding, inflammation, malabsorption (owing to their contained bacteria) and perforation. Occasionally fishbones or even non-steroidal anti-inflammatory tablets can become trapped in a diverticulum and cause local perforation. In symptomatic disease the affected segment of bowel may have to be locally resected, leaving other affected areas in situ.

Radiation injury

External beam irradiation or internal irradiation using radioactive implants can cause proctocolitis and enteritis. In the acute phase oedema, inflammation and ulceration may produce diarrhoea, lower abdominal pain, tenesmus, mucus discharge and rectal bleeding. Subsequently, the bowel may thicken, with fibrosis and stricture. Topical steroids or topical aminosalicylates such as a mesalasine enema may give symptomatic relief of proctitis. Stricture and fistula formation usually require resection of the affected bowel. If the fistula affects the rectum and vagina, excision of the whole rectum and replacement with fresh colon from outside the irradiated field, employing a coloanal J-pouch reconstruction, may be required. A defunctioning ileostomy has to be used with caution, as the small bowel itself often has been irradiated.

Ischaemia of the small intestine

In westernized countries small intestinal ischaemia is often due to atheromatous occlusion with superadded thrombosis of the superior mesenteric artery. Factors predisposing to mesenteric thrombosis include hypovolaemia or hypoperfusion of the gut resulting from trauma, cardiogenic shock, cardiac arrhythmia and septic shock. Arterial embolism can result from atrial fibrillation or recent myocardial infarction. In a third of patients dying from acute ischaemic necrosis of the midgut there is no demonstrable occlusion of a major vessel, and in these cases low perfusion is responsible. Other causes include polycythaemia, sickle cell disease and disseminated intravascular coagulation. Arteritis should be suspected where there are other stigmata or a history of disseminated arteritis, such as pre-existing renal failure. Impaired venous return from the gut can be due to hyperviscosity syndromes and prothrombotic tendency, but are also seen in the presence of malignancy and portal hypertension.

Ischaemic necrosis may progress to necrosis of all bowel layers with gangrene and perforation, but recovery may ensue if flow is restored within 6 hours. Slow resolution of a short segment of ischaemia may result in fibrosis and stricture formation in the longer term.

Acute mesenteric infarction

Acute occlusion of the superior mesenteric artery (SMA) is predominantly a disease of the elderly and is increasing in frequency. It leads to complete necrosis and gangrene of most of the midgut, and massive resection is inevitable unless flow can be restored within 6 hours. Even if the patient survives, the resulting nutritional problems may prove overwhelming.

Clinical features Early diagnosis is difficult as the symptoms and signs are non-specific. There may be a preceding history of chronic or episodic abdominal pain associated with meals, diarrhoea and weight loss. Cardiac arrhythmias, notably atrial fibrillation, are often present on initial presentation. Abdominal pain is a predominant symptom and may be associated with vomiting. In a third of cases there is watery or bloody diarrhoea. The pain varies in its location but is generally central, severe and constant in nature. Abdominal tenderness, guarding and rigidity are late signs denoting gangrene and perforation, and cardiovascular collapse signifies hypovolaemia and sepsis.

Investigation and diagnosis In almost all cases the diagnosis is made on the basis of clinical suspicion. As many affected patients are old and frail, with multiple comorbidities, a decision must be taken early as to whether active management is indicated. Plain abdominal films may reveal calcified atheroma in the mesenteric arteries and aorta, and there may be dilated thickened gas-filled small bowel loops. Gas in the bowel wall or in the peritoneal cavity is a grave sign. Leukocytosis and hyperamylasaemia are common, but the finding of metabolic acidosis on blood gas analysis should raise suspicion of bowel ischaemia. Arteriography is seldom helpful in practice because of the late presentation of most cases. The decision to undertake laparotomy should be taken on clinical grounds.

Treatment Following vigorous resuscitation gangrenous bowel requires resection, but this may be futile in elderly patients with extensive midgut involvement. In some instances of acute occlusion arterial flow can be restored by embolectomy or thrombectomy. A 'second-look' laparotomy 24 hours later may be useful. The prognosis is poor, with an overall mortality of 70–90%. Survival is restricted almost exclusively to patients in whom a defined vascular occlusion is treated early. Mesenteric venous occlusion has an equally bad prognosis, and treatment is usually confined to resection of the gangrenous bowel and anticoagulation.

Chronic mesenteric ischaemia

Chronic mesenteric ischaemia results in repeated bouts of ill-defined colicky central abdominal pain commencing 20–30 minutes after eating. Weight loss may be present as the patient is frightened to eat for fear of initiating the pain. Diagnosis is often elusive and frequently requires the exclusion of large bowel cancer and Crohn's disease. Mesenteric arteriography may be conclusive but must be taken in the context of symptoms, as athcromatous change in mesenteric vessels is common.

Paralytic ileus

Paralytic ileus is a term that refers to lack of propulsive contractions of the small intestine, affecting both jejunum and ileum, although the ileus can be localized in some instances. Treatment is usually focused on the underlying cause. Ileus is common after surgery owing to handling of

Table 22.4 Aetiology of intestinal obstruction		
	Small intestine	Large intestine
Intraluminal	Food bolus obstruction Gallstone ileus Trichobezoar/hairball (rare and restricted to mentally handicapped or psychiatrically disturbed patients)	Constipation
Intramural	Crohn's disease Radiation stricture Tumour Ischaemic stricture (Caecal cancer)	Colorectal cancer Diverticular stricture Crohn's disease Ischaemic stricture Volvulus (sigmoid colon or caecum) Ulcerative colitis (rare)
Extramural	Adhesions Incarcerated hernia Extrinsic compression by tumour Intussusception (usually predisposing cause in adults, e.g. caecal tumour)	Extrinsic compression by tumour

the bowel and in the presence of peritonitis due to any cause, such as perforated duodenal ulcer, pancreatitis, appendicitis and mesenteric ischaemia. Metabolic and electrolyte abnormalities, such as hypokalaemia, hyponatraemia, uraemia and diabetic ketoacidosis, can result in ileus. Drugs such as tricyclic antidepressants and lithium may be implicated in some cases.

Mechanical obstruction

Both large and small bowel obstruction can be classified into intraluminal, intramural and extramural (Table 22.4), but the most common cause of small intestinal obstruction in developed countries is adhesions and obstructed hernia. The most common cause of large bowel obstruction is colorectal cancer. Treatment usually requires operation and should be focused on the underlying cause of obstruction.

NON-NEOPLASTIC DISORDERS OF THE COLON AND RECTUM

Colonic diverticular disease

Colonic diverticular disease is an acquired condition which is extremely common in developed countries. Although there is a rare congenital solitary diverticulum of the caecum, which arises from the medial wall close to the ileocaecal valve and can extend upwards retroperitoneally, the aetiology of this condition is not related to that of the common type of acquired diverticular disease. Caecal diverticulum may become obstructed by a faecolith and inflamed, producing a clinical picture indistinguishable from appendicitis. Colonic diverticular disease is rare before the age of 35, but by 65 at least one-third of the population are affected. The diverticula are most common in the sigmoid colon and emerge between the mesenteric and antimesenteric taeniae. The diverticulum results from the herniation of mucosa through the circular muscle at the sites of penetration of blood vessels. Diverticular disease is associated with increased intraluminal pressure in the large bowel, and muscular hypertrophy can be detected radiologically before diverticula develop. The disease is rare in populations whose staple diet is high in roughage.

Uncomplicated diverticular disease

The disease may be asymptomatic or give rise to intermittent lower abdominal and left iliac fossa pain, altered bowel habit (usually constipation) and occasional minor rectal bleeding. The sigmoid colon is sometimes tender. Barium enema reveals muscle thickening and multiple diverticula (Fig. 22.13).

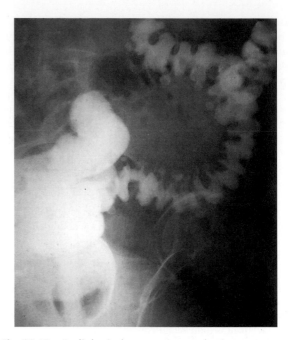

Fig. 22.13 Radiological appearance on barium enema of diverticular disease of the sigmoid colon.

Patients should be advised to take a high-fibre diet, supplemented if necessary by bran or a bulk laxative such as methylcellulose. Stimulant laxatives and purgatives are to be avoided. Antispasmodics such as propantheline may be useful if there is smooth muscle spasm and colicky pain. Sigmoid colectomy with primary anastomosis is indicated

Table 22.5 Complications of colonic diverticular disease
Inflammation
Peridiverticulitis
Pericolic abscess
Intestinal obstruction
Colonic fibrous stricture
Stricture and inflammatory mass
Adherent small bowel loops
Perforation
Purulent peritonitis
Faecal peritonitis
Fistula formation
Colovesical
Colovaginal
Enterocolic
Cutaneous (rare in modern practice)
Bleeding
Chronic intermittent blood loss
Massive lower GI haemorrhage

if there are persistent symptoms, or when carcinoma cannot be excluded by radiology or colonoscopy.

Complicated diverticular disease

Complications of diverticular disease are listed in Table 22.5. Faeces inspissated in a diverticulum may produce stasis and inflammation. Infection spreads locally and results in peridiverticulitis, producing a low-grade pyrexia and left iliac fossa pain. Persistent infection may cause necrosis and the formation of a peridiverticular abscess. Patients presenting with established diverticular abscess are usually toxic and may not respond to antibiotics. In the less acute setting, peridiverticular abscess may result in adherence to the vault of the bladder and the formation of a colovesical fistula. Free perforation of the peridiverticular abscess may result.

Diverticulitis

Peridiverticulitis presents with pyrexia, leukocytosis, nausea and vomiting, and there is often a history of alteration in bowel habit. Pain and tenderness in the left iliac fossa are almost universal and a mass may be palpable. The diagnosis is primarily a clinical one, with the typical presentation being sufficient to treat the patient expectantly. Confirmation of the diagnosis requires a barium enema, but this is best avoided for 4–6 weeks to allow the infection to settle. Treatment comprises bed rest, intravenous fluids and broad-spectrum antibiotics such as cephalosporin and metronidazole. Failure to settle suggests that a pericolic abscess is developing and that surgical drainage may be needed. Around a third of all patients admitted with acute diverticular disease undergo surgery during the index admission. The remainder settle and have no further attacks, but 10% eventually require surgery, which comprises sigmoid colectomy, preferably with full bowel preparation to allow primary anastomosis.

Perforation

Rupture of a pericolic abscess gives rise to purulent peritonitis, whereas free perforation of the bowel produces faecal peritonitis. The patient is usually profoundly ill, with septic shock, dehydration, marked abdominal pain, tenderness and distension. The patient is resuscitated vigorously and treated urgently by peritoneal lavage and resection of the affected bowel. Specialist colorectal surgeons may elect to perform an anastomosis in view of the fact that only 30% of colostomies are ever closed, and the patient would avoid the risk of a second laparotomy. If peritoneal contamination is severe and there is poor bowel perfusion of the gut, a colostomy may be preferable. The most common approach is to bring the proximal end on to the surface and oversew

the rectum (Hartmann's procedure), although the distal end may be exteriorized as a mucous fistula. Continuity can be restored after bowel preparation, but this should not be for at least 3 months. The mortality of perforated diverticular disease is 10–20% and may be as high as 50% in the elderly with faecal peritonitis.

Stricture formation and obstruction

Long-standing diverticular disease may cause stricture formation and subacute intestinal obstruction. Such strictures are often very difficult to distinguish from malignant strictures, particularly as diverticular disease coexisting with a cancer is almost universal. In many instances, a resection is undertaken without a firm diagnosis of cancer being established.

Fistula

Diverticular disease can give rise to fistulae to the skin or other viscera, notably the bladder, small bowel and vagina. Colovesical fistula is less common in women because the uterus is interposed between bladder and sigmoid colon. The patient usually complains of dysuria and the passage of a cloudy urine, with bubbling on micturition (pneumaturia). The diagnosis may be confirmed by barium enema but may not reveal the fistula in every case, because it is often intermittent. A CT or MRI scan may reveal air in the bladder and may show the fistulous tract itself. Treatment consists of sigmoid colectomy and synchronous repair of the bladder.

Bleeding

Diverticular disease may present with persistent fresh rectal bleeding or massive haemorrhage, which should be differentiated from angiodysplasia, haemorrhoids and fulminant inflammatory bowel disease. Colonoscopy seldom allows the bleeding site to be identified. Angiography may be helpful but the bleeding must be at the rate of 1 mL/min to be visible. In some cases of unremitting torrential haemorrhage, operation has to be undertaken when a source of bleeding has not been localized. On-table lavage and colonoscopy may be helpful in allowing a segmental resection of the affected bowel. However, in some cases a blind total colectomy and ileorectal anastomosis may be required.

Ischaemia of the large intestine

The aetiology of ischaemia of the large bowel is similar to that of the small intestine. Atheroma at the origin of the inferior mesenteric artery results in relative insufficiency of the arterial supply from the marginal artery (Fig. 22.2).

Colonic infarction may complicate aortic surgery if the inferior mesenteric artery is ligated. Untreated colonic ischaemia often progresses to gangrene and perforation. Some cases present with an acute bloody diarrhoeal illness known as ischaemic colitis, but others may declare symptoms from a chronic stricture.

Ischaemic colitis

In almost 50% of cases ischaemia of the large intestine is transient and necrosis is confined to the mucosa and submucosa. The patient presents with lower abdominal pain, nausea, vomiting and bloody diarrhoea. Coexisting cardiovascular disease should raise suspicion of the diagnosis. Examination reveals tenderness and guarding, often maximal in the lower left abdomen. There is usually a leukocytosis and pyrexia. Plain abdominal radiography may reveal a thickened segment of colon and thumbprinting due to submucosal oedema, which may be evident on barium enema (Fig. 22.14). Contrast studies should be carried out with water-soluble contrast such as gastrografin, because of the risk of perforation. The splenic flexure and sigmoid colon are most often affected. Ischaemic colitis is treated conservatively in the first instance unless abdominal signs reveal peritonitis, but symptoms should resolve after a few days of supportive therapy. A barium enema is indicated once the acute episode has settled to exclude diverticular disease.

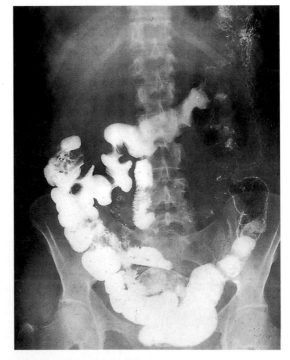

Fig. 22.14 Barium enema in a patient with ischaemic colitis showing oedema and appearance of thumbprinting in transverse colon.

Gangrenous ischaemic colitis

The clinical presentation is localized or even generalized peritonitis. Laparotomy is mandatory and resection with colostomy formation is the rule, as poor blood supply militates against a primary anastomosis.

Ischaemic stricture of the colon

Persistent bleeding and pain after an attack of bloody diarrhoea may suggest the diagnosis of ischaemic stricture. Barium enema reveals a smooth narrowing of a segment of bowel, with a funnelled appearance at either end which lacks the shouldered appearance of a malignant stricture (Fig. 22.15). Resection may be required, but some cases never come to medical attention and are revealed by chance during a barium study at a later date.

Other benign conditions

Volvulus

Volvulus of the colon principally affects the sigmoid or the caecum. Caecal volvulus is a misnomer, as it involves the caecum and the small intestine as the twist occurs around the superior mesenteric artery. The presence of a congenital intraperitoneal caecum predisposes to the volvulus. Sigmoid volvulus is more common and involves only the sigmoid itself, with the twist occuring around a narrow origin in the sigmoid mesentery. This acquired condition is the most common cause of large bowel obstruction in Nigeria. In the

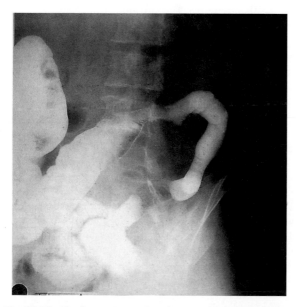

Fig. 22.15 Barium enema showing resolving ischaemic stricture at the splenic flexure.

UK patients are usually elderly and chronic constipation is associated. The clinical presentation is of a bowel obstruction with lower abdominal pain, abdominal distension, nausea, vomiting and absolute constipation. Occasionally the patient may present with sepsis owing to an established visceral perforation.

Sigmoid volvulus exhibits a characteristic Y-shaped shadow surrounded by a grossly distended colon arising out of the pelvis on a plain radiograph. Caecal volvulus is usually suggested by an anticlockwise rotation of dilated small bowel loops around a grossly distended caecum. Contrast studies or CT may help in atypical cases. Sigmoid volvulus can be treated conservatively in the emergency situation by reduction and deflation, using rigid sigmoidoscopy and the placement of a large-bore tube into the sigmoid. Elective sigmoid colectomy following full bowel preparation is curative in the fit patient. Caecal volvulus usually requires emergency laparotomy and resection of any infarcted bowel. The caecum is sutured to the posterior abdominal wall or resected by a limited right hemicolectomy. The narrow root of the small intestinal mesentery must be corrected by anchoring sutures.

Angiodysplasia

Angiodysplasia is an important cause of massive lower GI haemorrhage and may coexist with diverticular disease. The acquired submucosal arteriovenous malformations commonly affect the caeum and sigmoid colon, but any part of the large bowel can be affected. The diagnosis may be secured by visualization of a bleeding point at colonoscopy. Bleeding angiodysplastic lesions can be treated by angiographic embolization, by laser treatment or injection sclerotherapy at colonoscopy, or by resection at emergency laparotomy.

Pseudo-obstruction

This condition, also known as Ogilvie's syndrome, is of particular importance as part of the differential diagnosis of mechanical large bowel obstruction: 25–30% of patients presenting with symptoms, signs and radiological features conducive with obstruction have a pseudo-obstruction. Contrast radiography is therefore essential in all cases of suspected mechanical large bowel obstruction. Operative mortality from pseudo-obstruction is high and surgery should be avoided wherever possible. Pseudo-obstruction is a functional disorder of the large bowel and usually arises in the elderly and frail. The underlying mechanism is not fully understood, but there is frequently other comorbidity or active disease such as chest infection. Other specific associated aetiological factors include hypokalaemia, hypocalcaemia, lithium therapy for manic depression, retroperitoneal haematoma or tumour, and diabetes.

Management is conservative and involves stimulant enemas. Colonoscopic deflation may be required in cases where caecal distension causes concern about impending caecal perforation. Erythromycin has been shown to bind to the motilin receptors in the colon and can be effective in non-resolving cases. In a minority of cases colectomy and ileorectal anastomosis may be required.

Pseudomembranous colitis

Pseudomembranous colitis is associated with the use of oral broad-spectrum antibiotics in particular. *Clostridium difficile* is the organism responsible in almost all cases, and can be diagnosed by stool culture or by assays for the presence of *Cl. difficile* toxin in stool or blood. Necrosis of the colorectal mucosa causes watery diarrhoea, toxaemia, shock and collapse. The stools are watery, green, foul-smelling and bloodstained, and often contain fragments of mucosal slough. A pseudomembrane is often visible on sigmoidoscopy and a biopsy confirms the diagnosis. Treatment consists of intravenous fluid replacement and vancomycin (125 mg orally every 6 hours for 10 days). In rare instances a toxic megacolon may develop that is indistinguishable from that associated with inflammatory bowel disease.

Hirschsprung's disease

Hirschsprung's disease affects 1 in 5000 live births and is due to the absence of ganglion cells in Auerbach's and Meissner's plexuses. It is an inherited disorder showing incomplete penetrance and variable expressivity. In some cases there is a strong familial component and mutations of the *RET* oncogene on chromosome 10 are responsible for most of these cases. *RET* gene mutations are also associated with multiple endocrine neoplasia type 2. In most cases 5–20 cm of the distal large bowel is affected. The disease usually presents in childhood, but late presentation in adult life is not unknown. Loss of peristalsis in the affected segment leads to large bowel obstruction with gross distension of the colon proximal to the aganglionic segment. The differential diagnosis in the neonate includes imperforate anus and meconium ileus, and in older children megacolon acquired as a result of chronic constipation. Ischaemic colitis and necrotizing enterocolitis due to superinfection with *Staphylococcus aureus* have been reported.

Barium enema reveals dilated bowel above the narrowed aganglionic segment, and lack of ganglia can be confirmed by full-thickness biopsy of the abnormal area. In neonates treatment consists of irrigation of the bowel with saline, followed by operation at about 6 weeks to bring ganglionated bowel down to the anal verge. In older children a preliminary colostomy may be needed to allow bowel decompression. In the rare instance where the disease is not diagnosed until adulthood, the proximal colon is usually dysfunctional due to chronic megacolon and proctocolectomy, and ileoanal pouch reconstruction may be preferable to anterior resection.

Acquired megacolon and idiopathic slow-transit constipation

In some children chronic constipation may result in megacolon and is associated with behavioural problems and difficulty with toilet training. The initial complaint is often faecal soiling, but a vicious cycle of constipation and anal fissure may ensue. In adults defaecatory problems ranging from idiopathic slow-transit constipation to adult megacolon and megarectum may arise. Electrophysiological studies have shown changes reminiscent of Hirschsprung's disease affecting the whole of the large bowel, and there may be associated gastric motility dysfunction. Examination reveals gross faecal loading of the colon and rectum. Barium studies reveal a capacious and poorly contracting bowel with huge redundant loops. Transit studies with radio-opaque markers or with radiolabelled enema typically show that transit is delayed.

Initial conservative management with aperients, bulk laxatives and regular enemas is successful in many cases, but faecal disimpaction under general anaesthesia may be required. In resistant cases colectomy may be indicated, but careful specialist consideration should be sought as severe cases are often due to neuropathy of the whole gut and surgery may not be curative.

Irritable bowel syndrome

Irritable bowel disease is a functional bowel disease that is relevant to surgical practice because it presents with symptoms that are often indistinguishable from structural bowel disease, such as inflammatory bowel disease and cancer. Because of the lack of discriminatory clinical features, the diagnosis is largely one of exclusion, once appropriate investigation has ruled out other disorders.

POLYPS AND POLYPOSIS SYNDROMES OF THE LARGE INTESTINE

The terms 'polyp' and 'tumour' are not synonymous, as metaplastic polyps are commonly mistaken for adenomas. The histological classification of colorectal polyps into four groups has clinical relevance (Table 22.6).

Colorectal adenoma

True neoplastic epithelial polyps are classified as tubular, tubulovillous and villous adenomas. These affect 70% of

Table 22.6   Classification of benign intestinal polyps

Type	Solitary	Multiple
Neoplastic	Adenoma	Familial adenomatous polyposis
Hamartomatous	Juvenile polyp	Juvenile polyposis
	Peutz–Jeghers polyp	Peutz–Jeghers syndrome
		Cronkhite–Canada syndrome
		Cowden's disease
Inflammatory	Benign lymphoid polyp	Benign lymphoid polyposis
		Pseudopolyposis
		in ulcerative colitis
Unclassified	Metaplastic (hyperplastic)	Multiple metaplastic polyps

people aged 65–69 years and 40% of asymptomatic individuals over 50 years of age. Tubular adenomas are usually pedunculated but occasionally are sessile. Tubular adenomas account for 75% of all adenomas, villous adenomas for 10%, and tubulovillous types for 15%. However, villous adenomas account for 60% of lesions larger than 2 cm. Villous tumors are most common in the rectum and some may carpet the rectum. Around 50% of such tumours have a focus of carcinoma at presentation. Villous adenomas greater than 1 cm in diameter have an approximately 30% chance of malignancy, whereas the risk in a similar-sized tubular adenoma is around 10%. Multiple adenomas are common, with 24% of patients having two tumours.

Clinical features   The majority of polyps are asymptomatic. They may cause rectal bleeding or large bowel colic, especially when a large polyp has caused intussusception. Occasionally a rectal polyp may prolapse through the anus. Patients with rectal villous adenomas can present with severe watery diarrhoea, with water and electrolyte depletion due to excessive mucus loss. Rectal adenomas may be palpable, but villous tumors are soft and may be missed. Distal polyps are detected readily by sigmoidoscopy, but there is a need for full colonoscopy (Fig. 22.16) in view of the risk of synchronous lesions. Colonoscopy is superior to barium enema as it affords the opportunity for polypectomy.

Clinical management   The rationale for removal of asymptomatic polyps is to prevent malignancy. Colonoscopy with polypectomy enables histological assessment of the polyp, and advanced colonoscopic techniques such as lasering or submucosal resection are now well established for difficult cases. Smaller adenomas can be biopsied and a current applied to destroy the polyp site ('hot' biopsy). However, polypectomy using an electrocautery snare may be the only treatment required. Polyps demonstrating malignant change may be managed in this way if there are no features of poor differentiation, stalk invasion at the resection margin, or invasion of submucosal lymphatics. It may be necessary to surgically excise larger polyps per-anally or by bowel resection. Transanal endoscopic microsurgery (TEM) allows resection of large rectal villous adenoma and suture of the rectum using an operating microscope.

Follow-up colonscopy is recommended 6–12 months later and after 2–3 years. The current view is not in favour of long-term follow-up once the colon has been shown to be clear of any further polyps, unless the original polyp was large or there are recurrent lesions at the 3-year screen.

Familial adenomatous polyposis

Familial adenomatous polyposis (FAP) is one of the most common single gene disorders predisposing to cancer and is inherited as an autosomal dominant trait. The gene responsible is the *APC* gene, which is located on the long arm of chromosome 5. Almost every sporadic colorectal cancer has a defect in the *APC* gene or in other components of the involved pathway. The annual incidence of FAP is 1/6670 live births and the population prevalence is 1 in 13 528. Around 25% of affected individuals have no family history of FAP, the disease arising in these sporadic cases as a result of a new germline mutation.

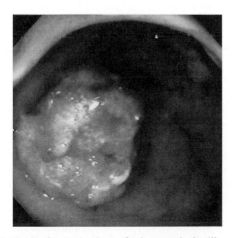

Fig. 22.16   Endoscopic view of a large tubulovillous adenoma of rectum.

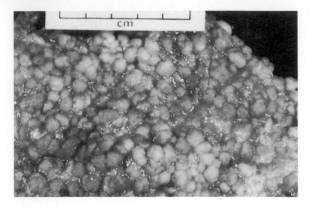

Fig. 22.17 Operative specimen of gross colonic polyposis in FAP.

Although the direct testing from the *APC* gene is possible, clinicopathological diagnosis requires the presence of >100 adenomatous polyps of the large bowel (Fig. 22.17). Polyps usually develop during the teenage years and early adulthood, with a virtual certainty of colorectal cancer by the third or fourth decade if prophylactic colectomy is not undertaken. Because of effective surgical prophylaxis, FAP now accounts for less than 0.2% of all cases of colorectal cancer in the UK. Furthermore, the prevalence of colorectal cancer at diagnosis is 65% for symptomatic 'sporadic' cases and only 5% for screened family members.

Extracolonic features Most of the gastric polyps detected in 70% of FAP patients show cystic enlargement of the fundic glands rather than adenomatous change. Duodenal adenomas are almost universal and malignant degeneration of periampullary adenoma is now the major cause of death, with 7% of patients eventually developing periampullary cancer. Ileal adenomas also occur in FAP, but the risk of progression to malignancy appears to be very low. Craniofacial and long bone osteomata, when associated with epidermoid cysts, give rise to Gardner's syndrome.

Intra-abdominal desmoid tumours arise in around 10% of FAP cases. Although benign, these lesions expand and compress adjacent structures. Intra-abdominal and retroperitoneal disease may be amenable only to surgical palliation. Treatment with teromiphene, tamoxifen, sulindac, indomethacin, chemotherapy and radiotherapy provides benefit in a few cases.

An epidermoid cyst arising in a prepubescent child should raise suspicion of FAP. Pigmented lesions of the retina, known as congenital hypertrophy of the retinal pigment epithelium (CHRPE), are well described in association with FAP. The lesions are asymptomatic but frequently affect both eyes. Women aged < 35 years with FAP are at 160 times greater risk of papillary thyroid carcinoma than non-FAP counterparts, but there is no excess risk in

men. Other rare associations with FAP include hepatoblastoma, carcinoma of the gallbladder, bile duct and pancreas, and an increased risk of brain tumors.

Diagnosis and clinical management The diagnosis can be established by sigmoidoscopy and biopsy. Screening of affected individuals by direct *APC* gene mutation analysis is used to define the optimal timing of prophylactic surgery. All FAP patients should be referred to a regional genetics service for registration and gene analysis.

Presymptomatic detection of FAP allows prophylactic colectomy before malignancy supervenes. The preferred treatment is restorative proctocolectomy with the formation of an ileal pouch reservoir. However, total colectomy with ileorectal anastomosis or proctocolectomy with ileostomy are also options. The upper GI tract should be screened for duodenal adenoma or carcinoma.

Peutz–Jeghers syndrome

This is discussed above in the section on small intestinal disorders.

Juvenile polyposis

Juvenile polyps are usually classified as hamartomas, although some regard them as inflammatory, with blockage of crypts resulting in retention cysts. Single juvenile polyps occur in around 1% of westernized populations and multiple juvenile polyposis is uncommon. The disorder usually manifests in childhood as volvulus or bleeding of the polyps. Occasionally children present with rectal prolapse, with the polyp as the head of the intussusception. The condition is inherited in an autosomal dominant fashion and the overall cumulative risk of colorectal cancer if there are any associated adenomas present is 68% at 60 years of age. Colonoscopic surveillance and prophylactic colectomy should be considered if adenomatous polyps are detected. Symptomatic polyps can be removed by polypectomy.

Other rare polyposis syndromes

Turcot's syndrome comprises adenomatous colorectal polyposis in association with astrocytoma (also medulloblastoma or glioblastoma) of the brain or spinal cord. In some families there is an autosomal recessive pattern of inheritance.

Cowden's disease is a rare disseminated form of gastrointestinal hamartomatous polyposis with an autosomal dominant pattern of inheritance, but most cases are due to mutations. There is a greater risk for benign and malignant disease of the breast and thyroid. All patients have warty tricholemmomas around the eyes, and these lesions are diagnostic when present with oral fibromas and keratoses of the hands and feet.

Cronkhite–Canada syndrome is a rare syndrome comprising intestinal polyposis with alopecia, atrophy of the nails and brown macular hyperpigmentation. Histological examination shows cystic dilatation of the crypts similar to that seen in juvenile polyposis. The condition does not seem to be inherited.

Metaplastic (hyperplastic) polyps

Large intestinal metaplastic polyps are usually less than 5 mm in diameter and occur in increasing numbers with age, being present in some 75% of the population over the age of 40 years. They tend to be pale, flat-topped, sessile plaques, mainly in the rectum and often on the crest of mucosal folds. There is no evidence of premalignant potential, and histologically the crypts are elongated, dilated and lined by columnar epithelium which has a sawtooth pattern. These polyps are often indistinguishable from adenomatous polyps and require no specific treatment. Some cases resemble multiple polyposis because the metaplastic polyps are both multiple and large.

Other colorectal polyps

Benign lymphoid polyps are round, smooth, sessile tumours, usually in the lower rectum, and vary in diameter from a few millimetres to 3 cm. They consist of an aggregate of normal lymphoid tissue covered by attenuated epithelium. They are most common in the third and fourth decades and usually present with rectal bleeding, anal pain and tenderness, or prolapse of the polyp. Treatment consists of local excision. Other polypoid conditions include pseudopolyps in chronic ulcerative colitis, submucosal lipoma, lymphosarcoma, carcinoid tumor and leiomyoma. Neurofibromatosis rarely results in colonic polyps. Mucosal ganglioneuromatosis has been described in association with multiple adenomatous or juvenile polyps and multiple endocrine neoplasia (MEN) type IIb.

MALIGNANT TUMOURS OF THE LARGE INTESTINE

Colorectal adenocarcinoma

Large bowel adenocarcinoma is the commonest gastrointestinal malignancy and is second only to lung cancer as a cause of cancer death in westernized countries. Of all cancer registration in the USA 18% are due to colorectal cancer, but only 2% in Nigeria. In the UK the lifetime risk of colorectal cancer is 5.1%, resulting in 32 000 cases each year. The male:female ratio for colon cancer is close to unity, whereas that for rectal cancer is 1.7:1 in high-incidence populations. The highest incidence rates are in the oldest popula-

---

> **SUMMARY BOX**
>
> **Neoplastic polyps of the large bowel**
>
> - Adenomatous polyps:
>   - account for 90% of large bowel polyps
>   - may bleed, prolapse or intussuscept
>   - carry a 5% risk of malignancy when over 1 cm in diameter.
> - Villous adenomas:
>   - account for 10% of all large bowel polyps
>   - are most common in the rectosigmoid region
>   - may produce a profuse mucous discharge (causing hypokalaemia)
>   - in one-third of cases are associated with carcinoma.
> - Familial adenomatous polyposis:
>   - is transmitted as an autosomal dominant trait in which the inherited defect is located in the *APC* gene on chromosome 5
>   - gives rise to polyps of the colon and rectum in late childhood
>   - is associated with a 100% risk of malignant transformation (although this is exceptional before the age of 20)

tion. The rectum and sigmoid are particularly common sites for tumours (Fig. 22.18), but in low-incidence countries tumours are more evenly distributed. Around 3% of patients present with synchronous tumours, and another 3% develop a metachronous tumour at a later date.

Aetiology

Diet A diet high in fibre is associated with lower cancer rates in certain populations, whereas the consumption of a diet high in fat and in red meat is associated with higher cancer rates. A low-fibre, high-fat diet appears to increase faecal pH, and this may enhance bile acid toxicity. Brassica vegetables, such as broccoli, contain antioxidants and other potential antineoplastic compounds. A deficiency of dietary calcium and vitamin D is associated with increased colorectal cancer risk.

Smoking, alcohol and exercise Smoking and alcohol excess are risk factors for men but women appear not to be subject to the excess risk. An association between lack of physical exercise and colorectal cancer has been observed. Colonic transit time may be reduced by exercise, but alterations in the levels of prostaglandins and antioxidant enzymes may also occur.

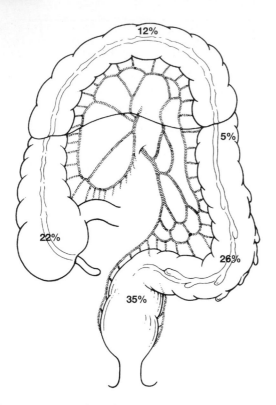

Fig. 22.18 Large bowel cancer: tumour distribution within the colon and rectum.

Inflammatory bowel disease The risk of colorectal cancer in ulcerative colitis and Crohn's disease is discussed in the relevant section.

Genetics Around 35% of all colorectal cancers can be accounted for by a substantial genetic contribution, which ranges from an ill-defined increased risk in individuals with a positive family history, to well defined autosomal dominant genetic traits in which the genes involved have been identified and mutations characterized. FAP and other polyposis syndromes are discussed above. The more common autosomal dominant syndrome, hereditary non-polyposis colorectal cancer (HNPCC), accounts for around 5% of all cases of colorectal cancer and is associated with only small numbers of adenomas. HNPCC is associated with an elevated risk of other malignancies, such as endometrial, gastric, ovarian, upper urinary tract and small intestinal. The minimum criteria for HNPCC diagnosis are (1) three or more relatives with histologically proven colorectal cancer, one being a first degree relative of the other two; (2) two or more generations affected; and (3) at least one family member affected before the age of 50 years. One case can be endometrial cancer rather than colorectal cancer. HNPCC is of major interest because of its prevalence and the potential to identify gene carriers by mutation analysis of blood samples, and so target those at risk for colonoscopic screening.

HNPCC is due to mutation of one of the genes that participate in DNA mismatch repair. Mutations are most common in *hMSH2* on chromosome 2p and *hMLH1* on chromosome 2q. Around 90% of large dominant HNPCC families from research studies have identifiable mutations. However, in clinical genetics practice only 30% of selected families have mutations in one of the genes responsible. A quarter of all patients aged under 40 years at diagnosis of colorectal cancer carry a DNA mismatch repair gene mutation, irrespective of family history.

Pathology and staging

Colorectal cancer may be polypoidal, ulcerating and stenosing (Fig. 22.19). Two-thirds are ulcerating and a typical lesion has raised everted edges, a slough-covered floor and indurated base. Tumours of the caecum tend to be large

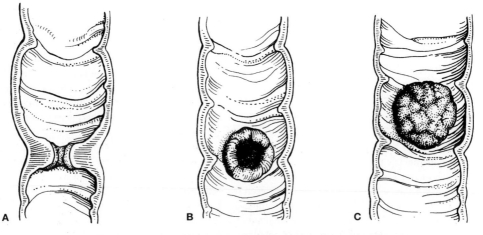

Fig. 22.19 Pathological types of large bowel cancer. **A** stenosing; **B** ulcerating; **C** polypoidal.

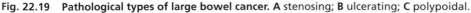

Table 22.7 Dukes' and TNM staging for colorectal cancer

Dukes' staging		Proportion of colorectal cancers
A	Spread into, but not beyond, muscularis propria	10
B	Spread through full thickness of bowel wall	30
C	Spread to involve lymph nodes	30
D*	Distant metastases	20

*Dukes' stage D is a misnomer as Dukes restricted staging to local and lymphatic spread.

TNM staging

Tx	Primary tumor cannot be assessed
Tis	Carcinoma in situ
T1	Cancer invades submucosa
T2	Cancer invades into muscularis propria
T3	Cancer invades through muscularis propria and into subserosa or adjacent non-peritonealized tissues
T4	Cancer perforates the visceral peritoneum or directly invades adjacent organs
Nx	The regional lymph nodes cannot be assessed
N0	No regional lymph nodes involved
N1	Metastases in 1–3 pericolic or perirectal lymph nodes
N2	Metastases in 4 or more pericolic or perirectal lymph nodes
N3	Metastases in lymph node along the course of a major named blood vessel
Mx	The presence of distant metastases cannot be assessed
M0	No distant metastases
M1	Distant metastases

exophytic growths. Tumour differentiation may be classified as good, moderate or poor. Around 10–20% of tumours have mucinous histology and a poor prognosis. There is an increasing proportion of proximal tumours in the UK, as right colonic cancer is more common in the elderly.

Colorectal cancer spreads by lymphatic invasion and via the portal blood to the liver. Once the peritoneum is breached, dissemination throughout the abdominal cavity is likely. Invasion of lymphatics results in regional lymph node involvement. Very low rectal tumours may also involve the inguinal nodes. Systemic metastases are unusual but do occur in the later stages of the disease. Tumours can be assessed using Dukes' and TNM staging systems (Table 22.7). Pathological staging has important implications for prognosis, but also for directing clinical management. Thus a decision on whether or not to offer patients adjuvant chemotherapy is made solely on the basis of staging.

Clinical features of established disease

There are no specific symptoms that discriminate cancer from benign intestinal diseases, or from symptoms common in healthy individuals. Presentation may include intermittent rectal bleeding, blood mixed with mucus, altered bowel habit, iron deficiency anaemia and colicky lower abdominal pain. Tenesmus occurs in over 50% of patients with low rectal cancers. Massive lower GI haemorrhage is rare and benign disease should be suspected. Perianal or sciatic type pain are ominous signs suggesting locally advanced rectal cancer. Sinister symptoms are often ignored by young patients, but 3% of presenting patients are under the age of 35. Around 15% of all patients present with obstruction and 3% have a perforation at presentation. Such complications significantly worsen the prognosis for a given tumour stage and increase the likelihood of the patient requiring a colostomy. Abdominal wall invasion may manifest as parietal pain and occasionally leads to abscess formation.

A full history is essential as clinical examination is often negative. There may be signs of anaemia and abdominal examination may reveal hepatomegaly or an abdominal mass, especially in right-sided colon cancer. There may be signs of bowel obstruction. Digital rectal examination is mandatory to detect low cancers and assess fixity and sphincter involvement. An FOB test will not alter the decision to investigate the symptomatic patient.

Population screening for colorectal cancer

Early detection of colorectal cancer by population screening may result in improved outcome and survival benefit. The most extensively studied screening test is the guaiac-

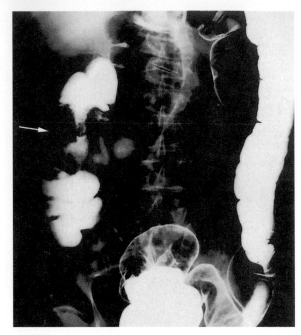

Fig. 22.20 Barium enema showing malignant 'apple-core' stricture in ascending colon (arrowed).

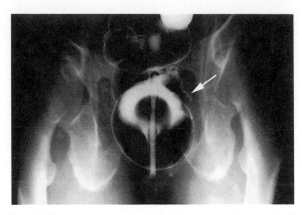

Fig. 22.21 Barium enema showing polypoidal cancer of the rectum (arrowed).

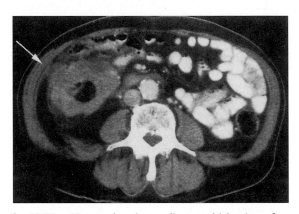

Fig. 22.22 CT scan showing malignant thickening of caecum (arrowed).

impregnated paper test for faecal occult blood (FOBT) – Haemoccult – but sensitivity is only 50–60%. The predictive value is around 10% for cancer and 50% for adenomas >1 cm. Specificity is the main problem with the test, as it generates large numbers of people with positive slides but no cancer. Screening by colonoscopy seems unlikely in view of the massive cost implications.

Diagnostic investigations

Barium enema is effective in identifying tumours throughout the colon and rectum (Fig. 22.20). In most instances with typical features of shouldering and mucosal destruction it is not necessary to visualize the tumour before operation. Sigmoidoscopy or colonoscopy allow visualization and biopsy of the tumour, particularly when the barium enema is inconclusive. Polypoidal tumours (Fig. 22.21) are easily visualized and snare polypectomy should be considered. In some very elderly patients colonoscopy or barium enema may not be tolerated and oral contrast-enhanced CT scans of the abdomen may be useful (Fig. 22.22).

Staging

Preoperative staging of colonic cancer requires an ultrasound or CT scan of the liver. For rectal cancer digital examination and rigid sigmoidoscopy allow assessment of the degree of tumour fixity, and this should be undertaken

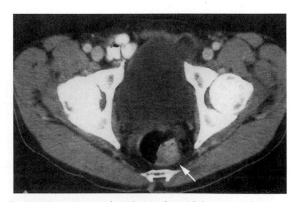

Fig. 22.23 CT scan showing polypoidal cancer of the rectum (arrowed) restricted to rectal wall.

in every case. Assessment may require an examination under anaesthetic (EUA). CT or MRI scan of the pelvis assesses the degree of local spread (Fig. 22.23). Endoanal ultrasound is also useful for staging at the time of an EUA.

Treatment

Surgery *En bloc* resection of the primary tumour and locoregional nodes is the principle of radical surgery for large bowel cancer and achieves cure in 75% of cases undergoing intended 'curative' resections. The ligation of the feeding vessel to the segments of bowel achieves lymphadenectomy of all locoregional nodes (Fig. 22.24). Resection offers cure for patients with localized disease and palliation for those with hepatic or other metastases, by preventing distressing features of advanced local disease. For rectal cancer, excision of the entire mesorectum reduces local recurrence rates to 5%. Wherever possible, bowel continuity should be restored. In specialist hands low rectal cancer should be treated by low anterior resection and coloanal anastomosis, and this can be combined with a small colonic J-pouch to improve defaecatory function. However, for a very low rectal cancer it may be necessary

to remove the anal sphincter as part of an abdominoperineal resection and fashion a permanent end-colostomy.

Local treatment of rectal cancer Rectal cancer can be excised peranally under direct vision or with a resectoscope. TEM is particularly applicable to small low-lying cancers (< 3 cm). Peranal excision gives acceptable results and avoids major abdominal surgery but should not be used in fit, potentially curable patients, as the recurrence rate is 25–30%.

Emergency surgery for obstruction or perforated colorectal cancer In cases of perforation or obstruction of colorectal cancer there is a substantially increased risk of perioperative mortality. The patient should be resuscitated before laparotomy is undertaken. For obstructed right-sided colon cancer, right hemicolectomy is the operation of choice. An ileotransverse anastomosis can be safely performed as the ileum has an excellent blood supply and the distal colon is not obstructed. Treatment of obstructed left colon cancer is best achieved by a one-stage resection with anastomosis whenever possible. Measures to reduce the risk of anastomotic leakage in such cases include on-table colonic lavage to remove faecal residue before anastomosis. Resection of the entire colon and ileorectal anastomosis avoids a colocolic anastomosis and also removes any syn-

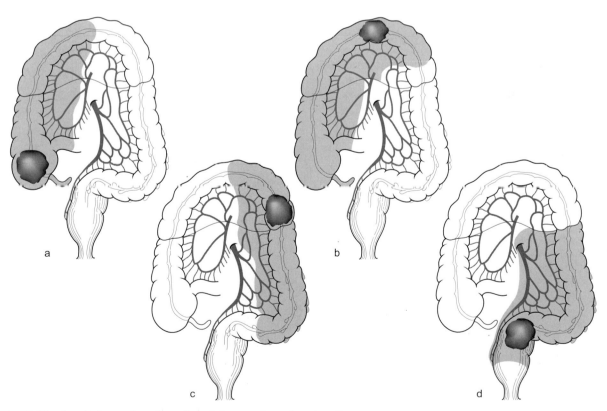

Fig. 22.24 Surgical resections for colorectal cancer in various locations.

chronous tumour. Patients with gross faecal peritonitis secondary to perforation of left colon cancer usually require resection, with the creation of an end-colostomy (Hartmann's procedure). If contamination is minimal, a specialist surgeon may elect to carry out primary resection and anastomosis.

Radiotherapy Adjuvant preoperative radiotherapy has an important place in the management of rectal cancer. It reduces local recurrence rates and also improves survival, but the practice of specialist surgeons in the UK is to offer selective preoperative radiotherapy. Either a 5-day short-course regimen of 45 Gy daily or a long-course regimen of 52 Gy given weekly over 3 months is administered. The former is reserved for patients with operable but tethered tumours, very low or anterior tumours, or if extrarectal spread is evident. Fixed, inoperable tumours are best dealt with by radical radiotherapy over 3 months, and this may be combined with 5-fluorouracil-based chemotherapy. Postoperative radiotherapy results in poor bowel function and may damage the small intestine, but has a role in palliation of local recurrence and in alleviating bone pain from metastases. Radiotherapy for colonic cancer is restricted in palliation as the fields are difficult to define and damage to adjacent bowel is likely.

Adjuvant chemotherapy Systemic adjuvant chemotherapy using 5-fluorouracil (5-FU) alone or in combination has been shown to improve survival for Dukes' C colorectal cancer after surgical resection, with an overall 30% improvement in survival. In the UK it is now routine practice to offer 5-FU-based chemotherapy to all patients with stage C cancers who do not have significant comorbidity. Suitable patients with Dukes' B tumours are invited to recruit to randomized trials, as it is not clear whether or not such patients benefit from the addition of chemotherapy. Newer agents are currently under trial, including irinotecan (CPT-11), temozolamide and oxiplatin, either alone or in combination with 5-FU.

Prognosis of colorectal cancer

Operative mortality rises from around 4% for elective resections to 25% in patients with obstructed colon going to theatre as an emergency. The overall 5-year survival for colorectal cancer in Scotland is 41%. However, overall 5-year survival is 75% for curative resections.

Local recurrence of colorectal malignancy may require further surgical intervention to deal with local symptoms, including obstruction. Both chemotherapy and radiotherapy may be required as palliation. It is also now evident that some patients with isolated hepatic metastases may be candidates for 'curative' resection of these (Chapter 19).

Other malignant tumours of the large intestine

Colorectal adenocarcinoma so dominates the incidence of large bowel cancer that all other malignant tumours are very rare in comparison.

> **SUMMARY BOX**
>
> **Large bowel cancer**
>
> - It is the second commonest cause of cancer death in western countries and has a particularly high incidence in Scotland.
>
> - Aetiological factors include diet, bile salts and a positive family history; recognized premalignant conditions are ulcerative colitis, pre-existing, adenomatous and villous polyps, and Crohn's disease.
>
> - Two-thirds of all large bowel cancers occur in the rectum and sigmoid colon, and the commonest clinical features are alteration in bowel habit and the passage of blood per rectum.
>
> - Presymptomatic diagnosis may be achieved by testing the stool for occult blood and by regular colonoscopy. With the identification of the genetic abnormalities associated with a high risk of colorectal cancer, genetic screening is becoming feasible.
>
> - The overall 5-year survival rate is 40% and the Duke's staging system is a useful prognostic index. If liver metastases are present survival beyond 2 years is exceptional.

Squamous cancer of the large bowel

Such tumours are not simply metastatic anal carcinomas but may arise in the caecum and proximal colon from an area of squamous metaplasia in long-standing ulcerative colitis. In the absence of chronic inflammation an adenosquamous pattern may be seen and the prognosis is poor.

Carcinoid tumors of the large bowel

Large bowel carcinoid tumours are rare but benign lesions which may be found incidentally during rectal examination as solitary, spherical, hard, sessile, yellowish submucosal nodules. Malignant carcinoid tumors of the colon may give rise to the carcinoid syndrome, and 60% have metastasized by the time of diagnosis.

Lymphoma of the large intestine

Primary lymphomas usually arise in the rectum or caecum but are occasionally multicentric. Secondary involvement of the large bowel in generalized disease is more common. Barium enema shows a long rigid segment with intramural thickening. The diagnosis is established by endoscopic or operative biopsy. Primary lymphomas are treated by resection followed by chemotherapy and radiotherapy.

Secondary malignant lymphoma and malignant lymphomatous polyposis are treated by systemic chemotherapy and targeted radiotherapy.

Leiomyosarcoma

These are tumors arise from the muscle of the bowel wall and are usually diagnosed by sigmoidoscopy. Benign and malignant forms are often impossible to distinguish clinically, and so resection is advisable. Metastasis occurs via the bloodstream to the liver and lungs.

23 Anorectal conditions

M.G. Dunlop

Table 23.2   Disorders of the anorectum
Anorectal abscess
Fistula-in-ano
Anal fissure
Haemorrhoids
Perianal haematoma
Rectal prolapse
Anal neoplasms
Functional disorders of sphincters and pelvic floor
Pilonidal disease

are often ignored or hidden from relatives and doctors alike. It is important that the perianal symptoms are elicited without embarrassment to the patient or clinician. The more common disorders of the anus and rectum that are encountered in clinical practice in the UK are listed in Table 23.2. Symptoms due to anorectal conditions overlap with those due to conditions affecting the large bowel, and so documentation of a full GI history is essential.

INTRODUCTION

Anorectal complaints are extremely common: approximately 2–3% of the population have anorectal symptoms at any given time. A basic understanding of the principles of applied anatomy and pathophysiology will help to differentiate patients who merit specialist assessment from those who can be treated symptomatically in the first instance. There remains a great deal of social taboo, and so the symptoms associated with anorectal disorders (Table 23.1)

Table 23.1   Symptoms associated with disorders of the anorectum
Bleeding
Perianal pain
Discharge
Pruritus ani
Anal incontinence
Prolapse

APPLIED SURGICAL ANATOMY

The anus is a remarkable structure which is capable of allowing (when socially convenient) the passage of between 25 000 and 80 000 formed stools during a lifetime, but it is also capable of maintaining continence to gas, fluid and solid at almost all other times. Knowledge of the anatomy is essential if effective treatment is to be instigated for many anorectal conditions, such as perianal fistula.

Anal musculature and innervation

The anal canal is 3–4 cm long in males and slightly shorter in females. It consists of two muscle layers (Fig. 23.1) known as the internal and the external sphincters. The internal sphincter is a condensation of the circular smooth muscle of the rectum and is continuous with the circular muscle of the whole of the GI tract. It is controlled by the autonomic nervous system with fibres from the pelvic sympathetic nerves, the lower lumbar ganglia and the pre-aortic/inferior mesenteric plexus. The parasympathetic fibres arise from the sacral plexus. The smooth muscle of the inter-

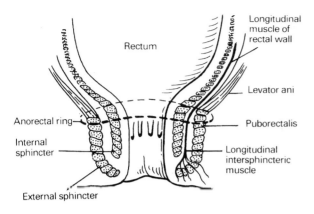

Fig. 23.1 Musculature of the anorectum.

nal sphincter maintains tone and contributes to resting pressure within the anal canal, and so plays an important role in maintaining anal continence. The longitudinal muscle of the gut ends at the anus as a series of fibrous bands which radiate to the perianal skin, and so is of little surgical or pathological consequence in perianal disease. The striated muscle of the external sphincter is under voluntary control, being innervated by the right and left internal pudendal nerves and the fourth branch of the sacral plexus. The circular muscle tube of the external sphincter blends with the lower part of the levator ani, known as the puborectalis sling (Fig. 23.2). The puborectalis fibres of the levator ani originate from the posterior aspect of the public symphysis and pass backwards to join with the external sphincter. The levator ani muscles themselves are also important in maintaining the relationship of the anus and rectum during defaecation.

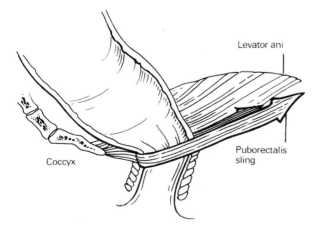

Fig. 23.2 The puborectalis sling establishing the anorectal angle.

Anal continence can be adversely affected by structural damage to the musculature, disruption of the nerve supply, or a combination of both. Damage to the internal or external sphincters can occur during childbirth. It can also occur as a consequence of perianal sepsis or the surgery required to treat it. Peripartum nerve injury or neurodegenerative disease can affect the pudendal nerves, eventually leading to denervation and atrophy of the striated muscle of the external sphincter, the puborectalis sling and the levator ani.

SUMMARY BOX

Anal continence

Continence is dependent on:
- Intact anorectal and pelvic floor sensation
- Intact anal sphincters and levator ani
- Preservation of the anorectal angle
- The bulk provided by the anal 'cushions'
- The anal 'flutter valve' effect.

The lining of the anal canal

The cell type of the anal canal epithelium determines why certain diseases, such as tumours and viral infections, affect only particular levels of the canal. The epithelium of the anal canal is specialized and contains three distinct zones. The external zone (from the pectinate line to the anal verge) is keratinized, stratified squamous epithelium, and is also known as the 'pecten'. There is a short anal transitional zone which lies above the pectinate line and is modified, non-keratinized squamous epithelium, separated from the columnar epithelial of the anal canal which is continuous with the rectal epithelium. The anal valves are crescentic mucosal folds that form a serrated or 'pectinate' line around the lumen of the mid anal canal (Fig. 23.3). The pectinate line, which is also known as the 'dentate' line, represents the line of fusion between the endoderm of the embryonic hindgut and the ectoderm of the anal pit. Thus, the epithelium is innervated by the autonomic nervous system and is insensate with respect to somatic sensation. The canal lining below the pectinate line is innervated by the peripheral nervous system and so conditions affecting this region, such as abscess, anal fissure or tumour, result in anal pain.

The composition of the epithelium of the anorectum determines the type of tumour that affects the region. Thus, squamous cell carcinoma of the anal canal arises from the epithelium *below* the pectinate line or in the transitional zone of non-keratinized squamous epithelium. Because the canal above the anal transition zone contains columnar

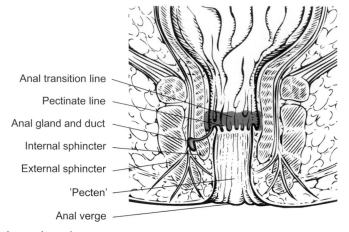

Fig. 23.3   The lining of the anal canal.

glandular epithelium, tumours of the upper anal canal are adenocarcinoma and best considered as a low rectal cancer and treated accordingly (see Chapter 22).

There are no epidermal appendages in the anal transitional zone, but there are specialized anal glands which are relevant to the aetiology of perianal abscess and fistula-in-ano. The precise function of the anal glands is unclear, but they secrete mucus and probably lubricate and protect the delicate epithelium of the anal transition zone. There are four to eight glands situated within the substance of the internal sphincter or in the space between the internal and external sphincter, known as the intersphincteric space (Fig. 23.4). The ducts from these glands open into the folds of mucosa at the pectinate line. The relevance of these glands lies in the fact that they are the source of most perianal abscesses. When an anal gland duct becomes occluded the obstructed gland may become infected with gut organisms such as coliforms, and anaerobic bacteria such as bacteroides. The fact that many glands are situated in the intersphincteric space explains the relationship of the tract of perianal fistulae: downwards to point at the perianal skin; upwards to the pelvirectal space between rectum and levator; or laterally through the external sphincter to point in the ischiorectal space (Fig. 23.4). The relationship of perianal fistulae to the sphincters is discussed below.

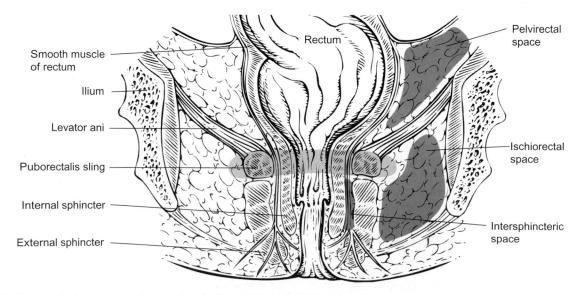

Fig. 23.4   Principal anorectal spaces in relation to the anal sphincters and rectum.

The anal (haemorrhoidal) cushions

Although the internal and external sphincters, the pubo-rectalis sling and the anorectal angle play important roles in maintaining anal continence, fine control is imparted by the anal 'cushions' that lie in the submucosa within the anal canal, partly above and partly below the pectinate line. The anal cushions are specialized vascular structures comprised of fibroconnective tissue containing arteriovenous communications, fed by the terminal branches of the superior rectal artery with inconstant anastomoses to the middle and inferior rectal arteries. There are usually three anal cushions, because there are three terminal branches of the artery. The position of the arteries determines the position of the anal cushions and also the position of haemorrhoids, which are caused by distension and prolapse of the anal cushions. There are two right (one anterior and one posterior) and one left lateral cushions.

The pathophysiology of haemorrhoids involves degeneration of the supporting fibroelastic tissue and smooth muscle, with enlargement and protrusion of the cushions. As the cushions prolapse, there is keratinization and hypertrophy of the overlying anal transitional zone and eventually prolapse of the columnar epithelial component in advanced stages. The anatomical relationship of the feeding arteries explains the position of haemorrhoids at the 3, 7 and 11 o'clock position (when the patient is viewed from below with the legs in the lithotomy position). From the above, it should be clear that haemorrhoids are not 'varicose veins' of the anal canal, but prolapse of the specialized anal cushions fed by arterial supply. Indeed, haemorrhoids are uncommon in patients with portal hypertension, despite the fact that the anal canal represents a potential porto-systemic anastomosis.

Lymphatic drainage of the anal canal

The majority of the lymphatic drainage of the rectum passes superiorly through the mesorectum to follow the superior rectal artery and on to the inferior mesenteric and aortic chains. There are also some lymphatic channels that follow the course of the middle rectal arteries to drain to the nodes around the internal iliac arteries. Lymphatic drainage of the anus below the pectinate line is to the inguinal lymph nodes. This anatomical distinction between the anus and the rectum has important implications for the management of tumours of the rectum and anus. As part of surgical resection of a tumour of the rectum, the lymph nodes clearance generally only involves removal of the mesorectum and the nodes along the inferior mesenteric artery. However, tumours of the anus frequently metastasize to the inguinal lymph nodes, and so treatment must include these nodes. Thus, the initial treatment modality for most anal squamous cancer is radiotherapy, and the inguinal nodes may be included in the irradiated field because of the importance of lymphatic drainage in recurrent disease.

ANORECTAL DISORDERS

Haemorrhoids

The terms haemorrhoids and 'piles' are used interchangeably, although patients tend to use the latter. Despite the fact that the condition is very common, the aetiology remains obscure. Almost all haemorrhoids are primary, with only a tiny proportion due to other factors, such as a cancer in the distal rectum. As discussed above, haemorrhoids are enlarged, prolapsed anal cushions resulting from degeneration and stretching of the supporting fibroelastic tissue and smooth muscle. However, the underlying cause of the stretching is unknown. Constipation and straining at stool are a common feature. This may be aggravated by a high anal sphincter pressure, with further entrapment of prolapsed piles. Haemorrhoids during pregnancy are very common and are probably due to hormonal effects inducing connective tissue laxity, combined with constipation and pressure from the baby's head. Sitting on the toilet for long periods, such as when reading, is also held to be an associated aetiological factor. However, as with other putative aetiological factors there is no real evidence for cause and effect. There may be some genetic component to the development of piles, but families share diet as well as other habits, and so the true cause will probably never be fully understood.

Presentation

Bleeding and prolapse are the cardinal features and may occur in isolation or together. The bleeding is typically intermittent 'outlet-type' bleeding, separate from the stool and evident in the pan or only on wiping. There may also be aching or dragging discomfort on defaecation, and patients may report having to reduce their piles to obtain relief after each bowel motion. Severe constant pain is unusual and in such cases other pathology should be suspected. In the later stages haemorrhoids remain prolapsed at all times and there is staining of the underwear with mucus and faecal fluid. However, it is very unusual for patients to present with incontinence of solid faeces and a sphincter defect should be suspected in such cases. In cases of constant prolapse there is often pruritis due to the discharge, with irritation of the perianal skin.

Haemorrhoids can be staged according to the degree of prolapse, but it is important to note that this classification does not necessarily relate to the amount of trouble that symptoms cause the patient. *First-degree* piles are those that bleed, are visible on proctoscopy but do not prolapse.

Second-degree piles are those that prolapse during defaecation but reduce spontaneously. *Third-degree* piles are prolapsed constantly but can be reduced manually. *Fourth-degree* piles are chronically and irreducibly prolapsed.

Patients may present as an emergency with a complication of haemorrhoids, such as thrombosed prolapsed piles or torrential haemorrhage. Thrombosed prolapsed piles are large, swollen, irreducible haemorrhoids which are dark blue or even black owing to necrosis and submucosal haemorrhage. They are acutely painful and tender and the diagnosis is easily made on inspection, but a rectal examination will be impossible because of pain. Major haemorrhage resulting in significant hypovolaemia and anaemia is unusual but should be excluded in any patient presenting with a major fresh rectal bleed. Presentation with a significant rectal bleed is more common in younger patients because of better sphincter tone.

Clinical assessment

It is important to stress that the assessment of suspected piles must always include consideration of other potential differential diagnoses, as the symptoms of piles and colorectal cancer can be so similar. However, piles are so common that it is important to take a sensible approach to the investigation of rectal bleeding. Indiscriminate large bowel investigation for a common complaint such as rectal bleeding, due most commonly to haemorrhoids and not to cancer, is inappropriate. A careful history is essential to guide further clinical assessment and investigation. If the bleeding is of the outlet type, there is no alteration in bowel habit and the patient is under 50 years of age, then the chance of rectal cancer is extremely remote. In such cases, digital rectal examination combined with proctoscopy and rigid sigmoidoscopy should secure the diagnosis. If piles are confirmed, then treatment can be instigated without recourse to imaging the rest of the colon by barium enema or colonoscopy. If the patient is older, or if there is a change of bowel habit, or if there is no evidence of piles on proctoscopy, then further colonic investigation is indicated.

Examination of the perianal region should be carried out in the left lateral position. Prolapsed piles will be apparent at this stage and evidence of associated anal skin tags should be noted. Digital rectal examination is essential to assess sphincter tone and the canal should be gently opened to check for other anal conditions. First or second-degree piles are rarely palpable as they compress on pressure, and are diagnosed by proctoscopy. The proctoscope should be gently inserted to the hilt and withdrawn. The bulging haemorrhoids will be visible at the right anterior, right posterior and left lateral positions, as discussed above. Rigid sigmoidoscopy should be performed to exclude other rectal pathology, even when the diagnosis is secured by proctoscopy.

Treatment

In many cases the patient is simply concerned to exclude cancer and reassurance after appropriate evaluation is all that many will require. Many patients will require no specific treatment, as symptoms are minor and intermittent. A high-fibre diet with plenty of vegetables is commonly recommended, although there is no good evidence that this actually provides any benefit at all. However, if constipation is a feature it does seem reasonable advice, and in some cases bulk laxatives or stool softeners may be indicated. Patients often self-medicate with proprietary ointments and creams. There is no good evidence from controlled trials that these are effective, but if patients find they help then it seems reasonable to advise their intermittent use.

Non-operative approaches

There are many non-operative approaches to the treatment of haemorrhoids, the aim of which is to cause fibrosis and shrinkage of the protruding haemorrhoidal cushion in order to prevent bleeding and prolapse. The available treatment approaches include the application of small rubber bands to strangulate the pile (using a special Barron's bander); submucosal injection of sclerosant; the application of heat by infrared photocoagulation; and the application of extreme cold using a cryoprobe. All of these can be carried out in the outpatient clinic, but cryotherapy is rarely used nowadays. A number of randomized trials have found that none of the approaches is much better than doing nothing at all. In the long term the symptoms of *untreated* piles tend to wax and wane, and the recurrence of symptoms after any of these procedures is much the same as without any treatment. However, of all the non-operative treatments rubber band ligation (Fig. 23.5) is normally preferred, but injection sclerotherapy is quite effective in the short term where bleeding is the predominant symptom. Where there is a significant cutaneous component to the piles, any of the outpatient treatments is likely to be painful because of the cutaneous nerve supply, and is also unlikely to succeed. In these circumstances the decision is to do nothing but reassure the patient, or to offer an operation.

Operative approaches

The principle of traditional haemorrhoidectomy involves total removal of the haemorrhoidal mass and secure haemostasis of the feeding vessel. The wound can be left open or can be closed, but there are rarely problems with healing or infection. In some cases there are secondary haemorrhoids between the main right anterior, right posterior and left lateral positions, and these are also removed as part of the operation. Recently, a different surgical

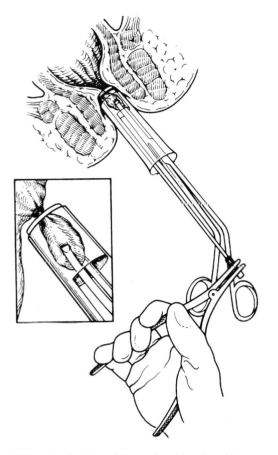

Fig. 23.5 Application of Barron's rubber band to haemorrhoids.

SUMMARY BOX

Haemorrhoids

- Internal haemorrhoids originate as bulges within the upper anal canal and consist of thickened mucosa and connective tissue which contains the internal haemorrhoidal plexus.

- Haemorrhoids are usually classified as:

  - first degree (visible in the lumen on proctoscopy but do not prolapse)

  - second degree (prolapse on defaecation but return spontaneously)

  - third degree (remain prolapsed but can be replaced digitally)

  - fourth degree (long-standing prolapse, cannot be replaced in anal canal).

- Manifestations of haemorrhoids include bleeding (usually on defaecation), prolapse, mucus discharge, discomfort and thrombosis.

- Treatment depends on the degree: first-degree piles are usually left alone with advice on avoiding constipation and straining, whereas symptomatic piles of a higher degree can be treated by injection, banding, photocoagulation or haemorrhoidectomy.

- Thrombosed piles are usually treated conservatively in the first instance but interval haemorrhoidectomy is usually needed to avoid further problems.

approach using a circular stapler has been developed. This technique aims to divide the mucosa and haemorrhoidal cushions above the dentate line in order to transect the feeding vessels and hitch up the stretched supporting fibro-elastic tissue, rather than removing the whole haemorrhoidal mass as in the standard haemorrhoidectomy. This 'stapled haemorrhoidectomy' is currently undergoing clinical trials in the UK and may have a place for the treatment of symptomatic first- and second-degree piles. With all surgical approaches to treating piles it is important to consider that the haemorrhoidal cushions contribute to fine control of continence. Hence, an element of anal incontinence can be one of the long-term sequelae of any haemorrhoidectomy. Surgery should not be considered lightly.

Fissure-in-ano

Fissure-in-ano is a common condition characterized by a linear anal ulcer, often with the internal sphincter visible in the base, affecting the anal canal below the dentate line from the anal transition zone to the anal verge (Fig. 23.6).

There is often little in the way of granulation tissue in the ulcer base. Owing to failed attempts at healing there may be a tag of skin at the lowermost extent of the fissure, known as a 'sentinel pile'. At the proximal extent of the fissure there may be a hypertrophied anal papilla. Sometimes fissures will heal incompletely and mucosa will bridge the edges of the fissure. This results in a low perianal fistula and may present years later. Fissures are most frequently observed in the posterior midline of the anal canal, although anterior fissures may occur in women following childbirth; they are rarely seen in males.

The condition most commonly affects people in their 20s and 30s, with a slight male preponderance. Most fissures are idiopathic, but it is clear that the pathophysiology involves ischaemia in the base of the ulcer associated with marked anal spasm and a significantly raised resting anal pressure. Successive bowel motions result in further trauma, pain and anal spasm, resulting in a vicious cycle of anal pain and sphincter spasm that causes further trauma to the anal mucosa during defaecation. Fissures may be acute and settle spontaneously, but chronic anal fissure is defined as an ulcer that has been present for at least 6 weeks. Recurrent, multiple or unusually extensive fissures affecting areas other than the midline should raise the suspicion of Crohn's disease, which can occasionally present with anal fissure as the sole initial complaint. Occasionally anal fissure may be associated with ulcerative colitis. Fissure is an uncommon complication of haemorrhoidectomy and results from a non-healing wound combined with anal spasm.

Fissure-in-ano is one of the most common causes of constipation in infants and children. The pain associated with the fissure leads to a pattern of behaviour where the child tries to avoid defaecation. This results in stool retention and rectal stool bolus formation. The rectum becomes overdistended and the child becomes unaware of the need to pass stool. Overflow incontinence and soiling results. Treatment includes stool softeners, aperient medication and, rarely, manual disimpaction under anaesthetic. Anal stretch, while having fallen into disrepute in adult practice, is still a widely used and successful treatment for resistant cases. Topical nitrate preparations are currently the subject of controlled trials in children and are not yet in widespread use.

Clinical presentation and diagnosis

The most common symptoms are pain on defecation in a young patient. There is often associated rectal bleeding of the outlet type, with blood on the paper or dripping into the pan after passing the motion. The amount of bleeding is usually minor and there may be some staining or mucous

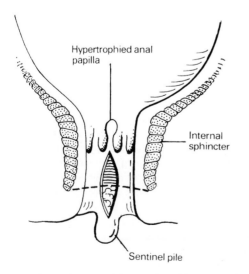

Fig. 23.6 Fissure-in-ano with associated hypertrophy of the anal column and a sentinel pile.

discharge in the underwear. Patients often report it is painful to wipe the anus after moving the bowels. Pain is the predominant symptom and may be burning, tearing or sharp in nature. It may last a few hours after defecation. There may be history of constipation, which could be aetiologically responsible for the tear but is more likely a response to the pain.

The diagnosis should be suspected from the history alone and is confirmed by gently parting the superficial part of the anal sphincter with the gloved fingers to reveal the characteristic linear ulcer. There may be an associated 'sentinel pile', which consists of heaped-up skin at the lowermost extent of the linear ulcer (Fig. 23.6). It is often too painful to perform a digital rectal examination or a proctoscopy and so this is best left until after treatment is instigated. However, it is important to complete clinical assessment with rigid sigmoidoscopy at a later date. A full history is important to exclude previous perianal surgery, perianal abscess, trauma during childbirth or symptoms conducive with Crohn's disease.

Treatment

It is only necessary to treat chronic symptoms that have been present for 6 weeks or more. Having established that the fissure is primary, treatment is aimed at alleviating pain and anal spasm in order to break out of the vicious cycle. It is important to document reproductive history for females, as surgery may have implications for future anal continence.

The optimal approach is conservative in the first instance. Stool softeners have a place but will rarely effect a cure as the sole treatment. Chemical sphincterotomy is the first-line treatment of choice. This can be achieved using topical nitrates (0.2–0.5%) as a cream applied twice daily to the anal canal. The rationale for treatment with topical nitrates follows on from understanding that the principal neurotransmitter that initiates relaxation of the internal sphincter is nitric oxide. Topical nitrates serve as a nitric oxide donor and can achieve healing in 50–70% of chronic fissures. Unfortunately, headaches can be a dose-limiting side-effect. Other means of chemical sphincterotomy include calcium channel blockers such as nifedipine, and also direct injection of the sphincter with botulinus toxin, which temporarily paralyses the sphincter.

Until the relatively recent advent of chemical sphincterotomy as first-line treatment, surgery was the only option. Surgery still has a major role in the management of patients who have fissures resistant to medical treatment, or who have recurrence. Anal stretching has largely been abandoned as it is associated with significant sphincter damage and the risk of incontinence. Lateral sphincterotomy is the most common operation for anal fissure and involves controlled division of the lower half of the internal sphincter at the lateral position (3 o'clock or 9 o'clock with the patient in lithotomy position). There is a small but appreciable risk of late anal incontinence following lateral sphincterotomy. This is usually only to gas, but occasionally faecal incontinence to liquid or solid can occur, particularly in women who have had birth-related anal sphincter damage. In women it may therefore be more appropriate to avoid further division of any sphincter muscle, and this can be achieved using an anal advancement flap or a rotation flap to cover the ulcerated base of the fissure and allow new, well vascularized skin to heal the ulcer and reduce the associated anal spasm.

SUMMARY BOX

Fissure-in-ano

- Most anal fissures are primary but fissures are also common as manifestations of Crohn's disease and ulcerative colitis.

- The typical primary anal fissure extends in the midline posteriorly from the pectinate line to the anal verge, and is associated with an oedematous skin tag (sentinel pile) and hypertrophied anal papilla.

- Pain on defaecation is the outstanding symptom of primary anal fissure. Fissures secondary to conditions such as Crohn's disease may be less painful, indolent and multiple.

- Operative division of the lower part of the internal sphincter (lateral subcutaneous internal sphincterotomy) is the treatment of choice.

Perianal abscess

Perianal abscess is a generic term encompassing the collection of pus to form an abscess in the perianal, intersphincteric, ischiorectal or pelvirectal spaces (Fig. 23.7). Perianal suppuration is common, affecting men three times more frequently than women. Conditions that predispose to perianal abscess include ulcerative colitis and Crohn's disease, as well as any cause of immunosuppression such as haematological disease, diabetes mellitus, chemotherapy and HIV infection. Occasionally, patients with established sepsis elsewhere may develop metastatic suppuration in the perianal region. However, most patients who present with perianal abscess have no predisposing factors and most abscesses are initiated by blockage of the anal gland ducts that lead into the anal canal (Fig. 23.3). The obstructed anal gland becomes secondarily infected with large bowel organisms such as *Bacteroides*, *Streptococcus faecalis* and coliforms. The fact that the anal glands are situated in the intersphincteric space (Fig. 23.4) explains why perianal abscess presents in various ways, depending on the route that the infection takes as pus tracks along the line of least resistance through the tissue spaces.

Presentation

In cases where the abscess remains localized within the intersphincteric space, the patient presents with acute anal pain and tenderness. There is usually no evidence of suppuration on inspection of the perianal region. Pain often prevents digital examination, and so an anaesthetic is required for proper assessment. The main differential diagnosis in such cases is of acute anal fissure. The diagnosis is confirmed by demonstration of a localized pea-sized lump in the intersphincteric space and will exclude acute anal fissure.

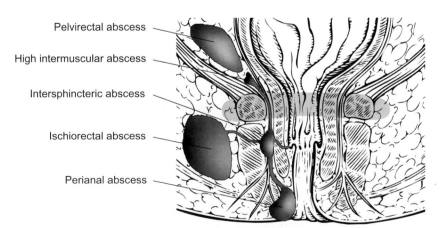

Pelvirectal abscess

High intermuscular abscess

Intersphincteric abscess

Ischiorectal abscess

Perianal abscess

Fig. 23.7 Spread of infection from anal gland to anorectal spaces and resultant abscess formation.

The most common perianal abscess is the simple type where pus tracks inferiorly to appear at the perianal margin between the internal and external sphincters (Fig. 23.7). The patient may have had symptoms for 1 or 2 days and the abscess may even have discharged spontaneously. Systemic upset is usually minimal and anal pain is the predominant presenting complaint.

In cases where infection tracks through the external sphincter, an abscess can become established in the ischiorectal space. Ischiorectal abscess is uncommon and may be associated with uncontrolled diabetes. Diabetes should be excluded in all cases of perianal abscess, particularly with ischiorectal abscess. As the ischiorectal space is horseshoe shaped and there are no fascial barriers within it, infection can track posteriorly around the anus to affect the contralateral space. In such cases the patient is toxic and pyrexial with a large, painful, fluctuant, brawny swelling affecting both buttocks, owing to the presence of large volumes of pus. There is a history of perianal pain for several days associated with difficulty in sitting.

Infection tracking upwards from the infected anal gland through the upper part of the intersphincteric space may result in a high intersphincteric (high intermuscular) abscess or a pelvirectal abscess. As these spaces encircle the anorectum above the levator muscles, abscesses can be bilateral and often present with a major systemic upset. It can be seen that these are complex problems that merit specialist assessment and treatment. With high abscesses it is also important to consider an abscess due to pelvic sepsis from diverticular abscess.

Treatment

By the time most patients present, an abscess has become established and antibiotics alone will not be effective. The treatment of perianal abscess is usually straightforward and involves drainage of the pus under general anaesthetic. Most cases are adequately dealt with by incising and deroofing the abscess at the point of maximal fluctuance, or where the pus can be seen pointing. However, anatomical considerations are important, as inappropriate incision of sphincter muscle can result in incontinence in the long term. Furthermore, drainage of pus through the wrong space will create a perianal fistula (see below). At operation, pus should be sent for bacteriological assessment to determine the causative organism(s). However, in uncomplicated cases antibiotics have no place after incision and drainage. Where there is extensive cellulitis, as is often the case with ischiorectal abscess, parenteral antibiotics should be administered. Broad-spectrum cephalosporins and metronidazole should be given on an empirical basis, in view of the likelihood that gut organisms are involved. Parenteral antibiotics should be given to diabetic patients with perianal sepsis.

Unusually complex perianal sepsis or recurrent abscess should raise suspicion about underlying inflammatory bowel disease, particularly Crohn's disease. Sigmoidoscopy and rectal biopsy should be performed and the roof of the abscess sent for histology. A full GI investigation may be indicated, particularly when there is a relevant history of GI upset.

SUMMARY BOX

Anorectal infection

- Most cases of anorectal infection are thought to originate in infection of an anal gland.
- Perianal and ischiorectal abscesses are the commonest forms of abscess in the anorectal region.
- Anorectal abscesses (and fissures and fistulae) are commonly associated with underlying Crohn's disease or ulcerative colitis, and may also be associated with rectal carcinoma, tuberculosis and HIV infection.
- Perianal and ischiorectal abscesses are treated by incision and drainage, taking care to exclude underlying bowel pathology or fistula, particularly in patients with recurrent abscesses.

Fistula-in-ano

There is a relationship between perianal abscess and fistula because suppuration is the common aetiological factor for both. Obstruction of the duct and infection of the anal glands is thought to be the underlying pathogenesis for both conditions. Frank abscess precedes some cases of fistula and inappropriate surgical drainage of perianal abscess is responsible for a small but significant proportion of fistulae. Figure 23.8 is a simplified diagram of different types of fistula. In each case the anal gland in the intersphincteric space is implicated in the original sepsis. There are many variations of the types of fistula and associated collections that are not discussed here for the sake of clarity and brevity. In patients with recurrent perianal abscesses a fistula tract may be identified. However, there is no need to search routinely for a fistula when draining straightforward perianal abscesses because probing may actually inadvertently cause a fistula. It is important to allow acute perianal abscesses to settle after incision and drainage before attempting to delineate a fistula. Some fistulae develop without any known perianal abscess, in which case the patient may present with a small abscess that intermittently points and discharges pus on to the perianal skin.

Perianal fistula may complicate Crohn's disease. Around 10% of patients with Crohn's disease of the small intestine, without colorectal involvement, also have perianal recurrent fistula or fissures. Hence, it is important to consider Crohn's disease in all patients with perianal fistula or sepsis that is resistant to treatment. Other rare causes of perianal fistula include ulcerative colitis, carcinoma of the anus or rectum, HIV infection, trauma and tuberculosis.

Clinical presentation and assessment

In most cases the patient presents with a chronically discharging opening in the perianal skin associated with pruritus and perianal discomfort. A careful clinical history is essential to ensure there are no predisposing factors and also to determine whether there has been any previous surgery.

Investigation requires examination under anaesthetic and the fistula tract should be probed by an experienced surgeon. When the fistula opens on the perianal skin of the anterior anus, the tract passes radially directly to the anal canal. However, when the opening is posterior to a line drawn between the 3 o'clock and 9 o'clock positions (Fig. 23.9), then the tract usually passes circumferentially backwards to the midline and enters the anal canal at the 6 o'clock position. This is known as *Goodsall's rule* and can help define the extent of the course of a fistula. It is essential to avoid inducing further fistulae by ill-advised probing of the region. It is important to determine whether the fistula is low or high (Fig. 23.8) as the prognosis and treatment are different for each. Low fistula is the more common type. Fistulae that involve only the lower part of the internal sphincter are termed low intersphincteric fistulae. Those tracking through the lower part of both the internal *and* the external sphincters are low transsphincteric fistulae. High fistulae are complex and may track through the upper part of both (high trans-sphincteric fistula), or can even pass directly through the levator ani to enter the high rectum (pelvirectal fistula). In any of these fistulae there may be an extension of the tract into the spaces shown in Figure 23.4; and such extension further complicates the management. The classification of fistula-in-ano is not merely academic, but determines the type of surgical management required.

Whereas most fistulae require no investigation other than a formal examination under anaesthesia (EUA), some

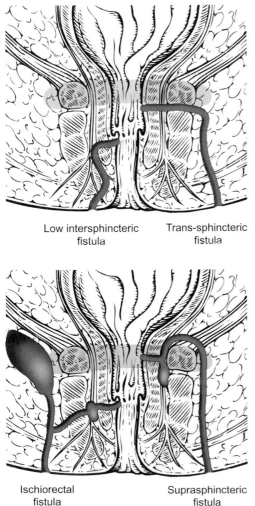

Low intersphincteric fistula   Trans-sphincteric fistula

Ischiorectal fistula   Suprasphincteric fistula

Fig. 23.8 Types of fistula-in-ano.

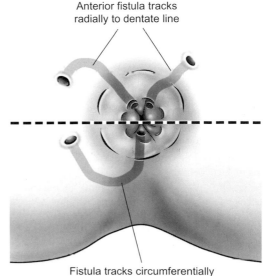

Anterior fistula tracks radially to dentate line

Fistula tracks circumferentially to posterior midline

Fig. 23.9 Goodsall's rule.

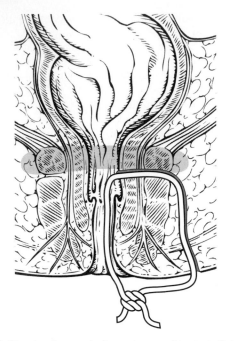

Fig. 23.10   A seton encircling a trans-sphincteric fistula.·

complex cases merit further investigation to define the extent of the tracts. Magnetic resonance imaging (MRI) is increasingly used for such cases, as is endoanal ultrasound. A full GI barium series may be indicated when inflammatory bowel disease is suspected.

Treatment

Treatment is determined by the course of the fistula tract. Low fistulae can usually simply be laid open and allowed to heal. However, where a significant proportion of the internal and/or external sphincter is involved then laying open the tract will result in faecal incontinence. In such complex cases the fistula tract can be probed and a 'seton' passed along its length (Fig. 23.10) to allow the fistula to drain. Once it is drained, a tighter seton can be applied that will gradually cut out through the sphincters, allowing them to heal behind the seton. This approach keeps the ends of the sphincters together and so minimizes the chances of inducing incontinence. Another approach to high fistulae is to raise a flap of the rectal wall and upper internal sphincter. The flap is advanced downwards to close the internal opening and the external part simply heals, as it has no faecal stream maintaining the sepsis and the tract. This is known as an anorectal advancement flap. In some complex cases a defunctioning colostomy may be necessary.

MISCELLANEOUS BENIGN PERIANAL LUMPS

Perianal haematoma

Perianal haematoma is a painful condition caused by the pressure of thrombus in the subcutaneous superficial space between the anoderm and the anal sphincter. A localized lump forms at the anal verge, due to blood tracking subcutaneously from haemorrhoids after the passage of a hard bowel motion or after prolapse of a haemorrhoid. It can also arise in patients with a bleeding diathesis or those on anticoagulants. It is important to recognize the condition because it is readily treated by surgical drainage under local anaesthetic. When the haematoma is deroofed, the relief is almost instantaneous. The condition will settle eventually without surgical intervention, but recognizing the haematoma will spare the patient several days of an exquisitely tender anus.

Perianal haematoma is easily recognized by the presence of a well circumscribed, bluish domeshaped lump under the perianal skin. The main differential diagnosis is prolapsed, thrombosed haemorrhoids, and so it is essential to make an accurate diagnosis as inappropriate incision of haemorrhoids will result in considerable bleeding. Perianal haematoma should be readily differentiated from perianal abscess by nature of the colour and by the surrounding erythema and induration.

Anal warts

Anal warts cause discomfort, pain, pruritus ani and difficulty with perianal hygiene. Warts are also associated with an increased risk of squamous carcinoma because they are usually associated with human papillomavirus (HPV). The lesions may be very extensive or relatively sparse.

After viral infection and the development of an initial crop of warts, they may be spread extensively by scratching caused by the associated pruritus ani. Many cases resolve spontaneously, but those requiring treatment can usually be managed effectively by the application of podophyllin. More extensive cases may require surgical excision, and very extensive cases associated with dysplasia may require excision and skin grafting, combined with a temporary colostomy.

Fibroepithelial anal polyp

Anal fibroepithelial polyp is not a neoplasm. The lesions are hypertrophic epithelium arising on a stalk from the anal canal itself, and histologically are comprised of keratinized squamous epithelium supported by scarred, fibrotic subcutaneous tissue. The clinical history may suggest haemorrhoids as the main differential diagnosis, but this is easily discounted by examination which will reveal the polyp on a stalk. Sometimes there are associated haemorrhoids. The main differential diagnosis on digital examination and proctoscopy is of a prolapsing rectal polyp on a long stalk. Rectal polyps are adenomas and so arise above the pectinate line. Biopsy will confirm the nature of the polyp, as rectal polyp is comprised of adenomatous glandular tissue, rather than the squamous epithelium of the fibroepithelial polyp.

Patients with fibroepithelial polyp may present with a prolapsing anal lesion, discomfort on defaecation, or with pruritus ani associated with faecal-stained mucus causing irritation to the delicate perianal skin. Anal polyps are usually associated with a previous history of perianal disease such as haemorrhoids or fissure-in-ano. Occasionally there is no preceding history and in these circumstances it is likely that the patient has had asymptomatic haemorrhoidal disease. Treatment of symptomatic polyps is by simple excision under general anaesthetic.

Anal skin tags

Prolapse of haemorrhoids is usually followed by a degree of regression, and this leaves behind irregular skin at the anal verge which are known as anal skin tags. Haemorrhoids often present with minor anal skin tags, but it is important to stress that the tags themselves are not haemorrhoids. Although the anus may not look particularly tidy, there is no indication to operate unless the patient is having significant problems with perianal hygiene or the lesions are causing pruritus. Anal tags associated with haemorrhoids that merit surgery can be removed at the same time as haemorrhoidectomy.

ANAL CANCER

Compared to colorectal cancer, anal cancer is uncommon. The ratio of anal to colorectal cancer is around 1:25, although the incidence of anal cancer is increasing. It is important to detect anal cancer at an early stage, as extensive local invasion and metastatic disease are associated with a poor outcome and usually require major surgery and a colostomy. Conversely, early disease is best treated non-operatively with radiotherapy, and a stoma can usually be avoided.

Over 80% of anal cancer is squamous carcinoma. Most anal cancers arise from the keratinized squamous epithelium of the anal margin, or of the pecten or from the non-keratinized squamous epithelium of the anal transitional zone immediately above the pectinate line. Anal verge tumours often present earlier than canal tumours because the patient becomes aware of a mass or irregular area at the anal

margin. Around 10% of tumours are adenocarcinomas and these arise from the glandular epithelium of the upper anal canal. Most patients with anal cancer present in the sixth and seventh decades, but younger cases are well recognized, particularly in females. Other rarer tumours include melanoma, lymphoma and sarcoma. Adenocarcinoma can rarely arise from the anal glands, rather than the lining of the canal itself.

The aetiology is not fully defined, but in population studies there is an association between anal and cervical cancer, as well as with penile tumours. Anogenital warts are also a risk factor for anal cancer, as is anal intercourse. HIV infection is also a predisposing factor, owing to immunosuppression and susceptibility to viral infection. All of this evidence points to a common aetiological factor which probably relates to viral infection, particularly with human papillomaviruses (HPV). HPV types 16 and 18 have been identified in more than 50% of anal carcinomas and also in anal intraepithelial neoplasia (AIN). AIN is probably the precursor of most anal carcinomas and is analogous to CIN, the precursor lesion of cervical cancer, which is also associated with HPV infection. It is important to perform a cervical smear in patients with proven anal cancer.

Clinical presentation and assessment

Given that anal cancer is uncommon, whereas symptoms due to benign anal conditions are highly prevalent, it is not surprising that a high proportion of anal cancers are misdiagnosed in the early stages. Early cancers may be confused with fissures, piles and warts. None the less, because of their accessibility anal tumours are readily detected by careful clinical examination.

Patients present with anal pain, bleeding or discharge into the underwear, and pruritus ani. Advanced tumours that have spread to the anal sphincters may present with incontinence. Clinical examination of anal cancer at the margin reveals an ulcerated discoid lesion at the anal verge which is hard to the touch (Fig. 23.11). Cancer of the anal canal may not be visible, although extensive lesions may protrude to the anal verge by direct spread. Examination under anaesthetic is necessary in almost all cases to allow tumour biopsy and sigmoidoscopy. Biopsy is essential to confirm the diagnosis, but also to determine the tissue of origin, as the treatment for squamous carcinoma varies from that for adenocarcinoma.

Staging

Staging is important for prognosis and may also direct treatment approaches. The most widely used staging system is shown in Table 23.3. The lymph nodes most commonly involved are the inguinal groups, particularly for anal verge cancers. Canal tumours may spread proximally to the

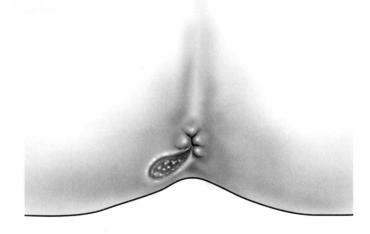

Fig. 23.11 Squamous carcinoma of the anal verge.

Table 23.3	Staging system for anal cancer
T1	< 2 cm
T2	2–5 cm
T3	> 5 cm
T4a	Invading vaginal mucosa
T4b	Invading other structures other than skin, rectal or vaginal mucosa (i.e. local spread to muscle or bone)

mesorectal nodes or to the internal iliac nodes via the middle rectal lymph nodes.

Lymphadenopathy alone is not sufficient to confirm lymph node spread, and accessible nodes should be biopsied because reactive changes due to infection are common.

Examination under anaesthetic is an important part of clinical staging as the tumour is often painful and the anus tender to digital examination. Endoanal ultrasound can also be performed under anaesthetic. Cross-sectional imaging techniques such as CT and MRI are now standard because they are widely available and highly accurate.

Treatment

Modern treatment of anal cancer is multidisciplinary, with surgeon and radiotherapist working collaboratively in the assessment and treatment on an individual basis. The current standard treatment for anal squamous cell cancer is radiotherapy to the anal canal and inguinal lymph nodes, combined with 5-fluorouracil and mitomycin C. The usual approach is external beam radiotherapy, but radioactive implants such as selectron wires are also used in selected cases. Surgery plays an important part in the management of advanced disease, but it is not the primary treatment modality. It is reserved for radiotherapy treatment failures, when 'salvage' abdominoperineal excision of the anus and rectum may afford a cure in some cases and alleviate symptoms in others. Surgery also has a place in the treatment of small anal verge cancers, when a local excision is all that may be required. This may avoid a protracted course of radiotherapy and chemotherapy for these good-prognosis tumours.

Prognosis

Chemoradiation has probably not affected the overall survival rate after a diagnosis of anal cancer, compared to cure rates achievable by surgery alone. However, the morbidity is substantially reduced and a permanent colostomy can be avoided in many cases. The 5-year survival rate is around 60%.

RECTAL PROLAPSE

Rectal prolapse is a distressing condition that can affect young and older adults as well as children. The term rectal prolapse encompasses three types of abnormal protrusion of all, or part of, the rectal wall. A *full-thickness* rectal prolapse includes the mucosa and the muscular layers. *Mucosal prolapse*, as the name suggests, involves only the mucosal lining of the rectum. *Occult* rectal prolapse refers to intussusception of the rectal wall but without the prolapse protruding through the anal canal. This term also refers to the much rarer condition of *solitary rectal ulcer syndrome*, which is a prolapse of the full thickness of only the anterior rectal wall, although the terms occult rectal prolapse and solitary rectal ulcer syndrome are not synonymous.

The pathological process that results in rectal prolapse is incompletely understood. However, certain factors are clearly implicated in predisposing to the condition. The majority of cases of full-thickness rectal prolapse occur in elderly women, with no obvious aetiological basis. Occasionally, there is a clear history of childbirth injury but many patients are nulliparous. There may be a history of previous anal surgery, such as haemorrhoidectomy, which may indicate past sphincter muscle damage, but sphincter injury is not a prerequisite for the development of rectal prolapse. Chronic constipation and straining at stool, combined with the weight loss that often accompanies old age, are probably related. The loss of fat supporting the rectum, combined with degeneration of collagen fibres and weakness of the musculature of the pelvic floor, results in loss of the anorectal angle and laxity of the rectal wall (Fig. 23.2). In many cases there is a deep rectovaginal pouch with a long loop of sigmoid colon that pushes down into the rectovaginal pouch and contributes to the prolapse.

In children the lack of a sacral hollow, combined with constipation and excessive straining at stool, is responsible for evagination of the rectum and protrusion of the prolapse through the anus. In children with cystic fibrosis, excessive coughing contributes to elevated intra-abdominal pressure. In adults, specific neurogenic causes include multiple sclerosis because of the combination of constipation and denervation of the pelvic floor. Spinal injuries and tumour are also predisposing factors. Mucosal prolapse is often associated with a degree of haemorrhoids, but whether these are causal or simply a result of a common aetiology is not understood.

Clinical presentation and assessment

Patients present with an uncomfortable sensation of 'something coming down' the back passage. Initially this is only on defaecation, but eventually the rectum remains constantly prolapsed and will not reduce spontaneously. The patient may be able to reduce the prolapse digitally. Constipation is usually an accompanying feature. There is often a degree of faecal incontinence and there may be mucous discharge into the underwear. Bloodstained mucus is also common when the rectum remains prolapsed. The prolapse may become ulcerated and in rare instances the rectum may become strangulated. In extreme cases there may be associated uterine prolapse, alluding to the fact that the underlying aetiology relates to weakness of the entire pelvic floor.

Examination may confirm the diagnosis in some cases. However, it is more common that there is no evidence of a prolapse on direct inspection of the anus. Digital examination reveals a patulous anus, poor sphincter tone and evidence of a weak pelvic floor on straining. Asking the patient to strain down will usually deliver the prolapse through the anus. Rigid sigmoidoscopy will reveal cases of occult prolapse. Usually there is no need for further investigation, but if the history is of short duration consideration should be given to the presence of a spinal tumour or spinal stenosis, or a prolapsed intervertebral disc. In occult rectal prolapse

radiological assessment using a defaecating proctogram may help secure the diagnosis. Conditions that might be mistaken for a rectal prolapse include large fourth degree haemorrhoids, prolapsing rectal neoplasia, anal warts, anal skin tags, and fibroepithelial anal polyp. On the basis of symptoms alone, the differential diagnosis of rectal prolapse includes rectal cancer and inflammatory bowel disease, and these should be excluded by appropriate investigations.

Treatment

Childhood prolapse Rectal prolapse in children is effectively treated in almost all cases by attention to maintaining a regular bowel habit with stool softeners, combined with digital reduction of the prolapse by the parents. The condition is self-limiting and surgery is rarely indicated.

Mucosal rectal prolapse In adults mucosal rectal prolapse can be treated by submucosal injection of sclerosant, by photocoagulation, or by applying Barron's bands to the prolapsed area. In resistant cases a limited excision of the area, similar to a haemorrhoidectomy, is effective.

Full-thickness rectal prolapse Surgery is the only effective treatment for established full-thickness rectal prolapse. However, the fact that there are numerous described operations points to the fact that none of the available surgical options is wholly satisfactory. The aim of surgery is to treat the prolapse and improve the associated incontinence. Operations for rectal prolapse can be undertaken employing perineal or abdominal approaches. **Perineal approaches** aim to surgically fixate or excise the prolapse from below. 'Delorme's procedure' involves the excision of the mucosa lining the prolapse, with plication of the muscle tube, and 'perineal rectosigmoidectomy' entails excision through the anus of the prolapsed rectum and lower part of the sigmoid. The latter may be combined with a repair of the pelvic floor. **Abdominal approaches** aim to fix the rectum to the sacral wall with sutures or foreign material. The abdominal approach may also include resection of the redundant sigmoid colon, particularly when constipation is a predominant feature, because rectal fixation usually aggravates the constipation.

Solitary rectal ulcer syndrome This rare condition is difficult to treat effectively because there is usually a psychological overlay. Patients with solitary rectal ulcer syndrome tend to be aged 20–40 years and are often professional men or women. The condition is associated with an introspective and anxious personality. Patients with this condition spend an inordinate amount of time in the toilet trying to move their bowels. The diagnosis is confirmed by visualizing the anterior ulcer in the low rectum, and biopsy shows the typical features of submucosal fibrosis, hypertrophy of the muscularis mucosae and overlying ulceration. Management involves the use of stool softeners and other conservative measures, along with input from a psychologist. Biofeedback may have a place in suitable patients who are compliant, but surgery should be avoided if at all possible.

ANAL INCONTINENCE

Anal or faecal incontinence is both distressing and socially disabling and yet patients are often very reluctant and embarrassed to discuss it with their relatives or their GP. The prevalence of incontinence is probably underestimated, although it has been variously documented as 2–5% in population studies and as high as 10% of all adult females. There are a variety of specific aetiological factors but the majority of cases are 'idiopathic', most commonly affecting older parous women. Aetiological factors associated with anal incontinence are listed in Table 23.4.

The substantial majority of patients presenting to colorectal surgeons are women with a past history of obstetric problems and difficult deliveries. The underlying mechanism of subsequent incontinence in such cases is complex. Although full-thickness obstetric tears are rare, significant sphincter defects have been observed in 10–30% in a number of recent prospective endoanal ultrasound studies in which the sphincters were scanned in women before and after childbirth. Prolonged labour has been implicated in damage to the nerve supply to the pelvic floor, principally the internal pudendal nerves. Denervation of the pelvic floor results in atrophy of the sphincter complex and the levator ani in later life. Most incontinent women have a combination of sphincter muscle damage and the secondary effects of denervation.

Clinical presentation and assessment

A full history is essential, with particular reference to obstetric history and any past perianal operations. The degree and frequency of incontinence should be established. Incontinence may be to gas, liquid or stool. Any coexisting disease should be documented and neurological symptoms sought. A defaecation history, including questions about the urgency of defaecation, should be sought as they are helpful for subsequent management. A history of coexisting urinary incontinence suggests a generalized problem, most likely neurogenic in origin. Examination to determine sphincter tone, the presence of previous scars and the state of the rectovaginal septum should be undertaken. Poor anal sensation suggests a neurogenic basis for the incontinence. Other anorectal causes of incontinence listed in Table 23.4 should be excluded where possible, and by rigid sigmoidoscopy in all cases. It is important to remember that any cause of intestinal hurry (such as colonic cancer) can render incontinent a patient who had been coping previously with a more formed stool. Colonoscopy or barium enema is therefore indicated in older patients. Endoanal ultrasound scanning of the sphincters is routine and allows delineation of the presence and extent of any sphincter defect. Anorectal physiology studies allows documentation of resting and squeeze anal sphincter pressures, and also define whether there is a predominant neurogenic element. Where there is any concern from the history or clinical examination about a spinal lesion, MRI should be performed.

Treatment

The underlying causes of incontinence listed in Table 23.4 should be managed appropriately. However, it is women with 'idiopathic' faecal incontinence who constitute the majority of cases dealt with by colorectal surgeons. Where there is clear evidence of sphincter defect in a young woman, overlapping sphincter repair is often highly successful in selected patients. However, those with an element of denervation tend to have poorer results. In older women, who almost universally have a combination of sphincter and nerve damage, conservative measures should be instigated in the first instance. Stool-bulking agents should be combined with loperamide to give the patient a degree of consti-

---

Table 23.4   Aetiology of anal incontinence

Trauma
Sphincter injury during childbirth (including episiotomy)
Accidental trauma (e.g. RTA. bicycle injury)
Surgical trauma (injudicious fistual surgery, drainage of perianal abscess or haemorrhoidectomy)
Perianal sepsis

Congential
Anorectal atresia (usually treated surgically in childhood)
Spina bifida

Miscellaneous
Rectal prolapse
Haemorrhoids
Rectal cancer invading sphincter
Perianal Crohn's disease
Faecal impaction
Relative incontinence due to intestinal hurry (e.g. inflammatory bowel disease)
Psychiatric or behavioural problems (including encopresis)

Neurological
Denervation of pelvic floor following childbirth
Multiple sclerosis
Low spinal or sacral tumour
Spinal trauma
Dementia

pation. When there is a predominant neurogenic basis, there is often rectal irritability resulting in faecal urgency. This can be damped using 25 mg of amitriptyline at night. Such conservative measures should be combined with regular emptying of the rectum with stimulant suppositories or enemas. In many cases these simple measures have a dramatic effect on the patient's quality of life, and although minor degrees of incontinence will continue, this approach is acceptable and effective for many patients.

In a minority of patients with idiopathic faecal incontinence, further surgery is indicated. The results of anterior sphincter repair alone are disappointing in this group, but posterior repair of the levators and even complex total floor repairs have been performed with some success in a limited proportion of patients. Other surgical approaches include transferring the gracilis muscle on a proximal pedicle to wrap it subcutaneously around the anal canal. An electrical stimulator is implanted which delivers an electrical signal to convert the muscle to a slow twitch type. This allows long-term tonic contraction of the gracilis muscle to maintain continence. The procedure has an acceptable level of success in around 50% of patients, but at a cost of major surgery and potentially major complications. Implantable artificial anal sphincters have been developed and these are placed to encircle the anorectal region. Results from the use of the available devices are encouraging but, as with any foreign material, there is a propensity for infection and many have to be removed. None the less, prosthetic devices have great potential for the future management of anal incontinence and much development work is in progress.

Another surgical option for the patient with anal incontinence is the creation of a permanent colostomy. Although this might be seen as an admission of failure, a well sited stoma and professional input from a stoma care specialist can transform a patient's life, from being afraid to leave the house to leading a virtually normal existence.

The management of anal incontinence remains imperfect, but it is clear that patients should be managed by specialist surgeons. This allows a full investigative work-up and tailoring of management for individual patients. In such a setting the management of anal incontinence can be highly successful. Improvements in obstetric practice are needed to avoid sphincter and nerve damage during childbirth. There is a real need for research to determine risk factors for obstetric injury. Unfortunately, progress in this area is hampered by the fact that it is many decades after the initial insult before patients present with anal incontinence.

PRURITUS ANI

Although distressing to patients, pruritus ani often receives only scant assessment and attention from clinicians. The condition can be a minor, short-lived episode but may be an all-consuming obsession for some patients. It is particularly a problem at night and some patients may unconsciously scratch the perianal region during sleep, resulting in further trauma and irritation.

Pruritus ani is a common complaint and may be a symptom of many anorectal disorders, including haemorrhoids, fistulae, fissures, faecal incontinence, anal carcinoma and rectal prolapse, to name but a few. Dermatological conditions can also be associated with pruritus ani, and these include psoriasis, dermatitis, lichen planus and anal warts; skin infections can also be responsible. Fungal infections are important to consider, including candida and tinea, and this is a particular problem if the patient is diabetic.

Treatment

Underlying conditions such as perianal fistula or haemorrhoids should be treated and diabetes mellitus should be excluded. If there is evidence of fungal infection this should be treated with antifungal creams. It may be necessary to take fungal scrapings in resistant cases. If the condition is idiopathic, full explanation and support for the patient is essential. The cycle of trauma to the delicate perianal skin followed by irritation and subsequent scratching should be explained in detail. Strong advice on avoiding scratching and a requirement for a great deal of willpower is essential. In some cases it may be necessary for the patient to wear cotton gloves in bed, to avoid subconscious nocturnal scratching. The use of perfumed soap and strong antiseptics or lotions should be avoided. The avoidance of nylon undergarments is important to minimize sweating. Particular attention should be paid to the diet, as certain foods (e.g. spicy foods or alcohol) may be responsible. Explanation should be given of the need to avoid overzealous cleansing of the perianal region after defecation. Gentle cleaning with toilet paper followed by washing with gentle soap may be necessary, but it is important to take care to avoid trauma during drying. A simple barrier cream such as is used for nappy rash may be appropriate in some patients, but generally it is best to avoid relying on creams in favour of avoiding trauma caused by scratching and overzealous cleansing. Overall it is possible to improve the symptoms of idiopathic pruritus ani in almost all patients, but it requires a commitment to continued support and advice to achieve this. It may take several months before symptoms come under control.

PILONIDAL DISEASE

Pilonidal disease is a chronic inflammatory condition characterized by the presence of one or more sinuses in the midline of the natal cleft that contain hair and debris (Fig. 23.12). The superficial part of the midline sinus is

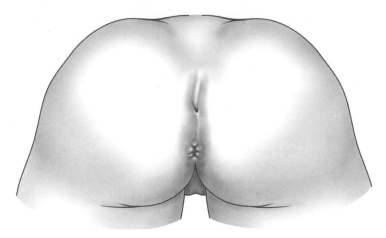

Fig. 23.12 Midline pit in the natal cleft indicating the superficial opening of a pilonidal sinus.

lined with squamous epithelium, but the tracts themselves are not lined with granulation tissue resulting from the associated infection. Pilonidal disease is more common in males than females and affects around 2% of the population between the ages of 15 and 35. However, it is exceedingly rare after the age of 40, suggesting that there is some fundamental aetiological relationship with age. The disease starts at puberty, when sex hormones act on hair follicles and sebaceous glands. There is enlargement of a hair follicle, which allows the accumulation of extraneous hairs that are caught in the natal cleft itself. A foreign-body reaction is set up, with the result that there is a chronic discharging sinus which attracts other debris and hairs. A sedentary occupation, particularly where sweating is common, is a predisposing factor. The condition was described in large numbers of American troops in the Vietnam war owing to the use of Jeeps in the warm climate.

Presentation

Many people have asymptomatic pilonidal sinuses and so it is important only to treat the condition if it is causing problems, in view of the high prevalence and the fact that it seldom presents after the fourth decade. When symptomatic, the disease is characterized by midline pits in the natal cleft discharging mucopurulent material, which may smell mildly offensive and may be bloodstained. There is often tenderness on pressure and the patient may avoid long periods of sitting, such as car journeys. When a sinus becomes infected and the pus is loculated, the disease presents as pilonidal abscess, with the abscess typically pointing just off the midline. However, there is invariably a communication with a midline sinus containing hair and granulation tissue. Occasionally pilonidal sinus may present with extensive and complex branching sinus tracts. In these cases it is

important to consider perianal Crohn's disease, and careful examination of the anal canal is essential.

Treatment

The treatment of pilonidal disease includes conservative and surgical management. Conservative management comprises attention to natal cleft hygiene and hair removal by depilatory creams or by careful shaving. Antibiotics have a place in the early stages of abscess formation and may avert the need for incision and drainage of an established abscess. Some advocate removing hairs from the sinus tract itself on a regular basis to allow the sinus to drain and avoid the collection of hair and debris that causes establishment of the infection.

The reasons for surgical treatment are the presence of an established abscess and chronically discharging sinus tracts that are debilitating the patient. Surgical drainage is required for an abscess, and it is best to incise it away from the midline as this minimizes the likelihood of recurrence. There are a number of surgical options for sinus tracts. The tracts can be laid open, the granulations removed with a curette and the resultant defects dressed until they heal from the base. Tracts can also be excised and closed primarily with sutures, although the wound is prone to break down and heal by second intention. Unfortunately, the treatment of pilonidal disease is characterized by frequent recurrence, due partly to inadequate or inappropriate surgery in some cases, but mostly to the fact that the underlying aetiology is still present, namely the natal cleft and a predisposed skin type. Recurrent disease can be treated using rotation flaps to replace the pitted skin with fresh skin from the buttock. For complex recurrent disease ablation of the natal cleft using a flap procedure is highly effective but leaves a fairly large unsightly scar. It is important to advise the patient to keep the natal cleft free of hair by depilation

SECTION 6
SURGICAL SPECIALTIES

24 Plastic and reconstructive surgery

J.D. Watson

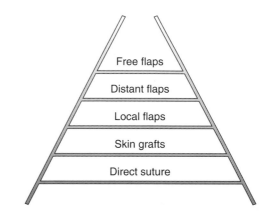

Fig. 24.1   Reconstructive ladder.

Plastic and reconstructive surgery is concerned with the restitution of form and function after trauma and ablative surgery. The techniques by which this is achieved are applicable to virtually every surgical subspecialty and are not limited to any single anatomical region or system. The 'reconstructive ladder' is broad, simple and widely applicable at its base, but narrow, technically demanding and complex at its top (Fig. 24.1). It is important to distinguish plastic and reconstructive surgery from cosmetic, or aesthetic, surgery. In the latter the techniques of the former are applied to improve appearance but not physical function, though there may be considerable psychological benefit.

STRUCTURE AND FUNCTIONS OF SKIN

Skin consists of epidermis and dermis. The epidermis is a layer of keratinized, stratified squamous epithelium (Fig. 24.2) that sends three appendages (hair follicles, sweat glands and sebaceous glands) into the underlying dermis. Because of their deep location the appendages escape destruction in partial-thickness burns and are a source of new cells for reconstitution of the epidermis. Its basal germinal layer generates keratin-producing cells (keratinocytes), which become increasingly keratinized and flattened as they migrate to the surface, where they are shed. The basal layer also contains pigment cells (melanocytes) that produce melanin, which is passed to the keratinocytes and protects the basal layer from ultraviolet light.

The dermis is composed of collagen, elastic fibres and fat. It supports blood vessels, lymphatics, nerves and the epidermal appendages. The junction between the epidermis and the dermis is undulating where dermal papillae push up towards the epidermis.

Three types of epidermal appendage extend into the dermis and, in some places, into the subcutaneous tissues. Hair follicles produce hair, the colour of which is determined by melanocytes within the follicle. The sebaceous glands secrete sebum into the hair follicles, which lubricates the skin and hair. The sweat glands are coiled tubular glands lying within the dermis and are of two types: eccrine

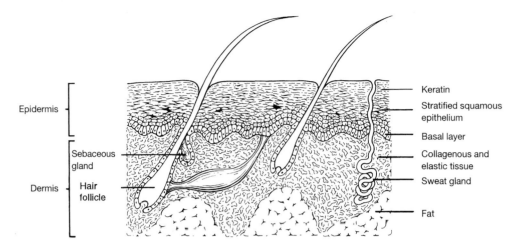

Fig. 24.2 Structure of skin.

sweat glands secrete salt and water on to the entire skin surface; apocrine glands secrete a musty-smelling fluid in the axilla, eyelids, ears, nipple and areola, genital areas and the perianal region. Hidradenitis suppurativa affects the latter.

The nails are flat, horny structures composed of keratin. They arise from a matrix of germinal cells, which can be seen as a white crescent (lunula) at the nail base. If a nail is avulsed, a new nail grows from this matrix. If the matrix is destroyed nail regeneration is impossible, and the layer of epidermal cells covering the nailbed thickens to form a keratinized protective layer.

WOUNDS

A wound may be defined as disruption of the normal continuity of bodily structures due to trauma, which may be penetrating or non-penetrating. In both cases, inspection of the body surface may give little indication of the extent of underlying damage.

Types of wound

Wounds can be classified according to the mechanism of injury.

- *Incised wounds* A sharp instrument causes these; if there is associated tearing of tissues the wound is said to be lacerated.
- *Abrasions* These result from friction damage to the body surface and are characterized by superficial bruising and loss of a varying thickness of skin and underlying tissue. Dirt and foreign bodies are frequently embedded in the tissues and can give rise to traumatic tattooing, for example in coal miners.

- *Crush injury* These are due to severe pressure. Even though the skin may not be breached there can be massive tissue destruction. Oedema can make wound closure impossible. Increasing pressure within fascial compartments can cause ischaemic necrosis of muscle and other structures (compartment syndrome).
- *Degloving injury* These result from shearing forces that cause parallel tissue planes to move against each other, for example when a hand is caught between rollers or in moving machinery. Large areas of apparently intact skin may be deprived of their blood supply by rupture of feeding vessels.
- *Gunshot wounds* These may be low velocity (e.g. shotguns) or high velocity (e.g. military rifles). Bullets fired from high-velocity rifles cause massive tissue destruction after skin penetration.
- *Burns* These are caused not only by heat but also by electricity, irradiation and chemicals.

Principles of wound healing

The essential features of healing are common to wounds of almost all soft tissues, and result in the formation of a scar. Soft tissue healing can be subdivided into three phases (Table 24.1) according to the development of tensile strength (Fig. 24.3).

Lag phase

The lag phase is the delay of 2–3 days that elapses before fibroblasts begin to manufacture collagen to support the wound. It is characterized by an inflammatory response to injury during which capillary permeability increases and a protein-rich exudate accumulates. It is from this exudate that collagen is later synthesized. Inflammatory cells

Table 24.1 Phases of wound healing

Lag phase (2–3 days)
    Inflammatory response
Incremental or proliferative phase (approximately 3 weeks)
    Fibroblast migration
    Capillary ingrowth (granulation tissue)
    Collagen synthesis with rapid gain in tensile strength
    Wound contraction
Plateau or maturation phase (approximately 6 months)
    Organization of scar
    Slow final gain in tensile strength (80% of original strength)

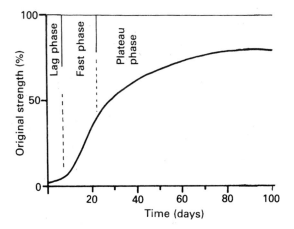

Fig. 24.3 Phases of wound healing.

migrate into the area, dead tissue is removed by macrophages, and capillaries at the wound edges begin to proliferate.

Incremental phase

During the incremental or proliferative phase there is progressive collagen synthesis by fibroblasts and a corresponding increase in tensile strength. Fibroblasts arise from perivascular mesenchymal cells and migrate into the wound in response to the high lactate levels that result from ischaemia. Increased collagen turnover in areas remote from the wound suggests that there may also be a systemic stimulus for fibroblast activity. Collagen synthesis increases over a period of about 3 weeks, during which the gain in tensile strength accelerates. Old collagen undergoes lysis and new collagen is laid down.

Proline and lysine are essential for collagen formation. They are hydroxylated by oxygen and ascorbic acid and

incorporated into tropocollagen, which polymerizes to form collagen. The energy needed for collagen synthesis is supplied by oxygen and nutrients brought into the wound by the ingrowth of capillary buds, which form fragile capillary arches. In unapposed wounds the excessive formation of new capillaries, mixed with fibroblasts, macrophages and leukocytes, results in granulation tissue. To the naked eye healthy granulation tissue is red, granular and friable. Fibroblasts also synthesize the mucopolysaccharide ground substance, which forms an ideal environment for the alignment and approximation of tropocollagen monomers prior to polymerization. Some fibroblasts, known as myofibroblasts, contain myofibrils, which pull in the wound margins. This wound contraction reduces the size of the defect in unapposed wounds and must be distinguished from contracture, which can be the unfortunate result of healing when a wound crosses a joint and there is a shortage of skin. The resultant scar restricts mobility. The gain in tensile strength during the incremental phase allows the removal of skin sutures without wound disruption at times ranging from 4–5 days on the face to 10–14 days on the trunk and lower limbs.

Plateau or maturation phase

After 3 weeks the gain in tensile strength levels off as the rate of collagen breakdown first approaches and then temporarily surpasses its synthesis. Excess collagen is removed during this final clearing-up process and the number of fibroblasts and inflammatory cells declines. Orientation of collagen fibres in the direction of local mechanical forces increases tensile strength for some 6 months. However, skin and fascia usually recover only 80% of their original tensile strength.

At the time of suture removal the edges of the newly healed wound should be directly apposed and flat. Thereafter, for up to 3 months the scar may become progressively raised, red and thickened. It can then remain static for a further 3 months, before slowly improving to become narrow, flat and pale. These changes vary with age, race, the direction of scar and the degree of dermal damage.

 In children, scars take longer to resolve, whereas in the elderly they tend to mature and fade very quickly.

Hypertrophic scars

This is an exaggeration of the normal maturation process. Such wounds are very raised, red and firm, but never continue to worsen after 6 months. They are particularly common in children and after deep dermal burns. Unless under tension they eventually resolve, often after several years. Resolution can be hastened by elastic pressure garments, steroid injections or the application of silicone gel; these scars should not be excised.

Keloids

These are similar to hypertrophic scars except that they continue to enlarge after 6 months and invade neighbouring uninvolved skin. They are most likely to occur across the upper chest, shoulders and earlobes, and are common in black patients. They are difficult to treat successfully. If the measures described above fail, intralesional excision followed immediately by low-dose radiotherapy is sometimes considered.

Epidermis

Epithelium heals by regeneration and not by scar formation. Epithelial cells at the edge of the wound lose their adhesion to each other and migrate across the wound until they meet cells from the other side. As they migrate, they are replaced by new cells formed by the division of basal cells near the wound edge. The cells that have migrated undergo mitosis and the new epithelium thickens, eventually forming normal epithelial cover for the scar produced by the dermis.

Primary and secondary intention

Wounds may heal by primary intention if the edges are closely approximated, for example by accurate suturing. In this situation epithelial cover is quickly achieved and healing of the apposed dermis produces a fine scar (Fig. 24.4). If the wound edges are not apposed the defect fills with granulation tissue and the restoration of epidermal continuity takes much longer. The advance of epithelial

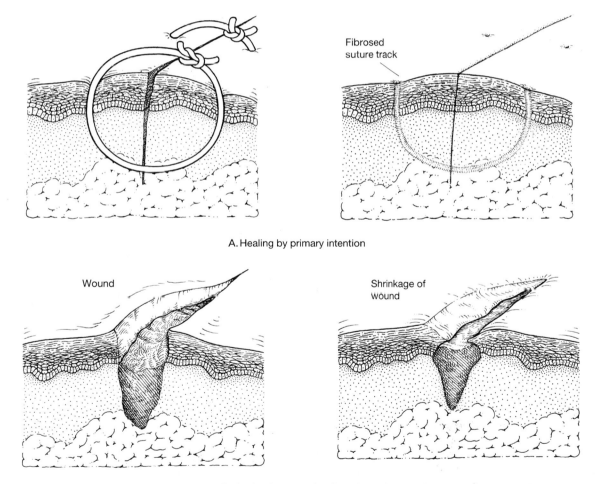

A. Healing by primary intention

B. Healing by secondary intention

Fig. 24.4 Wound healing by **A** primary intention and **B** secondary intention, showing shrinkage of the wound.

cells across the denuded area may also be hindered by infection. This is known as healing by secondary intention and usually results in delayed healing, excessive fibrosis and an ugly scar. If a wound has begun to heal by second intention it may still be possible to speed healing by excising the wound edges and bringing them into apposition, or by covering the defect with a skin graft.

SUMMARY BOX

Classification of wound healing

- Healing by *first intention* is the most efficient method and results when a clean incised surgical wound is meticulously apposed and heals with minimal scarring.

- Healing by *second intention* occurs when wound edges are not apposed and the defect fills with granulation tissue. In the time taken to restore epithelial cover, infection supervenes, fibrosis is excessive and the resulting scar is unsightly.

- The term 'healing by *third intention*' describes the situation where a wound healing by second intention (e.g. a neglected traumatic wound or a burn) is treated by excising its margins and then apposing them or covering the area with a skin graft. The final cosmetic result may be better than if the wound had been left to heal by second intention.

Factors influencing wound healing

Many of the factors influencing healing are interrelated, for example the site of the wound, its blood supply, and the level of tissue oxygenation. Although some adverse factors, such as advanced age, cannot be influenced, others, such as surgical technique, nutritional status and the presence of intercurrent disease, can be modified or eliminated.

Blood supply

Wounds in ischaemic tissue heal slowly or not at all. They are prone to infection and frequently break down. When this occurs the ischaemic wound may not be able to sustain the metabolic demands of healing by second intention. Arterial oxygen tension (Pao_2) is a key determinant of the rate of collagen synthesis. Anaemia per se may not affect healing if the patient has a normal blood volume and arterial oxygen tension. Poor surgical technique, such as crushing tissue with forceps, approximating wound edges under tension and tying sutures too tightly, can render well vascularized tissue ischaemic and lead to wound breakdown.

Infection

The general risks of wound infection depend upon age, the presence of intercurrent infection, steroid administration, diabetes mellitus, disordered nutrition, and cardiovascular and respiratory disease. Local factors are also important. Bacterial contamination can be minimized by careful skin preparation and meticulous aseptic technique, but some wounds are more likely to be contaminated than others. Despite every precaution, bacteria may enter wounds from the atmosphere, from internal foci of sepsis or from the lumen of transected organs. In some cases contamination occurs in the postoperative period. Provided contamination is not gross and that local blood supply is good, natural defences are usually able to prevent and contain overt infection. Devitalized tissues, haematomata and the presence of foreign material such as sutures and prostheses favour bacterial survival and growth. Common infecting organisms are staphylococci, streptococci, coliforms and anaerobes. Overcrowding of wards and excessive use of operating theatres increase the bacterial population of the atmosphere and hence the risk of wound infection. The failure of medical and nursing staff to wash their hands before and after touching and examining each patient is perhaps the greatest source of cross-contamination. Such handwashing is absolutely mandatory.

When wound contamination is anticipated, topical antibacterial chemicals or topical and systemic antibiotics can be used prophylactically. For example, a short course of systemic antibiotics (often a single dose) is normally used to reduce the risk of infection during gastrointestinal surgery and when prosthetic material (hip joint, cardiac valves, arterial bypass) is being inserted. In acute traumatic wounds tetanus prophylaxis is routine, but antibiotics are not normally necessary provided prompt and thorough surgical treatment is undertaken. However, if there has been a delay in the treatment of such a wound antibiotic prophylaxis may be necessary.

Age

Wounds in the elderly may heal poorly because of impaired blood supply, poor nutritional status or intercurrent disease. However, as mentioned above, they tend to form 'good' scars.

Site of wound

Surgical incisions placed in the lines of least tissue tension are subject to minimal distraction and should heal promptly, leaving a fine scar. On the face these lines run at right-angles to the direction of underlying muscles and form the lines of facial expression.

Nutritional status

Malnutrition has to be severe before healing is affected. Protein availability is most important, and wound dehiscence and infection are common when the serum albumin is low. Healing problems should be anticipated if recent weight loss exceeds 20%. Vitamin C is essential for proline hydroxylation and collagen synthesis. The number of fibroblasts is not reduced in scorbutic states. Zinc is a cofactor for important enzymes involved in healing, and its deficiency retards healing. Supplements of ascorbic acid and zinc are effective in patients with known deficiencies, but do not improve healing in normal subjects.

Intercurrent disease

Healing may be affected by the disease itself or by its treatment. Cachectic patients with severe malnutrition (as seen in advanced cancer) have marked impairment of healing. Diabetes mellitus impairs healing by reducing tissue resistance to infection and by causing peripheral vascular insufficiency and neuropathy. Haemorrhagic diatheses increase the risk of haematoma formation and wound infection. Obstructive airway disease lowers arterial Po_2 and so affects healing. Abdominal wound dehiscence is commoner in patients with respiratory disease, because of the strain put on the wound during coughing. Corticosteroid therapy reduces the inflammatory response, impairs collagen synthesis and decreases resistance to infection. The effect of steroids on wound healing is most marked if they are given within 3 days of injury. Immunosuppressive therapy impairs healing by reducing resistance to infection. Such patients are already compromised by their underlying disorder. As radiotherapy greatly reduces the vascularity of the tissues the healing of wounds in irradiated areas is often impaired. Chemotherapy also inhibits wound healing.

Surgical technique

Where possible, skin incisions are placed in the line of least tissue tension. Meticulous aseptic technique and gentle handling are mandatory. Crushing with tissue forceps, failure to achieve haemostasis, excessive use of diathermy and crude ligatures all contribute to wound devitalization. Accurate apposition of wound edges favours healing by first intention. Dead spaces in the depth of the wound must be avoided, as bleeding and the accumulation of exudate encourage infection. Correct suturing of the deeper layers often allows the skin edges to fall together without tension, so that superficial sutures or adhesive tape can achieve skin apposition. Deep sutures should obliterate any potential dead space. If this is not possible, the space must be drained. Drains should also be used in contaminated wounds and those where exudate is expected. Drains may be connected to a suction apparatus or allowed to empty by gravity. The drain site is a potential portal of entry for infection and drains should be removed as soon as possible, especially when prosthetic material has been implanted.

Choice of suture and suture materials

The choice of suture materials is important. Foreign material in the tissues predisposes to infection. The finest sutures that will hold the wound edges together should be used. A wound must never be closed under tension. Wounds are often subjected to stress postoperatively and, whereas 5/0

> **SUMMARY BOX**
>
> *Factors affecting wound healing*
>
> - The site of the wound and its orientation relative to tissue tension lines is a major determinant of healing.
> - Wounds with a good blood supply (e.g. head and neck wounds) heal well.
> - Infection is a major adverse factor and the risk of infection is influenced by:
>   - general factors such as the patient's age, presence of intercurrent infection, nutritional status, and cardiorespiratory disease.
>   - local factors including bacterial contamination, antibacterial prophylaxis, aseptic technique, degree of trauma, presence of devitalized tissue, haematoma and foreign bodies.
> - Intercurrent disease may impair healing. Important factors include:
>   - malnutrition
>   - diabetes mellitus
>   - haemorrhagic diatheses
>   - hypoxia (e.g. obstructive airways disease)
>   - corticosteroid therapy
>   - immunosuppression
>   - radiotherapy.
> - Surgical technical factors which have a major influence on wound healing include:
>   - gentle tissue handling
>   - avoidance of undue trauma
>   - accurate tissue apposition
>   - meticulous haemostasis
>   - appropriate choice of suture material.

or 6/0 sutures are appropriate for the face, stronger ones (3/0 or 4/0) are needed for incisions near joints and still stronger ones for the abdominal wall. The suture should be strong enough to support the wound until tensile strength has recovered sufficiently to prevent breakdown. Absorbable materials are preferred for buried layers, but non-absorbable sutures may be needed in some situations, for example in the aponeurotic layer of an abdominal wound. Non-absorbable sutures should be inert, retain strength and preferably be monofilaments, that is, without interstices that might favour bacterial growth.

Wound infection

Classification

Surgical procedures can be classified according to the likelihood of contamination and wound infection as 'clean', 'clean-contaminated' and 'contaminated'.

Clean procedures are those in which wound contamination is not expected and should not occur. An incision for a clean elective procedure should not become infected provided no infective focus is encountered and no viscus is entered. In clean operations the wound infection rate should be less than 1%.

Clean-contaminated procedures are those in which no frank focus of infection is encountered but where a significant risk of infection is nevertheless present, perhaps because of the opening of a viscus, such as the colon. Infection rates in excess of 5% may suggest a breakdown in ward and operating theatre routine.

Contaminated or 'dirty' wounds are those in which gross contamination is inevitable and the risk of wound infection is high; an example is emergency surgery for perforated diverticular disease, or drainage of a subphrenic abscess.

Antibiotic prophylaxis is appropriate for the latter two types of operation.

Clinical features

Wound infection usually becomes evident 3–4 days after surgery. The first signs are usually superficial cellulitis around the margins of the wound, or swelling of the wound with some serous discharge from between the sutures. Fluctuation is occasionally elicited when there is an abscess or liquefying haematoma. Crepitus may be present if gas-forming organisms are involved. In some cases of deep infection there are no local signs, although the patient may have pyrexia and increased wound tenderness. Systemic upset is variable, usually amounting to only moderate pyrexia and leukocytosis. Toxaemia, bacteraemia and septicaemia can complicate serious wound infection, especially where there is an accumulation of pus. The differential diagnosis includes other causes of postoperative pyrexia, wound haematoma and wound dehiscence. Wound haematoma may result from reactive bleeding during the first 24–48 hours after operation. It causes swelling and discomfort, but only minimal pyrexia and few systemic signs.

Prevention

The risk of wound infection is reduced by careful patient preparation, the prophylactic use of antibiotics in high-risk patients, and meticulous attention to good operating theatre techniques. Severely contaminated wounds are sometimes best closed by delayed primary suture: most gunshot wounds are treated in this way. Skin sutures may be inserted at this time but are not tied for several days, by when it should be clear that infection has been avoided. Antibiotic therapy is essential for grossly contaminated wounds. The aim is to achieve high tissue concentrations as soon as possible. The choice of antibiotics is determined by the nature of the infection. Topical agents such as povidone-iodine may also be used to combat infection in contaminated wounds. Radical excision of the wound margins, thorough mechanical cleansing and delayed suture may also be required.

Management

A wound swab or specimen of pus is sent routinely for bacteriological culture and sensitivity determination. In urgent cases a Gram stain may be useful. The state of immunity against tetanus is assessed and appropriate action taken. Trivial superficial cellulitis can be managed expectantly. The area of redness is 'mapped out' with an indelible pen so that its extent can be monitored. Spreading cellulitis is an indication for antibiotic therapy. Many infected wounds heal rapidly without further surgery, particularly if the original skin incision is placed in the line of least tissue tension. The problem is often to keep the wound open, rather than to achieve closure. If it appears that spontaneous wound closure will take a long time, secondary suture or skin grafting can be considered to speed healing, but only once it is clear that infection has been eradicated. The presence of clean healthy granulation tissue in the wound is usually a good indication that closure can be undertaken.

Involvement of other structures

All wounds must be inspected carefully in good light to assess the extent of devitalization and injury to other structures. However, it is important to appreciate that a small, apparently innocent wound may conceal extensive damage to deeper structures. Body cavities may have been penetrated, or tendons, nerves and blood vessels divided. Damage to muscles, tendons or nerves is assessed by checking relevant motor and sensory function. If the injury involves a limb, the distal circulation must be checked. Where appropriate, X-rays will help to establish whether peritoneal, pericardial or pleural cavities have been entered, and whether there is underlying bony injury.

Provided there is no deep damage, small, relatively uncontaminated wounds can be treated under local anaesthesia in the A&E department on an outpatient basis. The wound margins are cleaned with a mild antiseptic such as cetrimide and the wound is irrigated copiously with sterile saline. Any devitalized tissue is removed, deep tissues are sutured with absorbable material and the skin margins are closed.

If there is any possibility of damage to deep structures requiring more extensive exploration then this should also be conducted under general anaesthesia in an operating theatre by appropriately experienced surgeons.

More extensive or severely contaminated wounds also usually require inpatient treatment, with exploration and debridement under general anaesthesia. The wound and its margins are cleansed, and pieces of grit, soil and other obvious foreign material picked out. All devitalized tissue is trimmed back until bleeding occurs. This process is known as debridement. In areas of poor vascularity such as the leg,

or if there is severe contamination, crushing or a fracture, the wound margins are formally excised (Fig. 24.5). Bleeding from the wound margin is not a certain indication of its ultimate survival, as impaired venous drainage can lead to progressive necrosis, particularly after a crushing or degloving injury. If there is any doubt, the wound should not be sutured and a 'second-look' dressing change undertaken under anaesthesia after 48 hours.

Primary closure should also be avoided if there is significant delay in treating a grossly contaminated wound, that is, more than 6 hours without antibiotic cover. If this is attempted, wound infection and breakdown are likely and there is a risk of anaerobic infection, which may threaten both life and limb. It is also too late for formal excision, as bacteria will have penetrated the tissues, but foreign bodies and dead tissue should be removed in the usual way. The wound is dressed and antibiotics are started. The dressing is changed daily, and if the wound is clean in 2 or 3 days delayed primary suture may be carried out. If closure is delayed until granulation tissue has formed, this is usually excised and sec-

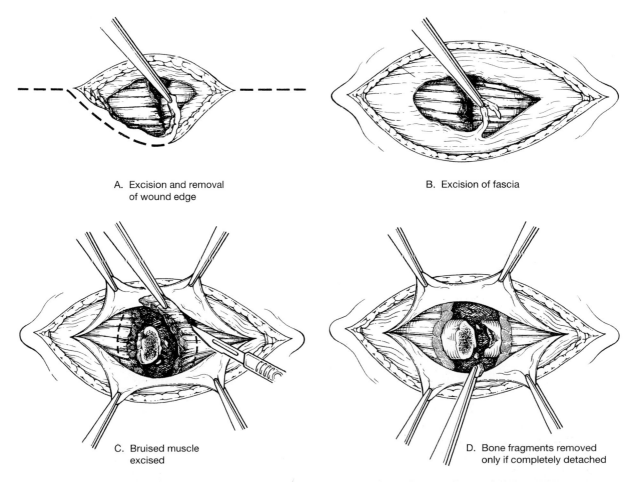

A. Excision and removal of wound edge

B. Excision of fascia

C. Bruised muscle excised

D. Bone fragments removed only if completely detached

Fig. 24.5 Technique of wound excision in the presence of a compound fracture.

ondary suture performed. If this is not possible, split skin grafts (see below) can be applied to the granulations.

Provided that surgical treatment is carried out early, prophylactic antibiotics are only required for deeply penetrating wounds, especially those from dog and human bites or those caused by nails, where adequate debridement may be impossible. However, the early use of antibiotics in situations where a delay in surgical treatment is anticipated may allow primary suture of wounds after 8–12 hours, an interval that is normally considered safe.

Devitalized skin flaps

A common emergency problem is posed by the patient, usually an elderly woman, who falls and raises a triangular flap over the surface of the tibia (pretibial laceration). In some cases the flap is blue-black in colour and obviously non-viable, but in most cases viability is uncertain. Similar injuries can occur elsewhere in the body. The wound must be cleansed and all non-viable tissue excised. No attempt should be made to suture the flap back into place: because of the post-traumatic oedema this would only be possible under tension, and would lead to death of the flap. If the defect is small it can be treated conservatively on an outpatient basis. The wound is dressed, an elastic supporting bandage is applied to the leg (providing the arterial circulation is normal;

SUMMARY BOX

Principles of management of contaminated traumatic wounds

- Contaminated wounds should be debrided under general anaesthesia.

- The contaminated wound and its margins must be cleansed thoroughly, and grit, soil and foreign bodies/materials removed.

- Devitalized tissue is formally excised until bleeding is encountered.

- Primary closure is avoided if there has been gross contamination and when treatment has been delayed for more than 6 hours. Inappropriate attempts to achieve primary closure increase the risk of wound infection and expose the patient to the risks of anaerobic infection (tetanus and gas gangrene).

- Wounds left open may be suitable for delayed primary suture after 2–3 days, or for later excision and secondary suture (with or without skin grafting).

- Appropriate protection against tetanus must be afforded and the use of antibiotics should be considered.

---

see Ch. 27) and the patient is kept ambulant. The wound will normally take several weeks to heal. Alternatively – and this is essential if the defect is large – a split skin graft can be applied, either immediately or as a delayed primary procedure. The patient is usually kept in bed with the leg horizontal until the graft has taken. It must be remembered that this latter approach is not without risk, for example DVT and chest complications. Recently there has been a trend to mobilize these patients early using supportive bandages.

Wounds with skin loss

The aim of wound care is to obtain skin cover and healing as soon as is safely possible, by either primary or delayed primary closure. If skin has been lost as a direct result of trauma, or following the excision of a tumour or necrotic tissue, direct suture may not be possible. If the skin defect is small and at a functionally or aesthetically unimportant site, it may be allowed to heal by secondary intention. However, it is often better to speed healing by importing skin to close the wound. This may be achieved by means of a skin graft, which requires a vascular bed as it has no blood supply of its own, or a flap.

Skin grafts

These may be split skin or full thickness. Split-skin grafts are cut with a special guarded freehand knife or an electric dermatome. The donor site heals by re-epithelialization from epithelial appendages in the dermis (the bases of hair follicles and sweat ducts) within 2–3 weeks, depending on the thickness of the graft. To cover very large areas the graft can be expanded by 'meshing'. The thinner the graft, the more easily it will take on a bed of imperfect vascularity, but the poorer the quality of skin the more it will shrink. Split-skin grafts are used to cover wounds after acute trauma, granulating areas and burns, or when the defect is large. A full-thickness graft leaves a donor defect (which needs to be sutured or grafted) as large as the one to be filled and requires a well vascularized bed to survive. However, such grafts are strong, do not shrink, and look better than a split-skin graft. They are rarely advisable after acute trauma but are commonly used in reconstructive surgery to close small defects where strength is needed (e.g. on the palm of the hand) or where a good functional and/or cosmetic result is important (e.g. on the lower eyelid). An area where there is skin to spare is chosen for the donor site (e.g. the groin for the former and the area behind the ear or upper eyelid for the latter).

Flaps

Whereas grafts require a vascular bed to survive, flaps bring their own blood supply to the new site. They can therefore be thicker and stronger than grafts and can be

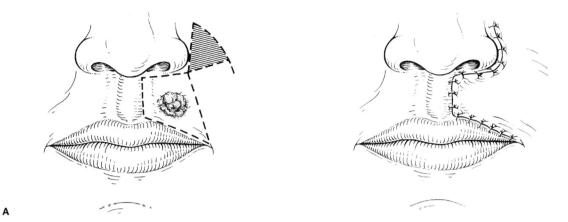

A   B

Fig. 24.6   Local skin flap used to repair a defect after the excision of a skin lesion.

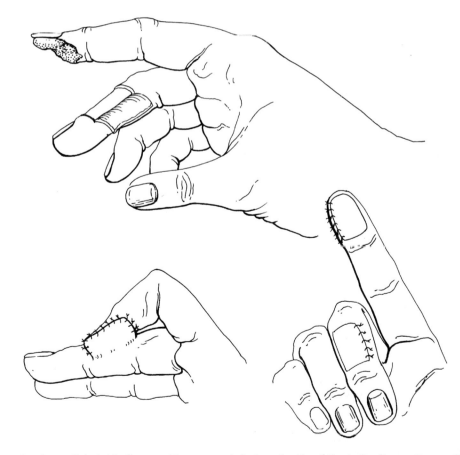

Fig. 24.7   Example of a pedicled skin flap used to cover a defect on the tip of the index finger. Once a blood supply is established, the pedicle is divided.

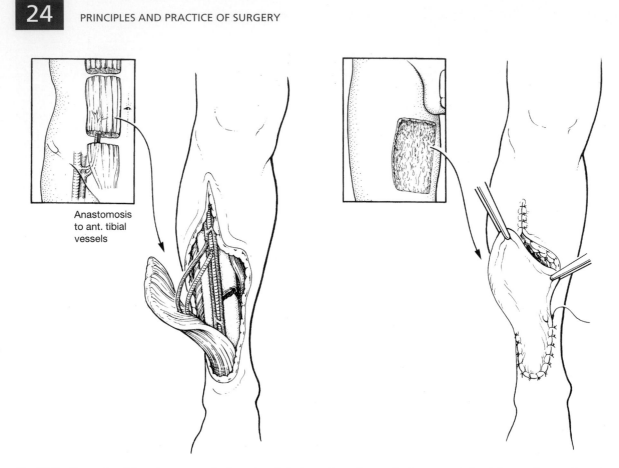

Anastomosis
to ant. tibial
vessels

Fig. 24.8 Example of free tissue transfer based on inferior epigastric vessels. **A** Rectus abdominis muscle transferred to shin and its vessels (inferior epigastric vessels) anastomosed to anterior tibial vessels; **B** Muscle covered by split-skin graft.

applied to avascular areas such as exposed bone, tendon or joints. They are used in acute trauma only if closure is not possible by direct suture or skin grafting, and are more usually reserved for the reconstruction of surgical defects and for secondary reconstruction after trauma. The simplest flaps use local skin and fat (local flaps) and are often a good alternative to grafting for small defects such as those left after the excision of facial tumours (Fig. 24.6). If not enough local tissue is available a flap may have to be brought from a distance (distant flap) and remain attached temporarily to its original blood supply until it has picked up a new one locally (Fig. 24.7). This usually takes 2–3 weeks, after which the pedicle can be divided. Advances in our knowledge of the blood supply to the skin and underlying muscles have led to the development of many large skin, muscle and composite flaps, which have revolutionized plastic and reconstructive surgery. One example is the use of the transverse rectus abdominis musculocutaneous (TRAM) flap for reconstruction of the breast. The ability to join small blood vessels

under the operating microscope now allows the surgeon to close defects in a single stage, even when there is no local tissue available, by free tissue transfer (Fig. 24.8). Other tissues, such as bone, cartilage, nerve and tendon, can also be grafted to restore function and correct deformity after tissue damage or loss.

Crushing and degloving injuries, gunshot wounds

Wounds of this type should never be closed primarily as the tissue destruction is always much greater than at first appears. After thorough irrigation and the removal of any obviously dead tissue and foreign material, such wounds should be lightly packed and dressed. Dressings are removed 48 hours later under anaesthesia and further excision is carried out if necessary. The wound is closed by suture, skin grafting or flap cover once it is clear that all dead tissue has been removed.

BURNS

Mechanisms

Burn injuries range from the trivial to severe burns that pose a threat to life, involve a long hospital stay, and carry the risk of permanent disfigurement or impaired function. Most burns follow accidents in the home and could be prevented. They may be caused by flames, hot solids, hot liquids or steam, irradiation, electricity or chemicals. Toddlers are particularly liable to scalding by hot liquids in kitchen accidents, and unguarded fires are a threat to all children. Severe disfigurement of the face and neck can result from the combustion of clothing, although this has become less common with the increased use of fire-resistant materials. Burns sustained in house fires are often accompanied by smoke inhalation, with injury to the lungs. Alcohol is a common contributing factor in burn injury. In the elderly and infirm impaired mobility, poor coordination and diminished awareness of pain increase the incidence of burns. Sunburn is the most common irradiation injury but is rarely serious. Industrial accidents account for most physicochemical burns, although the accidental or deliberate ingestion of caustic or corrosive chemicals is still an occasional cause of domestic burns.

Local effects of burn injury

The local effects result from destruction of the more superficial tissues and the inflammatory response of the deeper tissues (Table 24.2). Fluid is lost from the surface or trapped in blisters, the magnitude of loss depending on the extent of injury. Loss is greatly increased by leakage of fluid from the circulation (see below) where, instead of the normal insensible loss of 15 mL/m^2 body surface/h, as much as 200 mL/m^2 may be lost during the first few hours. With deeper injuries the epidermis and dermis are converted into a coagulum of dead tissue known as eschar. In its least severe form the dermal inflammatory response consists of capillary dilatation, as in the erythema of sunburn. With deeper burns the damaged capillaries become permeable to protein, and an exudate forms with an electrolytic and protein content only

Table 24.2   Effects of burn injury
Destruction of tissue (depth depends on heat of causative agent and contact time)
Loss of barrier to infection
Fluid loss from surface
Red cell destruction
Increased capillary permeability
Oedema
Loss of circulating fluid volume
Hypovolaemic shock
Increased metabolic rate

slightly less than that of plasma. Lymphatic drainage fails to keep pace with the rate of exudation and interstitial oedema leads to a reduction in circulating fluid volume. An increase of 2 cm in the diameter of the leg represents the accumulation of over 2 L of excess interstitial fluid. Exudation is maximal in the first 12 hours, capillary permeability returning to normal within 48 hours. Destruction of the epidermis removes the barrier to bacterial invasion and opens the door to infection. The burn surface may become contaminated at any time, and wound care must commence when the patient is first seen. Sepsis delays healing, increases energy needs, and may pose a new threat to life, just when the early dangers of hypovolaemia have been overcome.

General effects of burn injury

The general effects of a burn depend upon its size. Large burns lead to water, salt and protein loss, hypovolaemia and

---

SUMMARY BOX

Consequences of burns

- The morbidity and mortality of burns depend on the site, extent and depth of the burn and on the age and general condition of the patient.

- Early consequences include:

  - hypovolaemia (loss of protein, fluid and electrolytes)

  - metabolic derangements (hyponatraemia followed by risk of hypernatraemia, hyperkalaemia followed by hypokalaemia)

  - sepsis, which may be both local and generalized

  - haemolysis with anaemia and need for transfusion

  - hypothermia.

- Short-term consequences include:

  - renal failure (acute tubular necrosis due to hypovolaemia, haemoglobinuria and myoglobinuria)

  - respiratory failure (smoke inhalation, airway obstruction, ARDS)

  - catabolism and nutritional depletion

  - venous thrombosis

  - Curling's ulcer and erosive gastritis.

- Long-term consequences include permanent disfigurement, prolonged hospitalization, psychological problems and impaired function.

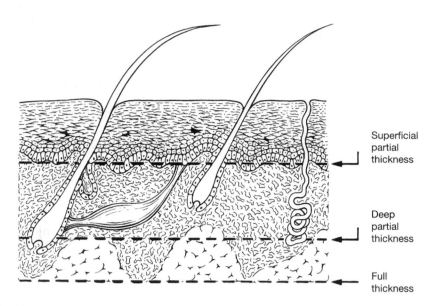

Fig. 24.9 Depth of burn injury.

increased catabolism. Circulating plasma volume falls as oedema accumulates, and fluid leaks from the burned surface. With large burns the effect is compounded by a generalized increase in capillary permeability, with widespread oedema. Some red cells are destroyed immediately by a full-thickness burn, but many more are damaged and die later. However, red cell loss is small compared to plasma loss in the early period, and haemoconcentration, reflected by a rising haematocrit, is the norm. The shifts in water and electrolytes are ultimately shared by all body tissues, and if circulatory volume is not restored hypovolaemic shock ensues. Large burns increase metabolic rate as water losses from the burned surface cause expenditure of calories to provide the heat of evaporation. In severe burns some 7000 kcal may be expended daily, and a daily weight loss of 0.5 kg is not unusual unless steps are taken to prevent it.

Classification

Burns are classified according to depth as either partial or full thickness (Fig. 24.9). In a partial-thickness burn epithelial cells survive to restore the epidermis. Full-thickness burns destroy all of the epithelial elements.

Superficial partial-thickness burns

Superficial partial-thickness burns involve only the epidermis and the superficial dermis. Pain, swelling and fluid loss can be marked. New epidermal cover is provided by undamaged cells originating from the epidermal appendages. The burn will usually heal in less than 3 weeks, with a perfect final cosmetic result.

Deep partial-thickness burns

In deep partial-thickness (also known as deep-dermal) burns the epidermis and much of the dermis are destroyed. Restoration of the epidermis then depends on there being intact epithelial cells within the remaining appendages. Pain, swelling and fluid loss are again marked. The burn takes longer than 3 weeks to heal, as fewer epithelial elements survive, and often leaves an ugly hypertrophic scar. Infection often delays healing and can cause further tissue destruction, converting the injury to a full-thickness one.

Full-thickness burns

A full-thickness burn destroys the epidermis and underlying dermis, including the epidermal appendages. The destroyed tissues undergo coagulative necrosis and form an eschar that begins to lift after 2–3 weeks. Unless the raw area is grafted, epidermal cover can only occur through the inward movement and growth of cells from intact skin around the burn, and by contraction of its base. Fibrosis and ugly contracture are thus inevitable in all but small ungrafted injuries.

Determination of burn depth

There is no foolproof method for the early determination of burn depth: even experienced plastic surgeons may not be able to make an accurate assessment for days or even weeks after injury. However, a number of pointers are valuable.

Mechanisms Burn depth is proportional to the temperature of the causal agent and to the length of contact time. Scalds from liquids below boiling point usually produce partial-thickness injury, whereas scalds from boiling water and burns due to prolonged contact with hot metal often produce full-thickness damage. Flame burns can be of mixed depth but nearly always include areas of full-thickness loss. Electrical burns are almost always full thickness, and high-tension electricity can cause devastating necrosis of muscles and other deep tissues.

Appearance Erythema means that epidermal damage is superficial, and blanching on pressure confirms that dermal capillaries are intact and that the injury is partial thickness. Blisters are accumulations of fluid superficial to the basal layer of the epidermis and suggest partial-thickness injury. They are often broken by the time the patient is seen by a doctor, but may continue to appear several hours after injury. A dead-white appearance frequently indicates full-thickness injury, although at least some of these burns prove to be deep dermal. A dry, leathery mahogany-coloured eschar with visible thrombosed veins denotes full-thickness destruction.

Sensation Intact cutaneous sensation implies that the epidermal appendages have survived, as they lie at the same level as cutaneous nerve endings in the dermis. Superficial burns are thus very painful. In practice, anaesthesia to pinprick does not always indicate full-thickness loss.

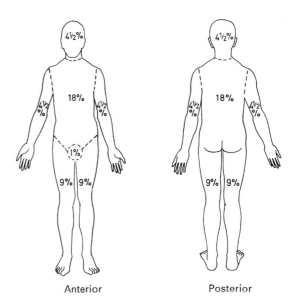

Fig. 24.10 Rule of nines for calculating surface areas of a burn.

Prognosis

Prognosis depends on the following factors.

Age and general condition

Infants, the elderly, alcoholics and those with other co-morbidity fare less well than healthy young adults.

Extent of the burn

The approximate extent of the burn can be quickly calculated in adults by using the 'rule of nines' (Fig. 24.10). Tables are available for more accurate estimations of burn area. The patient's hand with fingers together is about 1% of body surface area (BSA). Hypovolaemic shock is anticipated if more than 15% of the surface is burned in adults, or more than 10% in a child. If the sum of an adult patient's age and the percentage area of full-thickness burn comes to more than 80, death is probable.

Extent of burned area

- The 'rule of nines' as used in adults cannot be used for children because of the relatively large head size (about 20% of body surface at birth) and the relatively small limbs (legs are about 13%).
- Hypovolaemic shock is to be anticipated if more than 10% of body surface is burned.

Depth of burn

Superficial burns of whatever size should heal without scarring within 3 weeks if properly treated. Deep dermal burns take longer and produce hypertrophic scarring. Full-thickness burns inevitably become infected unless excised early, and in the case of large burns infection may prove life-threatening.

Site of the burn

Burns involving the face, neck, hands, feet or perineum are particularly liable to threaten appearance or function. They require inpatient management.

Associated respiratory injury

This is now extremely common in house fires and usually results from the inhalation of smoke from burning plastic foam upholstery. It is frequently fatal.

Management
First aid

Prompt effective action prevents further damage and may save life or prevent months of suffering. The key principles are to arrest the burning process, ensure an adequate airway and avoid wound contamination (Table 24.3).

Table 24.3   First aid for burns

Arrest the burning process
    Extinguish flames
    Remove clothing
    Cool with water
Ensure adequacy of airway
Avoid wound contamination
    'Clingfilm'

Transfer for definitive treatment as soon as possible

Arrest the burning process

Burning clothing is extinguished by smothering the flames in a coat or carpet. The victim is laid flat to avoid flames rising to the head and neck, with inhalation of smoke and fumes. Heat within clothing can continue to burn for many seconds after flames have been extinguished; clothing must therefore be removed or doused with cold water. The same applies to clothing soaked in scalding water, which will continue to cause damage until removed. Cool water is an excellent analgesic and dissipates heat, but common sense must be applied: immersing a child in cold water or covering a patient with cold soaks can cause hypothermia. Cooling counteracts the heat of a burn only if applied immediately after injury. Chip-pan fires are common. It is dangerous to attempt to remove the burning pan from the kitchen. Instead, the source of heat should be turned off and the pan covered with a lid, fibreglass firemat or damp dish-towel to exclude air and extinguish the flames. Do not throw water over a chip-pan fire as it will lead to an explosion of burning fat, boiling water and steam. Chemical burns require copious irrigation. If the eyes are involved, prompt and prolonged irrigation may save the patient's sight. Electrical burning is arrested by switching off the current, not by pulling the patient free. If this is not feasible, the patient should be pushed free from the contact with a non-conductor such as a wooden chair.

Ensure an adequate airway

The patient must be moved as quickly as possible into a smoke-free atmosphere. Smoke and fumes can cause asphyxia, often contain poisons and can precipitate respiratory arrest. Mouth-to-mouth mouth ventilation is commenced if necessary. If cardiac arrest follows electrocution, resuscitation is instituted.

Avoid wound contamination

The burn should be covered with a clean sheet or 'cling-film'. Traditional household remedies must be avoided: at best they are messy and interfere with subsequent care; at worst they are destructive, converting a partial injury to a full-thickness one.

Transfer to hospital

The patient should be transferred to hospital as quickly as possible, unless the burn is obviously trivial. Severe burns are best treated in a specialized burns unit from the outset. Hypovolaemia takes time to become manifest and it is easy to misjudge the severity of injury, thereby missing the opportunity for uncomplicated early transfer. Patients embarking on a journey expected to take more than 30 minutes should be accompanied by a trained person. An intravenous infusion should be commenced if the burn is extensive. Transfer between hospitals of patients with large burns should be avoided between 8 and 24 hours after injury. Full-thickness burns are often relatively painless. Partial-thickness injuries can be excruciating and opiates are usually needed. Analgesics must be given intravenously and the dose and route of administration noted.

Adequate ventilation

On arrival at hospital the maintenance of an adequate airway remains the first priority. Lack of respiratory symptoms on admission is no guarantee that the patient will remain free from airway problems. Every patient who has been exposed to smoke in a closed room should be admitted for observation. Respiratory tract injury is suggested by dyspnoea, cough, hoarseness, cyanosis, coarse crepitations on auscultation and the presence of soot particles around the nostrils, in the mouth or in the sputum. Endotracheal intubation is advisable if there is anxiety about airway patency, and assisted ventilation may be needed. Tracheostomy is never undertaken lightly in view of the danger of infection of burned tissues around the stoma.

Initial assessment and management

Once airway patency is assured, the time of injury, the type of burn and its previous treatment, and its extent and depth are established. If the burn is over 15% in extent (10% in children), establishing an intravenous infusion takes priority over a detailed history and physical examination. Intravenous therapy may be needed for many days, but there may be few veins available and they must be treated with great respect. It is best to start with the most peripheral vein available in the upper limb, but in shocked patients with vasoconstriction cannulation of the internal jugular or subclavian vein may be needed. Blood is withdrawn for cross-matching and determination of haematocrit and urea and electrolyte concentrations. Arterial blood gas analyses are performed and carboxy-haemoglobin levels measured if there is concern about the airway and smoke inhalation. Once an infusion has been established, the pulse rate, blood pressure and core/peripheral temperature difference are monitored. In patients with burns of more than 20% a catheter is inserted to measure hourly urine output. Severe pain is relieved by intravenous opiates. Tetanus can complicate burns, and tetanus toxoid is given if the patient has not received it recently. In general, patients with burns involving more than 5% of body surface should be admitted to hospital, as should all those with significant full-thickness injury or burns in sites likely to pose particular management problems.

Prevention and treatment of burn shock

The aim of management is to prevent hypovolaemic shock by prompt and adequate fluid replacement (Table 24.4). Opinions vary as to the relative amounts of colloid and crystalloid that should be used. Various formulae are available to help calculate replacement needs, but all are merely guides and the amounts of fluid given must be adjusted in the light of the patient's response to resuscitation. In a formula commonly used in the UK, the first 36 hours after injury are divided into six successive periods of 4, 4, 4, 6, 6 and 12 hours. The volume of colloid, for example purified protein solution (PPS), to be infused in each period is calculated from the equation:

$$\text{Burn area (\%)} \times \text{body weight (kg)}/2$$

i.e. 0.5 mL/kg for each percent burn. There are other resuscitation formulae that use crystalloids rather than colloid. The need for fluid is greatest in the early hours, but excessive losses may persist for 36–48 hours.

Despite renal retention of sodium after injury, there is a tendency to hyponatraemia in the first 2–3 days owing to the secretion of antidiuretic hormone and the sequestration of sodium in oedema. As inflammatory oedema is reabsorbed the serum sodium concentration returns to normal, and unless water intake is maintained there is now a danger of hypernatraemia. Tissue destruction releases large amounts of potassium into the extracellular fluid (ECF), but hyperkalaemia is largely prevented by increased renal excretion as part of the metabolic response to injury. Once the first few days have passed, continuing potassium

losses can produce hypokalaemia in a patient unable to eat and drink normally.

Water replacement

Daily water losses are replaced using 5% dextrose solution, taking care to avoid water intoxication, especially in young children, in the first few days following injury. Excessive evaporation continues until the burn has re-epithelialized, and a high water intake must be maintained. Although most patients are thirsty, paralytic ileus may occur during the first 48 hours in those with very large burns, so that giving oral fluids too soon can cause gastric distension, vomiting and aspiration. Most patients are able to drink normally after 48 hours and should be encouraged to do so.

Blood transfusion

Blood should not be given in the first 24 hours but may be needed thereafter in patients with large full-thickness burns. Continuing red cell destruction in deep burns with bone marrow suppression can necessitate repeated transfusion. Haemoglobin concentration and haematocrit should be monitored regularly.

Organ failure and burn shock

Organ failure and shock are discussed in detail in Chapter 3, and only those respiratory and renal problems specific to burn shock are considered here.

Respiratory complications Inhalation of smoke and fumes can cause direct heat damage, carbon monoxide poisoning and damage from other chemicals, all of which predisposes to infection. Patients with head and neck burns are best nursed sitting up to encourage the dispersal of oedema. Continued observation is mandatory and physiotherapy is essential to clear bronchial secretions. Chest X-rays and blood gas analyses are repeated regularly in patients with ventilation problems. Arterial hypoxaemia and carbon monoxide poisoning require oxygen therapy, and may necessitate early endotracheal intubation and assisted ventilation. Antibiotics should be prescribed. Tracheostomy is occasionally unavoidable despite the problems associated with its management. Encircling eschar impairing chest or abdominal expansion must be incised (escharotomy) or excised.

Renal failure Acute tubular necrosis may complicate extensive burns, especially in the elderly, those with pre-existing renal disease and those who develop haemoglobinaemia or myoglobinuria. These pigments appear in the urine after massive red cell destruction or extensive muscle damage (particularly after electrical injury), and can damage the tubules and obstruct urine flow by forming casts. Hourly urine output should be maintained at 30–50 ml in adults. Falling output reflects inadequate resuscitation or impending

Table 24.4	Hypovolaemic shock and burns
Anticipate if burn more extensive than 15% (10% in children)
Prevent by early intravenous resuscitation
Control pain by adequate intravenous administration of opiates
Fluid requirements assessed from patient's response 'Formulae' for fluid replacement provide rough guides only

renal failure (acute tubular necrosis). Measurement of urine osmolality and the response to a test infusion will distinguish between them. Diuretics are used only if oliguria persists despite adequate fluid replacement, when 20% mannitol (1 g/kg) may be infused over 30 minutes.

Nutritional management

Evaporation from open wounds and sepsis is an important cause of increased energy expenditure following a severe burn. Energy expenditure can be reduced by nursing in an environmental temperature of 30–32°C. A high-calorie intake is impractical during the period of hypovolaemic shock, but is encouraged as soon as the patient can drink. The daily caloric intake in adults can be calculated as 20 kcal/kg body weight plus 70 kcal/percent burn. It is particularly important to provide sufficient protein intake (1 g/kg body weight plus 3 g/percent burn). In large burns oral intake can usually be supplemented at 48 hours by enteral feeding using a fine-bore nasogastric tube. If the patient's total calculated energy and protein requirements are supplied in this way, weight loss can be limited to less than 10%. Vitamin supplements and iron must also be provided. It is unusual, and often considered undesirable, to use parenteral nutrition in burned patients.

Sepsis

Septicaemia is a constant threat until skin cover has been fully restored, as resistance to infection is low. The wound provides a reservoir of infecting organisms. Catheters, cannulae and tracheostomy wounds are all potential sources of infection. The incidence of septicaemia has been reduced by topical antibacterial agents and early excision and grafting. However, in large burns the risk remains high. Regular monitoring by means of blood cultures is advisable. Systemic antibiotics are not prescribed routinely for fear of producing superinfection with resistant organisms. Their use is reserved for invasive infection and for patients with positive blood cultures.

Curling's ulcer and gastric erosions

Acute duodenal ulceration (Curling's ulcer) and multiple gastric erosions may follow major burns. Early resumption of feeding reduces their incidence, and H_2-receptor antagonists such as ranitidine are prescribed prophylactically.

Local management of burns

Care of the burn wound commences at the time of injury and continues until epithelial cover has been restored. Infection poses the main threat to life once the first 48 hours have passed.

Initial cleansing and debridement

The wound is cleansed meticulously with a mild detergent containing antiseptic and saline as soon as possible after admission. Adherent clothing and loose devitalized tissues are removed. Cleansing must be carried out in an operating theatre or clean dressing room using aseptic technique. Blisters are punctured and serum expressed. Broken blisters are completely deroofed. General anaesthesia may be necessary, but in most cases pain can be relieved by intravenous opiates. In shocked patients the wound is covered with a sterile drape and further local care is postponed until the circulatory state has stabilized.

Prevention of contamination

Destruction of the epidermis removes the normal barrier to infection. In full-thickness injury, thrombosis of cutaneous vessels impairs the normal response to infection. In large burns both cellular and humoral immune mechanisms are depressed. Organisms readily colonize the burn wound. If dead tissue is present they multiply rapidly and invade the surrounding tissues. Staphylococci remain by far the commonest infecting organism. *Pseudomonas aeruginosa* remains troublesome in most burn units. Haemolytic streptococci are feared because they can convert superficial into deep burns, and can cause a severe systemic illness. Once contaminating organisms have been cleared, further contamination can be prevented in a number of ways. The methods described below are not mutually exclusive, and more than one may be used as the patient's needs alter. All dressings are applied using meticulous aseptic technique.

Exposure After cleansing and debridement, burns of a single surface may be exposed to the air. Evaporation of the protein-rich exudate leaves a dry, adherent crust that is an effective barrier to bacteria as long as it remains intact. Exposure is particularly useful for burns to the face and neck, but can be used on the trunk and extremities. The technique is difficult and should only be practised by units familiar with it: badly performed 'exposure' is a recipe for infection.

Evaporative dressings These dressings prevent contamination, allow exudate to evaporate and provide comfortable support. After the initial cleansing, the wound is covered by a layer of sterile non-adherent dressing, e.g. paraffin gauze or Mepotil, a layer of cotton gauze swabs, a bulky layer of cotton wool or Gamgee, and an outer retaining crepe bandage. The dressing is reviewed daily but left in place for 8–10 days, unless exudate soaks through to the outside. The dressing is then changed down to the inner layer, as bacteria can traverse a soaked dressing in only a few hours.

Semiocclusive and occlusive dressings 'Clingfilm' is useful in first aid but leaks and is too messy for use as a definitive dressing. OpSite is an adhesive film that is effective for small burns; it may also leak initially, and should be covered with a well-padded dressing for 48 hours, after when it can be patched or replaced as necessary. Many new dressings are now available. Hydrogels and hydrocolloids absorb exudates but offer no particular advantages in acute management. Commercial polythene bags are cheap, sterile when taken from the roll, and useful for treating superficial hand burns. The hands are smeared with liquid paraffin for the first 24–48 hours until a decision as to depth is made. If the decision is made to continue with a conservative regimen then silver sulfadiazine cream is applied. The bags are kept in place with a bandage at the wrist. They must be changed at least daily after washing the hand and reapplying the antibacterial cream. Such 'hand bags' allow the patient to continue to use the hand and so prevent stiffness.

Topical antibacterial agents Silver sulfadiazine cream (Flamazine) and povidone-iodine (Betadine) are valuable local antibacterial agents for large burns. To be effective they must be reapplied daily. They are not necessary or cost-effective for minor burns given proper initial surgical debridement and the use of evaporative dressings.

'Biological' dressings Freeze-dried xenografts such as porcine skin can be reconstituted for use as temporary occlusive 'biological' dressings, but are very expensive. Amnion or stored homograft skin are now used rarely because of the danger of infection with human immunodeficiency virus (HIV). Sheets of keratinocytes grown in tissue culture are fragile and easily destroyed by infection, limitations which may be overcome in the future by growing the cells on sheets of collagen or synthetic 'dermis'. As yet this type of dressing is of little value in current practice.

Relief of constriction (escharotomy)

The danger of progressive respiratory embarrassment from encircling eschar has already been mentioned. Increasing oedema beneath encircling eschar in the limbs may also imperil the circulation. Relieving incisions (escharotomy) which run from the top to the bottom of circumferential deep burns may be needed in the first few hours after injury. As these wounds can bleed profusely it is important to have available methods for controlling haemorrhage, e.g. diathermy and dressings at hand.

Restoration of epidermal cover

Full-thickness and deep dermal burns of less than 10% are suitable for primary excision of eschar and grafting under general anaesthesia within 48–72 hours of injury. Tangential excision is used for deep dermal burns. The dead outer layers of skin are shaved away down to the deep dermal layer and a split-skin graft is applied immediately. More extensive burns can be partially excised and grafted

soon after injury, and the remaining areas of skin destruction treated by delayed grafting. After some 2 weeks eschar begins to separate spontaneously. The process is accelerated by infection and delayed by topical antibacterial agents. As the slough separates healthy granulation tissue should be revealed, and when all the slough has gone or been excised the burn should be ready for grafting. Haemolytic streptococci are a troublesome cause of graft loss, and when such infection is present grafting must be deferred until the patient has been treated with intravenous penicillin and barrier nursed until three successive wound swabs are negative.

Free skin grafts may be full or partial thickness (split skin), but only split-skin grafts are used to cover acute burns. The grafts may vary in thickness from epidermis only to almost full thickness; medium-thickness grafts are most commonly used. The donor site forms a new epidermis from residual islands of epithelium, and more skin can be harvested after 14 days. Excess skin can be stored at 4°C for up to 3 weeks.

Full-thickness grafts are used for secondary reconstruction in cosmetically important areas where contraction has to be avoided, or in areas such as the palm of the hands, which are subject to repeated trauma.

Functional and cosmetic result

With energetic treatment it is usually possible to restore skin cover to even the most extensive injury within 3 months, but wound closure is not the end point. Skin grafts and donor sites must be kept soft and supple by applying moisturizing cream several times a day for many months. Splints may be needed to prevent contractures, and physiotherapy is essential to mobilize joints. Elastic pressure garments help to prevent the build-up of hypertrophic scars. In spite of all this care, reconstructive procedures may be required for many years to correct contractures or rebuild missing or distorted features. Severely burned patients often have difficulty coming to terms with their disfigurement and limitations to their way of life. Long-term support with counselling from surgeon and supporting staff is invaluable.

SKIN AND SOFT TISSUE LESIONS

Diagnosis of skin swellings

In addition to describing the site and size of the lesion it is necessary to determine whether it arises from the skin or is deep to it. If it comes from the skin then it arises from either the epidermis or the dermis. Surface changes indicate an epidermal origin, whereas over dermal lesions the surface is stretched but remains normal. Ulceration may occur later as a result of pressure necrosis. The colour of a skin lesion is also an important feature in its diagnosis.

Cysts

Sebaceous cysts

Sebaceous (or epidermoid) cysts are dermal swellings covered by epidermis (Fig. 24.11). They have a thin wall of flattened epidermal cells and contain cheesy white epithelial debris and sebum. They form soft smooth hemispherical swellings over which the skin cannot be moved. A small surface punctum is often visible. If infection supervenes the cyst becomes hot, red and painful. Infected cysts are incised to allow the infected material to escape. Excision is deferred until the inflammation has settled. In some cases the inflammation destroys the cyst lining so that excision is not necessary.

Dermoid cysts

Dermoid cysts (Fig. 24.11) arise from nests of epidermal cells that have been sequestered in the dermis during development or implanted as a result of trauma. Congenital dermoid cysts are found at sites of embryonic fusion, notably on the face, the base of the nose, the forehead and the occiput. External angular dermoid is the commonest congenital dermoid cyst and lies at the junction of the outer and upper margins of the orbit, in the line of fusion of the maxilla and frontal bones. Implantation dermoid cysts are found at sites of injury, notably the palmar surfaces of the hands and fingers. They are lined by squamous epithelium and contain sebum, degenerate cells and, in some cases, hair. A soft rubbery swelling forms deep to the skin. The cyst may be fixed deeply, particularly when situated on the face. Implantation dermoids can be removed under local anaesthesia. Congenital dermoids usually require formal dissection under general anaesthesia, as they may extend deeply for example, an external angular dermoid can extend within the cranium.

Table 24.5 Classification of skin tumours	
Cell/tissue of origin	Type of tumour
Epidermal neoplasms (common)	
From basal germinal cells	Papillomas
	Infective warts
	Senile warts
	Pedunculated papilloma
	Keratoacanthoma
	Premalignant keratoses
	Carcinoma in situ
	Epidermoid cancer
	Basal cell cancer
	(rodent ulcer)
	Squamous cell cancer
From melanocytes	Benign pigmented moles
	Common mole
	Giant hairy mole
	Blue naevus
	Halo naevus
	Malignant melanoma
	Melanotic freckle
	(lentigo maligna)
	Superficial spreading melanoma
	Nodular melanoma
	Other forms of melanoma
Dermal neoplasms (rare)	Fibroma
	Lipoma
	Neurofibroma

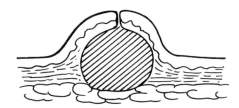
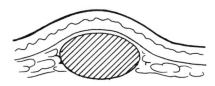

Fig. 24.11   Types of cyst. **A** Sebaceous (epidermoid) cyst; **B** dermoid cyst.

Tumours of the skin

Skin tumours may arise from the epidermis or the dermis (Table 24.5). Epidermal tumours are common and can arise from basal germinal cells or melanocytes. Dermal tumours arising from connective tissue elements are rare. The remainder of this section will be devoted to the commoner epidermal neoplasms.

Epidermal neoplasms arising from basal germinal cells

Papillomas

Papillomas (or warts) are common benign skin neoplasms.

Infective warts These are common and caused by viral infection. They are found most commonly on the hands and fingers of young children and adults. They spread by direct inoculation and are often multiple. They form greyish-brown, round or oval elevated lesions with a filiform surface and keratinized projections (Fig. 24.12) and may be studded with spots of blood. They often regress spontaneously but can be removed by caustics (acetic acid) or freezing (liquid nitrogen or CO_2 snow). Plantar warts (verruca plantaris) are particularly troublesome infective warts acquired in swimming pools and showers. They are found under the heel and metatarsal heads. They are flush with the surface (Fig. 24.13) and may be intensely painful. If persistent they are treated by curettage or freezing. Infective warts in the perineum and on the penis may be of venereal origin and are associated with gonorrhoea, syphilis, human immunodeficiency virus (HIV) infection and lymphogranuloma. Infective warts are also common in immunosuppressed patients.

Senile warts These are basal cell papillomas and are common in the elderly. They form a yellowish-brown or black greasy plaque (synonym: seborrhoeic keratosis) with

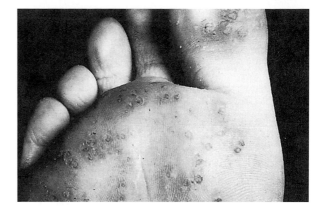

Fig. 24.13   Verruca plantaris (plantar warts) affecting the sole of the foot.

a cracked surface that falls off in pieces. Senile warts are often multiple, commonly affect the upper back and trunk, and are best treated by curettage.

Pedunculated papilloma These simple non-infective papillomas form a flesh-coloured spherical warty mass on a stalk of normal epithelium. If small, they can be dealt with by grasping with fine forceps, pulling out from the skin surface and cutting off with scissors: a stitch is rarely required. If they are large the papilloma and its pedicle are removed formally with an ellipse of normal skin.

Keratoacanthoma (molluscum sebaceum) This lesion can be confused with squamous cancer because of its clinical appearance. It grows rapidly over 4–6 weeks and then involutes. Histologically it has a well defined 'shoulder', but even under the microscope it may resemble a squamous carcinoma. The distinction between the two is the history. Keratoacanthoma occurs most commonly on the face as a hemispherical nodule with a friable red centre crusted with keratin (Fig. 24.14). It is found mainly in those over 50 years of age. It heals after shedding its central core, but can also be eradicated by curettage.

Actinic (solar) keratosis This is a premalignant keratosis and is characterized by small, single or multiple, firm warty spots on the face, back of the neck and hands. Such keratoses are particularly common in older, fair-skinned people who have been exposed to excessive sunlight. The scaly lesions drop off periodically to leave a shallow premalignant ulcer. The keratoses should be biopsied to exclude frank malignancy, and then treated by freezing.

Intraepidermal cancer (carcinoma in situ)

This non-invasive form of skin cancer forms a discrete, often solitary, raised brown or red fissured plaque which is keratinized. Histologically, the plaques are composed of hyperplastic atypical epithelial cells, but there is no evi-

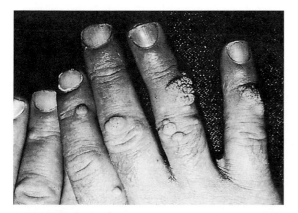

Fig. 24.12   Verruca vulgaris. Infective warts affecting the hands.

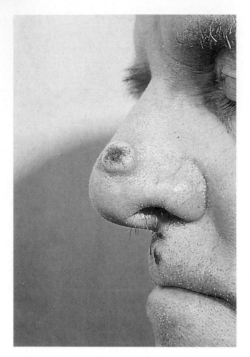

Fig. 24.14 Keratoacanthoma affecting the nose of an elderly man.

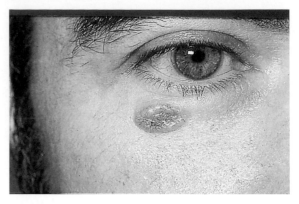

Fig. 24.15 Basal cell carcinoma (rodent ulcer). Note the raised pearly edge.

dence of invasion through the basement membrane. Intra-epidermal skin cancer is also known as Bowen's disease and, when it affects the penis or vulva, as erythroplasia of De Queyrat.

Cancer of the epidermis

Epidermal cancer occurs primarily on exposed areas and in those with poor natural protection against sunlight. Albinos and patients with xeroderma pigmentosa (a congenital defect leading to undue sensitivity to sunlight) are at particularly high risk, whereas skin cancer is rare in black, brown and yellow-skinned races. Chronic skin irritation by chemicals (e.g. arsenic, tar and soot), chronic ulceration (e.g. old burns or varicose ulcers), and exposure to other forms of radiation, are also established causes. Epidermoid cancer is particularly common in those over 50 years of age. There are two distinct pathological forms: basal cell and squamous cell carcinoma.

Basal cell carcinoma (rodent ulcer)

Rodent ulcers are slow-growing, locally invasive and, for all practical purposes, never metastasize. They almost all arise in the skin of the middle third of the face, typically on the nose, inner canthus of the eye, forehead and eyelids (Fig. 24.15). The earliest lesion is a hard pearly nodule, dimpled in its centre and covered by thin telangiectatic skin. Cystic degeneration may make the lesion raised and translucent. A number of clinical types are recognized, being described as cystic, nodular, sclerosing, morpheoic, centrally healing and 'field fire'. Over a period of years the rodent ulcer repeatedly scales over and breaks down. Growth is extremely slow. Occasionally the tumour is highly invasive and can burrow deeply, despite little apparent surface activity. All suspicious lesions must be biopsied. Surgical excision or radiotherapy can be used for definitive treatment, but the latter is contraindicated if the lesion is close to the eye or overlies cartilage. Complex reconstructive surgery may be needed to restore structure and function in patients who present late.

Squamous cell carcinoma

This tumour may affect any area (Fig. 24.16) but is particularly common on exposed parts such as the ear, cheeks, lower lips and backs of the hands. It commonly develops in an area of epithelial hyperplasia or keratosis. In mucosa, such as the lips, the analogous change is leukoplakia. The lesion starts as a hard erythematous nodule, which proliferates to form a cauliflower-like excrescence or ulcerates to form a malignant ulcer with a raised fixed hard edge. The cancer grows more quickly than a rodent ulcer but more slowly than a keratoacanthoma. The regional nodes can be involved early and become enlarged, hard and fixed. The choice of treatment (surgery or radiotherapy) depends on the tumour's size, site and aggressiveness. Palpable lymph nodes are an indication for regional lymphadenectomy by block dissection. This may be followed by adjuvant radiotherapy if histology shows extracapsular spread. Chemotherapy is of limited value.

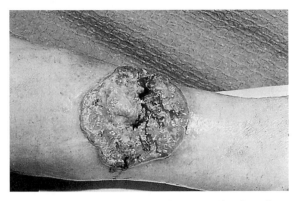

Fig. 24.16 A squamous cell carcinoma at the site of long-standing leg ulceration.

Epidermal neoplasms arising from melanocytes

Benign pigmented moles

The number of melanocytes is relatively fixed (approximately 2000 million) regardless of the colour of the individual, but the amount of pigment produced obviously varies greatly. As a developmental abnormality, conglomerates of melanocytes may migrate to the dermis or epidermis to form a melanocytic naevus or mole. The naevus cells can cause a variety of pigmented spots and swellings (naevi) according to their site and activity (Fig. 24.17). Moles showing melanocyte activity at the junction of epidermis and dermis (junctional change) are common in childhood:

all moles on the soles and palms are of this type. Migration of sheets of naevus cells to the dermis produces a dermal naevus; migration to both dermis and epidermis produces a compound naevus.

Common moles

The common mole is a flat or slightly raised brown-black lesion covered by normal epidermis. It has a period of active growth during childhood as a result of junctional activity, but usually becomes quiescent at puberty and may later atrophy. If naevus cells migrate to the dermis the lesion becomes firm and raised, and there is often aberrant hair growth. The epidermis remains smooth if it remains uninvolved, but can become soft and roughened in a compound naevus. As only one in 100 000 moles becomes malignant they need not normally be removed. Active growth in childhood need not cause concern, but growth after puberty demands removal. An increase in pigmentation, scaliness, itching and bleeding may also give rise to anxiety about malignancy and indicate the need for excision. Any mole that develops these characteristics should be removed. Further treatment depends on the histological appearances (see below).

Giant hairy naevus

Unlike the common mole this lesion is present at birth. It can cover a large area, which may correspond to a dermatome. Typical sites are the bathing-trunk area and face. The risk of malignant change is small but such moles

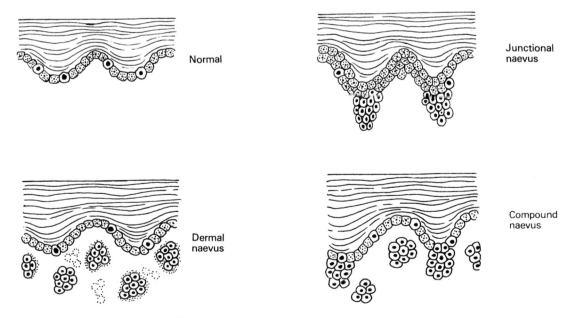

Fig. 24.17 Histopathological types of benign moles.

should be kept under observation, and in some cases there may be cosmetic indications for excision.

Blue naevus

This intradermal naevus can appear blue because the melanin-containing cells are deep in the dermis. It can develop at any time from birth to middle age.

Halo naevus

This pigmented naevus is surrounded by a white circle of depigmentation associated with lymphocytic infiltration.

SUMMARY BOX

Epidermal neoplasms arising from melanocytes

- A mole is due to a conglomeration of melanocytes.

- Melanocyte activity at the junction of epidermis and dermis (i.e. junctional activity) is common in childhood.

- Migration of melanocytes into the dermis produces a dermal naevus while migration to both dermis and epidermis produces a compound naevus.

- Only 1 in 100 000 moles becomes malignant, so that the presence of a mole is not in itself an indication for removal. Active growth in childhood need not cause concern, but growth thereafter should.

- Excision is indicated if a mole shows an increase in pigmentation, scaliness, itching or bleeding. A 3-mm excision margin is adequate in the first instance.

Malignant melanoma

Malignant melanomas predominantly affect fair-skinned people. They are rare in blacks but can occasionally affect the depigmented areas such as the palms, soles and mucosa. Exposure to sunlight is the major precipitating factor. In Scotland the incidence is 8 per 100 000 individuals per year, compared to 40 per 100 000 in Queensland, Australia. The incidence has increased worldwide, and in Scotland there has been a 100% increase over the last 10 years. Malignant melanomas are commoner in females with a higher incidence on the legs presumably because of greater exposure. About half of all malignant melanomas are thought to arise in pre-existing naevi. The average individual has 14 melanocytic naevi and the risk of any one of

them becoming malignant is very small. However, the greater the number of moles the greater the risk, particularly in those with a family history of malignant melanoma. The essential feature of malignant melanoma is invasion of the dermis by proliferating melanocytes with large nuclei, prominent nucleoli and frequent mitoses. Three distinct clinicopathological types of malignant melanoma are described.

SUMMARY BOX

Malignant melanoma

- Malignant melanomas are predominantly but not exclusively a disease of fair skinned individuals.

- Exposure to sunlight is the key aetiological factor.

- The lesion is commoner in females, reflecting the higher incidence of malignant melanomas of the lower leg.

- 50% of all malignant melanomas arise in a pre-existing naevus.

- The essential feature of malignancy is invasion of the dermis by proliferating melanocytes (which show large nuclei, prominent nucleoli and frequent mitoses).

- Malignant melanoma spreads rapidly by the lymphatic system and the bloodstream. 'In transit' metastases may develop in the lymphatics of the skin and subcutaneous tissues.

Hutchison's melanotic freckle (lentigo maligna)

One in 10 malignant melanomas arises in a melanotic or senile freckle. These occurs most commonly on the face of elderly women (Fig. 24.18), beginning as a brown-red patch which grows slowly, advancing and receding over the years. The edge of the lesion appears serrated but its margin with normal skin remains abrupt. Kaleidoscopic pigmentation of the surface is typical. This premalignant phase may last for 10–15 years. The first sign of malignancy is a brownish-red papule that develops eccentrically within the freckle and indicates vertical extension of melanocytes into the dermis in the form of a lentigo maligna melanoma.

Superficial spreading melanoma

This is the commonest type of malignant melanoma (Fig. 24.19). It occurs on the trunk and exposed parts, and is most common in middle age. During a preinvasive phase, which lasts for at most one or two years, malignant cells spread outwards (horizontal growth phase) in the epidermis

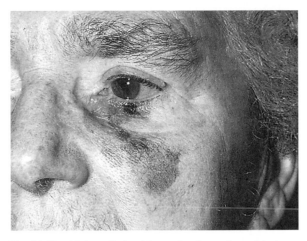

Fig. 24.18 Melanotic freckle on the face of an elderly woman.

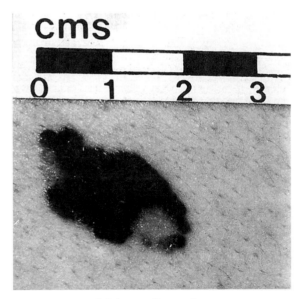

Fig. 24.19 Superficial spreading melanoma.

in all directions. The surface is slightly raised, the outline indistinct, pigmentation is patchy and there may be a wide range of colours. Invasion of the dermis (vertical growth phase) occurs while the lesion is still relatively small and produces an indurated nodule, which soon ulcerates or bleeds.

Nodular melanoma

These elevated, deeply pigmented melanomas can occur at any site and at any age. They are particularly common in females on the leg. They may occur at the site of a pre-existing benign naevus. Nodular melanomas are vertically invasive from the start and there is no initial intraepidermal spread and therefore no surrounding pigmented macule. The nodule enlarges steadily, both centrifugally and on the surface. Surface spread is detected by the destruction of normal skin lines. The lesion darkens progressively and the surface over the area of active growth becomes jet black and glossy. Bleeding may follow trivial injury and is noted as spots of blood on clothes. Crusting, scab formation, itching, irritation and ulceration are typical. Satellite nodules may form around neglected lesions.

Other types of malignant melanoma

Not all melanomas are deeply pigmented. Amelanotic melanomas are rare, pale-pink lesions that can grow rapidly. Careful histological examination will demonstrate pigment in virtually every case. Acral lentiginous melanoma is seen on the soles and palms (Fig. 24.20). It resembles superficial spreading melanoma in its behaviour, although the thick skin of the affected regions may mask some of the features and cause late presentation, with nodularity and ulceration. Subungual melanomas typically affect the thumb or great toe of the middle-aged and elderly, causing chronic inflam-

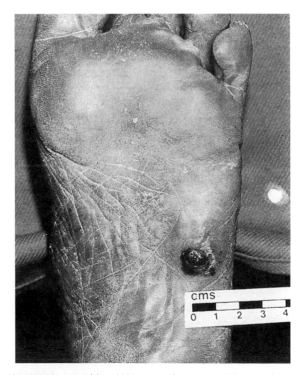

Fig. 24.20 Acral lentiginous melanoma arising on the sole of the foot.

mation beneath the nail. Pigmentation is not usually visible in the early stages and the lesion is often misdiagnosed as a paronychia or ingrowing toenail.

Spread of malignant melanoma

Malignant melanomas spread readily via the lymphatics and bloodstream. In-transit metastases may develop in the subcutaneous or intracutaneous lymphatics, and form painless discoloured nodules in the line of the lymphatics between the primary and the regional nodes. Lymph node metastases often present as firm enlargement of a node that remains untethered and mobile. The disease then spreads to adjacent regional and central nodes. Bloodborne metastases can occur at any site but are common in the brain, liver, lungs, skin and subcutaneous tissues. Extensive metastatic growth may be associated with the excretion of melanin or its precursor (5-S-cystine L-dopa) in the urine. In about 5% of cases metastases are present in the absence of a recognizable primary site.

Clinical and pathological staging

Three clinical stages are recognized and staging has major prognostic implications (Table 24.6). For lesions in clinical stage I the most reliable prognostic indicator is the depth of the lesion (Fig. 24.21): the more superficial the lesion, the better the prognosis. Depth can be measured by reference to the normal layers of skin (Clark) or by a micrometer gauge (Breslow). As the skin layers may be distorted by the tumour, the Breslow system is usually preferred. Mitotic activity also influences prognosis, and tumours can be graded according to the number of mitotic figures in each field. Lymphocytic response and features of regression can also influence prognosis. Melanotic freckles and superficial spreading melanomas tend to remain superficial and so have a better prognosis than do nodular melanomas.

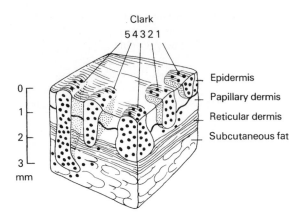

Fig. 24.21   Methods of grading malignant melanoma according to depth of invasion.

Treatment of malignant melanoma

A biopsy is essential to confirm the diagnosis. Thereafter, the depth and stage of the disease are assessed to define the most appropriate form of treatment. Small pigmented lesions are excised with a margin of 3 mm of normal skin, usually under local anaesthesia. Surgical excision is used to treat stage I lesions. Wide excision with a margin of normal skin of at least 5 cm was once routine but has been shown

---

SUMMARY BOX

Management of malignant melanoma

- The depth of the lesion is a key prognostic factor and can be assessed by micrometer (Breslow) or by reference to normal layers of the skin (Clark). Superficial spreading melanomas and melanotic freckles have a better prognosis than nodular melanomas.

- Excision biopsy is essential to confirm malignancy, assess depth and stage, and define the optimal method of treatment.

- Once malignancy is confirmed, an excision margin of 1 cm for every 1 mm of Breslow depth is advised. The lesion is excised down to the deep fascia to remove all subcutaneous fat. Skin grafting may be required to close the defect.

- Lymph node or satellite deposits reduce 5-year survival rates from 70% to 30%, but patients with distant metastases are not expected to survive for 5 years.

- Block dissection of regional lymph nodes is no longer practised routinely but may be indicated if the nodes are obviously involved or located close to the primary lesion.

Table 24.6   Prognosis in relation to the stage and depth of malignant melanoma

Clinical stage	5-year survival rate (%)
I Primary lesion only	70
Breslow depth (mm)	
<1.5	93
1.5–3.5	60
>3.5	48
II Primary lesion + regional lymph node or satellite deposit	30
III Metastatic disease	0

to be unnecessary, particularly for the more superficial melanomas. Breslow depth is now used as the determinant of clearance margin, using a formula of 1 cm clearance for every millimetre of depth up to 3 cm. A smaller margin may be acceptable to avoid mutilation, for example on the face. The tumour and surrounding skin are excised down to the deep fascia so that the entire depth of subcutaneous fat can be removed. Smaller defects can usually be closed primarily. Large defects have to be covered with a split-skin graft or flap. A block dissection of regional lymph nodes carries significant morbidity and is no longer carried out routinely. However, if the nodes are involved (clinical stage II), or if the primary tumour overlies the nodes, block dissection can be performed at the time of primary surgery. Isolated limb perfusion with cytotoxic drugs can be used in patients with recurrent disease in a single limb. The treatment of metastatic melanoma remains unsatisfactory. The key to the successful management of malignant melanoma is early diagnosis and appropriate surgical excision, with reconstruction as appropriate.

Vascular neoplasms (haemangiomas)

The histological classification of haemangiomas is complex and they are best differentiated by their clinical behaviour; that is, whether they are regress or persist.

Involuting haemangiomas

These true neoplasms arise from endothelial cells. They appear at or within weeks of birth, and affect predominantly the head and neck. Superficial involuting haemangiomas form a bright-red raised mass with an irregular bosselated surface (strawberry naevus); deeper lesions form a soft, blue-black tumour covered by normal skin. Active growth continues for about 6 months. The tumour then remains static until the child is 2 or 3 years of age, when it shrinks and loses its colour. The lesion usually disappears before the child is 7 years of age and should be left alone unless it involves the periorbital skin.

Non-involuting haemangiomas

These hamartomas are due to abnormal blood vessel formation, and are of two main types.

Port-wine stain This bright-red patchy lesion often overlies the area of distribution of a peripheral nerve. The lesion neither grows nor involutes, and good cosmetic results can be achieved by laser therapy.

Cavernous haemangioma This bluish-purple elevated mass appears in early childhood. It empties on pressure and then refills, and histologically consists of mature vein-like structures. It is treated by excision. Cirsoid aneurysm is a variant in which the mass of vein-like structures is fed

directly by arterial blood and becomes tortuous, dilated and pulsating. The scalp is a common site and the mass may erode the skull. Penetrating channels may connect the scalp lesion with a similar malformation in the extradural space. Angiography is essential to show the extent of the lesion and outline its arterial supply. Angiographic embolization may be useful prior to ligation of the feeding vessels and excision of the lesion.

Tumours of nerves
Neurilemmoma

This is an encapsulated solitary benign tumour that originates from the Schwann cells of a nerve sheath and forms a subcutaneous swelling in the course of the nerve. It is laterally mobile but fixed in the direction of the nerve. It may cause radiating pain in the distribution of the involved nerve. Most neurilemmomas occur superficially in the neck or limbs. They grow slowly, have no malignant potential, and are readily treated by excision. Excision can result in loss of nerve function.

Neurofibroma

This is regarded as a hamartoma of nerve tissue. Such lesions may be solitary, but more commonly they are multiple in von Recklinghausen's disease (neurofibromatosis). This autosomal disorder is present at birth or becomes apparent in early childhood. Multiple dermal and subcutaneous nodules arise from peripheral nerves in association with patches of dermal pigmentation ('*café-au-lait*' spots). The tumours can cause bony deformities, particularly of the spine. They are potentially malignant, transforming to neurofibrosarcoma. An increase in size of existing swellings, or the appearance of new swellings suggests malignant change.

Tumours of muscle and connective tissues
Lipoma

A lipoma is a slow-growing benign tumour of fatty tissue that forms a lobulated soft mass enclosed by a thin fibrous capsule. Large lipomas rarely undergo sarcomatous change. Although lipomas can occur in the dermis, most arise from the fatty tissue between the skin and deep fascia. Typical features are their soft fluctuant feel, their lobulation, and the free mobility of overlying skin. Lipomas may also arise from fat in the intermuscular septa, where they form a diffuse firm swelling under the deep fascia which is more prominent when the related muscle is contracted. They may cause discomfort. Unless it is small and asymptomatic a lipoma should be removed, either by surgical excision or by liposuction.

Liposarcoma

Liposarcoma is the commonest sarcoma of middle age. It may occur in any fatty tissue but is most common in the retroperitoneum and legs. Wide surgical excision is recommended but can be difficult for retroperitoneal tumours, and postoperative radiotherapy and chemotherapy are advised but are of doubtful worth. Most liposarcomas grow slowly and recurrence may take a long time to develop.

Fibrosarcoma

This tumour arises from fibrous tissue at any site but is most common in the lower limbs or buttocks. It forms a large, deep firm mass. Wide excision is the initial treatment of choice; radiation therapy may be indicated in the palliation of recurrence.

Rhabdomyosarcoma

This greyish-pink, soft, fleshy lobulated or well-circumscribed tumour arises from striated muscle. It is more common in children, is highly malignant, and requires treatment by radical excision and/or radiotherapy. Amputation of a limb may be unavoidable.

Disorders of the nails

Onychogryphosis (hooked nail)

This overgrowth of the nail resembles an ox or goat horn. The big toenail is most commonly affected (Fig. 24.22). Simple avulsion of the nail does not prevent recurrence, and excision of the nailed is required. A flap of skin is reflected from the base of the nail and the germinal layer removed. Care must be taken to excise the edges of this layer completely or troublesome spikes of nail continue to grow. An alternative to excision of the nailbed is to cauterize it with phenol.

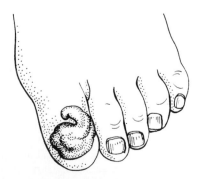

Fig. 24.22 Onychogryphosis.

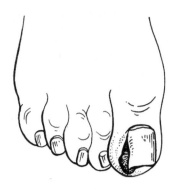

Fig. 24.23 Ingrowing toenail.

Ingrowing toenail

This is caused by the sharp edges of the nail impinging on the surrounding skin folds (Fig. 24.23). The skin is split and infection follows. The condition is painful and made worse by misguided attempts to cut the nail back at the corners. The patient usually comes for help once infection has occurred. An attempt is made to 'lift out' the ingrowing portion of the nail with a pledget of gauze soaked in antiseptic. The patient is then instructed to cut the nail square, or shorter in the centre than at the edges, and to avoid wearing narrow shoes. Once infection has spread under the nail, or the nail has become deeply embedded, it is best to

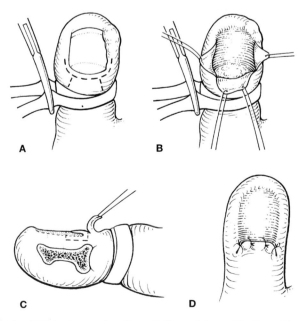

Fig. 24.24 Operation for ablation of the nailbed. **A** skin incision; **B** nail avulsed and skin flaps raised; **C** excision of nailbed; **D** skin flaps sutured.

avulse it under general anaesthesia. Antiseptic footbaths then allow the infection to resolve rapidly. The patient is instructed on the correct way to cut the new nail. If the condition recurs, the nailbed must be ablated surgically or with phenol (Fig. 24.24).

Nailfold infections (paronychia)

Pain, redness and swelling at the side and base of a nail are the first signs of paronychia. This may extend around the nail to produce a horseshoe swelling of the nailfold. Extension under the nail and into the underlying pulp space may occur (Fig. 24.25). A minor paronychia will usually resolve spontaneously, but if the infection is spreading an antibiotic should be prescribed. The development of a tense shiny swelling indicates suppuration and the need for surgical drainage. A single unilateral incision may suffice, but if the infection extends under the nail a flap of skin should be reflected from the nailbase, which is then excised to allow free drainage (Fig. 24.26). A simple vaseline gauze dressing is applied. Failure of an acute paronychia to resolve leads to chronic thickening of the nailfold. Fungal infection is a common cause of chronic paronychia, and nail scrapings are essential for diagnosis. The possibility of a subungual melanoma must always be kept in mind.

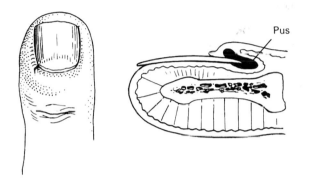

Fig. 24.25 Paronychia. The longitudinal section shows relation of pus to the nailbed.

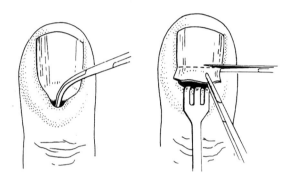

Fig. 24.26 Surgical treatment of paronychia.

25 The breast

J.M. Dixon

ANATOMY AND PHYSIOLOGY

Overview

The breast is an appendage of skin and is a modified sweat gland. It is composed of glandular tissue, fibrous or supporting tissue and fat. The functional unit of the breast is the terminal duct lobular unit, and any secretions produced in the terminal duct lobular unit drain towards the nipple into 12–15 major subareolar ducts. Although often described as being segmental like an orange, the glandular and ductal structures of the breast interweave to form a composite mass. In the resting state the terminal duct lobular unit secretes watery fluid which is reabsorbed as it passes through the ductules and ducts. This rarely reaches the surface of the nipple because the nipple ducts are blocked or plugged by keratin. If the keratin becomes dislodged then this physiological secretion can be seen on the surface of the nipple. It varies in colour from white to yellow to green to blue/black, and can be produced in up to two-thirds of non-pregnant women by gentle cleaning of the nipple and massage of the breast.

Anatomy

The breast lies between the skin and the pectoral fascia, to which it is loosely attached. It extends from the clavicle superiorly down on to the abdominal wall, where it extends over the rectus abdominis, external oblique and serratus anterior muscles. The axillary tail of the breast runs between the pectoral muscles and latissimus dorsi to blend with the axillary fat. The breast is supplied by the lateral thoracic artery or the lateral thoracic branch of the axillary artery superolaterally, and by perforating branches of the internal mammary artery superomedially. The functioning unit of the breast is the terminal duct lobular unit and this is lined, as are the draining ducts, by a single layer of columnar epithelial cells surrounded by myoepithelial cells. The major subareolar ducts in their terminal portion are lined by stratified squamous epithelium.

The main route of lymphatic spread of breast cancer is to the axillary nodes, which are situated below the axillary vein. On average, there are 20 nodes in the axilla situated below the axillary vein (Fig. 25.1). These are separated into three levels by their relation to the pectoralis minor muscle. Nodes lateral to the pectoralis minor are considered level I, those beneath are classified as level II, and the nodes medial to pectoralis minor are level III. Level I nodes, which are nearest the breast, are usually affected first by breast cancer. In less than 5% of patients levels II or III nodes are involved without level I nodes being affected. Lymph also drains to the internal mammary nodes. Occasionally, the main route of lymph drainage of a cancer is to the interpectoral nodes situated between the pectoralis major and pectoralis minor muscles.

Congenital abnormalities

These are most commonly the result of persistent extramammary portions of the breast ridge. In the sixth week of embryonal development a bilateral ridge called the 'milk line' develops and extends from the axilla to the groin. Segments coalesce into nests of cells and, in humans, all but one of these nests opposite the fifth intercostal space disappear. In 1–5% of people one or more of the other nests persists as supernumerary or accessory nipples or, less frequently, as breasts. The commonest site for an accessory

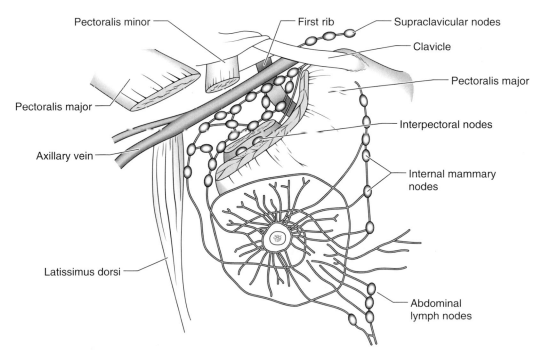

Fig. 25.1 Lymph node drainage of the breast.

nipple is between the normal breast in the milk line and the umbilicus; the commonest site for an accessory breast is the lower axilla. Supernumerary nipples or breasts rarely require treatment unless they are unsightly. Accessory breast tissue is subject to the same diseases found in normally placed breasts.

Some degree of breast asymmetry is normal, the left usually being the larger of the two. One breast can be absent or hypoplastic, and this is often associated with pectoral muscle defects. Some patients have abnormalities of the pectoralis muscle and absence of or hypoplasia of the breast, associated with a characteristic deformity of the upper limb; this cluster of anomalies is called Poland's syndrome. Abnormalities of the chest wall, such as pectus excavatum and scoliosis of the thoracic spine, can make normal breasts look asymmetric. True asymmetry can be treated by augmentation of the smaller breast, reduction or elevation of the larger breast, or a combination of the two

HORMONAL CONTROL OF BREAST DEVELOPMENT AND FUNCTION

Enlargement of the breast bud in the first week or two of life occurs in approximately 60% of newborn babies, when the gland may reach several centimetres in size before regressing. This is because circulating maternal oestrogens cause one or both breasts to enlarge and secrete a colostrum-like fluid (witch's milk) from the nipple. The swelling usually subsides within a few weeks and the breasts then normally remain dormant until puberty, when the onset of cyclical hormonal activity stimulates growth.

The lifecycle of the breast consists of three main periods: development (and early reproductive life), mature reproductive life and involution. Development occurs at puberty and involves the proliferation of ducts and ductules associated with very rudimentary lobule formation. The breast then undergoes regular changes in relation to the menstrual cycle. During pregnancy the breast approximately doubles in weight and the lobules and ducts proliferate in preparation for milk production. Lobular development only becomes marked during pregnancy. Milk production during pregnancy is inhibited by ovarian and placental steroids. Delivery reduces the amount of circulating oestrogen and increases the sensitivity of the breast epithelium to prolactin. Suckling stimulates the release of prolactin and oxytocin, with oxytocin stimulating the myoepithelial cells to eject milk into the terminal ducts. By the age of 30, ageing or involution is evident and continues to the menopause and beyond. During involution, glandular tissue and fibrous tissue atrophy and the shape of the breasts changes as they become more ptotic or droopy. Microscopic changes in the glandular tissue that occur during involution include fibrosis, the formation of small cysts (microcysts) and an increase in the number of glandular elements (adenosis). These changes were previously considered abnormal and called fibrocystic disease or fibroadenosis. However, they occur as part of normal breast ageing or involution and should not be considered as disease.

EVALUATION OF THE PATIENT WITH BREAST DISEASE

Symptoms

Approximately 25% of all surgical referrals relate to breast problems. In the UK one in four women will attend a breast clinic, and one in 10 will develop breast cancer at some point in their lives. The commonest symptoms are a breast lump, which may or may not be painful; an area of lumpiness; pain alone; nipple discharge; nipple retraction; a strong family history of breast cancer; breast distortion; swelling or inflammation; or a scaling nipple or eczema. The most important pointer to the diagnosis is the age of the patient. Although malignant disease can occur in young women, benign conditions are much more common. The duration of any symptom is important – breast cancers

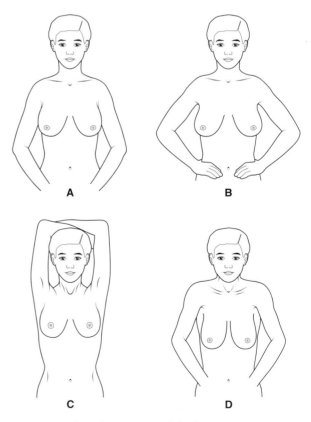

A   B

C   D

Fig. 25.2 Clinical inspection of the breast.

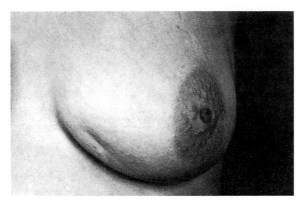

Fig. 25.3 Skin dimpling in the lower inner quadrant of the left breast associated with breast cancer.

Clinical examination

The patient is asked to undress to the waist and sit facing the examiner. Inspection should take place in good light with the patient's arms by her side, above her head, and pressing on her hips (Fig. 25.2). Skin dimpling or a change

usually grow slowly, but cysts may appear overnight. Details of risk factors, including family history and current medication, can be obtained using a simple questionnaire that the patient can complete while waiting to be seen in the outpatient clinic.

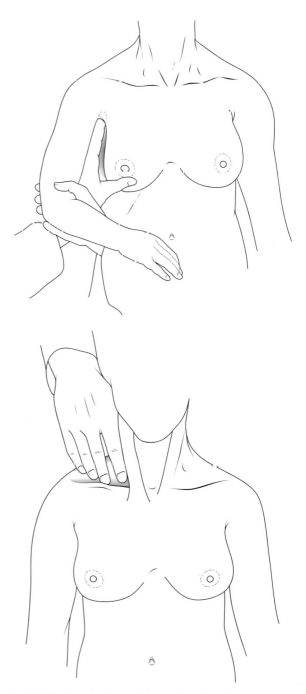

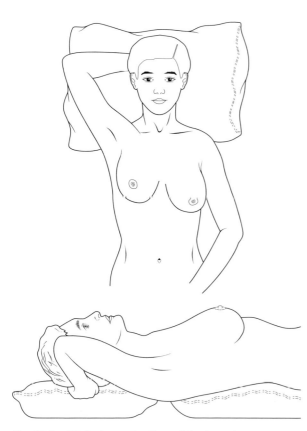

Fig. 25.4 Clinical examination of the breast.

Fig. 25.5 Examination of the regional nodes.

of contour is present in a high percentage of patients with breast cancer (Fig. 25.3). Breast palpation is performed with the patient lying flat with her arms above or under her head. All the breast tissue is examined, keeping the hand flat but using the fingertips to detect any abnormality (Fig. 25.4). Any abnormal area is then examined in more detail, once again using the fingertips, to determine the texture and outline of the mass. Deep fixation is assessed by asking the patient to tense the pectoralis major muscle, which is accomplished by asking her to press her hands on her hips. All palpable lesions should be measured with callipers and the size and site (using the clock, with 13 representing the nipple area and 14 the axillary tail) recorded in the hospital notes.

If the patient complains of a nipple discharge an attempt should be made to reproduce the discharge and to determine whether it arises from a single or multiple ducts. Any discharge should be tested for haemoglobin. Only marked or moderate amounts of haemoglobin in a nipple discharge are significant.

Assessment of regional nodes

Once the breast has been palpated the nodal areas are checked (Fig. 25.5). Clinical assessment of axillary nodes is not always accurate. Palpable nodes can be identified in up to 30% of patients with no clinically significant breast disease, and up to 40% of patients with breast cancer who have no palpable nodes on examination will be found histologically to have metastatic disease in the axillary nodes. The supraclavicular nodes are best examined from behind.

Mammography

This requires compression of the breast between two plates and is uncomfortable. By using high-resolution films and X-rays of low penetrating power, the radiation dose is kept as low as possible (0.5–1.5 mGy per film). A single oblique view or two views, an oblique and a craniocaudal, can be obtained. Mammography allows the detection of mass lesions, areas of parenchymal distortion and microcalcification. Because the breasts are relatively radiodense in women under 35 years of age, mammography is rarely of value in this group.

Ultrasonography

High-frequency waves are beamed through the breast and reflections are detected and turned into images. Cysts show up as transparent objects (Fig. 25.6), and other benign lesions tend to have well demarcated edges (Fig. 25.7), whereas cancers usually have an indistinct outline and absorb sound, resulting in a posterior acoustic shadow (Fig. 25.8).

Magnetic resonance imaging

This is an accurate way of imaging the breast. It has a high sensitivity for breast cancer and may be of value in demon-

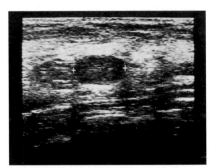

Fig. 25.7   Ultrasound of a fibroadenoma.

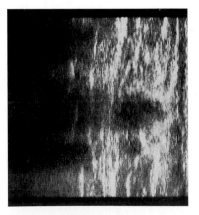

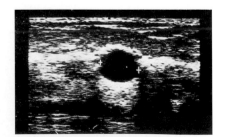

Fig. 25.6   Ultrasound of a cyst.

Fig. 25.8   Ultrasound of a cancer.

strating the extent of both invasive and non-invasive disease. It is particularly useful in the conserved breast to determine whether a mammographic lesion at the site of previous surgery is due to scar or to recurrence. It is currently being evaluated as a screening tool for high-risk women between the ages of 35 and 50. MRI is the optimum method for imaging breast implants and detecting implant leakage or rupture.

Fine-needle aspiration cytology

Needle aspiration can differentiate between solid and cystic lesions. If the lesion is cystic, the fluid is aspirated and, providing it is not bloodstained, discarded. Aspiration of solid lesions requires skill to obtain sufficient cells for cytological analysis and expertise is needed to interpret the smears. Aspiration is usually performed with a 21- or 23-gauge needle attached to a syringe. The needle is introduced into the lesion and suction applied by withdrawing the plunger; multiple passes are then made through the lesion (Fig. 25.9). The plunger is then released and the material spread on to microscope slides. These are then either air-dried or fixed in alcohol and later stained. In some units a report is available within 30 minutes.

Core biopsy

Several cores are removed from a mass or an area of microcalcification by means of a cutting needle technique. A 14-gauge needle combined with a mechanical gun produces satisfactory samples and allows the procedure to be performed single-handed. The mammotome vacuum 11-gauge core biopsy device allows several large cores to be removed

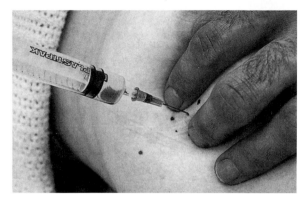

Fig. 25.9 Fine-needle aspiration cytology being performed.

without withdrawing the needle from the breast, and is currently being evaluated.

Open biopsy

An open biopsy should only be performed in patients who have been appropriately investigated by imaging, fine-needle aspiration cytology and, if appropriate, core biopsy. Breast biopsy is a morbid procedure and a fifth of patients who have a biopsy performed develop a further lump under the scar, or pain specifically related to the operation site. Biopsy can be performed under local or general anaesthesia. The removal of impalpable lesions requires localization by a hooked wire. Following excision the specimen is X-rayed to confirm that the appropriate area has been removed.

Table 25.1 Accuracy of investigations in the diagnosis of symptomatic breast disease in specialist clinics

	Clinical examination (%)	Mammography (%)	Ultrasonography (%)	Fine needle aspiration cytology (%)	Core biopsy (%)
Sensitivity for cancers*	86	86	85	95	85–95‡
Specificity for benign disease†	90	90	88	95	95
Positive predictive value for cancers§	95	95	90	99.8	100

*Percentage of cancers detected by test as malignant or probably malignant (that is, complete sensitivity).
†Percentage of benign disease detected by test as benign.
§Percentage of lesions diagnosed as malignant by test that are cancers (that is, absolute positive predictive value).
‡Sensitivity increases if core biopsy is image guided.

Frozen section

The routine use of frozen sections to diagnose breast cancer is no longer acceptable. It has been used to assess lymph nodes, but in this situation the sensitivity (the ability to detect cancer in the lymph nodes) is only 80%.

One-stop clinics

The combination of clinical examination, imaging (mammography with or without ultrasonography for women over 35 years, and ultrasonography for women under 35 years) and fine-needle aspiration cytology is known as triple assessment. Patients presenting with breast symptoms can now have triple assessment performed and reported during a single clinic visit. This allows patients with benign disease to be reassured, and in many cases discharged.

Accuracy of investigations

False positive results occur with all diagnostic techniques. The sensitivity of clinical examination and mammography varies with age, and only two-thirds of cancers in women aged under 50 are considered suspicious or definitely malignant on clinical examination or mammography (Table 25.1).

DISORDERS OF DEVELOPMENT

Most benign breast conditions occur during either development, cyclical activity or involution, and are so common that they are best considered as aberrations rather than true disease (Table 25.2).

Juvenile hypertrophy

Uncontrolled overgrowth of breast tissue occurs occasionally in adolescent girls, whose breast development initially

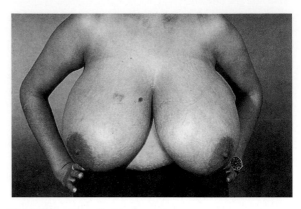

Fig. 25.10   Juvenile hypertrophy.

begins normally at puberty and is followed by rapid breast growth. These changes are usually bilateral, but may be limited to one breast or part of one breast. This process is often referred to as virginal or juvenile hypertrophy (Fig. 25.10). However, it is not hypertrophy, as there is an increase in the amount of stromal tissue rather than in the number of lobules or ducts. This excessive growth is an aberration rather than a true disease, and presenting symptoms are large breasts and pain in the shoulder, neck and back or under the bra straps. Treatment is by reduction mammoplasty.

Fibroadenoma

Fibroadenomas are classified in most texts as benign tumours, but are best considered as aberrations of development rather than true neoplasms. The reasons are that fibroadenomas develop from a single lobule rather than from a single cell, and show hormonal dependence similar to that of normal breast tissue, lactating during pregnancy and involuting in the perimenopausal period. Fibroadenomas are most commonly seen immediately following the period of

Table 25.2	Aberrations of normal breast development and involution	
Age (years)	Normal process	Aberration
<25	Breast development	
	Stromal	Juvenile hypertrophy
	Lobular	Fibroadenoma
25–40	Cyclical activity	Cyclical mastalgia
		Cyclical nodularity
		(diffuse or focal)
35–55	Involution	
	Lobular	Macrocysts
	Stromal	Sclerosing lesions
	Ductal	Duct ectasia

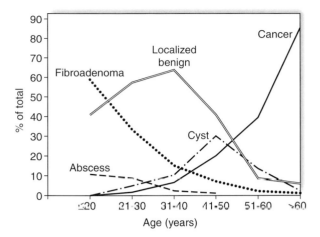

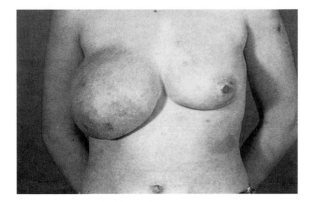

Fig. 25.12 Juvenile fibroadenoma

Fig. 25.11 Percentage of patients in 10-year age groups with a discrete breast lump who have common benign conditions and breast cancer.

breast development and growth in the 15–25-year age group (Fig. 25.11). They are usually well circumscribed, firm, smooth, mobile lumps, and may be multiple or bilateral. Although a small number of fibroadenomas increase in size, the majority do not and over a third become smaller or disappear within 2 years. Fibroadenomas have a characteristic appearance with easily visualized margins on ultrasound (Fig. 25.7). Large or giant fibroadenomas (>5 cm) are infrequent but are more commonly seen in women from certain African countries. Occasionally a fibroadenoma in an adolescent girl undergoes rapid growth, a condition called juvenile fibroadenoma (Fig. 25.12). Once a diagnosis of fibroadenoma has been established on triple assessment, and provided the lesion measures less than 4 cm, options for management include observation or excision; fibroadenomas over 4 cm in diameter should be excised to ensure that phyllodes tumours are not missed (see below). A carcinoma arising in a fibroadenoma is rare, and patients with simple fibroadenomas are not at significantly increased risk of developing breast cancer.

DISORDERS OF CYCLICAL CHANGE

Premenstrual nodularity and breast discomfort are so common that they are considered part of the normal cyclical changes. When premenstrual pain is severe, interferes with daily activities and influences quality of life, then this is classified as moderate or severe cyclical mastalgia. There is no association between cyclical breast pain and any underlying histological abnormality. The cause of cyclical mastalgia is unknown. Another common and significant problem is non-cyclical mastalgia. Differentiation between the two types of pain is best achieved by using a breast pain chart.

Cyclical mastalgia

More than 85% of cyclical breast pain is of a minor degree and, once cancer has been excluded, no specific treatment is required. Some women gain relief from simple measures such as wearing a soft support bra 24 hours a day. Treatment should be considered for women who have moderate or severe cyclical mastalgia that interferes with daily activity. Antibiotics, vitamin B_6, progestogens and diuretics are not

Table 25.3 Response of cyclical and non-cyclical mastalgia to drug treatment

	Useful response to treatment (%)		
	Cyclical mastalgia	Non-cyclical mastalgia	Side effects
Danazol	79	40	30
Gamolenic acid	58	38	4
Bromocriptine	54	33	35

effective in the treatment of breast pain. The three drugs that do have a product licence for the treatment of cyclical mastalgia are evening primrose oil (prescribed as Efamast), danazol and bromocriptine (Table 25.3). The effective agent in evening primrose oil is gamolenic acid and the correct dose is 240–320 mg/day. A trial of treatment should last at least 4 months. Danazol is used in a dose of 100 mg/day. Bromocriptine is rarely used because of its side-effects. Occasionally tamoxifen in a dose of 10 mg/day is used for breast pain. Although it does not have a product licence for this condition it improves pain in 80%.

Nodularity

Lumpiness and nodularity in the breast can be diffuse or focal. Diffuse nodularity is normal, particularly pre-menstrually. It is now appreciated that the normal breast is lumpy. In the past women with lumpy breasts were regarded as having fibroadenosis or fibrocystic disease, but this diffuse nodularity is not associated with any underlying pathological abnormality and so these terms are inappropriate. Focal nodularity is a common cause of a breast lump and is seen in women of all ages (Fig. 25.11). Patients with focal nodularity often report that the lump fluctuates in size in relation to the menstrual cycle. Breast cancer should be excluded in patients with localised asymmetric areas of nodularity, using triple assessment.

Non-cyclical breast pain

Localized pain in the chest wall, referred pain and diffuse true breast pain must be differentiated. Examining a patient on her side to move the breast away from the chest wall is the best way of demonstrating that the ribs or chest wall muscle are the site of origin of the pain. Oral non-steroidal anti-inflammatory agents are usually effective in improving chest wall pain. Up to 60% of patients with a persistent localized painful area in the chest wall can be effectively treated by infiltration of local anaesthetic and steroid (2 ml 0.5% marcaine and 1 ml containing 40 mg of methylprednisolone).

DISORDERS OF INVOLUTION

Aberrations of the normal ageing process include cyst formation, areas of scarring (sclerosis) and epithelial hyperplasia.

Palpable breast cysts

Approximately 7% of women in western countries develop a palpable breast cyst at some time in their life. Cysts consti-tute approximately 15% of all discrete breast masses. They

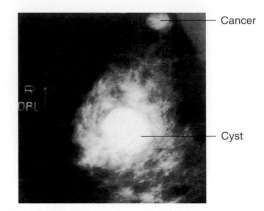

Fig. 25.13   Mammogram of a cyst and a cancer.

are distended involuted lobules and are most frequently seen in the perimenopausal period (Fig. 25.11). Clinically they are smooth discrete lumps that can be painful and are sometimes visible. Mammographically they have character-istic halos and are easily diagnosed by ultrasonography (Fig. 25.6). Symptomatic palpable cysts are treated by aspi-ration and, provided the fluid is not bloodstained, it can be discarded. If aspiration results in the disappearance of the mass then the patient can be reassured. Any residual mass should be investigated by fine-needle aspiration cytology. Cysts that rapidly and persistently refill, or contain blood-stained fluid, require excision to exclude an associated cancer. Most cysts are asymptomatic and, provided they are appropriately investigated by ultrasound, do not need aspira-tion. All patients with cysts should have mammography, preferably before cyst aspiration, as between 1 and 3% will have a cancer, usually remote from the cyst, visible on mam-mography (Fig. 25.13). Patients with cysts have a slightly increased risk of developing breast cancer, but the magni-tude of this risk is not considered of clinical significance.

Sclerosis

Areas of excessive fibrosis or sclerosis can occur as part of stromal involution. These lesions are of clinical importance only because they produce stellate lesions that mimic breast cancer mammographically, and so can cause diagnostic problems during screening.

Duct ectasia

The major subareolar ducts dilate and shorten with age and, when symptomatic, this is known as duct ectasia. By the age of 70 40% of women are affected, some of whom present with nipple discharge or retraction. The discharge is usually cheesy and the retraction is classically slit-like (Fig. 25.14), which contrasts with breast cancer, when the whole nipple is pulled in (Fig. 25.15). Surgery is indicated

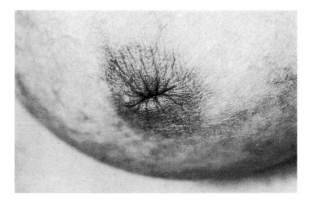

Fig. 25.14 Duct ectasia showing slit-like nipple retraction.

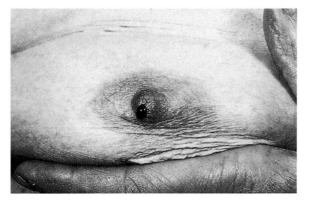

Fig. 25.16 Bloodstained nipple discharge.

if the discharge is troublesome or if the patient wishes the nipple to be everted.

Epithelial hyperplasia

An increase in the number of cells lining the terminal duct lobular unit is known as epithelial hyperplasia, the degree of which is graded as mild, moderate or florid. If the hyperplastic cells show cellular atypia the condition is called atypical hyperplasia. Women with atypical hyperplasia have a significant increase in their risk of breast cancer. The absolute risk for a woman with atypical hyperplasia without a first-degree relative with breast cancer is 8% at 10 years; for women with a first-degree relative with breast cancer it is 20–25% at 15 years.

BENIGN NEOPLASMS

Duct papillomas

These can be single or multiple, are very common, and should be considered as aberrations rather than true neo-

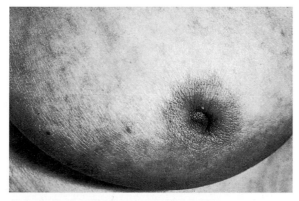

Fig. 25.15 Symmetrical whole nipple inversion characteristic of breast cancer.

plasms as they show minimal malignant potential. They cause persistent and troublesome nipple discharge, which is frankly bloodstained (Fig. 25.16) or serous and contains moderate or large amounts of blood on testing. Treatment comprises removal of the discharging duct (microdochectomy), which removes the papilloma (if this is the cause) and allows the exclusion of an underlying neoplasm, which is seen in approximately 5% of women who present with a bloodstained nipple discharge.

Lipomas

These are soft, lobulated, radiolucent lesions and are common. Interest lies in their confusion with pseudolipoma (a soft mass that can be felt around a cancer, caused by indrawing of surrounding fat).

Phyllodes tumours

These rare fibroepithelial neoplasms may be malignant in their behaviour, although most are benign. They are localized discrete masses which clinically feel like fibroadenomas, although they tend to be larger (> 4 cm). Up to 20% of benign phyllodes tumours recur locally following simple excision. In the more malignant lesions it is the sarcomatous element that recurs; approximately one-quarter of lesions reported as malignant by the pathologist metastasize. Treatment of phyllodes tumours, whether malignant or benign, is wide excision or, if necessary because of the size of the lesion, mastectomy.

Other benign tumours that occur in the breast are granular cell myoblastoma and neurofibroma.

BREAST INFECTION

Breast infection is less common than it used to be. It is seen occasionally in neonates but most commonly affects women between the ages of 18 and 50. In this age group, infection

SUMMARY BOX

Benign breast disease

- Is commoner than breast cancer

- Can be difficult to differentiate from breast cancer

- Inappropriate treatment of benign conditions is associated with significant morbidity

- Occurs against the background of breast development (age <25), cyclical activity (up to menopause) and involution (following the menopause)

- The only benign condition associated with a significant increased risk of subsequent breast cancer is atypical hyperplasia

can be divided into lactational and non-lactational. Infection can also affect the skin overlying the breast, when it can be a primary event or secondary to a lesion in the skin (such as a sebaceous cyst or an underlying condition such as hidradenitis suppurativa).

The principles in treating breast infection are:

1. Give appropriate antibiotics early to reduce the formation of abscesses (Table 25.4).
2. If an abscess is suspected, confirm pus is present by aspiration before considering surgical drainage.
3. Exclude breast cancer using imaging and cytology in an inflammatory lesion which is solid on aspiration and which does not settle despite adequate antibiotic treatment.

Most breast abscesses can be managed by repeated aspiration combined with oral antibiotics or incision and drainage under local anaesthetic. Few abscesses, except those in children, require drainage under general anaesthesia. Placement of a drain or packing the abscess cavity after incision and drainage is unnecessary.

Lactating infection

Improvements in maternal and infant hygiene have considerably reduced the incidence of infection associated with breastfeeding. When it does occur it usually develops within the first 6 weeks or, occasionally, during weaning. Presenting features are pain, swelling, tenderness and a cracked nipple or skin abrasion. *Staphylococcus aureus* is the most common organism, although *Staph. epidermidis* and streptococci are occasionally implicated. Drainage of milk from the affected segment is often reduced, with the resultant stagnant milk becoming infected. Early infection is treated with flucloxacillin or co-amoxiclav. An established abscess should be treated by recurrent aspiration, or by incision and drainage (Fig. 25.17). Women should be encouraged to breastfeed as this promotes milk drainage from the affected segment.

Non-lactating infection

This can be separated into infections that occur centrally in the periareolar region and those affecting the periphery of the breast.

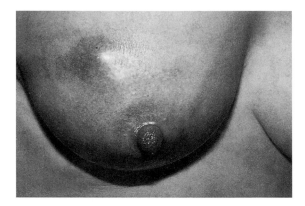

Fig. 25.17 Lactating breast abscess.

Table 25.4 Antibiotics most appropriate for treating breast infections*		
Type of infection	No allergy to penicillin	Allergy to penicillin
Neonatal Lactating and skin-associated Non-lactating	Flucloxacillin (500 mg four times daily) Co-amoxiclav (375 mg thrice daily)	Erythromycin (500 mg twice daily) Combination of erythromycin (500 mg twice daily) with metronidazole (200 mg thrice daily)
*Doses are for adults.		

Central (periareolar) infection

This is most commonly seen in young women (mean age 32 years). The underlying cause is periductal mastitis. It used to be thought that recurrent infection was related to duct ectasia and that the contents of ectatic ducts leaked into the surrounding tissue to cause periductal inflammation. This is now known to be incorrect. Current evidence suggests that smoking is an important factor in the aetiology of non-lactational infection, with 90% of women who present with periductal mastitis or its complications being smokers. Substances in cigarette smoke either directly or indirectly damage the subareolar breast ducts, and the damaged tissue then becomes infected by either aerobic or anaerobic organisms. Initial presentation may be with periareolar inflammation, with or without an associated mass, or with an established abscess. Clinical features include breast pain, erythema, a periareolar swelling and tenderness, and/or nipple retraction that occurs in relation to the affected duct.

Treatment is with appropriate antibiotics (Table 25.4). Abscesses are managed by aspiration or incision and drainage. Infection associated with periductal mastitis is commonly recurrent because treatment does not remove the damaged subareolar duct(s). Following drainage of a non-lactating abscess, up to a third of patients develop a mammary duct fistula. Recurrent episodes of periareolar infection require excision of the diseased ducts (total duct excision).

Mammary duct fistula

This is a communication between the skin – usually in the periareolar region – and a major subareolar duct (Fig. 25.18). Treatment is by excision of the fistula and diseased duct or ducts under antibiotic cover.

Peripheral non-lactating abscesses

These are less common than periareolar abscesses and are often associated with an underlying condition, such as dia-

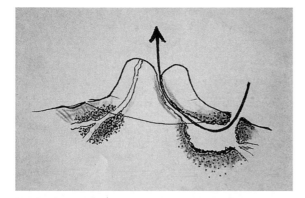

Fig. 25.18 Diagram of a mammary duct fistula and periductal mastitis.

betes, rheumatoid arthritis, steroid treatment, granulomatous lobular mastitis or trauma. Infection associated with granulomatous lobular mastitis can be a particular problem as there is a strong tendency for this condition to persist and recur despite surgery. This condition usually affects young parous women, who develop large areas of infection with multiple simultaneous peripheral abscesses. Peripheral abscesses should be treated by recurrent aspiration with antibiotics (Table 25.4) or incision and drainage.

Skin-associated infection

Primary infection of the skin most commonly affects the lower half of the breast and can be recurrent in women who are either overweight or have large breasts. It is more common after previous surgery or radiotherapy. Treatment is with antibiotics (Table 25.4) and drainage or aspiration of abscesses. Women with recurrent infection should be advised about weight reduction and keeping the area as clean and dry as possible.

Sebaceous cysts are common in the skin of the breast and may become infected. Some recurrent infections in the inframammary fold are due to hidradenitis suppurativa. This condition, which affects the apocrine glands of the breast, is difficult to treat. Excision of the affected skin is effective at stopping further infection in about half of patients.

> **SUMMARY BOX**
>
> *Breast infection*
>
> - Antibiotics should be given early to abort abscess formation.
> - Hospital referral is indicated if the infection does not settle rapidly on antibiotics.
> - If an abscess is suspected, this should be confirmed by aspiration.
> - If the lesion is solid on aspiration, a sample of cells should be obtained for cytology to exclude an underlying inflammatory carcinoma.

BREAST CANCER

Epidemiology

Approximately 1 million new cases of breast cancer are diagnosed each year worldwide. It is the commonest malignancy in women and comprises 18% of all female cancers. In the UK, approximately one in 10 women will develop breast cancer. The known risk factors for breast cancer are shown in Table 25.5.

Table 25.5   Established and probable risk factors for breast cancer

Factor	Relative risk	High-risk group
Age	>10	Elderly
Geographical location	5	Developed country
Age at first full pregnancy	3	First child in early 40s
Previous benign disease	4–5	Atypical hyperplasia
Cancer in other breast	> 4	
Socioeconomic group	2	Social class I and II
Diet	1.5	High intake of saturated fat
Exposure to ionizing radiation	3	Abnormal exposure in young females after age 10
Taking exogenous hormones		
Oral contraceptives	1.24	Current use
Hormone replacement therapy	1.5	Use for ≥10 years
Family history	≥2	Breast cancer in first-degree relative

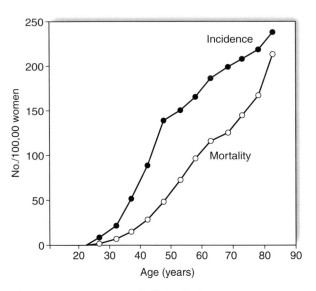

Fig. 25.19 Percentage of all deaths in women attributable to breast cancer.

The incidence of breast cancer increases with age, doubling every 10 years until the menopause, when the rate of increase slows dramatically (Fig. 25.19). Compared with lung cancer, the incidence of breast cancer is higher at young ages. There is a variation in incidence by up to a factor of 5 between different countries. Studies of migrants from Japan, a low-risk area, to Hawaii show that the rates of breast cancer in migrants become the same as the rate in the host country within one or two generations. This suggests that environmental, rather than genetic, factors are important in the aetiology. Women who start menstruating early in life, or who have a late menopause, have a slightly increased risk of developing breast cancer. Young age at first delivery protects against breast cancer. The risk of breast cancer in women who have their first child after the age of 30 is twice that of women who have their first child before the age of 20. Breast cancer is also increased in nulliparous women, who have a risk of approximately 2.4 times that of women having their first child before the age of 20. The highest risk is in women who have a first pregnancy over the age of 40 years (Table 25.5).

Table 25.6 Relationship of HRT to breast cancer development

Time on HRT (years)	Breast cancers over the 20 years from age 50 to 70 (per 1000)	Extra breast cancers in HRT users (per 1000)	Individual risk in women over 20 yrs
None	45	–	1:22
5	47	2	1:21
10	51	6	1:9
15	57	12	1:17–18

Women with severe atypical hyperplasia have a four to five fold higher risk of developing breast cancer than women who have no proliferative changes. A doubling of breast cancer was observed among teenage girls exposed to radiation during the second world war. Although there is a close correlation between the incidence of breast cancer and dietary fat intake in populations, the true relationship does not appear to be particularly strong or consistent. Patients who take the oral contraceptive pill have an increased relative risk of breast cancer while they are on the pill of 1.24 times that of the general population. This rapidly falls to normal after stopping the pill. Hormone replacement therapy increases breast cancer risk by a factor of 1.023 for each year of use. The excess of breast cancers only becomes clinically relevant after 10 years use (Table 25.6). Combined oestrogen and progestogen HRT is associated with a greater risk than oestrogen alone preparations.

Up to 10% of breast cancers in western countries are due to genetic predisposition. The genetic contribution is mainly through single genes inherited as autosomal dominants but with limited penetrance. Not all gene carriers develop breast cancer. Four human breast cancer genes have been identified that affect different families: *BRCA1* on chromosome 17, *BRCA2* on chromosome 13, *p53* on chromosome 17 and *PTEN* on chromosome 10. Throughout the USA and most of Europe, germline mutations in *BRCA1* and *BRCA2* are believed to occur in just over one per 1000 of the population.

In some populations, e.g. Askanazy Jews and Icelanders, particular mutations in *BRCA1* and *BRCA2* may be relatively common. In breast cancer families there is also an increased risk of other tumours, notably ovarian cancer. Most *BRCA1* and *BRCA2* mutations confer a 50–60% lifetime risk of breast cancer. Environmental factors probably modify inherited breast cancer risk, and other genes probably interact with *BRCA1* and *BRCA2* to modify the risk. Pointers to an inherited disposition are a first-degree relative who developed breast cancer under the age of 40 years, numerous female relatives with breast cancer, or a close female relative who has had ovarian cancer. Options for high-risk women include regular screening, prevention using the agents tamoxifen or raloxifene, or prophylactic bilateral mastectomy. Tamoxifen appears to reduce the risk of developing breast cancer by 40–50%, whereas surgery reduces the risk by 90%.

TYPES OF BREAST CANCER

Breast cancers are derived from the epithelial cells that line the terminal duct lobular unit. Cancer cells that remain within the basement membrane of the unit and the draining ducts are classified as in situ or non-invasive. An invasive cancer is one in which cells have moved outside

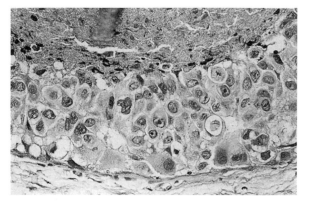

Fig. 25.20 Ductal carcinoma in situ. This is characterized by cells with irregularly shaped and often angular nuclei with variable amounts of chromatin. The cells themselves are variable in size and the necrosis seen in the lumen is a frequent finding.

the basement membrane of the ducts and lobules into the surrounding adjacent normal tissue. Both in situ and invasive cancers have characteristic patterns by which they are classified.

Non-invasive

Two main types of non-invasive cancer can be recognized on the basis of cell type. Ductal carcinoma in situ (DCIS) is the most common form (Fig. 25.20), making up to 3–4% of symptomatic and 17–25% of screen-detected cancers. Screen-detected DCIS is most commonly associated with microcalcifications (Fig. 25.21), which can either be localized or widespread. Lobular carcinoma in situ (LCIS) (Fig. 25.22) is usually an incidental finding and is generally treated by observation.

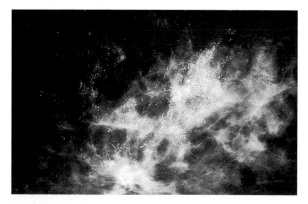

Fig. 25.21 Diffuse microcalcification in the breast affected by ductal carcinoma in situ.

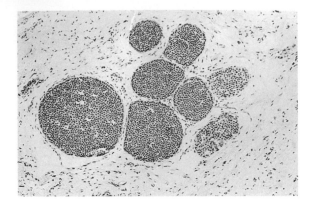

Fig. 25.22 Lobular carcinoma in situ. This is characterized by regular cells with regular round or oval nuclei (contrast this with DCIS).

Invasive

The most commonly used classification of invasive cancers divides them into ductal and lobular types, based on the belief that ductal carcinomas arise in ducts and lobular carcinomas in lobules. This is now known to be incorrect, as almost all cancers arise in the terminal duct lobular unit. Certain tumours show distinct patterns of growth and are classified separately as tumours of special type, including tubular, cribriform, mucinous, medullary and lobular. Tubular and mucinous cancers are well differentiated and have a better than average prognosis. Mucinous cancers are rare circumscribed tumours characterized by tumour cells that produce mucin; these also have a good prognosis. Medullary cancers are circumscribed and soft and consist of aggregates of high-grade pleomorphic cells surrounded by lymphoid cells. Invasive lobular cancer, which accounts for up to 10% of invasive cancers, is characterized by a diffuse pattern of spread that causes problems with clinical and mammographic detection. These tumours are often large at diagnosis and have an increased rate of bilaterality.

Tumours of 'no special type' are graded on the presence or absence of glands, the extent of nuclear pleomorphism and the mitotic rate of the tumour. Grade I are the most differentiated and have the best prognosis, grade II have an intermediate prognosis and grade III or high grade cancers have a poor prognosis. The presence of tumour cells in lymphatics or blood vessels is a marker of aggressive disease and of both local and systemic recurrence.

Screening for breast cancer

Randomized controlled trials have shown that screening by mammography can significantly reduce mortality from breast cancer. Mortality is reduced by up to 40% in women who attend for screening, with the greatest benefit being seen in women aged over 50. Published data from the com-

bined Swedish trials have shown an overall reduction in breast cancer mortality of 29% in the first 12 years after screening of women aged 50, with a smaller, 13% reduction in younger women. To be effective, attendance at screening programmes has to be greater than 70%. Ideally, screening should incorporate the 50–70-year age group, but in the UK screening is currently available only for women aged 50–64 years of age, but plans are underway to include women to age 70.

The most appropriate interval between mammographic screens is yet to be determined. In the UK screening takes place every 3 years but the rate of cancers diagnosed between the second and third years after the initial screen climbs rapidly, suggesting that this interval is too long.

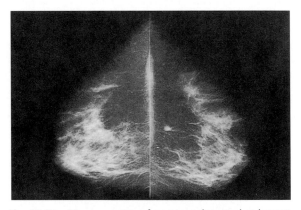

Fig. 25.23 Mammogram of a cancer detected at breast screening: small lesion at back of left breast

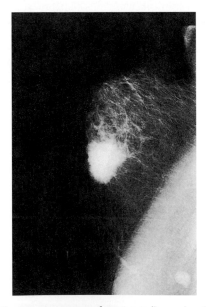

Fig. 25.24 Mammogram of a cancer (irregular dense mass) and involved axillary nodes (see localized density in axillary tail).

Patients are currently screened by two-view mammography, with a single oblique view at follow-up. Ongoing studies are evaluating the use of two views at all screens.

About two-thirds of screen-detected abnormalities are shown to be unimportant on further mammographic or ultrasound imaging. Among women aged 50–64 approximately 60 cancers are detected for every 10 000 attending for their initial screen. At subsequent screens, 35 cancers should be identified for every 10 000 attenders. Up to 70% of important abnormalities are impalpable, and for these image-guided (ultrasound or stereotactic radiography) fine-needle aspiration or core biopsy is necessary to establish a diagnosis. Compared with symptomatic cancers, screen-detected cancers are smaller and more likely to be non-invasive. The ability of screening to influence mortality from breast cancer indicates that early diagnosis identifies the cancer at an earlier stage of evolution, when metastasis is less likely to have occurred.

Mammographic features of breast cancer

Mammographically, a cancer most commonly appears as a dense opacity with an irregular outline from which spicules pass into the surrounding tissue (Fig. 25.23). Associated features include microcalcifications, which can occur within or outside the lesion, skin tethering or thickening, distortion of the shape of the breast or overlying skin, and tenting or direct involvement of underlying muscle. Involved lymph nodes can also sometimes be seen (Fig. 25.24).

Staging

When invasive cancer is diagnosed the extent of the disease should be assessed. The currently used TNM (tumour, nodes and metastases) system depends on clinical measurements and clinical assessment of lymph node status, both of which are inaccurate (Table 25.7). To improve the TNM

Table 25.7 TNM staging for breast cancer

Primary tumour (T)	
T_X	Primary tumour cannot be assessed
T_0	No evidence of primary tumour
T_{1s}	Carcinoma in situ; intraductal carcinoma, lobular carcinoma in situ, or Paget's disease of the nipple with no associated tumour mass*
T_1	Tumour 2.0 cm or less in greatest dimension†
T_{1a}	0.5 cm or less in greatest dimension
T_{1b}	more than 0.5 cm but not more than 1.0 cm in greatest dimension
T_{1c}	more than 1.0 cm but not more than 2.0 cm in greatest dimension
T_2	Tumour more than 2.0 cm but not more than 5.0 cm in greatest dimension†
T_3	Tumour more than 5.0 cm in greatest dimension†
T_4	Tumour of any size with direct extension to chest wall or skin
T_{4a}	extension to chest wall
T_{4b}	oedema (including *peau d'orange*), ulceration of the skin of the breast or satellite nodules confined to the same breast
T_{4c}	both of the above (T_{4a} and T_{4b})
T_{4d}	inflammatory carcinoma
Regional lymph nodes (N)	
N_X	Cannot be assessed (e.g. previously removed)
N_0	No regional lymph node metastasis
N_1	Movable ipsilateral axillary lymph nodes(s)
N_2	Ipsilateral lymph node(s) fixed to one another or to other structures
N_3	Ipsilateral internal mammary lymph node(s)
Distant metastases (M)	
M_X	Cannot be assessed
M_0	No distant metastasis
M_1	Distant metastasis present (includes metastasis to ipsilateral supraclavicular lymph nodes)

Note: Chest wall includes ribs, intercostal muscles and serratus anterior muscle, but not pectoral muscle.
*Paget's disease associated with tumour mass is classified according to the size of the tumour.
†Dimpling of the skin, nipple retraction or other skin changes may occur in T_1, T_2 or T_3 without changing the classification.

system, a separate pathological classification has been added. Patients with small breast cancers (<4 cm) have a low incidence of detectable metastatic disease and, unless they have specific symptoms, should not undergo investigations to search for metastases. Patients with larger or more locally advanced breast cancers are more likely to have metastases and should be considered for bone scans and liver ultrasounds. A simpler classification of breast cancer separates patients into three groups: operable, locally advanced and metastatic.

THE CURABILITY OF BREAST CANCER

Over half the women with operable breast cancer treated by surgery, with or without radiotherapy, die from metastatic disease. This suggests that in most cases the cancer has already spread at the time of presentation. Invasive breast cancers spread via the lymphatics and bloodstream. The first lymph node that drains the tumour (the sentinel node) is most commonly a level I axillary node. However, in 5% of women the sentinel node is in the internal mammary chain. In most patients with internal mammary node metastases, axillary nodes are also involved. Rarely (usually in medial tumours) the internal mammary nodes are the only regional nodes involved. It was believed that haemotogenous spread took place after lymph node involvement, but it is now appreciated that lymph nodes do not act as a filter and that the presence of nodal metastases usually means the cancer has spread systemically. Metastasis can occur at any site, but the most commonly affected organs are the bony skeleton, lungs, liver, brain, ovaries and peritoneal cavity.

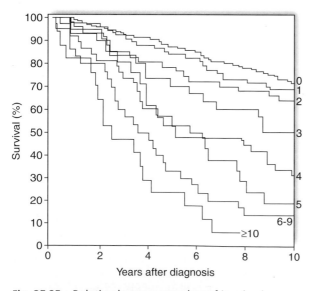

Fig. 25.25 Relation between number of involved axillary lymph nodes and survival after breast cancer.

Prognostic factors

Factors related to prognosis include:

1. The stage of the tumour at diagnosis – principally its size and the involvement of the axillary lymph nodes or the presence of clinically evident metastases;
2. Biological factors that relate to tumour aggressiveness. These include histological grade. histological type, the presence of lymphatic or vascular invasion, markers or proliferation, and hormone receptor content.

The single most important prognostic factor is the number of axillary lymph nodes involved (Fig. 25.25). It is possible to combine independent prognostic factors to form an index that allows the identification of groups with different prognoses. The Nottingham Prognostic Index (Table 25.8) is the most widely used and incorporates three factors: tumour size, node status and histological grade.

- Tumour size is the pathological size of the tumour in centimetres.
- Node status is scored 1 if no nodes are involved, 2 if one to three nodes are involved, and 3 if four or more nodes are involved.
- Grade I tumours are scored as I, grade II tumours are scored as 2 and grade III tumours are scored as 3.

Then, Nottingham Prognostic Index = (0.2 × size (cm)) + score of lymph node stage + score of grade.

PRESENTATION OF BREAST CANCER

The most common presentation is with a breast lump, which is usually painless. Any discrete lump, no matter how small or mobile, can be a cancer. The investigation of a breast lump is shown in Figure 25.26. Malignant lesions are usually firm and irregular and often produce visible signs of breast asymmetry, such as flattening, dimpling or puckering of the overlying skin, or retraction or alteration in nipple contour. Approximately 50% of breast cancers are located in the upper outer quadrant of the breast. Diagnosis of breast lumps is a particular problem in young women, where the breasts are dense and lumpier and cancer is rare. Some

Table 25.8 Nottingham Prognostic Index (NPI) and survival		
Prognostic group	NPI value	10 year survival (%)
Excellent	≤ 2.4	94
Good	2.4–≤ 3.4	83
Moderate I	3.4–≤ 4.4	70
Moderate II	4.4–≤ 5.4	51
Poor	> 5.4	19

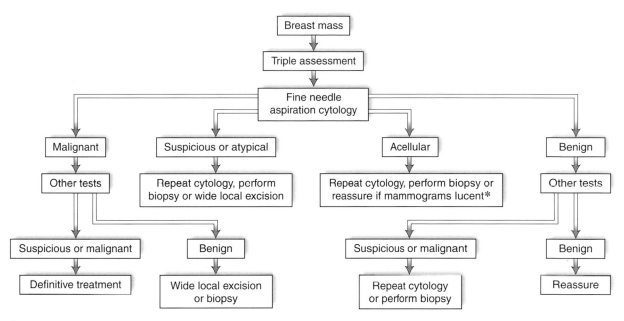

Fig. 25.26 Investigation of a breast mass.

* An acellular cytological report is acceptable in the presence of lucent mammograms

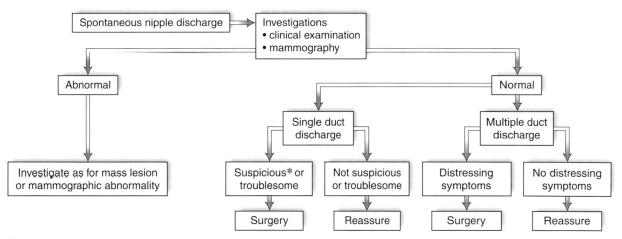

* Bloodstained or persistent

Fig. 25.27 Investigation of nipple discharge.

patients present with skin ulceration, direct infiltration of the skin by tumour or with oedema (*peau d'orange*) of the overlying skin. These are features of locally advanced breast cancer.

Breast pain alone is a rare presenting feature of breast cancer: 2.7% of patients with breast pain have breast cancer, whereas 4.6% of patients presenting with breast cancer have pain as their only symptom. Nipple discharge, which is either bloodstained or contains moderate or large amounts of blood on testing, can be a presenting feature of breast cancer. However, only 5–10% of patients who have a bloodstained or blood-containing discharge will have an underlying malignancy. The investigation of patients who present with nipple discharge is shown in Figure 25.27. Patients with breast cancer occasionally present with a dry scaling or red weeping appearance of the nipple known as Paget's

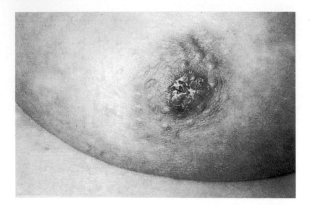

Fig. 25.28   Paget's disease.

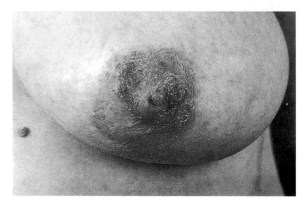

Fig. 25.29   Eczema of the nipple.

disease; this signifies an underlying invasive or non-invasive cancer (Fig. 25.28) and should be differentiated from eczema (Fig. 25.29). Paget's disease always affects the nipple and only involves the areola as a secondary event, whereas eczema primarily involves the areola and only secondarily affects the nipple. Approximately 1–2% of patients with breast cancer present with Paget's disease. In half of these it is associated with an underlying mass lesion, and 90% of such patients will have an invasive cancer. Of the patients without a mass lesion, 30% have an invasive cancer and the rest have in-situ disease alone.

Patients can also present with palpable axillary nodes or signs and symptoms of distant metastatic disease, for example palpable supraclavicular nodes, bone pain, a cough or breathlessness, lethargy and tiredness, jaundice and headaches, or a sudden onset of *grand-mal* seizures. Less than one in 300 patients with breast cancer presents with nodal metastases and an occult primary cancer. Up to 70% of women shown histologically to have metastatic adenocarcinoma in the axillary nodes will have an occult breast cancer, and most of these will be visible on mammography.

TREATMENT OF OPERABLE BREAST CANCER

In situ breast cancer

Localised DCIS (less than 4 cm in maximum dimension) should be treated by complete wide excision, ensuring that surrounding normal tissue is present at all lateral margins. Following wide excision alone, approximately 2% per year will develop recurrence, half of which will be further in situ disease, the other half being invasive. For this reason, following wide excision the majority of patients should receive postoperative radiotherapy. Only in patients with small areas of DCIS which have been widely excised should radiotherapy be omitted. Tamoxifen may reduce both the risk of recurrence and the rate of development of contralateral cancer. Only patients who present with palpable areas of DCIS do not appear to benefit from tamoxifen, although it is likely that those who have oestrogen receptor-positive disease gain most from this treatment. DCIS that is incompletely excised requires re-excision or mastectomy. Widespread (> 4 cm) or multi-focal DCIS should be treated by mastectomy, with or without reconstruction.

SUMMARY BOX

DCIS

- Localized disease is treated by wide local excision to clear margins.

- All patients other than those at low risk of recurrence should receive adjuvant radiotherapy to the breast following wide local excision. Tamoxifen reduces all breast cancer events following wide excision, but its exact role in reducing local recurrence following conservative treatment is not clear.

- Widespread (> 4 cm) areas of DCIS are treated by mastectomy ± reconstruction.

Operable breast tumours

Operable breast tumours are those restricted to the breast or associated with mobile axillary lymph nodes on the same side: T_1, T_2, T_3, N_0, N_1, M_0. As only a minority of patients are cured by locoregional treatments alone, all patients should be considered for systemic therapy.

Local therapy

There are currently two accepted methods of local therapy for operable breast cancer.

Breast-conserving treatment (wide local excision and radiotherapy)

This involves excising the tumour with a 1 cm margin of macroscopically normal tissue. Breast conservation is usually only suitable for single cancers measuring less than 4 cm in diameter. Complete excision of all invasive and non-invasive cancer is necessary. Wide excision should be combined with an axillary node staging procedure. This involves either removing the first node draining the tumour (sentinel node biopsy), sampling (removing four nodes of the lower axilla) or axillary clearance (removing all nodes at levels I, II and III). To identify the sentinel node blue dye and/or radioisotope is injected around the cancer. The sentinel node can be seen on scintigraphy, identified with a handheld probe, or is stained blue. When blue dye and radioactively labelled sulphur colloid or albumin techniques are combined, approximately 97% of patients will have one or more sentinel nodes identified, and this sentinel node is accurate in determining the presence of any involved nodes in the axilla in approximately 98% of patients.

The cosmetic outcome following breast conservation relates to psychological wellbeing. Patients who have a good cosmetic result have low levels of anxiety and depression and improved body image and self-esteem. The larger the volume of tissue excised the poorer the cosmetic result. The aim is therefore, to completely remove the cancer in as small a volume of tissue as possible.

Wide excision should be followed by radical radiotherapy using megavoltage equipment to deliver 45–50 Gy to the whole breast. An additional boost of 10–15 Gy by electrons of appropriate energy, or an iridium-192 (^{192}Ir) implant, is given to the tumour bed. For patients with involved nodes following either a sentinel node biopsy or an axillary node sampling procedure, all axillary nodes are removed or radiotherapy is given to the axilla and/or supraclavicular nodes.

SUMMARY BOX

Breast conservation

- Localized, unifocal operable breast cancers in which there is no evidence of metastatic disease are suitable for breast conservation, where excision will leave a reasonable cosmetic result.

- Breast conservation includes wide local excision of the cancer to clear histological margins, axillary surgery (sampling or clearance of the axillary nodes), and whole-breast radiotherapy.

- 45–50 MV radiotherapy is applied to the breast, with an optional 10–15 Gy boost to the tumour bed.

Mastectomy

This is an alternative method of local treatment. It is indicated in patients:

- Where radiotherapy is not available or where there is a wish to avoid radiotherapy
- Who elect to have a mastectomy
- Who have more than one focus of cancer in their breast
- Who have a localized invasive cancer but a large area of surrounding non-invasive disease
- Where breast conservation would produce an unacceptable cosmetic result (this includes some central lesions directly underneath the nipple, and most cancers measuring more than 4 cm in diameter). Breast-conserving surgery is only possible in these women if they have shrinkage following initial systemic therapy, or if the breast defect is filled with a latissimus dorsi miniflap.

Mastectomy removes all breast tissue with some overlying skin (usually including the nipple), but leaves the chest wall muscles intact. If reconstruction is being performed minimal skin around the tumour is excised. Mastectomy should be combined with some form of axillary surgery. Radiotherapy is given after mastectomy to patients who are at high risk of local recurrence. Risk factors for local recurrence after mastectomy include axillary lymph node involvement, lymphatic or vascular invasion by tumour, a grade III cancer, a cancer more than 4 cm in diameter (pathological measurement), or a tumour that involves the pectoral fascia or pectoral muscle.

SUMMARY BOX

Mastectomy

- In large multifocal operable breast cancers or in patients with extensive non-invasive disease, an incomplete excision or some women with central tumour, mastectomy is appropriate treatment.

- Surgery consists of total mastectomy with axillary node sampling or axillary clearance.

- Chest wall radiotherapy should be restricted to those identified to be at increased risk of local recurrence.

Systemic therapy

Systemic treatment may be given as adjuvant therapy after surgery and/or radiotherapy, or as primary or neoadjuvant treatment before surgery and/or radiotherapy. The effectiveness of adjuvant treatment has been shown in clinical trials. Randomized studies comparing primary systemic treatment with adjuvant treatment have shown similar survivals, with a higher rate of breast-conserving surgery in patients having

Table 25.9   Reduction in recurrence and mortality in polychemotherapy trials

Age	Reduction in annual odds of recurrence (% ± SD)	Reduction in annual odds of death (% ± SD)
<40	37 ± 7	27 ± 8
40–49	34 ± 5	27 ± 5
50–59	22 ± 4	14 ± 4
60–69	18 ± 4	8 ± 4
All ages	23 ± 8	15 ± 2

initial medical treatment. Adjuvant treatments consist of chemotherapy or hormonal therapy. For chemotherapy, a combination of drugs is more effective than a single drug and the optimal benefit seems to come from at least four cycles of postoperative chemotherapy. The benefits of chemotherapy are greatest in women under the age of 50 (Table 25.9); a smaller but still significant benefit is seen in older women. Commonly used regimen's include CMF (cyclophosphamide, methotrexate and 5-fluorouracil) and the anthracycline-containing regimens AC (adriamycin, cyclophosphamide) or FEC (5-fluorouracil, epirubicin and cyclophosphamide). The taxanes (taxol and taxotere) are currently being evaluated in the adjuvant setting.

Adjuvant hormonal treatments consist of oophorectomy, tamoxifen and the aromatase inhibitors letrozole or anastrozole. Oophorectomy is only of benefit in women aged under 50 and produces survival benefits of similar magnitude to those obtained by polychemotherapy in younger women. It can be achieved surgically, by radiation or by the administration of gonadotrophin-releasing hormone (GnRh) analogues. Tamoxifen is a partial oestrogen agonist that is given in a dose of 20 mg once daily. At least 5 years of tamoxifen should be given. It reduces the risk of contralateral breast cancer by between 40 and 50%. The benefits of tamoxifen and oophorectomy are greatest in patients with tumours that are rich in oestrogen receptors. Tamoxifen is effective in both pre- and postmenopausal women. The aromatase inhibitors, which block the conversion of androgens to oestrogen in postmenopausal women, are currently being evaluated in adjuvant trials.

Adjuvant systemic therapy is effective in both patients at low and high risk of recurrence, but the absolute gains in survival are greatest in the latter. Risk can be calculated using the Nottingham Prognostic Index or can be based on individual factors (Table 25.10). An outline of the use of adjuvant treatment in different groups is presented in Table 25.11.

Primary systemic therapy

The use of primary medical (neoadjuvant) or preoperative treatment for operable breast cancer can allow large tumours which would otherwise require a mastectomy to become suitable for breast conserving surgery. Both the primary tumour and lymph node metastases can be shown to respond. With conventional chemotherapy regimens, approximately 70% of patients will demonstrate tumour shrinkage of over 50%. Although chemotherapy is most commonly used as preoperative treatment particularly in premenopausal women, primary hormonal therapy is becoming used increasingly in postmenopausal women with strongly oestrogen receptor positive breast cancers. Response rates of over 75% are reported. Randomised studies have suggested that the aromatase inhibitor, letrozole, produces significantly better responses in the neoadjuvant setting than tamoxifen and this is currently the first line agent of choice in this setting.

Table 25.10   Definitions of risk groups and associated risk of relapse

Risk group	Age and tumour characteristic	Survival without relapse at 5 years (%)
Node-negative patients		
Low	>35 y, tumour ≤1 cm in diameter	>90
Intermediate	≤35 y, tumour ≤1 cm in diameter >35 y, tumour >1 cm grade I or II	75–80
High	≤35 y, tumour >1 cm grade I or II Any age, tumour >1 cm grade III	50–60
Node-positive patients		
Low + intermediate	>35 y, 1–3 positive nodes	40–50
High	≤35 y, 1–3 positive nodes >35 y, 4–9 positive	20–30
Very high	≤35 y, 4+ nodes involved >35 y, 10+ nodes involved	10–15

Table 25.11 Adjuvant treatment for patients with breast cancer

Risk group	Premenopausal	Postmenopausal
Node-negative patients		
Low	Tamoxifen or no treatment	Tamoxifen or no treatment
Intermediate	Tamoxifen	Tamoxifen
High	Consider chemotherapy* (with or without tamoxifen) *or* ovarian ablation (with *or* without tamoxifen) if tumour is oestrogen receptor positive	Tamoxifen (with or without chemotherapy)
Node-positive patients		
Low & intermediate	Chemotherapy* (with or without tamoxifen) *or* ovarian ablation (with or without tamoxifen) if tumour is oestrogen receptor positive, *or* chemotherapy* and ovarian ablation (with or without tamoxifen)	Tamoxifen with or without chemotherapy
High & very high	Consider more intensive chemotherapy† (with or without tamoxifen)	Tamoxifen and chemotherapy if fit

*For example cyclophosphamide, methotrexate and fluorouracil.
†For example regimen containing anthracycline.

SUMMARY BOX

Adjuvant therapy

Following surgery and/or radiotherapy for operable breast cancer, patients should receive adjuvant systemic therapy, which can either be hormonal, e.g.:

- Premenopausal women: tamoxifen, goserelin, or both together
- Postmenopausal women: tamoxifen, aromatase inhibitors, or the two combined chemotherapy:

Or

- Commonly used regimens are CMF, AC, FEC, AT

The following factors positively influence the use of chemotherapy:

- Young age (especially less than 60)
- Axillary node positivity
- Large tumour size
- Histological features
  - Grade III
  - Lymphatic/vascular invasion
- Negative oestrogen receptor

Complications of treatment

Haematoma and infection are uncommon (less than 5%) after breast surgery. Removal of all the axillary nodes often damages the intercostobrachial nerve and these patients develop numbness and paraesthesia down the upper inner aspect of the arm. Other nerves that can potentially be damaged during axillary surgery are the long thoracic – damage to which causes winging of the scapula – and the thoracodorsal, which can lead to atrophy of the latissimus dorsi muscle and prominence of the scapula. Axillary surgery is associated with some short-term reduction in shoulder movement and about 5% of women develop a frozen shoulder. Approximately 5% of patients treated by a full axillary dissection develop lymphoedema. The treatment of lymphoedema is unsatisfactory and is best managed by bandaging and a supportive elastic arm stocking.

Radiotherapy

Following radiotherapy the skin develops an erythematous reaction, which often lasts for 3–4 weeks. Patients should avoid exposing the area to direct sunlight for several months. Subsequent exposure is possible with an appropriate sunscreen. Following radiotherapy to the axilla some patients develop fibrosis around the shoulder, which can lead to some restriction in their range of movement.

Chemotherapy

Although hair loss is the most common concern of patients before starting chemotherapy, 80% report fatigue and lethargy as the most troublesome side-effect. The occurrence of alopecia with some chemotherapy regimens may be reduced by scalp cooling. Nausea and vomiting are unpleasant side-effects but in most patients can be controlled with appropriate antiemetic drugs.

Hormonal treatments

The side-effects of hormonal treatments are greatest in pre-menopausal patients. Only 3% of patients stop taking tamoxifen because of side-effects, but vaginal dryness or vaginal discharge, loss of libido and hot flushes all have a considerable impact on quality of life.

PSYCHOLOGICAL ASPECTS

Most women who present with breast lumps are emotionally distressed. Up to 30% of women with breast cancer develop an anxiety state or depressive illness within a year of diagnosis, which is three to four times the expected rate. After mastectomy, 20–30% of patients develop persisting problems with body image and sexual difficulties. Breast-conserving surgery reduces problems with body image. Psychiatric morbidity is increased when radiotherapy or chemotherapy is used. Few patients mention psychological problems to their doctor because they think it is unacceptable to do so. Doctors can promote the disclosure of such problems by being empathetic, making educated guesses about how patients are feeling, and summarizing what they have disclosed.

When breaking bad news to the patient, the first step should be to check their idea about what is wrong. Almost two-thirds of patients with breast cancer already suspect that their lump is malignant. In patients with proven malignancy the doctor's role is to confirm to the patient that their diagnosis is correct, pause to let this sink in, and acknowledge their distress and establish what concerns are contributing to this distress. When a patient is unaware that she has cancer, the doctor should break the news more slowly. Only once her distress and concerns are addressed should reassurance, information and advice be offered. Counselling is essential and most specialist units employ nurse counsellors who ensure that the patient is fully informed about the nature of the disease and its treatment, provide advice on prostheses after surgery, and are trained to recognize and support patients with significant psychiatric problems.

There is evidence that patients benefit psychologically from immediate breast reconstruction. One option for reconstruction is to insert an implant behind the chest wall muscles at the time of mastectomy. The problem with this approach is that the size of implant that can be inserted is limited and symmetry is difficult to obtain. Another option is to place a tissue expander behind the pectoral muscles. Small amounts of fluid are injected regularly into the expander over a period of months before replacing it, at a second operation, with a permanent prosthesis. Alternative options include using myocutaneous flaps, the most commonly used being the latissimus dorsi flap with an implant, or the rectus abdominis myocutaneous flap alone.

Follow-up

Patients treated by wide local excision and radiotherapy have an approximate 1% per year rate of local recurrence in the treated breast. Patients with cancer in one breast are also at risk of cancer in the other breast (0.4–0.6% per year). The majority of local recurrences after mastectomy occur within the first few years. The aim of follow-up is to detect local recurrence at a stage when it is treatable, to support the patient psychologically and to discuss problems associated with adjuvant therapy. Patients should have an annual clinical examination and mammography of one or both breasts every 1–2 years. No investigations should be performed to detect asymptomatic metastases as there is no evidence that detecting such disease earlier influences survival.

TREATMENT OF LOCALLY ADVANCED BREAST CANCER

Locally advanced disease is characterized by features suggesting infiltration of the skin or chest wall by tumour or

---

Table 25.12   Clinical features of locally advanced breast cancer

Skin
Ulceration
Satellite nodules
Dermal infiltration
Peau d'orange
Erythema over tumour

Chest wall
Tumour fixation to
Ribs
Intercostal muscles
Serratus anterior

Axillary nodes
Nodes fixed to one another or to other structures

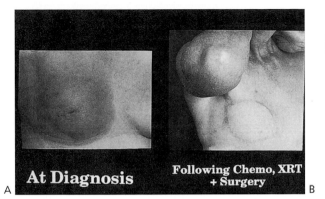

Fig. 25.30 **A** Patient with an inflammatory breast cancer prior to treatment. **B** Same patient with an inflammatory cancer treated initially by surgery and radiotherapy, but with residual tumour and treated by mastectomy with a latissimus dorsi flap which allowed wide excision of all remaining disease.

SUMMARY BOX

Locally advanced breast cancer

- For the majority consider systemic chemotherapy or, in the elderly or those who have indolent hormone sensitive cancers, initial hormonal therapy.

- Radiotherapy can be used following primary chemotherapy, or can be given concurrently with hormonal therapy.

- Consider surgery if the disease becomes operable following primary systemic therapy, or in patients with locally advanced breast cancers which have occurred either because of a delay in diagnosis or their position in the breast, e.g. superficial or at the breast margin.

---

matted involved axillary nodes (Table 25.12). Between 1 in 12 and 1 in 4 patients with breast cancer presents with locally advanced disease. It has a variable natural history, with reported 5-year survivals of between 1% and 30%. The median survival is about 2–2.5 years. Locally advanced breast cancer (LABC) may arise because of its position in the breast (for example peripheral), neglect (some patients do not present to hospital for months or years after they notice a mass) or biological aggressiveness. The latter includes inflammatory cancers that present with erythema and/or widespread *peau d'orange* affecting the breast skin. Inflammatory carcinomas are uncommon and are characterized by brawny, oedematous, indurated and erythematous skin changes (Fig. 25.30 A). They have the worst prognosis of all locally advanced breast cancers.

Local and regional relapse is a major problem in LABC and affects more than half of patients. By treating initially with systemic therapy, followed by surgery and radiotherapy or radiotherapy alone, improvements in local control have been achieved. Systemic treatment consists of either chemotherapy (inflammatory cancers, oestrogen receptor-negative tumours and rapidly progressive disease) or hormonal treatment (slow or indolent disease, oestrogen receptor-positive cancers, or women who are elderly or unfit). Following systemic therapy the disease may become operable, at which point surgery, usually mastectomy, is followed by radiotherapy. In women whose disease remains inoperable following systemic treatment, radiotherapy is given. This is followed by surgery in some women in whom viable resectable cancer remains following radiotherapy (Fig. 25.30 B).

BREAST CANCER IN PREGNANCY

Overall, 1–2% of breast cancers occur during pregnancy. It affects one to three of every 10 000 pregnancies. Although there is no evidence that breast cancer occurring during pregnancy is more aggressive, because the diagnosis is often delayed up to 65% have involved axillary nodes. Treatment during the first two trimesters is with mastectomy. Radiotherapy should not be delivered during pregnancy. Chemotherapy can be given but is associated with a small risk of fetal damage. Breast cancer during the third trimester can be managed either by immediate surgery or by monitoring the tumour and delivering the baby early at 32 weeks, and then instituting treatment after delivery.

Pregnancy after treatment for breast cancer

There is only limited information of the effect of pregnancy on the outcome of patients with breast cancer, but the available data show no detrimental effect.

TREATMENT OF METASTATIC OR ADVANCED BREAST CANCER

The average period of survival after a diagnosis of metastatic disease is 18–24 months, but this varies widely between patients. The survival of patients with bone-only disease is approximately 2 years, with a median survival of patients with lung, liver and brain metastases of 10, 8 and 3 months, respectively. A patient may present with metastatic breast carcinoma or can develop metastases following treatment of an apparently localized breast cancer. The aim of treatment is to produce effective symptom control with minimal side-effects. This ideal is only achieved in the 30% of patients whose cancers respond to hormonal or chemotherapy. There is no evidence that treating asymptomatic metastases improves overall survival, and chemotherapy is normally given only to symptomatic patients.

Chemotherapy

With chemotherapy a balance must be achieved between a high response rate and limiting side-effects. The best palliation is obtained with regimens that produce the highest response rates. The most commonly used drugs are the anthracyclines, adriamycin and epirubicin. Taxanes (taxol and taxotere) are also becoming commonly used. Overall rates of response to chemotherapy are approximately 40–60%, with a median time to relapse of 6–10 months. Subsequent courses have response rates of less than 25%.

Hormonal treatment

A variety of hormonal interventions are available for use in metastatic breast cancer (Table 25.13). In premenopausal women these include oophorectomy (surgical, radiation- or drug-induced by GnRh analogues). Tamoxifen can also be used in premenopausal women, usually combined with GnRh analogues. Options in postmenopausal women include the new aromatase inhibitors (anastrozole, letrozole and exemestane) and the progestogens (such as medroxyprogesterone acetate or megestrol acetate). Objective responses to hormonal treatments are seen in 30% of all patients and in 50–60% of those with oestrogen receptor-positive tumours. Response rates of 25% are seen when using second-line hormonal agents, although less than 15% of patients who show no response to first-line treatment will have a response to second-line agents. Approximately 10–15% of patients respond to third-line endocrine agents.

> **SUMMARY BOX**
>
> *Metastatic breast cancer*
>
> - The primary aim is to improve symptoms and quality of life.
> - Consider hormone therapy if long disease-free interval, tumour is hormone receptor positive and liver and lungs are not affected.
> - Consider chemotherapy if short disease-free interval, vital organs affected and tumour is oestrogen receptor negative.

Bone disease

Three-quarters of patients who develop secondary breast cancer will have disease involving the bony skeleton. Widespread bony disease responds well to hormonal treatment, but in young patients cytotoxic agents may be required. Treatment of localized pain includes external beam radiotherapy and analgesics, including non-steroidal anti-inflammatories and opiates. Pathological fractures due to bone disease should be avoided and can be predicted by a sharp increase in pain over a few days or weeks. When X-rays show that fracture is likely, a combination of internal fixation and radiotherapy should be used. Options for widespread bony pain include the use of bisphosphonates (which reduce osteoclast activity) and sequential upper and lower body hemiradiotherapy or radioactive strontium.

Hypercalcaemia

This is seen in up to 40% of patients with bony metastases. Symptoms include nausea, constipation, thirst, polyuria, personality change, muscle weakness and bone pain. Treatment

Table 25.13 Hormonal treatment of metastatic breast cancer	
Premenopausal	Postmenopausal
Gonadotrophin releasing hormone analogues	Aromatase inhibitor*, progestins, e.g. megestrol or medroxyprogestone acetate Tamoxifen (or new SERM)** 'Pure' antioestrogens***
Oophorectomy Radiation menopause Tamoxifen** Ovarian suppression + any postmenopausal agent	

These agents can be used in any order. There is weak evidence that combined ovarian suppression plus an antioestrogen may be superior to single agent treatment in premenopausal women.
  * Anastrazole or letrozole currently licensed for 1st line metastatic setting. Exemestane in clinical trials.
  ** Other tamoxifen-like agents – selective oestrogen receptor modifiers with slightly different selectivity c/w tamoxifen under trial
*** In clinical trials, not yet licensed	

consists of hydration with saline (about 3 L given over 24 hours) and the administration of intravenous bisphosphonates, followed by a change in systemic anticancer therapy.

Marrow infiltration

A leukoerythroblastic blood picture (immature cells in the peripheral blood) suggests extensive marrow infiltration. Chemotherapy is generally required, but should be given initially in reduced doses with careful monitoring and adequate supportive care.

Spinal cord compression

This is most often seen in patients with thoracic spinal metastases. It must be recognized early and treated promptly. Patients with isolated metastases causing cord compression, and who are fit, should be treated by surgery followed by postoperative radiotherapy and appropriate systemic therapy. In the remaining patients, treatment consists of steroids and fractionated radiotherapy.

Pleural effusion

Up to half of patients with metastatic breast cancer will develop a malignant pleural effusion. Cytological examination of aspirated fluid reveals malignant cells in only 85% of patients. Aspiration of pleural effusions is ineffective, as between 97 and 100% of patients will reaccumulate fluid. In contrast, tube drainage alone is effective in controlling effusions in over a third of patients. The instillation of bleomycin, tetracycline or talc to cause pleurodesis reduces recurrence.

Liver metastases

Right upper quadrant pain, general debility, tiredness, a feeling of nausea and lack of appetite or the onset of jaundice are all symptoms suggestive of liver infiltration. Chemotherapy is usually indicated in these patients. Where jaundice is due to nodal disease at the porta hepatis, a stent inserted in the common bile duct using an ERCP approach should be considered.

Brain metastases

These should be suspected in any patient with breast cancer who presents with focal neurological symptoms. CT or MRI can detect even small volumes of disease. Initial treatment consists of high-dose corticosteroids (16 mg daily of dexamethasone) followed by radiotherapy. The greatest benefits of radiotherapy are seen in patients whose neurological symptoms improve following steroid treatment, but the long-term results of treatment are disappointing. A small group of patients with solitary brain metastases, and without evidence of involvement at other sites, are suitable for local excision followed by post-operative radiotherapy and appropriate systemic treatment. A few of these patients remain well without other evidence of disease for many years.

SUMMARY BOX

Metastatic disease – specific problems

- Bone metastases may require local radiotherapy, bisphosphonates, or orthopaedic intervention, combined with systemic hormonal or chemotherapy.

- Hypercalcaemia causes nausea, constipation, thirst, polyuria, weakness, pain and personality change, and is treated by rehydration followed by bisphosphonates.

- Spinal cord compression should be treated by surgical decompression if appropriate, or by steroids and radiotherapy.

- Pleural effusions should be treated by tube drainage, followed by instillation of bleomycin, tetracycline or talc.

- Discrete lung metastases may not cause acute symptoms but lymphangitis carcinomatosa can cause severe bronchospasm and dyspnoea, which may be relieved by steroids, bronchodilators and chemotherapy.

- Liver metastases are usually treated by chemotherapy.

- Brain metastases are treated initially with steroids, followed by radiation. Surgery can be used for isolated single metastases.

MISCELLANEOUS TUMOURS OF THE BREAST

Lymphoma

This is rare in the breast. Staging investigations are necessary because patients will usually have disease outside the regional nodes. Characteristically it presents as a discrete smooth rubbery mass. Small localized breast lymphomas can be treated by wide excision, axillary node sampling, radiotherapy and chemotherapy. Larger lesions should be treated by radiotherapy and chemotherapy after biopsy.

Sarcomas

Sarcomas can develop in breast tissue and can affect the skin overlying the breast. Rarely, they are induced by radiotherapy to the chest wall. Sarcomas are treated by excision and, as many of these tumours are large at diagnosis, mastectomy is generally necessary. Radiotherapy should be given to the chest wall after excisional surgery, but there is no evidence that adjuvant chemotherapy is of benefit.

Malignant phyllodes tumours

Previously called cystosarcoma phyllodes, these present as large lobulated lesions that can involve the overlying skin. Initial treatment is by wide excision and mastectomy is often required. The role of radiotherapy and chemotherapy in these lesions in unclear.

Secondary tumours

Metastases from tumours elsewhere, e.g. bronchus, thyroid, melanoma or the opposite breast, produce a well defined mass both clinically and mammographically.

MALE BREAST

Gynaecomastia

Gynaecomastia (the growth of breast tissue in males to any extent in all ages) is entirely benign and usually reversible.

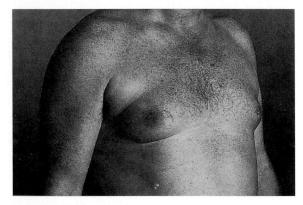

Fig. 25.31   Gynaecomastia.

It commonly occurs at puberty and in old age and is seen in 30–60% of boys aged 10–16. In this age group it usually requires no treatment, as 80% resolve spontaneously within 2 years (Fig. 25.31). Embarrassment or persistent enlargement is an indication for surgery. Senescent gynaecomastia usually affects men between 50 and 80, and in most cases does not appear to be associated with any endocrine abnormality. Causes include drugs, cirrhosis, hypogonadism and, rarely, testicular tumours. Rapidly progressive gynaecomastia is an indication for an assessment of hormonal profile. A history of recent progressive breast enlargement without pain and tenderness, or an easily identifiable cause, should raise the suspicious of breast cancer. If there is a localized mass then further investigations should be performed.

Male breast cancer

Less than 0.5% of all breast cancers occur in men, and breast cancer comprises 0.7% of all male cancers. The peak incidence in males is 5–10 years older than in women. Klinefelter's syndrome and a strong family history are the only known risk factors. It usually presents with an eccentric breast mass or retraction of the overlying skin. Direct involvement of the skin occurs more often in male breast cancer because of the smaller breast volume compared to the female breast, and so the disease is more likely to be advanced at diagnosis. Mammography, fine-needle aspiration cytology or core biopsy confirms the diagnosis. Treatment for localized breast cancer is by total mastectomy and the removal of axillary nodes, followed by postoperative radiotherapy to the chest wall. Wide local excision, axillary surgery and postoperative radiotherapy can treat some small breast cancers. Adjuvant tamoxifen is effective at reducing recurrence, but adjuvant chemotherapy should be considered for fit patients with tumours that have nodal involvement and are oestrogen receptor negative.

26 Endocrine surgery

J.R. Farndon

THYROID GLAND

Surgical anatomy and development

The thyroid gland develops from the thyroglossal duct, which grows downwards from the pharynx through the developing hyoid bone. On the front of the trachea the duct bifurcates and fuses with elements from the fourth branchial arch, from which the parafollicular (C cells) are derived. The duct is normally obliterated in early fetal life but can persist in part to produce a thyroglossal cyst. The upper end of the duct is identified in adults as the foramen caecum at the junction of the anterior two-thirds and the posterior third of the tongue. Arrest of descent of the duct may result in an ectopic thyroid (e.g. lingual thyroid).

There are two pairs of parathyroid glands. The upper glands arise from the fourth branchial arch and are usually found at the back of the thyroid above the inferior thyroid

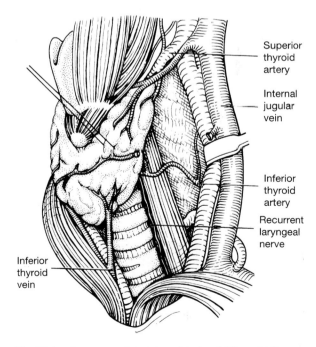

Fig. 26.1 Anatomy of the thyroid gland. The middle thyroid vein has been divided to allow forward rotation of the left lobe of the gland.

Superior thyroid artery

Internal jugular vein

Inferior thyroid artery

Recurrent laryngeal nerve

Inferior thyroid vein

artery. The lower glands arise from the third arch (in association with the thymus) and are less constant in position. They are usually found posterior to the lower pole of the thyroid lobes but can lie within the gland, some distance below it, in the upper mediastinum or within the thymus.

The right and left lobes of the thyroid lie on the front and sides of the trachea and larynx at the level of the 5–7th cervical vertebrae (Fig. 26.1). The two lobes are connected by a narrow isthmus, which overlies the second and third tracheal rings. The thyroid normally weighs 15–30 g and is invested by the pretracheal fascia, which binds it to the larynx, cricoid cartilage and trachea (Fig. 26.2). The strap muscles (sternohyoid and sternothyroid) lie in front of the pretracheal fascia and must be separated to gain access to the gland. It is difficult to feel the normal thyroid gland except at puberty and during pregnancy, when physiological enlargement occurs.

The superior thyroid artery runs down to the upper pole of the gland as a branch of the external carotid artery, whereas the inferior thyroid artery runs up to the lower pole from the thyrocervical trunk (a branch of the subclavian artery). As it nears the gland the inferior thyroid artery usually passes in front of the recurrent laryngeal nerve, but may branch around it. Blood from the thyroid drains through superior, middle and inferior thyroid veins into the internal jugular and innominate veins. Lymphatics drain laterally to the deep cervical chain and downwards to pretracheal and mediastinal nodes. The recurrent laryngeal nerve is a branch of the vagus, which passes upwards in the groove between the oesophagus and trachea to enter the larynx and supply all of its intrinsic muscles except the

cricothyroid. The superior laryngeal nerve (also a branch of the vagus) runs with the superior thyroid vessels and supplies the cricothyroid muscles (external branch), which tense the vocal cords. The recurrent nerve supplies sensation to the larynx below the vocal cords. The internal branch of the superior laryngeal nerve provides sensation above the cords. Normal sensory and motor function within the larynx is necessary for speech and coughing. Both nerves are at risk of damage during thyroid surgery and the consequences, if permanent, can be disabling.

Thyroid function

Histologically the gland is made up of follicles containing colloid, which on haemotoxylin and eosin staining appears pink (Fig. 26.3). The follicles are spheroids lined by cuboidal epithelium (thyrocytes). The parafollicular or C cells may be seen between follicles. The gland has an exceedingly rich blood supply. The thyrocytes secrete triiodothyronine (T_3) and thyroxine (T_4). T_3 is the active hormone and T_4 is converted to T_3 in the periphery. Synthesis involves the combination of iodine with tyrosyl groups to form mono- and diiodotyrosine, which are then coupled to form T_3 and T_4. The hormones are stored in the follicles bound to thyroglobulin and, when released, circulate free or bound to plasma proteins.

Secretion of T_3 and T_4 is controlled by thyroid-stimulating hormone (TSH), which is secreted by the anterior pituitary. TSH release is in turn controlled by thyrotropin-releasing hormone (TRH) from the hypothalamus. Circulating levels of T_3 and T_4 exert a negative feedback effect on the hypothalamus and anterior pituitary. The parafollicular cells produce calcitonin. This can be measured in the blood and is normally secreted in small amounts. Secretion is increased after food. Calcitonin lowers the serum calcium but it is not

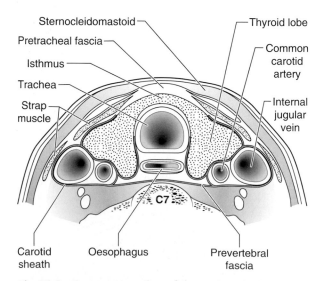

Fig. 26.2 Transverse section of the neck at the level of the seventh cervical vertebra to show the arrangement of the deep cervical fascia.

Labels (clockwise): Sternocleidomastoid, Pretracheal fascia, Isthmus, Trachea, Strap muscle, Carotid sheath, Oesophagus, C7, Prevertebral fascia, Internal jugular vein, Common carotid artery, Thyroid lobe.

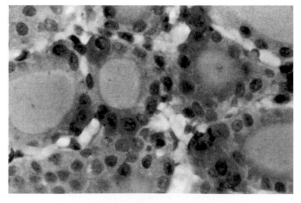

Fig. 26.3 Histology of the thyroid gland to show the follicular structure. Cells staining grey are positive for calcitonin and are the so-called parafollicular or C cells.

an essential hormone and does not require replacement after total thyroidectomy.

Assessment of thyroid disease

Measurement of T_3, T_4 and TSH gives a biochemical estimation of thyroid function. TSH is totally suppressed in thyrotoxicosis and elevated in hypothyroidism. Pregnancy or oestrogen administration increases the level of thyroid-binding globulin, so that estimation of the ratio of free to bound hormone may be needed. TRH and TSH stimulation tests may be required to determine the site of failure of production of thyroid hormones.

The thyroid can be imaged by plain films, ultrasonography or radioisotope scanning (^{99m}Tc-sodium pertechnetate behaves like iodine and is 'trapped' by the gland). The main value of scanning is to differentiate between 'hot' (actively functioning), 'cool' (normally functioning) and 'cold' (non-functioning) thyroid nodules. Total isotope uptake also reflects thyroid activity.

MRI and CT scanning provide excellent means of determining the extent of goitre. Fine-needle aspiration cytology is used to determine the nature of thyroid nodules. Thyroid antibodies detected in significant titre may indicate autoimmune thyroid disease.

ENLARGEMENT OF THE THYROID GLAND (GOITRE)

Clinical features

Goitre is a visible or palpable enlargement of the thyroid. The swelling appears in the lower part of the neck and retains the shape of the normal gland (*thyreos* – Greek for shield). The swelling characteristically moves upwards on swallowing because of the gland's attachment to the trachea. Careful observation usually allows this physical sign to be detected during a spontaneous swallow. Patients in consultation are often nervous and have a dry mouth, and to ask them to swallow repeatedly is unnecessary unless water can be provided.

'Physiological' enlargement

Transient enlargement may occur during puberty or pregnancy.

Non-toxic nodular goitre
Aetiology

This common disease occurs endemically in areas of iodine deficiency, but can be sporadic or a reaction to drugs. It occurs much more commonly in females. In the past lack of iodine in the diet was a common cause of thyroid enlargement, but 'endemic goitres' in areas such as Wales and Derbyshire are now rare because table salt is iodized. In areas of the world where iodine intake cannot be guaranteed, iodized oil emulsion can be injected.

Pathology

In iodine deficiency the gland initially enlarges diffusely as the follicles fill with colloid. Later, multiple nodules develop, some of which contain abundant colloid whereas others show degenerative changes, with the formation of cysts, areas of old and new haemorrhage, and even calcification. The goitre varies greatly in size, from little more than normal to weighing several hundred grams. The whole gland may be involved, or the changes may be confined to one lobe.

Clinical features

Most multinodular goitres are asymptomatic. Others cause tracheal compression and dyspnoea, particularly when they extend behind the sternum (retrosternal goitre). Oesophageal compression can cause dysphagia. Very rarely, bleeding into a nodule may cause pain and rapid enlargement and, in the case of retrosternal goitre, respiratory distress. The thyroid is visibly enlarged and multiple nodules are usually palpable (Fig. 26.4). Sometimes only one nodule is palpable, giving the erroneous impression of a solitary nodule.

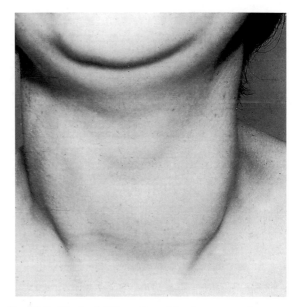

Fig. 26.4 Marked diffuse thyroid enlargement in a female patient with multinodular disease.

Investigations

In the case of retrosternal goitre plain films of the thoracic inlet may reveal tracheal deviation (Fig. 26.5). Only a CT scan will show tracheal compression. The presence of

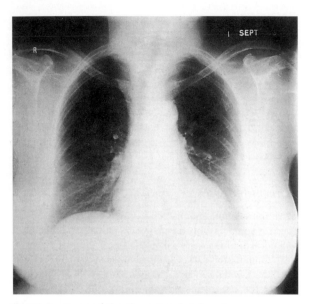

Fig. 26.5 X-ray of the thoracic inlet showing a retrosternal goitre with marked deviation of the trachea to the right.

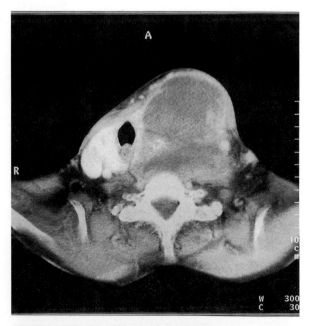

Fig. 26.6 CT scan of the neck of an 80-year-old woman with massive enlargement of the left thyroid lobe, causing marked tracheal deviation and narrowing.

stridor should alert the physician to the presence of compromise of the tracheal lumen (Fig. 26.6). T_3, T_4 and TSH are usually normal. Isotope scans are usually unhelpful.

Treatment

The administration of thyroxine occasionally prevents further enlargement by suppressing TSH secretion, but regression of the goitre is unusual. Large goitres and those causing symptoms of compression require total or subtotal thyroidectomy. Some patients request surgery for cosmetic reasons. If the gland is not functioning normally, the risk of hypothyroidism following operation is greater than after resection for thyrotoxicosis. Thyroxine may be used postoperatively to suppress TSH secretion and prevent the enlargement of any residual gland. Patients may be willing to accept total thyroidectomy and lifelong replacement therapy as preferable to the chance of recurrence and the need for reoperation.

Thyrotoxic goitre

Diffuse thyroid enlargement can result from stimulation by TSH or TSH-like proteins, resulting in increased production of T_3 and T_4 and thyrotoxicosis. However, most goitres occur in individuals who have normal function. The combination of goitre and hyperfunction is an indication for surgical treatment.

Thyroiditis

Subacute thyroiditis (De Quervain's disease)

This rare condition is associated with a flu-like illness during which there is painful diffuse swelling of the gland. Thyroid antibodies may appear in the serum. The disease may be due to a viral infection and usually resolves, although occasionally it runs an intermittent course.

Autoimmune thyroiditis (Hashimoto's disease)

Aetiology This condition is believed to be due to the destruction of thyroid follicles by immunocompetent lymphocytes. Antibodies are detected in the serum against thyroglobulin, thyroid cell cytosol and microsomes. Histologically, there is marked lymphocytic infiltration around destroyed follicles.

Clinical features The patient is usually euthyroid, but thyrotoxicosis can occur. In the long term the patient becomes hypothyroid. Postmenopausal women are most commonly affected (female:male ratio 10:1). The thyroid is diffusely enlarged and firm. A nodular form may be confused with multinodular goitre. Lymphoma may occur in a thyroid that has been affected by long-standing Hashimoto's disease.

Investigation The diagnosis depends on demonstrating high titres of circulating antithyroid antibodies, particularly to microsomal components of the follicle cells. Biopsy for cytology helps to confirm the diagnosis.

Treatment Thyroxine causes regression of small goitres, but subtotal thyroidectomy is needed when a large goitre is causing compression symptoms. Surgery can be difficult because of the firm nature of the gland and inflammation of the surrounding structures. There is a higher than normal risk of damage to the recurrent laryngeal nerves or parathyroid glands.

Riedel's thyroiditis

In this very rare condition the thyroid is replaced by dense fibrous tissue, resulting in a firm painless swelling and tracheal compression. The cause is unknown. Surgical decompression of the trachea may be required.

Solitary thyroid nodules

Slow-growing and painless 'solitary' nodules are common, although 50% of them are really part of a multinodular goitre. Of the true solitary nodules, half are benign adenomas and the rest are cysts or differentiated cancers. The pivotal diagnostic test is fine-needle aspiration cytology, complemented by ultrasonography, isotope scans and thyroid function tests (Fig. 26.7). Tru-cut biopsy can cause bleeding or nerve damage and is no longer used. Cysts can be aspirated and, provided that they do not refill, and that the cytology is negative for neoplastic cells, they need not be removed. Very rarely a cyst contains a carcinoma (often papillary) within its wall, and bloodstained aspirate or a residual swelling after aspiration should raise this possibility. A cytopathologist cannot distinguish between a follicular adenoma and follicular carcinoma: this can only be achieved on definitive histopathology by looking for capsular or vascular invasion. Surgery is needed if aspiration reveals a follicular neoplasm. Intraoperative frozen section does not always provide a definitive diagnosis, but the demonstration of carcinoma means that more extensive surgery is needed. In some patients carcinoma is only revealed on definitive histopathological examination, and reoperation may then be indicated.

Other forms of neoplasia

All forms of thyroid cancer can produce a goitre. Lymphoma and anaplastic tumours may cause diffuse thyroid swellings. Medullary and follicular tumours are often solitary swellings.

HYPERTHYROIDISM

Thyrotoxicosis results from the overproduction of T_3 and T_4 and, because of the feedback mechanism, serum TSH

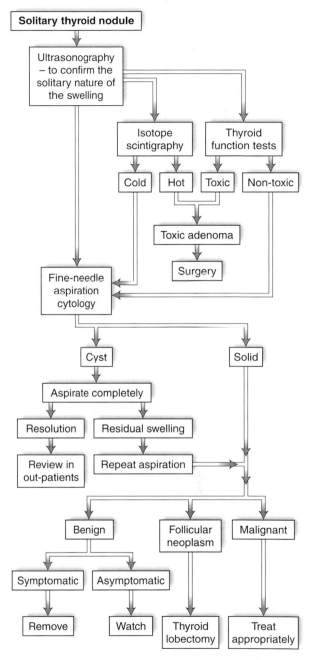

Fig. 26.7 Algorithm for the management of a patient with a suspected solitary thyroid nodule.

levels are reduced or undetectable. The three conditions that may produce thyrotoxicosis are primary thyrotoxicosis (Graves' disease), toxic multinodular goitre and toxic adenoma.

Primary thyrotoxicosis (Graves' disease)

Pathophysiology

This condition accounts for 75% of cases. It is an autoimmune disease in which TSH receptors in the thyroid are stimulated by circulating thyroid-stimulating immunoglobulins (TSI). The gland is uniformly hyperactive, very vascular and usually symmetrically enlarged, although not to a great degree. Histologically there is marked epithelial proliferation, with papillary projections into follicles devoid of colloid. TSI can cross the placental barrier, so that neonatal thyrotoxicosis can occur.

Clinical features

The patient is usually a young female (male: female ratio 1:8) and the condition can be familial. The thyroid is usually moderately and diffusely enlarged and soft and because of its vascularity a bruit may be audible. High circulating levels of T_3 and T_4 increase the basal metabolic rate and potentiate the actions of the sympathetic nervous system.

Metabolic effects The patient feels hot at rest and is intolerant of warmth. The skin is moist and warm because of peripheral vasodilatation and excess sweating. Weight loss is the rule, despite an increased appetite. Cardiac output is increased to meet the metabolic demands.

Sympathetic effects Tachycardia is present even during sleep. Palpitations can be troublesome, and cardiac irregularities and arrhythmias (especially atrial fibrillation) are common in older patients. The hands exhibit a fine tremor. The upper eyelids are retracted (the levator palpebrae superioris has some non-striated muscle which is innervated by the sympathetic nervous system) and there is lid lag. Gastrointestinal motility is increased. There is general hyperkinesia; anxiety and psychiatric disturbance may occur.

Other features Exophthalmos is usual but not invariable. Ophthalmoplegia, pretibial myxoedema, proximal muscle myopathy and finger clubbing are sometimes present. Menstrual irregularity and relative infertility can occur.

Diagnosis

The diagnosis is usually obvious clinically, although in patients with anxiety, distinction from neurosis can be difficult. Raised T_3 and T_4 levels, coupled with low TSH levels, are confirmatory. The TSH response to intravenous injection of TRH is absent owing to atrophy of the TSH-producing cells of the pituitary.

Treatment

Antithyroid drugs These drugs block the incorporation of iodine into tyrosine and so prevent the synthesis of T_3 and T_4. Carbimazole, given in full blocking doses (30–60 mg daily in four divided doses), can render the patient euthyroid within 4–6 weeks. Maintenance doses (5–15 mg daily) can then be used. If full blockade has to continue, T_3 (liothyronine sodium 10–20 g daily, increasing at weekly intervals to 60 g daily in divided doses) or T_4 (100 µg thyroxine daily) is added to provide hormone replacement. As primary thyrotoxicosis is likely to remit, carbimazole is normally stopped after 12–18 months. However, 60–70% of patients will relapse within 2 years of stopping treatment. Compliance may be low and sensitivity reactions (skin rash, gastrointestinal upset and agranulocytosis) can occur. Although radioactive iodine therapy or surgery have to be considered as second-line treatments, medical control is essential once relapse occurs.

Radioactive iodine Many consider this to be the treatment of choice. As long as it is not used in pregnancy, the risks of genetic damage are minimal in both patients and their offspring. If ablative doses of iodine are used, patients require thyroxine replacement, but can lead an otherwise normal life with little risk of recurrence.

Surgery Subtotal thyroidectomy is a highly successful form of treatment for many, especially younger, patients. In experienced hands operative mortality and morbidity are low. Patients may be cured by surgery, and recurrence is usually due to the removal of insufficient glandular tissue. Hypothyroidism occurs in 50% or more of patients, and low T_3 and T_4 levels with high TSH levels persisting for more than 6 months signals the need for lifelong thyroid hormone replacement.

Before surgery patients must be rendered euthyroid with antithyroid drugs. Iodine can be given before surgery to reduce vascularity. β-Adrenergic blocking drugs can be used as an alternative means of countering the effects of thyrotoxicosis before operation. They block sympathetic overactivity and make the gland less vascular. Cardiac failure, obstructive airways disease and diabetes (where they may mask hypoglycaemic symptoms) are contraindications to the use of β-blockers. Propranolol is given in a dose of 40–80 mg every 6 hours, the aim being to reduce the pulse rate below 80 beats per minute (bpm). Long acting preparations may be preferred. The drug is continued on the morning of operation and for 7 days thereafter to avoid 'thyroid storm' or 'thyrotoxic crisis'. Excessive sweating or tachycardia after operation is an indication to increase the dose.

Toxic multinodular goitre and toxic adenoma

Pathophysiology

A toxic multinodular goitre is responsible for thyrotoxicosis in about 25% of patients. There is usually a long-standing non-toxic goitre in which one or more nodules become hyperactive and begin to function independently of TSH levels. A single functioning adenoma is a rare cause of thyrotoxicosis (1–2% of patients). The adenoma secretes thyroid hormones autonomously, TSH secretion is completely suppressed, and the remainder of the gland is non-functional.

Clinical features

Toxic multinodular goitre is commoner in older women and cardiac complications such as arrhythmias are particularly frequent. Exophthalmos is rare. Patients with a toxic adenoma hardly ever have exophthalmos, ophthalmoplegia or myopathy.

Diagnosis

In a toxic multinodular goitre the isotope scan demonstrates one or more areas of increased uptake. In toxic adenoma the nodule is 'hot' and the remainder of the gland is 'cold'.

Treatment

Treatment consists of removal of the hyperfunctioning glandular tissue by subtotal thyroidectomy (multinodular goitre) or lobectomy (toxic adenoma).

MALIGNANT TUMOURS OF THE THYROID

Thyroid cancer accounts for less than 1% of all forms of malignancy. As with all thyroid disease, females are more often affected (male:female ratio 1:3). The two main types of thyroid carcinoma are papillary (50%) and follicular (30%), with the remainder comprising medullary carcinoma, anaplastic carcinoma and lymphoma. The incidence of thyroid cancer is increased by exposure to ionizing radiation, for example following the Chernobyl disaster.

Papillary carcinoma

Clinical features

This tumour is rare after the age of 40 years and presents as a slow-growing solitary thyroid swelling which is not particularly hard. Enlarged lymph nodes are palpable in one-third of patients and may be the only finding in some patients with a microscopic primary (a situation once misinterpreted as a 'lateral aberrant thyroid'). Distant metastases are rare. Occasionally, papillary carcinoma is discovered as an incidental finding in a gland that has been removed for other reasons. Histologically, complex papillary folds lined by several layers of cuboidal cells project into what appear to be cystic spaces.

Treatment

The disease is commonly multifocal, so that total or near-total thyroidectomy is indicated. Involved lymph nodes are removed but radical neck dissection is unnecessary. Hormone replacement therapy (T_3, 20 g three or four times a day, or thyroxine 100 µg/day) is given and its adequacy monitored by measuring TSH. Widespread metastases are rare but may be amenable to radioactive iodine therapy. The disease has an excellent prognosis, with 10-year survival rates approaching 90%.

Follicular carcinoma

Clinical features

This disease typically presents as a solitary thyroid nodule in patients aged 30–50 years. Lymph node metastases are much less common than haematogenous spread, and 20% of patients have deposits in the lungs, bone or liver. Histologically, malignant cells are arranged in solid masses with rudimentary acini. Vascular and capsular invasion characterize this neoplasm and distinguish it from a benign follicular adenoma.

Treatment

Treatment consists of total thyroidectomy with preservation of the parathyroids. All palpable lymph nodes are removed. If a postoperative radioisotope scan (tracer dose) reveals increased uptake in the skeleton or neck, therapeutic doses of radioiodine are given. T_3 is administered routinely to suppress TSH secretion. Plasma thyroglobulin levels should be undetectable after surgery and radioiodine therapy. Subsequent detection of thyroglobulin indicates recurrent disease. The disease is more aggressive than papillary carcinoma and the 10-year survival rate is 50%.

Anaplastic carcinoma

Clinical features

These rapidly growing, highly malignant tumours tend to occur in older patients. Local invasion may involve the recurrent laryngeal nerve(s) and cause hoarseness, compress the trachea and cause dyspnoea and stridor, and/or compress the oesophagus and cause dysphagia. Invasion of the cervical sympathetic nerves may cause Horner's syndrome (contraction of the pupil, enopthalmos, narrowing of the palpebral fissure and loss of sweating on the face and neck). Pulmonary metastases are common. Death usually occurs within 6 months of diagnosis.

Treatment

Resection is rarely possible but surgery can relieve tracheal compression. Radiotherapy and chemotherapy are of marginal value.

Medullary carcinoma

Clinical features

This tumour arises from the parafollicular C cells. There is hard enlargement of one or both thyroid lobes, and in 50% of patients the cervical lymph nodes are involved. The tumour may occur sporadically or as part of an inherited multiple endocrine neoplasia (MEN) syndrome type II (Sipple's syndrome). Calcitonin levels are elevated, although the serum calcium remains normal. Calcitonin can be used to monitor progress and to screen relatives. The gene causing the inherited form of this tumour is now identified as a *Ret* proto-oncogene, and the finding of this mutation allows the diagnosis to be made at any age. Prophylactic thyroidectomy for affected children is recommended from the age of 5 years.

Treatment

Treatment consists of total thyroidectomy and dissection of the lymph nodes in the central compartment of the neck. Medullary carcinoma in MEN IIb syndrome is particularly aggressive, and those affected rarely live beyond 30–40 years of age. Other forms, for example pure inherited medullary thyroid cancer occurring without other endocrine tumours, can be very indolent.

Lymphoma

Primary lymphoma of the thyroid is a rare complication of autoimmune thyroiditis. It can also occur as a primary tumour that originates in an otherwise normal gland. It is amenable to treatment by radiotherapy and chemotherapy, but patients often require an open biopsy of the gland to characterize the type of lymphoma. CT scanning is used to stage the disease fully.

SUMMARY BOX

Thyroid cancer

- Thyroid cancers may arise from the epithelium (papillary 50% or follicular 30%). Anaplastic parafollicular C cells (medullary carcinoma) or lymphoreticular tissue (lymphoma) make up the other tumours of the gland.

- Papillary cancers are rare after the age of 40 years, are often multifocal and spread to lymph nodes, but rarely disseminate widely. Total or near-total thyroidectomy with the removal of involved nodes is followed by T_4 replacement therapy. 10-year survival rates approach 90%.

- Follicular carcinoma occurs in the 30–50-year age group, spreads preferentially via the bloodstream, and is treated by total thyroidectomy. Involved nodes require removal, and residual neck or skeletal radioisotope uptake signals the need for radioiodine therapy. T_4 is used routinely to suppress TSH production. The 10-year survival rate is 50%.

- Anaplastic carcinoma occurs in older patients, spreads locally and frequently gives rise to pulmonary metastases. Curative resection is rarely possible, radiotherapy/chemotherapy are of little value, and most patients die within 1 year.

- Medullary carcinomas secrete calcitonin, may involve both lobes, and involve neck nodes. They may be sporadic or part of MEN II. Treatment consists of total thyroidectomy and node dissection, and prognosis can be poor.

THYROIDECTOMY

Technique

The gland is exposed through a transverse skin-crease incision placed 2–3 cm above the sternal notch. The deep cervical fascia is divided longitudinally in the midline and the strap muscles are separated. Each lobe is mobilized by dividing first the vessels supplying the superior pole, then the middle and inferior thyroid veins, and finally the inferior thyroid artery. The recurrent laryngeal nerves should be identified so that they can be protected from injury. The amount of thyroid tissue removed depends on the indication for operation. Care is taken to preserve the parathyroid glands. Haemostasis must be meticulous and drains are unnecessary. The layers of the neck are reconstituted with interrupted absorbable sutures and the skin is approximated with skin clips, a subcuticular suture or steristrips. Skin clips and steristrips can be removed on the second postoperative day. Minimally invasive techniques are being explored as a means of performing thyroidectomy, but at present the procedure takes an inordinate time using complex, expensive equipment, and there is no advantage to be gained.

Complications

Haemorrhage

Early secondary haemorrhage should not occur if meticulous haemostasis is achieved before closure. If bleeding does occur it can compress structures in the thoracic inlet, leading to venous engorgement, tracheal compression and asphyxia. The wound must be reopened urgently and the patient intubated and taken back to theatre for exploration of the wound, removal of haematoma and control of bleeding.

Nerve damage

The external branch of the superior laryngeal nerve may be damaged during ligation of the vascular pedicle at the upper pole of the thyroid. Inability to tense the vocal cord results in a weak, hoarse deep voice. Anaesthesia of the mucous membrane of the upper larynx allows foreign bodies to enter the larynx more readily. Damage to the recurrent laryngeal nerve is more serious. Traction or bruising of this nerve causes temporary paralysis of a vocal cord in 5% of patients undergoing thyroidectomy, but recovery within 3 months is the rule. Division of the nerve paralyses the cord in the 'cadaveric' position (i.e. midway between the closed and open positions). The normal cord on the other side compensates by crossing the midline in phonation, but the voice is altered in timbre and weak. Some degree of stridor, especially on exertion, may be noted.

Bilateral nerve injury results in stridor and ineffective coughing when the endotracheal tube is withdrawn at the end of the operation. The tube is reinserted immediately and, if there is no early improvement, tracheostomy may be required. The paralysis is originally flaccid, but fibrosis draws the cords together and, even if tracheostomy has been avoided, increasing dyspnoea on exertion may be troublesome. Laryngoplasty may be needed to reconstitute the cords, but if this fails permanent tracheostomy may be unavoidable.

The vocal cords must be examined to document their position and movement before and immediately after thyroid surgery, for medicolegal reasons. Sometimes an asymptomatic paralysis predates surgery: this would have very significant consequences if the opposite nerve were to be damaged.

Hypothyroidism

Thyroid function is monitored after surgery in case replacement therapy is needed. The risk of hypothyroidism depends on the type of disease and extent of surgery. After total thyroidectomy replacement therapy may commence the following day. A standard dose for adults is 100 µg thyroxine daily, adjusted according to clinical findings and thyroid function tests.

Hypoparathyroidism

Bruising or accidental removal of the parathyroid glands leads to hypoparathyroidism, manifest by hypocalcaemia and symptoms of increased neuromuscular excitability. Early symptoms are tingling or numbness around the mouth and in the fingers. Hypercontractility can be demonstrated in the muscles of facial expression by tapping the facial (VII) nerve over the parotid gland (Chvostek's sign). In extreme cases tetany may develop. Serum calcium must be checked 24 hours after thyroid surgery. Hypocalcaemic symptoms, or a serum calcium less than 2.0 mmol/L, require calcium supplements. Severe hypoparathyroidism may require vitamin D as well. Serum calcium checks are required, with gradual withdrawal of supplements as the parathyroids recover. If supplementation is still necessary at 12 months then the patient is likely to require lifelong treatment.

Scar complications

The scar can become hypertrophic or keloid, particularly when the incision has been placed low in the neck. Recurrent keloid formation is common after excision of the scar (with or without steroid infiltration), and reoperation is not advised lightly.

Informed consent

A forewarned patient is much less aggrieved than one who learns about previously unmentioned complications on the first postoperative day. Full informed consent should describe the potential complications and should be obtained by the surgeon who will carry out the procedure. Surgeons should be able to provide patients with their own complication rates, and how these compare with national averages. It is important to couch the advice in readily understood terms. Remember that the patient is unlikely to have heard of the parathyroid glands, let alone know what they do. The starting point must certainly be at the beginning, and in simple language. The advice must be full and honest, but without frightening the patient. Written advice may be provided for reading and digestion at home. The patient may be well informed, having 'surfed' the Internet, or may have obtained totally inaccurate and inappropriate information from this source.

PARATHYROID GLANDS

Surgical anatomy

The development of the parathyroid glands was considered earlier in the chapter. These glands receive a rich blood supply from the inferior thyroid artery, the branches of which are a valuable guide to their position. Histologically, the glands contain chief cells (classified as dark, light and water clear) which secrete parathormone (PTH). After the age of 5–7 years eosinophilic cells appear; their function is unknown.

Calcium metabolism

Plasma calcium levels are kept constant in the range 2.25–2.6 mmol/L by regulating the amounts absorbed from the intestine, deposited in or withdrawn from bone, and excreted in the urine. PTH and vitamin D are the main regulators, with minimal modulation by calcitonin.

Parathormone

PTH is an 84 amino acid polypeptide hormone. Its secretion is controlled by the level of ionized calcium in the plasma. This fraction normally makes up 50% of the total plasma calcium; the remainder is protein bound and not directly available. PTH:

1. Mobilizes calcium from bone by stimulating osteoclastic activity
2. Increases renal phosphate excretion and calcium reabsorption

3. Promotes renal conversion of less active forms of vitamin D to the highly active form 1,25-dihydroxy-cholecalciferol.

However, when there is excessive PTH secretion (hyperparathyroidism) the resulting hypercalaemia is associated with an increased urinary excretion of calcium, which predisposes to renal stone formation.

Vitamin D

The active form of vitamin D is 1,25-dihydroxycholecalciferol, which:

1. Promotes calcium absorption from the intestine
2. Augments the effects of PTH on osteoclasts.

Calcitonin

Calcitonin inhibits osteoclast activity. It may be used to treat conditions such as Paget's disease. It is doubtful whether it is significantly involved in normal calcium homeostasis for, although production increases in medullary carcinoma of the thyroid, hypocalcaemia does not occur.

Hypercalcaemia and hypocalcaemia

Hypercalcaemia is a common biochemical abnormality and may be due to many causes other than excess PTH secretion (Table 26.1). Similarly, hypocalcaemia may be due to causes other than parathyroid removal or damage (Table 26.2).

Primary hyperparathyroidism

Pathology

In 90% of patients primary hyperparathyroidism is due to an adenoma, in 10% it results from hyperplasia (usually

Table 26.1   Causes of hypercalcaemia
Hyperparathyroidism
Primary
Secondary
Tertiary
Increased calcium absorption
Vitamin D excess
Sarcoidosis
Drugs (e.g. diuretics, lithium)
Excessive bone breakdown
Metastatic disease (particularly breast cancer)
Myeloma
Immobilization following multiple fractures
Ectopic secretion of PTH-like hormone
Cancer of bronchus
Cancer of breast

Table 26.2	Causes of hypocalcaemia

Hypoparathyroidism
  Thyroid surgery
  Parathyroid surgery
Hypoproteinaemia
  Nephrosis (excessive protein loss)
  Malnutrition (inadequate intake)
  Cirrhosis (deficient synthesis)
  Severe inflammation (e.g. burns, acute
  pancreatitis)
Vitamin D deficiency
Pseudohypoparathyroidism

affecting all four glands), and in less than 1% it results from parathyroid carcinoma. Adenomas are normally small spherical brown nodules but can be 10 times larger than the normal gland (Fig. 26.8). Most are single, but 20% of patients have multiple adenomas. Histologically there is a mixed pattern of cells in which chief cells predominate. Hyperplasia is due to an increase in the number of chief cells and, by definition, the gland must be at least twice the upper limit of normal, that is, weigh more than 70 mg.

Clinical features

Women are affected twice as often as men. The disease usually presents in middle age and is increasingly being diagnosed in asymptomatic patients who happen to be found to have hypercalcaemia on routine biochemical estimations. If clinical manifestations occur, renal and bone effects predominate. Renal effects include nephrocalcinosis (speckled calcification) and the formation of urinary calculi owing to increased excretion of calcium and phosphate.

Polyuria is an early sign of hyperparathyroidism. Serum calcium levels must be checked repeatedly in all patients with urinary calculi, especially if recurrent, if hyperparathyroidism is to be diagnosed in time to avoid renal damage.

Bone damage used to be common but is now rarely seen as the disease is diagnosed earlier. Gross demineralization, subperiosteal bone resorption (seen typically in the middle and distal phalanges of the fingers), cysts in the long bones and jaw, and the moth-eaten appearance of the skull gave rise to the descriptive term 'osteitis fibrosa cystica' (Fig. 26.9). Multiple pathological fractures were also once common.

Other manifestations of hyperparathyroidism include peptic ulceration, acute and chronic pancreatitis, lethargy, muscle weakness and psychotic symptoms. The clinical picture of florid hyperparathyroidism is often summarized as one of 'bones, stones and groans'. Rarely, patients present with a hypercalcaemic crisis characterized by marked hypercalcaemia (> 3.5 mmol/L), mental confusion, nausea and vomiting. The vomiting increases pre-existing dehydration, leading to higher levels of serum calcium, more confusion and prostration, more dehydration, and so on. Urgent expert attention is required to reverse this vicious downward spiral. The most pressing need is to correct the dehydration. The calcium may be further reduced by the use of diphosphonates.

Diagnosis

If hyperparathyroidism is suspected, serum calcium and PTH levels must be measured on more than one occasion. PTH levels may be normal, but the detection of PTH in a patient

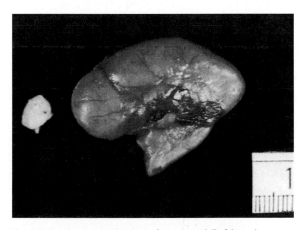

Fig. 26.8 Gross specimens of a normal (left) and adenomatous parathyroid gland (next to the scale). A normal parathyroid should weigh only 45 mg and be 3–4 mm in size.

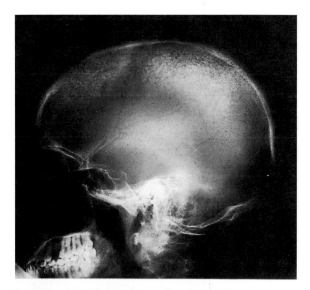

Fig. 26.9 Lateral skull X-ray of patient with hyperparathyroidism showing lytic lesions of osteitis fibrosa cystica.

with hypercalcaemia supports the diagnosis of primary hyper-parathyroidism. Other supportive findings include a low serum phosphate, hyperchloraemia (and an abnormal Cl/PO_4 ratio), and a raised 24-hour urinary calcium excretion. A low urinary calcium excretion should alert the clinician to the possibility of familial hypercalcaemic hypocalciuria, a disease of the renal tubules in which the parathyroids are normal. Alkaline phosphatase (skeletal) levels may be raised even if there is no radiological evidence of bone disease.

Treatment

The aim of treatment is to identify and remove overactive parathyroid tissue. The surgical approach is similar to that used for thyroidectomy. Each lobe of the thyroid is mobilized, and all four glands must be identified and inspected. Normal parathyroids are smooth and brownish-tan in colour. They are small, especially if suppressed by overproduction of PTH from an adenoma. Enlarged glands are nodular. Immediate frozen section examination is used to establish the diagnosis and make certain that parathyroid, rather than thyroid, thymus or fat, has been identified and removed.

Various methods have been used to localize abnormal glands in an attempt to make surgical exploration more efficient. These include ultrasonography, CT, MRI, isotope scintigraphy, arteriography and selective venous sampling for PTH assays. However, none is capable of bettering the results of bilateral neck exploration by an experienced parathyroid surgeon. As in thyroid surgery, some have used minimally invasive techniques to explore the neck and are willing to accept the less than satisfactory localization procedures to direct exploration to one or other side. The advantages to this approach are not apparent, as current methods of treatment are efficient, effective, and cause little morbidity.

In the majority of patients only one gland is enlarged and this is removed. If two or more glands are enlarged they should be removed. If all four glands are thought to be hyperplastic then all but a portion of one gland should be removed. The integrity of the recurrent laryngeal nerves must be assured. If exploration fails to identify an adenoma or hyperplasia, the incision is closed. Reoperation is considered after (re)confirming the diagnosis and attempting to localize the gland by thallium–technetium scan or Sestamibi scintigraphy (Fig. 26.10), MRI scans or selective venous catheterization with PTH measurement. Recurrent hyper-parathyroidism is approached in the same way.

SUMMARY BOX

Hyperparathyroidism

- Serum calcium levels are normally controlled by parathormone (mobilizes calcium from bone and increases renal calcium absorption and phosphate excretion) and vitamin D (promotes absorption from the intestine and augments effect of PTH on osteoclasts), with an uncertain contribution from calcitonin.

- Hyperparathyroidism may be primary (90% adenoma, 10% hyperplasia, 1% carcinoma), secondary to renal disease/malabsorption (low serum Ca^{2+} triggers PTH secretion) or tertiary (development of autonomous secretion in secondary hyperparathyroidism).

- Hyperparathyroidism is now normally diagnosed while asymptomatic, but can produce renal effects (nephrocalcinosis, calculi and failure), skeletal effects (demineralization), gastrointestinal upsets (peptic ulcer, pancreatitis) and psychotic symptoms, i.e. 'stones, bones and groans'.

- The diagnosis of primary hyperparathyroidism is supported by detection of circulating PTH in the presence of hypercalcaemia.

- Primary hyperparathyroidism is treated surgically by displaying all four glands and removing a gland enlarged by adenoma formation. If all four glands are involved by hyperplasia, all but a portion of one gland is removed.

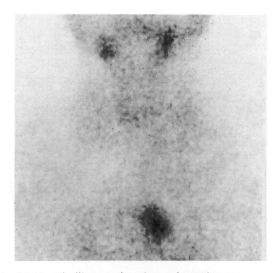

Fig. 26.10 Thallium–technetium subtraction scan showing excess thallium uptake in a mediastinal parathyroid adenoma.

Secondary and tertiary hyperparathyroidism

In secondary hyperparathyroidism there is oversecretion of PTH in response to low plasma levels of ionized calcium, usually because of renal disease or malabsorption. This is an increasing problem in patients on long-term dialysis for chronic renal failure. It is managed initially by giving 1-α-hydroxyvitamin D_3 (alfacalcidol) to increase calcium absorption and provide negative feedback on the parathyroids.

Excessive PTH secretion in secondary hyperparathyroidism may become autonomous: it is then termed tertiary hyperparathyroidism. This may occur after renal transplantation. Total parathyroidectomy may be needed, with autotransplantation of parathyroid tissue (equivalent in size to one normal gland) into an arm muscle (where it can be readily located if problems persist). Postoperatively, alfacalcidol and calcium are continued to heal bone disease and reduce the risk of recurrent hyperparathyroidism.

Hypoparathyroidism

Hypoparathyroidism may occur temporarily after parathyroidectomy until the suppressed residual glands assume normal function. A fall in ionized calcium levels gives rise to paraesthesiae ('pins and needles') in the hands and feet, and muscle cramps and spasms (tetany) which cause bunching and flexion of the fingers and toes. Respiratory obstruction with stridor due to spasm of the laryngeal muscles can prove fatal. Clinical signs include Chvostek's sign (twitching of the facial muscles on tapping of the facial nerve), Trousseau's sign (spasm of hand and forearm muscles after applying a tourniquet to occlude the pulse), and Erb's sign (hyperexcitability of muscles on electrical stimulation). The patient is lethargic and depressed. Blood levels of ionized calcium and PTH are low, and the electrocardiogram (ECG) shows a lengthened Q-T interval. Acute hypoparathyroidism is treated by intravenous calcium gluconate (20 mL of a 10% solution given 4-hourly until calcium levels rise). Oral calcium (effervescent calcium gluconate) and vitamin D (cholecalciferol 20 000 units daily) are prescribed for maintenance. Calcium levels must be monitored regularly.

Patient information

Patients may have heard of the thyroid gland and might have some understanding of its function. However, because parathyroid disease is rare, patients will not have heard of these glands and will have no understanding of their function. In providing informed consent it is important that patients understand several aspects about the glands and the disease; specifically:

- The variable position of the glands
- The function of the glands
- The results of hyperfunction: renal effects, bone disease and systemic effects

- That only one gland is likely to be diseased and over-active, and that this is not cancerous
- That surgery will attempt to remove the abnormal gland but may fail to locate it because it is in an ectopic position
- That there may be a need for calcium and vitamin D supplements after surgery.

PITUITARY GLAND

Surgical anatomy

The pituitary gland is small and weighs about 500 mg. It is enclosed within a bony shell, the sella turcica, which is sealed superiorly by a fold of dura mater, the diaphragma sellae. The pituitary stalk connects the pituitary to the hypothalamus. The pituitary has two parts: the anterior pituitary (adenohypophysis) and the posterior pituitary (neurohypophysis) (Fig. 26.11).

Anterior pituitary

The anterior pituitary develops from an epithelial outgrowth from the pharynx (Rathke's pouch). Some cells are thought to be of neural crest origin and belong to the APUD (amine and precursor uptake and decarboxylation) system. The anterior pituitary contains solid cords of secreting cells that used to be classified as acidophil, basophil or chromophobe on staining with haematoxylin and eosin. On the basis of immunofluorescence and other specific stains these are now subdivided into cell types that secrete:

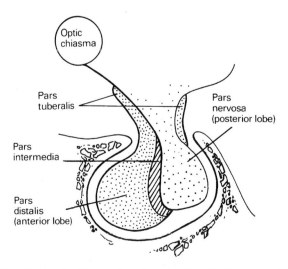

Fig. 26.11 Sagittal section through the pituitary gland.

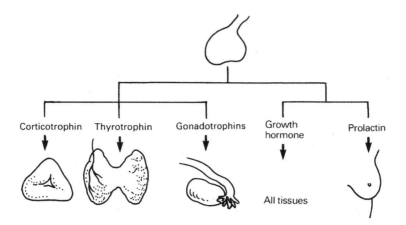

Fig. 26.12   The anterior pituitary hormones and their target organs.

1. The polypeptides: growth hormone (GH), prolactin (PRL) and adrenocorticotrophic hormone (ACTH)
2. The glycoproteins: luteinizing hormone (LH), follicle-stimulating hormone (FSH) and TSH (Fig. 26.12).

The hypophysial stalk contains a portal venous system that connects capillaries in the median eminence of the hypothalamus with capillaries and sinusoids of the anterior pituitary. This system carries neurosecretory hormones that stimulate or inhibit specific endocrine cells in the pituitary. The most important messengers are growth hormone-releasing and -inhibiting factors, corticotrophin-releasing factor (CRF), gonadotrophin-releasing hormone (GnRH), TRH and prolactin-inhibiting factor (PIF). If the portal tract is divided the secretion of all anterior pituitary hormones is suppressed, with the exception of prolactin, the secretion of which is increased. A number of feedback loops ensure that the secretion of pituitary hormones is adjusted to need.

Growth hormone GH has many functions besides growth regulation. It increases the uptake of amino acids, promotes protein synthesis and increases the size of muscles and viscera. Lipolysis is increased and utilization of fatty acids is enhanced, with the production of ketosis. It has an anti-insulin effect (increased gluconeogenesis and decreased peripheral utilization of glucose) and in large amounts it augments milk secretion. Some of its growth-promoting effects are due to increased secretion of somatomedin from the liver and kidney. Growth hormone release is stimulated by stress, fasting and hypoglycaemia, and inhibited by bromocriptine and phenothiazines, for example chlorpromazine.

Prolactin PRL is normally secreted in only small amounts and levels are highest at night. Secretion increases greatly in pregnancy, and PRL is essential for the lobuloalveolar development of the breast and the initiation of lactation. Release is increased by stress, oestradiol and phenothiazines, and inhibited by L-dopa and bromocriptine.

Corticotrophin (ACTH) This is a 39 amino acid polypeptide that shares a 4–10 amino acid sequence with melanocyte-stimulating hormone (MSH), which partly accounts for the pigmentation associated with excess ACTH production. ACTH is secreted as part of a larger molecule with three constituents: pro-γ-ACTH, ACTH and β-lipoprotein (LPH). Pro-γ-ACTH is thought to sensitize the adrenal cells to ACTH, whereas LPH mobilizes fat (and, by virtue of amino acid sequences shared with metencephalin and β-endorphin, it may bind to opiate receptors and have analgesic properties). ACTH itself stimulates the secretion of cortisol and adrenal androgens by the adrenal cortex. ACTH secretion is stimulated by CRF, which in turn is secreted in response to stress.

Glycoprotein hormones Each has α and β subunits. The α subunit is common to all three, whereas the β subunit is specific and determines the actions of each individual hormone. FSH stimulates follicle development towards the end of the menstrual cycle and the secretion of oestrogens by thecal cells. LH triggers ovulation and promotes formation of the corpus luteum and the secretion of oestrogens and progesterone. In males, FSH stimulates spermatogenesis and LH (known in males as interstitial cell-stimulating hormone) stimulates testosterone secretion by the Leydig cells (Fig. 26.13). TSH promotes thyroid growth and thyroid hormone secretion.

Tumours of the anterior pituitary

Pathophysiology

Functioning pituitary adenomas may result from overstimulation by hypothalamic factors. Initially small and confined within the gland (microadenomas), they grow slowly and can ultimately expand the sella turcica. Eccentric enlargement is common and asymmetry of the pituitary fossa can often be detected by lateral tomograms. Upward extension

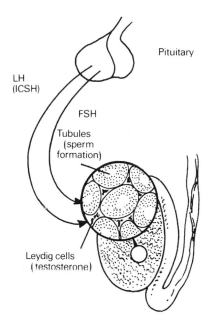

Fig. 26.13 The role of pituitary hormones in the control of male sexual function. ICSH = interstitial cell-stimulating hormone.

of the adenoma may stretch the diaphragm or herniate through it, to compress the optic chiasma and cause visual defects. It is therefore important that pituitary adenomas are detected before they enlarge the fossa or extend above it.

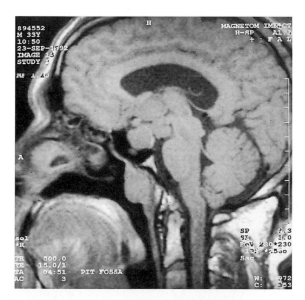

Fig. 26.14 MRI scan showing a pituitary tumour.

CT with contrast enhancement or MRI (Fig. 26.14) can be used to reveal the tumour and delineate its extent. Three endocrine syndromes caused by anterior pituitary disorders have surgical relevance.

Acromegaly

Excess secretion of GH occurs most often in early adult life and results in overgrowth of the soft tissues of the hands, feet and face. This gives the patient 'large extremities' and a characteristically coarse face, with bulging supraorbital ridges and a protruding jaw. Endochondral ossification and periosteal new bone formation account for some of these changes. All viscera are enlarged and there is muscle hypertrophy; although muscle weakness and cardiac failure develop later. The skin is coarse and greasy and acne is common. Headaches, sweating and the carpal tunnel syndrome often develop. Glucose tolerance is impaired and galactorrhoea can occur in females. GH and somatomedin levels are increased and glucose or a meal do not suppress their secretion.

Treatment is directed at restoring GH levels to normal. External radiation achieves this in 70% of patients, but only after 10 years. Radioactive implants act more quickly (see below). For small adenomas trans-sphenoidal removal is the treatment of choice. Although bromocriptine inhibits GH release, it achieves normal levels in only 20% of patients with acromegaly. Somatostatin analogues offer a more effective way of normalizing GH levels and can be used to reduce the size of macroadenomas or to treat recurrent or residual tumour.

Hyperprolactinaemia

Prolactin is the commonest hormone secreted by pituitary tumours. Hypersecretion results in galactorrhoea and amenorrhoea (owing to the suppression of gonadotrophin secretion) in young women, whereas in men gynaecomastia and impotence may occur. Basal levels of prolactin are high, the nocturnal increase is absent, and the response to TRH and metoclopramide is dimished. It is important to exclude other causes of hyperprolactinaemia, notably the administration of drugs such as metoclopramide.

To preserve pituitary function in younger patients, small adenomas are enucleated and larger tumours are treated by bromocriptine, with monitoring to ensure that tumour expansion does not threaten visual integrity.

Cushing's disease

This may be due to a functioning adenoma of ACTH-secreting cells. Only 15% of patients show expansion of the pituitary fossa. Removal of the microadenoma or its irradiation will relieve symptoms. Unsuccessful surgery

SUMMARY BOX

Tumours of the anterior pituitary gland

- The tumour may be detected while still small (microadenoma) or after it has expanded, often with upward extension to compress the optic chiasma.

- The three endocrine syndromes that have surgical importance are acromegaly, hyperprolactinaemia and Cushing's disease.

- Acromegaly is due to excessive secretion of growth hormone (GH). Somatostatin analogues (or bromocriptine) can be used to normalize GH levels, but small adenomas are treated by transsphenoidal removal; radiotherapy (usually by radioactive implants) can be used for larger tumours.

- Hyperprolactinaemia causes galactorrhoea and amenorrhoea in females and impotence and gynaecomastia in men. Small adenomas are usually enucleated, whereas larger tumours are treated by bromocriptine.

- Cushing's disease may result from a functioning adenoma of ACTH-secreting cells, which is treated by removal or irradiation.

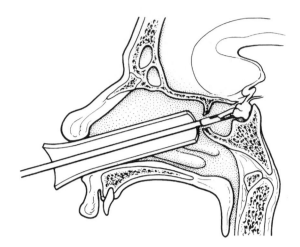

Fig. 26.15 Trans-sphenoidal removal of a pituitary adenoma.

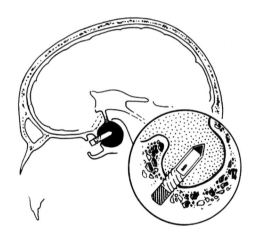

Fig. 26.16 Implantation of radioactive yttrium-90 into the pituitary fossa.

may require bilateral adrenalectomy (removal of end organs) to terminate the syndrome of hypercortisolism, with its widespread destructive systemic effects.

Surgical hypophysectomy

The trans-sphenoidal approach is preferred for the removal of a normal-sized gland or enucleation of a small adenoma. An operating microscope is used to approach the gland through the sphenoidal or ethmoidal sinuses (Fig. 26.15). The pituitary stalk is divided low, so that diabetes insipidus is rare. By placing a free flap of muscle in the fossa, cerebrospinal fluid (CSF) rhinorrhoea is prevented. The transcranial approach is a major neurosurgical procedure that results in loss of sense of smell and the development of diabetes insipidus. It is now reserved for the removal of large tumours with suprasellar extension, often in combination with a trans-sphenoidal approach.

Radiation therapy

External radiation

The pituitary is radioresistant and at least 100 Gy are needed to affect the function of a normal gland. Smaller doses (40–50 Gy) are used to treat acromegaly and Cushing's disease. A rotational technique avoids excessive irradiation of surrounding neural tissue. Larger doses can be delivered by the narrow focused beam of heavy particles that are generated by a cyclotron.

Internal irradiation

Radioactive sources can be implanted, under radiological control, via the trans-sphenoidal or transethmoidal routes (Fig. 26.16), although trans-sphenoidal surgery is now preferred. Yttrium-90 is a β-particle emitter of high energy and short half-life (64 hours) and was once commonly used. Diabetes insipidus followed only if the hypothalamic nuclei were irradiated; CSF rhinorrhoea was an occasional complication.

Maintenance therapy

After total hypophysectomy replacement therapy is required for life, that is, hydrocortisone 20 mg each morning and 10 mg each evening. All episodes of stress or trauma, including hypophysectomy itself, require additional cortisol or cortisone to cover the metabolic response. The patient is advised to wear a band or bracelet advising medical attendants that they are receiving steroid replacement therapy. Aldosterone secretion is unaffected and there is no need for mineralocorticoid replacement. TSH secretion is suppressed and hypothyroidism is avoided by giving thyroxine (0.1–0.2 mg daily). Diabetes insipidus is a common, but often transient, complication of pituitary surgery or the insertion of radioactive implants. Intramuscular injection, or intranasal delivery, of the vasopressin analogue desmopressin (DDAVP) relieves polyuria.

The posterior pituitary

Pathophysiology

The neurohypophysis is part of a secretory and storage unit that includes the nerve cells of the supraoptic and paraventricular hypothalamic nuclei (Fig. 26.17). Fibres pass from these nuclei via the hypothalamo–hypophysial tract to the median eminence of the hypothalamus and posterior pituitary. The nerve cells secrete arginine vasopressin (antidiuretic hormone, ADH) and oxytocin, both of which pass down the nerve fibres to be stored in vesicles in the pituitary. The close anatomical relationship of the anterior and posterior pituitary has functional significance in that oxytocin release during lactation is paralleled by increased TSH and prolactin production, and the posterior pituitary may influence prolactin secretion by dopamine release.

Vasopressin

This hormone increases permeability in the distal tubule, facilitating water reabsorption and reducing plasma osmolality. Its release is governed by osmoreceptors in the hypothalamus and baroreceptors in the heart and great vessels, which react to changes in arterial and venous pressure. Failure of vasopressin secretion results in diabetes insipidus and may follow trauma, irradiation, inflammation or neoplasia. Surgical hypophysectomy causes diabetes insipidus only if the hypothalamic nuclei are irreparably damaged by traction on the pituitary stalk or its high division. Diabetes insipidus produces thirst and polyuria, with the passage of 5–12 litres of dilute urine (osmolality 50–200 mmol/L) every 24 hours. Plasma osmolality is normal (270–290 mmol/L) or slightly increased. It is treated with DDAVP.

Inappropriate vasopressin secretion can occur in patients with bronchial carcinomas or other paraendocrine tumours, and results in hyponatraemia, increased extracellular fluid (ECF) volume and renal loss of sodium. It can also complicate positive-pressure ventilation.

ADRENAL GLAND

Surgical anatomy and development

Each adrenal gland weighs approximately 4 g and lies immediately above and medial to the kidneys. They are not easily accessible to the surgeon. The right adrenal lies in close contact with the inferior vena cava, into which it drains by a short wide vein that can be difficult to ligate at operation. The left adrenal vein drains into the left renal vein (Fig. 26.18). The glands are supplied by small vessels that arise from the aorta and the renal and inferior phrenic arteries.

Each gland has an outer cortex and inner medulla. The cortex, like the gonads, is derived from mesoderm, whereas the medulla is derived from the chromaffin ectodermal cells of the neural crest. The cortex secretes corticosteroids. The medulla is part of the sympathetic nervous system. Its APUD cells secrete the catecholamines adrenaline, noradrenaline and dopamine, and are supplied by preganglionic sympathetic nerves.

Adrenal cortex

Cortical function

Microscopically, the adrenal cortex has three zones (Fig. 26.19). The outer *zona glomerulosa* secretes the

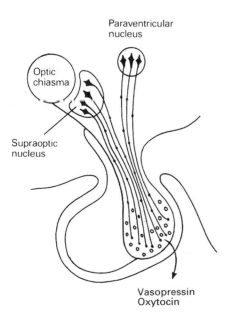

Fig. 26.17 The neurohypophysial system.

(labels: Paraventricular nucleus; Optic chiasma; Supraoptic nucleus; Vasopressin Oxytocin)

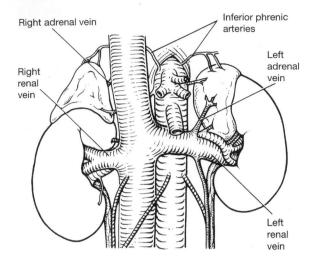

Fig. 26.18   Blood supply and venous drainage of the adrenal glands. IVC = inferior vena cava.

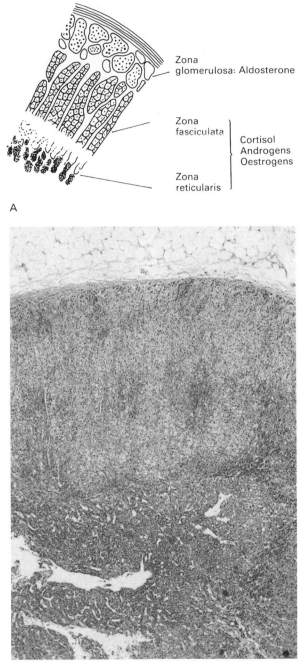

mineralocorticoid aldosterone. The *zona fasciculata* and *zona reticularis* act as a functional unit and secrete glucocorticoids (cortisol and corticosterone), androgenic steroids (androstenedione, 11-hydroxy-androstenedione and testosterone) and the inactive androgen and oestrogen precursor dehydroepiandrosterone sulphate (DHA-S). Precursors of aldosterone are also synthesized by the fasciculata–reticularis zone, as are small amounts of progesterone and oestrogen.

Only a fraction of the amount of hormone needed daily is stored in the cortex. The hormones are, therefore, secreted 'to order' and circulate either free (5%) or bound to α-globulin.

Cortisol   Cortisol secretion (15–20 mg/day) is controlled by pituitary ACTH through a feedback loop (Fig. 26.20). ACTH also stimulates the secretion of androgenic steroids and, if excessive, this can cause virilization. Output of testosterone and androstenedione is normally low while DHA-S output is high.

Cortisol is essential for life and has ill-defined but vital intracellular functions that protect the body against stress, maintain blood pressure and aid recovery from injury and shock. Important metabolic activities include protein breakdown (catabolic effect), increased gluconeogenesis and reduced glucose utilization (diabetogenic effect), and the mobilization and redistribution of fat stores and water. In excess, cortisol has mineralocorticoid activity (promotes the reabsorption of sodium and excretion of potassium) and can cause psychosis and mental instability. It has anti-inflammatory effects and reduces the number of circulating lymphocytes and eosinophils, inhibits fibroblastic activity and depresses antibody formation (effects employed in the

Fig. 26.19   **A** Functional zones of the adrenal cortex. **B** Histology of the normal adrenal gland with the outer cortex (steroid hormones) and central medulla (catecholamines). The cortex is subdivided into three layers, an outer glomerulosa (grape-like) producing mineralocorticoid, an inner fasciculata (bundles), and a reticularis (lattice) producing glucocorticoids and sex steroids.

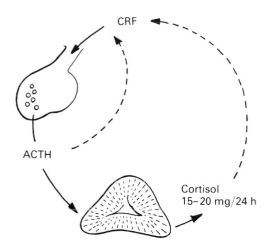

Fig. 26.20 Feedback loop in the control of cortisol secretion. CRF = corticotrophin-releasing factor.

treatment of rejection after organ transplantation and many other immunologically mediated conditions).

Aldosterone Aldosterone is secreted in small amounts (100–200 μg/day) and circulating levels are low. Angiotensin is the main determinant of aldosterone production and is controlled in turn by renin liberated from the juxtaglomerular apparatus of the kidney in response to diminished perfusion (Fig. 26.21). Aldosterone secretion is also influenced by the concentration of sodium and potassium in adrenal blood, and can increase in response to high levels of ACTH

Aldosterone conserves ECF sodium by facilitating its exchange for potassium or hydrogen in the kidney (and to a lesser extent in all cells). In low potassium states the urine may be acid despite extracellular alkalosis, because hydrogen ions are more available for exchange. Sodium retention increases plasma volume, but this is limited by an exchange mechanism that can override the effect of aldosterone.

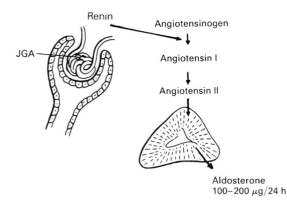

Fig. 26.21 Control of aldosterone secretion by the adrenal cortex. JGA = juxtaglomerular apparatus.

DHA-S This is biologically inactive but is converted in fat, liver and other tissues to testosterone, its 5-α-reduced products and oestrogen. Peripheral aromatization of DHA-S is the main source of oestrogen in postmenopausal women.

SUMMARY BOX

Adrenocortical hormones

- Cortisol secretion is controlled by pituitary ACTH. Cortisol protects against stress, maintains blood pressure and aids recovery from injury/shock. Its metabolic activities include protein breakdown, increased gluconeogenesis, reduced glucose utilization and mobilization/redistribution of fat and water.

- In excess, cortisol has mineralocorticoid activity, can cause psychosis, and has anti-inflammatory effects (used in transplantation immunosuppression).

- Aldosterone secretion is controlled mainly by angiotensin levels (and thus by renin release from the juxtaglomerular apparatus during decreased perfusion).

- Aldosterone conserves sodium (by facilitating its exchange for potassium and hydrogen ions in the kidney) and is a major determinant of ECF conservation.

- Androgenic steroids and dehydroepiandrosterone sulphate (DHA-S) are also secreted by the adrenal cortex. DHA-S is converted to testosterone and oestrogen by fat and liver, and this peripheral aromatization is the main source of oestrogen in postmenopausal women.

Cushing's syndrome

This syndrome was first described by the American neurosurgeon Harvey Cushing. It results from any prolonged and inappropriate exposure to cortisol and has the following causes.

Tumours of the adrenal cortex (20%)

Benign adenoma is the commonest adrenal cause of Cushing's syndrome. It is almost invariably unilateral and is more common in females. Histologically, the tumour contains clear cells like those of the zona fasciculata, or compact cells like those of the zona reticularis. Autonomous cortisol secretion inhibits ACTH production so that the contralateral gland becomes atrophic and ceases to function (Fig. 26.22).

Adrenal carcinoma is a rare cause of Cushing's syndrome that occurs more frequently in young adults and

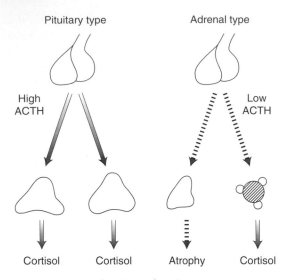

Fig. 26.22 Types of Cushing's syndrome.
A Overstimulation of the normal adrenal glands by excess ACTH. **B** Oversecretion of cortisol by a functioning tumour of the left adrenal gland, leading to suppression of function in the opposite gland.

children. The tumour grows to a large size and has frequently metastasized by the time of presentation.

Pituitary disease (80%)

Pituitary tumours causing Cushing's syndrome are usually basophil or sometimes chromophobe adenomas of ACTH-secreting cells. They range from tiny 'microadenomas' to large and even invasive tumours. Because of the continued ACTH secretion, both adrenals become hyperplastic. When Cushing's syndrome is caused by a pituitary tumour, it is referred to as Cushing's disease.

Ectopic ACTH production

Inappropriate secretion of ACTH-like peptide by tumours of non-pituitary origin (e.g. pancreas, bronchus, thymus) is a rare cause.

Iatrogenic

Cushing's syndrome can be a major side-effect of therapeutic steroid use. Adrenal atrophy occurs if the steroid dosage is considerable and prolonged in duration.

Clinical features

Cushing's syndrome occurs most frequently in young women. The most striking feature is truncal obesity, a 'buffalo hump' (due to redistribution of water and fat) and 'mooning' of the face. Cushing's original description was a

'tomato head, potato body and four matches as limbs' (Fig. 26.23). As a result of protein loss the skin becomes thin, with purple striae, dusky cyanosis and visible dermal vessels. Proximal muscle weakness is prominent. Other features include increased capillary fragility, purpura, osteoporosis, acne, loss of libido, hirsutism, diabetes, hypertension and amenorrhoea. The clinical signs develop insidiously over years and are best recognized by reviewing old photographs. In some cases the disease runs a fulminant course, particularly when due to an adrenal carcinoma or ectopic ACTH secretion. Electrolyte disturbances, cachexia, pigmentation, severe diabetes and psychosis are common in these patients.

Investigation

Before proceeding to adrenalectomy, the surgeon must be convinced that:

- Cortisol secretion is beyond normal control. In Cushing's syndrome plasma cortisol levels are high, diurnal variation is lost and secretion is not suppressed by low-dose dexamethasone or increased by insulin-induced hypoglycaemia.
- The primary problem is in the adrenal. In patients with a functioning adrenal tumour, ACTH cannot be detected in the plasma and urinary excretion of cortisol is not suppressed by high-dose dexamethasone (Fig. 26.24).
- Pituitary and ectopic sources of excessive ACTH production have been excluded. In Cushing's disease due to a pituitary adenoma, plasma ACTH levels are inappropriately high and urinary cortisol excretion is suppressed by dexamethasone. In ectopic ACTH syndrome the ACTH levels are often exceedingly high and there is an associated electrolyte disturbance. These patients may also have cancer cachexia.
- Attempts have been made to localize the lesion by techniques such as CT (Fig. 26.25) or isotope scintigraphy using radiolabelled iodocholesterol (Fig. 26.26).

Treatment

Adrenal adenoma Adrenal adenomas are rarely bilateral and unilateral adrenalectomy is indicated. As the other adrenal is suppressed and atrophic, cortisone replacement is needed until the pituitary–adrenal axis recovers. This may take up to 2 years, and steroids must not be reduced or discontinued until a low-dose dexamethasone test shows normal function in the remaining gland.

Adrenal carcinoma These should be completely removed whenever possible; debulking may be helpful if chemotherapy is to be used. Patients often present late, with large tumours and lung metastases (Fig. 26.27). Even if adrenalectomy appears curative, adjuvant systemic therapy is advisable and adrenal antagonists such as aminoglutethimide or metyrapone may help to control symptoms. Chemotherapy with mitotane or o-p'-DDD may be tried, but this is a toxic

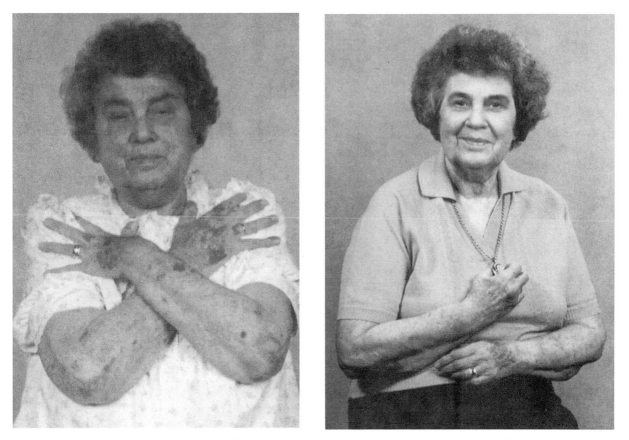

Fig. 26.23 Dramatic return to normality following the removal of an adrenal tumour causing Cushing's syndrome. Features of Cushing's (left panel) include thin, papery skin with bruising, moon face, puffy eyes, muscle wasting and lacklustre mood. Six months later (right panel), return to normal vigorous bright health. (courtesy of patient.)

drug and is often poorly tolerated. The therapeutic gain may be small.

Pituitary disease The symptoms of bilateral adrenal hyperplasia due to pituitary hyperfunction can be relieved by bilateral adrenalectomy, but at the price of lifelong steroid therapy. Furthermore, adrenalectomy removes all feedback control, so that overproduction of ACTH and MSH produces characteristic skin pigmentation and continued growth of the adenoma may compress the optic chiasma (Nelson's syndrome). Pituitary irradiation or surgery avoids the side-effects of adrenalectomy, and microsurgical removal of the adenoma is now the treatment of choice after preoperative preparation with adrenal antagonists.

Hyperaldosteronism

Primary hyperaldosteronism (Conn's syndrome)

This is usually due to a benign adenoma and is most common in young or middle-aged women. The adenoma is small,

single, canary yellow on bisection and composed of cells of the glomerulosa type. Only rarely is the syndrome due to bilateral adrenal hyperplasia or multiple microadenomas. The high circulating levels of aldosterone suppress renin secretion – a helpful biochemical diagnostic observation.

Clinical features Retention of sodium increases plasma volume and produces hypertension, often in association with headaches and visual disturbance (although serious retinopathy is uncommon). Potassium loss leads to worsening hypokalaemia, episodes of muscle weakness and nocturnal polyuria. Unrecognized, the syndrome progresses to severe hypokalaemic alkalosis, with periodic muscle paralysis, paraesthesia and tetany.

Diagnosis Low serum potassium in a hypertensive patient should signal the possibility of hyperaldosteronism. Diagnosis then rests on the following:

- *Confirm hypokalaemia.* This may require repeated blood sampling without an occluding cuff; 24-hour urine collections usually show increased potassium excretion.

PITUITARY DEPENDENT   AUTONOMOUS ADRENAL TUMOUR

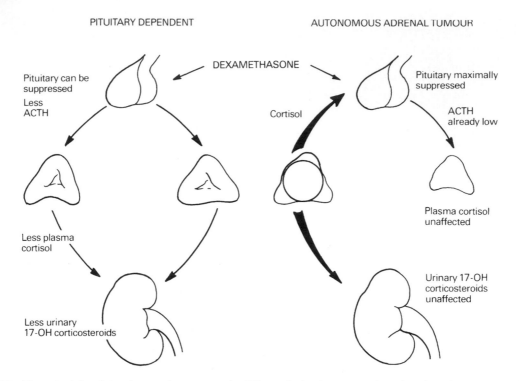

Fig. 26.24   The principle of the dexamethasone test in differentiating between adrenal and pituitary causes of excess cortisol secretion.

- *Demonstrate hypersecretion of aldosterone.* Plasma and/or urinary aldosterone levels are measured at 4-hourly intervals to allow for diurnal variations. Giving

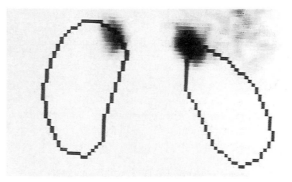

Fig. 26.26   Bilateral uptake of radio-labelled iodocholesterol in a patient with Cushing's disease.

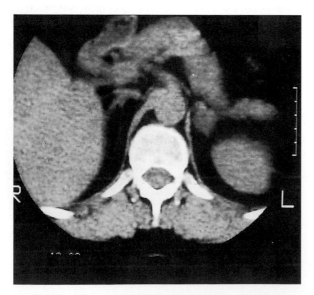

Fig. 26.25   CT scan of an adrenal tumour.

the aldosterone antagonist spironolactone should reduce blood pressure and reverse hypokalaemia.
- *Exclude secondary hyperaldosteronism.* Measurement of plasma renin is the critical investigation: renin levels are increased in secondary hyperaldosteronism but undetectable in the primary disease. Spironolactone causes further increases in renin levels in secondary hyperaldosteronism.
- *Localize the adenoma.* If primary hyperaldosteronism is confirmed biochemically, attempts should then be made to localize the adenoma by CT scanning (Fig. 26.25) or

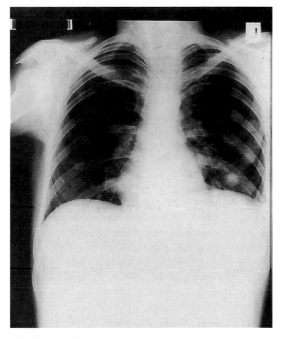

Fig. 26.27 Multiple pulmonary metastases in a patient with Cushing's disease caused by an adrenal carcinoma.

SUMMARY BOX

Cushing's syndrome

- Cushing's syndrome results from inappropriate secretion of cortisol.

- The syndrome may be caused by tumours of the adrenal cortex (20%), tumours of the anterior pituitary (80%), ectopic ACTH production (rare), or as a side-effect consequent upon the use of steroids for therapy.

- The main clinical features are truncal obesity, buffalo hump, mooning of the face ('tomato head, potato body, four matchsticks as limbs'), thinning of the skin, livid striae and proximal muscle weakness.

- An adrenal tumour is usually treated by unilateral adrenalectomy, but cortisone replacement is needed until the suppressed contralateral adrenal recovers.

- Before proceeding to adrenalectomy the surgeon should confirm that cortisol secretion is beyond normal control, that the primary problem is not pituitary or ectopic ACTH production, and that attempts have been made to localize the adrenal lesion (CT scan and radioisotope scan with iodocholesterol).

- Pituitary disease is best treated by pituitary surgery (or irradiation) rather than by bilateral adrenalectomy. This avoids continued growth of the pituitary tumour, problems due to ACTH and MSH production (pigmentation, Nelson's syndrome), and the side-effects of adrenalectomy.

scanning with radiolabelled iodocholesterol (Fig. 26.26). Failure to 'see' an adenoma may mean that there is no discrete tumour and that the patient has bilateral cortical hyperplasia. Plasma cortisol levels should always be measured to exclude Cushing's syndrome. Selective adrenal vein sampling to determine aldosterone levels may be required to help localize small adenomas to one or other gland.

Treatment Primary hyperaldosteronism due to an adenoma is treated by removal of the affected gland *after* correcting the hypokalaemia with oral potassium and spironolactone. Hyperaldosteronism due to adrenal hyperplasia can be cured by bilateral adrenalectomy, but at such a high price that long-term drug treatment with triamterene or amiloride (potassium-retaining diuretics) is preferable.

Secondary hyperaldosteronism

Hyperaldosteronism is most commonly secondary to excessive renin secretion (and stimulation of the zona glomerulosa by angiotensin) in chronic liver, renal or cardiac disease.

Adrenogenital syndrome (adrenal virilism)

Pathophysiology

This syndrome is due to one of a number of genetically determined enzyme defects that impair cortisol synthesis. The resultant increase in pituitary ACTH production causes adrenal hyperplasia and inappropriate adrenal androgen secretion.

Clinical features

The effects depend on the patient's sex and age. Female infants show enlargement of the clitoris and varying fusion of the labial folds. Later, other signs of virilism appear, leading to precocious heterosexual puberty. Young boys have precocious isosexual puberty. In both sexes growth is at first rapid, but the epiphyses fuse early so that the final height is stunted. Excess muscle growth produces an 'infant Hercules' appearance. Milder forms of the disease may affect older girls and cause hirsutism and acne.

Treatment

The patient is given cortisol for replacement purposes and to suppress ACTH production. Surgical correction of the genital abnormality may be needed. Rarely, virilism is due to an adrenal tumour, which is usually large and malignant.

Adrenal feminization

Exceptionally, a tumour of the adrenal cortex may secrete oestrogens. Such tumours are usually large and malignant. In the female there is sexual precocity; in the male there is feminization, with gynaecomastia, decreased libido and testicular atrophy. Treatment consists of removing the tumour, although recurrence and metastatic spread are usual.

Adrenal medulla

Pathophysiology

The adrenal medulla is not essential for life. There are other collections of chromaffin cells in paraganglia in the retroperitoneum, mediastinum and neck that release noradrenaline. The normal adrenal medulla secretes catecholamines in the ratio 80% adrenaline to 20% noradrenaline. It also secretes the noradrenaline precursor dopamine. Small amounts of catecholamines are excreted in the urine in free and conjugated form. Larger amounts are excreted as metnoradrenaline and 3-methoxy-4-hydroxymandelic acid (VMA).

Adrenaline This acts on α- and β-adrenergic receptors to redistribute blood flow. It constricts skin and splanchnic vessels and dilates those of the heart, skeletal muscles and brain. It causes tachycardia, induces anxiety, and has metabolic effects that include hepatic conversion of glycogen to glucose and increased levels of circulating free fatty acids.

Noradrenaline This acts mainly on α receptors to constrict all blood vessels and raise systolic and diastolic blood pressure.

Phaeochromocytoma

Pathology Phaeochromocytomas are tumours of the adrenal medulla (90%) that secrete large amounts of adrenaline and noradrenaline, or of the extra-adrenal paraganglionic tissue (10%) which secrete only noradrenaline. Virtually all (99%) arise within the abdomen, 10% are multiple and 10% are malignant. Benign tumours are usually about 5 cm in diameter, chocolate brown and highly vascular. Associated conditions are neurofibromatosis, medullary carcinoma of the thyroid (as part of MEN type II), duodenal ulcer and renal artery stenosis. If it presents in pregnancy, phaeochromocytoma can be mistaken for hypertension of pregnancy and may cause maternal and fetal mortality.

Clinical features Phaeochromocytomas usually present before the age of 50 years. Excess noradrenaline secretion causes hypertension; adrenaline excess has metabolic effects (e.g. diabetes and thyrotoxicosis) and may even give rise to hypotension. Paroxysmal hypertension is a very characteristic symptom, is due to the sudden release of catecholamines and may be precipitated by abdominal pressure, exercise or postural change. During an attack the blood pressure may rise to 200/100 mmHg and there is headache, palpitation, sweating, extreme anxiety, and chest and abdominal pain. Pallor, dilated pupils and tachycardia are prominent features. In some patients persistent and severe hypertension develops at the age of 30–40 years, often in association with severe retinopathy, which can cause optic atrophy and blindness. Glycosuria is common. The skin may be mottled, with tingling of the extremities. Extra-adrenal phaeochromocytomas are always associated with persistent hypertension. On rare occasions the tumour is in the bladder, and micturition may precipitate a syncopal attack. A few patients present with predominantly metabolic effects, such as those found in thyrotoxicosis. Occasionally, a phaeochromocytoma may cause sudden and unexplained death after trauma or during surgery, owing to severe hypertension causing a cerebrovascular accident or by precipitating a fatal arrhythmia.

Investigation All young hypertensive patients should be screened for a catecholamine-secreting tumour. The most reliable test is urinary VMA determination following a paroxysm. Twenty-four hour collections of urine should be analysed for free catecholamine, metadrenaline and VMA output. A CT scan may show the tumour. It may also be demonstrated by scintigraphy after giving radioiodine-labelled metaiodobenzylguanidine (MIBG), a substance which is taken up by catecholamine precursors (Fig. 26.28). Abdominal ultrasonography, intravenous urography with tomography, arteriography and selective venous sampling are no longer used for localization. Preliminary blockade (see below) is essential if invasive angiography is used.

Treatment Surgical removal of the tumour is the treatment of choice. The use of α- and β-blocking drugs has greatly reduced the risk of hypertensive attacks, tachycardia and arrhythmias during induction of anaesthesia or tumour handling. The patient should come to operation with blood pressure and pulse rate controlled. Adrenergic blockade also allows restoration of blood volume, so that sudden

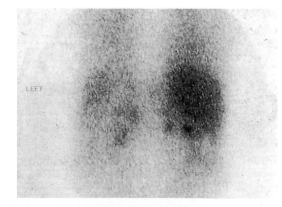

Fig. 26.28   Markedly excessive uptake of MIBG in a huge right-sided phaeochromocytoma.

hypotension after removal of the tumour is unusual. To achieve blockade the α-adrenergic receptor blocker doxazosin should be used. A typical starting dose would be 1 mg twice a day, building up to 6 or 8 mg a day until hypertension is controlled and postural symptoms occur. The benefit of this drug over longer-acting agents such as phenoxybenzamine is that once the tumour has been removed there is less residual hypotension.

Once α-blockade has been established unopposed β effects, such as tachycardia, may become evident and are treated with a β-blocker such as propranolol. β-Blockade should not be instituted first, as this may allow unopposed α-agonist effects, which may make hypertension worse and precipitate heart failure.

Atropine and thiopentone are best avoided and enflurane is the preferred anaesthetic. Pulse and blood pressure are monitored throughout surgery, and blood volume must be maintained. Short-acting α- and β-blocking agents and sodium nitroprusside (which acts directly on vessels independent of adrenergic receptors and gives additional control of hypertension) should be available.

> **SUMMARY BOX**
>
> *Phaeochromocytoma*
>
> - Phaeochromocytomas are usually benign tumours of the adrenal medulla (90% of patients) but 10% arise in extra-adrenal paraganglionic tissue, 10% are multiple and 10% are malignant (the '10% tumour').
> - Phaeochromocytomas may be associated with neurofibromatosis, medullary carcinoma of the thyroid (MEN II), duodenal ulcer and renal artery stenosis.
> - The tumour presents clinically with hypertension, which is often paroxysmal, and with metabolic effects such as diabetes mellitus.
> - All young hypertensive patients should be screened for phaeochromocytoma; urinary VMA, and catecholamine determination is the most reliable method of diagnosis.
> - The location of a phaeochromocytoma is best defined by CT scanning and radiolabelled MIBG scanning.
> - Treatment consists of adrenalectomy after careful preparation to control blood pressure and heart rate and to re-expand blood volume (by α-adrenergic blockade with β-blockade.

Non-endocrine adrenal medullary tumours

Ganglioneuromas These are benign, firm, well-encapsulated tumours of ganglion cells. They grow slowly, may become large and can cause diarrhoea. Surgical excision gives excellent results.

Neuroblastomas These are highly malignant tumours arising from sympathetic nervous tissue. They are one of the commonest malignant tumours of infancy and childhood, and metastasize widely. About 75% secrete catecholamines. Treatment by radical excision, radiotherapy and chemotherapy offers the only hope of cure, although spontaneous regression has been reported.

Adrenal 'incidentaloma'

The increasing use of imaging modalities such as CT or MRI has led to adrenal tumours being discovered incidentally in patients being investigated for other reasons. In such cases it is important to determine whether there is cortical or medullary hyperfunction, by the use of appropriate biochemical tests as detailed above. If there is no hyperfunction, the swelling is less than 5 cm in diameter and fine-needle aspiration excludes malignancy, further investigation and exploration are unwarranted. The lesion is likely to be a benign non-functioning cortical adenoma. Endocrine hyperfunction, a swelling larger than 5 cm or the suspicion of malignancy are indications for further assessment and exploration.

Adrenalectomy

Indications

Normal adrenal glands were once removed as palliative treatment in postmenopausal women with breast cancer (to remove the source of DHA-S and prevent its peripheral conversion to oestrogen). Aromatase inhibitors (e.g. aminoglutethimide) have made this approach obsolete.

Indications for adrenalectomy now include adrenal adenomas producing Cushing's syndrome, Conn's syndrome or excess catecholamines (phaeochromocytoma). Bilateral adrenalectomy may be needed for bilateral tumours, nodular hyperplasia producing Conn's or Cushing's syndromes, and if pituitary surgery fails to cure Cushing's disease.

Technique

Whether approached from in front, from the side or from behind, the adrenals are inaccessible. The anterior transperitoneal route requires a large incision, inevitably causes ileus, has a high incidence of wound and respiratory complications (especially in patients with Cushing's syndrome), and is now seldom used.

Large tumours may be malignant and are best approached through a flank incision, after removing a rib to allow access; if possible the diaphragm, pleura and peritoneum are left intact.

The posterior approach through the bed of the 11th or 12th rib is technically more difficult, but has lower morbidity and patients have a quicker return to normal activity. If the pleura is breached in the course of adrenalectomy it can be repaired on closing the wound, ensuring that the lung is fully inflated. There is no need for pleural or wound drains.

Adrenalectomy can be carried out using minimally invasive techniques. The usual route is anteriorly, beneath the costal margins, transperitoneally with reflection of liver and duodenum on the right and spleen, pancreas and colon on the left. The adrenal vein can often be divided early in laparoscopic surgery which, especially with phaeochromocytomas, means that dangerous levels of catecholamines are prevented from gaining access to the circulation, thereby reducing the perturbations in blood pressure that characterize open procedures with direct manipulation of the tumour. It is occasionally necessary to convert to an open procedure if bleeding is encountered or there are other technical or access problems.

Replacement therapy

Corticosteroid replacement is needed for life after bilateral total adrenalectomy, but may not be needed permanently after unilateral adrenalectomy. Replacement is best achieved by a combination of oral hydrocortisone (30 mg daily in divided doses) and the mineralocorticoid fludrocortisone acetate (0.1 mg daily). If both adrenals are removed, or the remaining adrenal is non-functional, the operation must be covered by commencing steroid replacement at the time of surgery. Adequacy of replacement is assessed by monitoring blood pressure in the erect and supine position, by serum electrolyte determinations and by patient well being.

Hydrocortisone sodium succinate is water soluble and can be given by intravenous infusion during the first 24 hours. Further doses are given intravenously until the patient can take oral steroid. It cannot be overemphasized that blood pressure is the best guide to therapy. If hypotension occurs, 100 mg hydrocortisone sodium succinate is given immediately by intravenous injection, followed by 100 mg every 6–8 hours in a saline infusion. All adrenalectomized patients must be warned to increase the dose of steroid if stress or infection occurs. Failure to anticipate the need for added steroid may precipitate an 'adrenal crisis', with acute hypotension and collapse. Such patients should carry a 'steroid card' giving details of dosage and possible complications, and should be able to recognize the symptoms of adrenal insufficiency (i.e. loss of appetite, nausea, cramps, muscle pains and malaise). If such symptoms occur, the patient should take an extra two tablets of hydrocortisone and seek urgent medical help.

Patient information

Although adrenal cortical function is vital for life, patients are unlikely to have heard of the adrenal glands. Patient awareness is to some extent governed by disease frequency, and so, for example, most will understand the rudiments of diabetes or cancer of the breast because these are very frequently encountered disorders. By contrast, adrenal tumours occur at a rate of about 1 per million population per annum. Patients may have an awareness of cortisone or adrenaline from contexts of other disease and fright/flight reactions, respectively.

In advising patients about adrenal or pituitary surgery, then, the starting point must be at the very beginning. Explain why they may not have heard of the adrenal glands, draw diagrams to show where the glands lie, and explain basic function in terms of the hormones produced and what effects they have.

It is necessary to discuss the technicalities of surgery and the approach to be used, and to forewarn patients that a laparoscopic procedure may have to be converted to an open one.

Complications should be minimal, but it is nevertheless worth mentioning blood loss and drains.

One of the most important features to describe will be any requirement for steroid replacement therapy (necessary after bilateral adrenalectomy, unilateral adrenalectomy for an adenoma producing Cushing's syndrome, and after pituitary surgery) and the need for dosage increase at times of stress (e.g. other surgery) or intercurrent illness (e.g. pneumonia).

OTHER SURGICAL ENDOCRINE SYNDROMES

Apudomas and multiple endocrine neoplasia

The APUD cell series

Distributed throughout the body are cells that have in common the capacity to store amines (e.g. catecholamines), take up their precursors (e.g. dopamine) and possess the decarboxylating enzymes necessary for their synthesis. The term APUD is an acronym denoting *Amine Precursor Uptake* and *Decarboxylation*. The cells can be demonstrated by specific histochemical and immunofluorescent techniques.

It is thought that these cells migrate from neural ectoderm to endocrine organs and to the respiratory and gastrointestinal tract. Examples of APUD cells in endocrine organs are the ACTH-secreting cells of the anterior pituitary, catecholamine-secreting cells of the adrenal medulla, and calcitonin-secreting cells of the thyroid. In the gastrointestinal tract APUD cells are present as single cells (e.g. argentaffin cells of the small intestine) or as large conglomerates, as in the pancreatic islets. The products of gastrointestinal APUD cells include 5-hydroxytryptamine and histamine, and a large number of polypeptide hormones (e.g. secretin, gastrin, cholecystokinin, enteroglucagon, somatostatin, vasoactive intestinal peptide).

Hyperplasia and tumour of any APUD cell can produce specific endocrine syndromes. Occasionally they give rise to ectopic hormone production, as in the secretion of ACTH by bronchial tumours.

Multiple endocrine neoplasia (MEN) syndromes

In MEN syndromes, patients develop benign or malignant tumours in more than one endocrine gland. The aetiology of the syndromes is uncertain, but they are inherited as autosomal dominant traits of variable penetrance and expression. The glands most often affected are the anterior pituitary, adrenal medulla, pancreas, and C cells of the thyroid. Although the cells that make up the parathyroid glands are derived from pharyngeal pouch endoderm, parathyroid hyperplasia and adenomas are also found in these syndromes.

MEN type I This syndrome is characterized by hyperplasia and/or tumours of the parathyroid, pancreatic islets and anterior pituitary. There may also be non-functioning tumours of the thyroid, pituitary, adrenal cortex and soft tissues (lipomas), and functioning carcinoid tumours of the gut or lungs. The earliest biochemical sign in affected individuals is hypercalcaemia from hyperparathyroidism or hyperprolactinaemia from an asymptomatic pituitary tumour. Families are often uncovered when an index patient presents dramatically, for example with small bowel perforation or bleeding due to the Zollinger–Ellison syndrome (see below), or hypoglycaemia due to an insulinoma of the pancreas. Family members should be screened by measurement of fasting serum calcium and other hormonal markers such as prolactin.

The mutational events have now been localized to chromosome 21, and it is possible to identify some of the mutations that produce the MEN I syndrome. Unlike the MEN II syndrome, however, biochemical tests will still be required to identify the earliest endocrine abnormalities, and these are likely to be hyperparathyroidism (hypercalcaemia) and a pituitary tumour (elevated prolactin). Although it is unlikely that 'prophylactic' surgery will be carried out 'at-risk' family members can be screened biochemically to allow the earliest discussions of treatment options. It also allows families to be informed of the more serious components of the syndrome – hyperinsulinism (hypoglycaemia) and hypergastrinaemia (fulminant peptic ulcer). A bracelet may be worn to alert medical attendants to the condition.

As confidence in the positive and negative genetic tests grows one of their most important functions will be to advise non-affected kindred members that they are not at risk, that they need no further testing, and that they will not pass the condition to their offspring.

Affected individuals may have mixed pancreatic tumours that produce a variety of hormones (e.g. gastrin, insulin and glucagon). Acromegaly is rare and prolactin-secreting tumours are more common. If a member of an affected kindred is shown to have hypercalcaemia, they must be kept under close surveillance for biochemical or clinical signs of other forms of endocrine overactivity. In some cases familial hyperparathyroidism occurs without the involvement of other endocrine glands.

Treatment is directed at the dominant clinical or biochemical feature. For example, pancreatic endocrine tumours are localized by ultrasonography or CT scanning and removed as necessary. Hypercalcaemia is treated by parathyroid surgery. Diseased glands are excised, and four-gland hyperplasia may be treated by excising all four glands and implanting small fragments from the most normal are into an accessible site, such as the foream. This allows easy identification and further removal of parathyroid tissue if hypercalcaemia recurs.

MEN type II This variant is also inherited as an autosomal dominant condition and is characterized by medullary carcinoma of the thyroid, phaeochromocytoma and parathyroid hyperplasia. Three subtypes are described:

- Familial medullary thyroid carcinoma alone.
- MEN type IIa, consisting of medullary thyroid carcinoma (all cases) with phaeochromocytomas and/or parathyroid hyperplasia. The phaeochromocytomas are often bilateral but rarely malignant.
- MEN type IIb, consisting of medullary thyroid carcinoma, bilateral phaeochromocytomas (but no parathyroid abnormality) and complex neural abnormalities, including mucosal neuromas, thickened nerves (e.g. corneal nerves) and ganglioneuromatosis of the gut. These patients have a typical facies, with thick blubbery lips, irregular dentition and a Marfanoid body habitus.

All of these syndromes were diagnosed by detecting high levels of circulating calcitonin, if necessary after provocation by calcium or pentagastrin. In some cases diagnosis would be achieved when the thyroid abnormality consisted of C-cell hyperplasia, the premalignant precursor of medullary thyroid cancer. The thyroid disorder is treated by total thyroidectomy and dissection of nodes from the central compartment of the neck (modified block dissection).

The mutation in chromosome 10 that 'causes' inherited MEN II syndromes is now identified and is due to altered base pairs in a *Ret* proto-oncogene. Genetic diagnosis is now possible on a single blood sample and, unlike in patients with MEN I, there is advantage in prophylactic surgery. If the mutation is identified thyroidectomy can be carried out at the age of 5 or earlier. At this age the thyroid tumour will be difficult to detect, except perhaps for the presence of C-cell hyperplasia on histology. Continued screening for phaeochromocytoma will be required by measurement of 24-hour urine collections for cate-cholamines.

Kindred members not showing the mutation can be dismissed from follow-up and can be reassured that they will not pass on the genetic abnormality to their off-spring.

Phaeochromocytomas are diagnosed by determination of urinary VMA and catecholamine excretion and localized by CT and metaiodobenzylguanidine (MIBG) scanning. Adrenal medullary hyperplasia is a precursor of phaeochromocytoma, which can be diagnosed by increased MIBG uptake. Surgical treatment of the adrenal medullary abnormality must take precedence over the treatment of thyroid and parathyroid disease, as anaesthesia and surgery in patients with undiagnosed or untreated phaeochromocytoma can be life-threatening.

Carcinoid tumours and the carcinoid syndrome

Carcinoid tumours can occur in any part of the gastro-intestinal tract or respiratory tree. They are found most frequently in the appendix as incidental findings in a patient presenting with acute appendicitis, and account for 85% of all appendiceal tumours. The carcinoid tumour is usually near the tip of the appendix, usually less than 1 cm in diameter, and dealt with by appendicectomy. Metastases are exceptional in this situation. Carcinoid tumours larger than 2 cm in diameter are rare, but may have spread to lymph nodes and are best treated by right hemicolectomy. Liver metastases are extremely rare in patients with appendiceal carcinoids. Carcinoids occurring in the small intestine frequently spread to lymph nodes, and in 10% of cases there are liver metastases by the time the patient presents with obstructive symptoms or bleeding.

Carcinoids in any site produce 5-hydroxytryptamine (5-HT) and other biologically active amines and peptides. In the case of gut carcinoids these products are normally inactivated by the liver, but liver secondaries secrete these substances directly into the systemic circulation, giving rise to a carcinoid syndrome: periodic flushing, diarrhoea, bronchoconstriction, wheezing and distinctive red-purple discoloration of the face. Right-sided heart disease, notably pulmonary stenosis, may result and can prove fatal.

The diagnosis of carcinoid syndrome is confirmed by detecting 5-hydroxyindoleacetic acid (a breakdown product of 5-HT) in the urine. If the primary tumour is causing symptoms it should be removed surgically if possible (e.g. right hemicolectomy, small bowel resection, lung resection). Hepatic metastases can be dealt with by excising the involved liver lobe or enucleating the deposits in an attempt to gain symptomatic relief. Alternatively, hepatic metastases may be de-arterialized by hepatic artery ligation or angiographic embolization.

Attempts have been made to relieve symptoms by blocking 5-HT synthesis (e.g. α-methyldopa) or action (e.g. methysergide), but the prevention of 5-HT release by somatostatin analogues or α-adrenergic antagonists may be more useful. Long-acting somatostatin analogues are now available and, instead of a need for once- or twice-daily injections of octreotide subcutaneously, 1 month's effective therapy can be achieved by an intramuscular injection of a depot preparation. Octreotide preparations are expensive but may bring dramatic symptomatic relief. Chemotherapy (e.g. 5-fluorouracil) is sometimes effective. Interferon is also sometimes used, but the side-effects can be troublesome.

27 Vascular and endovascular surgery

R.T.A. Chalmers, T.B. Buckenham, A.W. Bradbury

The management of patients with vascular disease requires a multidisciplinary approach involving vascular surgeons, vascular radiologists, anaesthetists, physicians (angiologists), nursing and rehabilitation specialists, physiotherapists, occupational therapists and orthotists. Standard surgical procedures have been complemented – in some cases replaced – by less invasive percutaneous endoluminal interventions. As the population ages and the risk factors for vascular disease show no sign of diminishing, the health and socioeconomic burden of arterial and venous disease will continue to increase.

PATHOPHYSIOLOGY OF ARTERIAL DISEASE

Pathology

Most patients presenting to vascular surgeons have atherosclerosis. This condition involves the following: endothelial cell injury; subendothelial deposition of lipids and inflammatory cells; smooth muscle cell migration and proliferation; and plaque haemorrhage, rupture and thrombosis (Fig. 27.1).

Endothelial injury

Chemical injury The main risk factor for the development of atherosclerosis is smoking. Hypercholesterolaemia and hypertriglyceridaemia are also important risk factors.

Arterial disease is also far commoner in diabetics, who have disordered glucose and lipid metabolism.

Physical injury Atheroma often first appears where blood flow exerts high levels of shear stress on the arterial wall, for example at bifurcations. Hypertension, which increases this stress, is an important predisposing factor for arterial disease.

Lipid deposition

Injury increases the permeability of the endothelium to lipids and inflammatory cells which become deposited in the subendothelial layer. At this point the atheroma forms a discoloured, but flat, yellow patch (fatty streak). In developed countries many young adults will have such lesions, which may progress to atherosclerosis.

Inflammatory cell infiltrate

Leukocytes adhere to the overlying damaged endothelium, migrate into the subendothelial space, digest lipid and

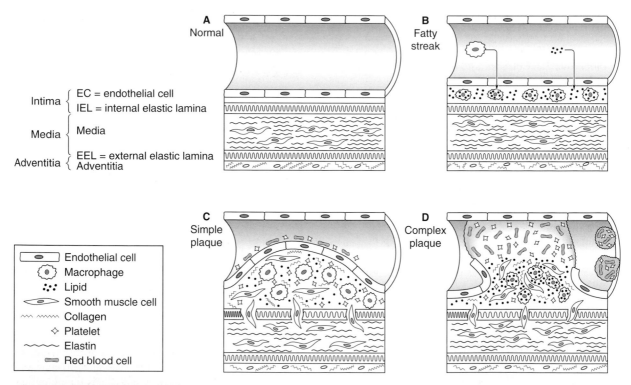

Fig. 27.1 Pathophysiology of atherosclerosis. **A** Normal arterial wall. The intima, comprising a single layer of endothelial cells, rests upon a basement membrane and the internal elastic lamina. The media comprises smooth muscle cells and elastin, and the adventitia of collagenous tissue and vasa vasorum. **B** Fatty streak. Injured endothelial cells permit the sequestration of lipids and macrophages in the subendothelial space. **C** Simple plaque. Smooth muscle cells enter the media though the internal elastic lamina where they proliferate, take on the characteristics of fibroblasts and produce collagen. **D** Complex plaque. The endothelial cap has ruptured, leading to acute thrombosis and distal embolization.

become 'foam' cells and liberate free radicals and proteases that destroy the arterial wall. They also liberate cytokines, which attract further leukocytes and smooth muscle cells from the media. The overlying endothelium becomes increasingly 'sticky', leading to platelet deposition and thrombosis.

Smooth muscle cells

Smooth muscle cells migrate from the media into the subendothelial space and begin to proliferate. They take on the properties of fibroblasts and lay down collagen. At this stage the atheroma is raised and encroaches upon the lumen of the artery.

Plaque rupture

At this point the plaque often comprises a thin 'cap' of endothelium stretched over a mass of lipid, inflammatory and smooth muscle cells. Intraplaque haemorrhage, from immature new blood vessels that infiltrate the lesion (angiogenesis), weakens the plaque. Further chemical and/or physical injury can lead to rupture and the exposure of highly thrombotic plaque contents to the flowing blood. This results in acute thrombotic occlusion of the vessel and/or distal embolization. It is important to appreciate that it is this sudden decompensation that leads to the most serious and dramatic clinical presentations of arterial disease, and that rupture can occur in a plaque which has hitherto been asymptomatic.

Clinical manifestations

The clinical manifestations of arterial disease depend upon:

- The site of the disease
- Whether the artery is an end-artery or well collateralized
- The speed with which the disease develops
- Whether the underlying process is haemodynamic, thrombotic, atheroembolic, thromboembolic or due to aneurysmal dilatation or dissection
- The presence of other comorbidity and the general condition of the patient.

Anatomic site

The patient's symptoms and signs will obviously depend upon the territory supplied by the affected artery:

- Coronary arteries: angina, myocardial infarction
- Cerebral circulation: stroke, transient ischaemic attack (TIA), amaurosis fugax, vertebrobasilar insufficiency (VBI)
- Renal arteries: hypertension, renal failure
- Mesenteric arteries: mesenteric angina, acute intestinal ischaemia

- The limbs: intermittent claudication (IC), chronic critical limb ischaemia (CLI), acute limb ischaemia.

Collateral supply

The clinical picture also depends upon whether the affected artery is essentially the only supply to the distal tissue (e.g. coronary artery, myocardium), or whether is it one of several arteries supplying the part (e.g. carotid artery, brain). This may vary between patients. For example, in a patient with a complete circle of Willis the occlusion of one carotid artery may be asymptomatic. In a patient where there is no cross-circulation occlusion is likely to cause a stroke.

Speed of onset

Where atheroma develops slowly over months or years a collateral supply to the distal part is likely to develop, such that when the main artery finally occludes there may be little change in the patient's clinical status. The commonest example is where the profunda (deep) femoral artery collateralizes around a diseased superficial femoral artery in patients with intermittent claudication (see below). By contrast, the sudden occlusion of a previously normal artery is likely to cause severe distal ischaemia.

Mechanism of injury

The mechanism of injury has a major influence on the clinical presentation, the prognosis and treatment of arterial disease (Fig. 27.2).

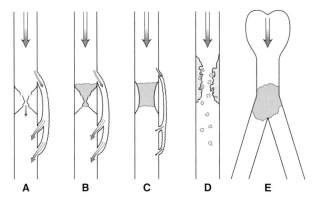

A	B	C	D	E

Fig. 27.2 Mechanisms of injury in atherosclerotic disease. **A** Critical stenosis of main artery compensated for by collateral vessels; only symptomatic on exercise. **B** Acute thrombosis of a critical stenosis; little change in clinical status because of well-developed collaterals. **C** Acute thrombosis of a non-critical stenosis; severe symptoms because collateral supply is poorly developed. **D** Atheroembolism from ruptured, ulcerated plaque. **E** Thromboembolism from the heart; severe ischaemia because of lack of collateral supply.

Haemodynamic An atheromatous plaque must reduce the cross-sectional diameter of an artery by about 70% to cause an appreciable drop in flow and pressure at rest, a so-called 'critical stenosis'. However, on exertion, for example walking, a much lesser stenosis may become 'critical'. The reason for this is that the pressure drop across a stenosis is proportional to the square of the velocity of the blood entering that stenosis; and, on exercise, blood velocity increases markedly. The clinical consequence of this is that the lesion only becomes flow limiting, and therefore symptomatic, on exertion. This type of mechanism tends to have a relatively benign course; intermittent claudication is a common example.

Thrombosis By the time a 'critical' stenosis occludes, the collateral supply may be so well developed that the event is clinically silent. However, if a plaque that has been causing little or no haemodynamic impairment suddenly ruptures, then acute thrombosis of the vessel can have severe consequences. Such an event can cause myocardial infarction (MI) or stroke in a previously asymptomatic patient.

Atheroembolism The effect that embolizing plaque contents (predominantly cholesterol) or adherent thrombus (predominantly platelets) have upon the distal circulation depends upon the factors outlined above, as well as the embolic load. Perhaps the best-known example is atheroembolism from a carotid plaque, which can cause small, discrete areas of cerebral and retinal ischaemia that manifest clinically as TIA and amaurosis fugax. If the embolic load is high, however, these emboli may cause irreversible occlusion of major distal vessels, leading to stroke and retinal infarction (monocular blindness).

Thromboembolism The most common source of thromboembolism is the left atrium, in association with atrial fibrillation (AF). The clinical consequences are usually dramatic, as the thrombus load is often large and tends to suddenly and completely occlude a large or medium-sized vessel that has previously been healthy, and for which there is therefore no collateral supply. This is an important cause of stroke and acute limb ischaemia.

LOWER LIMB ARTERIAL DISEASE

Anatomy

The lower limb arterial tree comprises the aortoiliac segment above the inguinal ligament ('inflow'), the femoropopliteal segment and the infrapopliteal segment ('outflow') (Fig. 27.3).

Clinical manifestations

Symptoms

Lower limb ischaemia presents as two distinct clinical entities: intermittent claudication (IC) and critical limb ischaemia (CLI). They have different epidemiologies, natural histories, treatments and prognoses (see below).

Examination findings

On examination, the chronically ischaemic limb is characterized by:

- Skin that is thin and dry
- Pallor, particularly on elevation. Upon dependency the foot becomes bright red; this is known as dependent

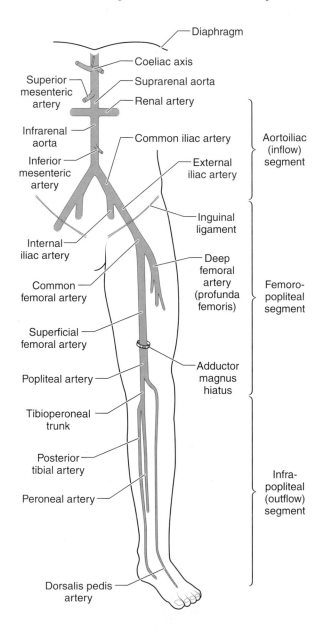

Fig. 27.3 Aortic and lower limb arterial anatomy.

rubor or 'sunset foot' and is due to reactive hyperaemia (Buerger's test)

- Superficial veins that fill sluggishly in the horizontal position and empty upon minimal elevation (venous guttering)
- Nails that are brittle and crumbly
- Muscle wasting
- Reduced temperature
- Pulses that are weak or absent and sometimes associated with bruits.

Pulse status

All patients admitted to hospital should have their pulse status recorded. In IC and CLI the popliteal and pedal pulses are usually absent. If there is aortoiliac disease, then one or both femoral pulses will be weak or absent. The presence of a bruit denotes turbulent flow.

Ankle: brachial pressure index

The severity of ischaemia can be estimated by determining the ratio between the ankle and brachial blood pressures. The latter is recorded in the normal way, the former using a cuff and a handheld Doppler device (Fig. 27.4). In health the ankle:brachial pressure index (ABPI) should be at least 1, that is, the pressure at the ankle should be at least as high as that in the arm. Patients with IC usually have an ABPI of 0.5–0.9, and those with CLI usually have an ABPI of less than 0.5.

Intermittent claudication

Clinical features

IC usually leads to pain in the muscles of the calf because the disease most often affects the superficial femoral artery (Fig. 27.5). If the iliac arteries are affected as well then the pain may also be felt in the thigh, even the buttock. The pain comes on after a reasonably constant 'claudication distance', and subsides rapidly and completely on cessation of walking. Resumption of walking returns the pain. These and other features distinguish it from neurogenic and venous claudication (Table 27.1).

Typically the earliest lesion is usually a stenosis in the superficial femoral artery in the region of the adductor canal (Fig. 27.5) and leads to IC after walking several hundred metres. Ankle pulses are palpable but diminished, and a bruit may be heard at or below the adductor canal. Ankle systolic pressures are often normal at rest but reduced following exercise.

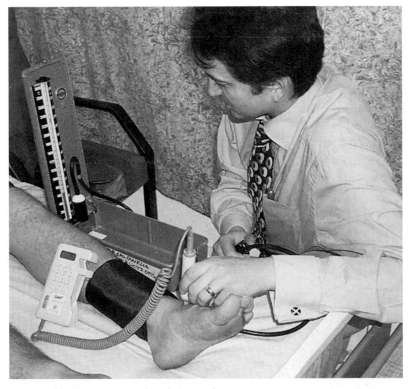

Fig. 27.4   Measurement of ABPI using Doppler ultrasound.

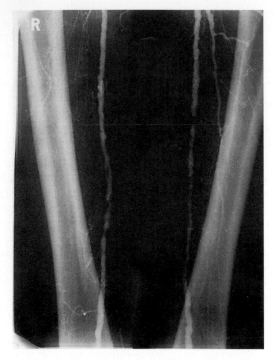

Fig. 27.5   Angiogram showing irregularity of outline of arteries with stenosis in left superficial femoral artery disease.

Over the next few months or years the collateral vessels of the profunda system enlarge to carry a higher proportion of the blood flow to the leg. In the majority of patients symptoms gradually improve or even disappear. Thrombotic occlusion (Fig. 27.6B) leads to a sudden deterioration in walking distance. Ankle and popliteal pulses are now absent.

Further development of the collateral circulation leads to an improvement in symptoms. This phase of moderate claudication may remain apparently stable for several years. However, unless there is a change in the patient's lifestyle the atherosclerosis may progress to involve other segments (Fig. 27.6C). Claudication is now severe, forcing the patient to stop every 50 metres or so and the scope for spontaneous improvement is steadily diminishing. As the disease spreads, symptoms may worsen (Fig. 27.6D) to a point where CLI develops.

An understanding of this cyclical pattern of exacerbation and resolution is important, as spontaneous improvement may mislead the patient into thinking all is well and that there is no longer a need to comply with medical advice (see below).

Epidemiology

IC affects 5% of middle-aged men. Provided patients comply with 'best medical therapy' (see below), only 1–2% per year will deteriorate to a point where amputation and/or

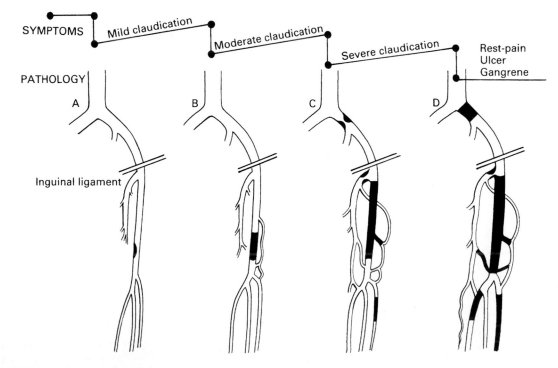

Fig. 27.6   Symptoms and pathology in intermittent claudication.

Table 27.1   Differential diagnosis of claudication

	Arterial	Neurogenic	Venous
Pathology	Stenosis or occlusion of major lower limb arteries	Lumbar nerve roots or cauda equina compression (spinal stenosis)	Obstruction to the venous outflow of the leg due to iliofemoral venous occlusion secondary to DVT
Site of pain	Muscles. Usually the calf but may affect thigh and buttock	Ill-defined. Whole leg. Shooting in nature. May be associated with tingling and numbness	Whole leg. Bursting in nature
Laterality	Usually unilateral if femoropopliteal, bilateral if aortoiliac disease	Often bilateral	Nearly always unilateral
Onset	Gradual onset after walking the 'claudication distance'	Often immediate upon walking, or even on standing up	Gradual onset but may be present from the moment walking commences
Relieving features	On cessation of walking the pain disappears completely in 1–2 minutes	On cessation of walking, the pain may gradually subside over 5–10 minutes. Often the patient has to sit down or lean against something to obtain relief	The subject usually needs to elevate the leg to obtain relief
Colour	Normal or pale	Normal	Cyanosed. Often visible varicose veins and venous skin changes
Temperature	Normal or cool	Normal	Normal or increased
Swelling	Absent	Absent	Always present
Pulses	Reduced or absent	Normal	Present, but may be difficult to feel because of swelling
Straight leg raising	Normal	Limited	Normal

revascularization is required. However, the annual mortality rate is over 5% per year, which is two to three times higher than an age- and sex-matched non-claudicant population. IC is a marker of widespread atherosclerosis, and most of these patients succumb to myocardial infarction (MI) or stroke. The emphasis is therefore on the preservation of life, as in most patients measures to reduce cardiovascular mortality will also improve the functional status of the limb.

Critical limb ischaemia

Whereas IC is usually due to single-level disease, CLI is caused by multiple lesions. These patients have tissue loss (ulceration or gangrene) with or without rest pain, and, by definition, have an ankle blood pressure of less than 50 mmHg. Without revascularization such patients will usually lose their limb – often their life – in a matter of weeks or months.

Subcritical limb ischaemia (SCLI)

The term SCLI is used to describe patients who have night and/or rest pain but not tissue loss. They are in an intermediate group between IC and CLI, and share features of both. A proportion of these patients may respond to book medical therapy (BMT), thereby obviating the need for arterial reconstruction to save the limb.

Severe limb ischaemia (SLI)

This term is sometimes used to describe all patients with chronic limb ischaemia that is more severe than IC, that is, CLI and SCLI.

Night and rest pain

Pain develops, typically in the forefoot, about an hour after going to bed. 'Night pain' is due to the accumulation of metabolites and occurs because the perfusion of the foot falls as a result of the loss of the beneficial effects of gravity, and because the patient's blood pressure and cardiac output also fall during sleep. It is severe and wakes the patient from sleep, but may at first be relieved by hanging the limb out of bed. As the disease progresses the patient has to get up and walk about to obtain relief. This happens increasingly frequently through the night, with resulting loss of sleep. The patient then takes to sleeping in a chair, which leads to dependent oedema. This increases interstitial tissue pressure and so further reduces arterial perfusion. The patient is then in a vicious cycle of increasing pain and sleep loss. At this point even a trivial injury will fail to heal, and the entry of bacteria leads to infection and an increase in the metabolic demands of the foot. The result is the rapid formation of ulcers and gangrene.

Diabetic vascular disease

Approximately 40% of patients with SLI have diabetes and such patients pose a number of unique problems for the vascular surgeon:

- Their arteries are often calcified, which *may* make surgery and angioplasty technically difficult.
- Measured ankle pressures may be spuriously high.

- Diabetics have a reduced ability to fight infection.
- Diabetics often have severe multisystem arterial disease (coronary, cerebral and peripheral), which increases the risks of intervention.
- In the lower limbs diabetic vascular disease has a predilection for the crural vessels. Although vessels in the foot are often spared, the technical challenge of performing a satisfactory bypass or angioplasty to these small vessels is considerable.
- Diabetics may have neuropathy, which may lead to foot ulceration in its own right but may also complicate peripheral ischaemia (see below).

The diabetic foot

This refers to the combination of ischaemia, neuropathy and immunocompromise that renders the feet of diabetic patients particularly susceptible to sepsis, ulceration and gangrene. Diabetic neuropathy affects the motor, sensory and autonomic nerves.

Sensory neuropathy This renders the patient incapable of feeling pain. Minor trauma – for example from a stone in the shoe – remains unnoticed. Even severe ischaemia and/or tissue loss that would lead a sensate patient to seek urgent medical advice may be completely painless. For this reason diabetic patients often present late, with extensive destruction of the foot. Sensory neuropathy also affects proprioception such that, upon walking, pressure is taken at unusual sites. This is thought to underlie the process of joint destruction (Charcot's joints) seen in severe cases and leads to ulceration.

Motor neuropathy The normal structure and function of the foot depend not only upon ligaments but also upon the long and short flexors and extensors of the calf and sole. The latter are affected more than the former by motor neuropathy, leading to weakness and atrophy. The result is that the long extensors of the toes are unopposed and the toes become increasing dorsiflexed. This exposes the metatarsal heads to abnormal pressure, and they are a frequent site of callus formation and ulceration (Fig. 27.7).

Autonomic neuropathy This leads to a dry foot deficient in the sweat that normally lubricates the skin and contains antibacterial substances. The result is scaling and fissuring of the skin, and the creation of a portal of entry for bacteria. Abnormal blood flow in the bones of the ankle and foot due to loss of autonomic control may also contribute to osteopenia and bony collapse.

Treatment If the blood supply is adequate then dead tissue can be excised in the expectation that healing will occur provided infection is controlled and the foot is protected from pressure. If there is ischaemia as well then the first priority is to revascularize the foot, if possible. Sadly, many diabetic patients present late with extensive tissue

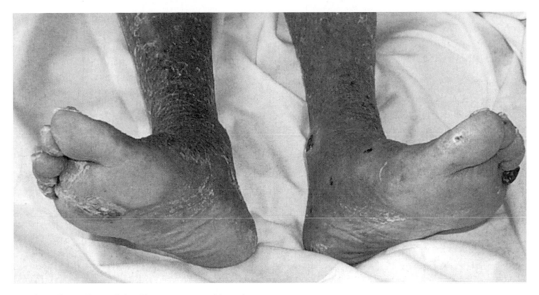

Fig. 27.7 Neuropathic ulceration of the first metatarsal head.

loss and 'unreconstructable' disease, which accounts for the very high amputation rate.

Treatment of lower limb ischaemia

Medical treatment

Patients should be urged to comply with best medical therapy (BMT), which comprises:

- Immediate, absolute and permanent cessation from smoking
- Control of hypertension
- Control of hypercholesterolaemia. In many cases this requires a combination of diet and drug therapy. The aim is to achieve a total cholesterol no higher than 5.0 mmol/L
- Prescription of an antiplatelet agent. This is normally aspirin (75 mg daily), but in the significant proportion of patients who state they are unable to tolerate this, clopidogrel is an equally effective alternative
- Regular exercise (if possible)
- Control of obesity. This will help to bring down blood pressure, cholesterol and the 'strain' of walking
- The identification and active treatment of patients with diabetes. This includes foot care (see below).

Compliance with BMT not only increases walking distance but also longevity. Unfortunately, many patients fail to comply and, in particular, continue to smoke. These patients have a guarded prognosis in terms of both limb loss and premature death. Active intervention, by either endovascular or open surgery, should not normally be considered until the patient has been compliant with BMT for

at least 6 months. Obviously, revascularization is in addition to, not instead of, BMT, a point that often has to be spelled out to patients anxious to return to their previous lifestyle.

By the time a patient develops CLI it is generally the case that without revascularization the limb will be lost. However, this does not in any way undermine the value of instituting BMT. This may not only improve the condition of the leg, but may also reduce the overall risk of intervention. Prostacyclin analogues may relieve rest pain and augment ulcer healing in some patients. Apart from this, however, there is no specific medical treatment.

Endovascular management

Percutaneous transluminal (balloon) angioplasty (PTA) has been used successfully in the iliac, femoral, popliteal and crural arteries. PTA is performed under local anaesthesia. The lesion is identified on arteriography and crossed with a wire. A balloon catheter is introduced over the wire and the balloon inflated (Fig. 27.8). This ruptures the atheromatous plaque, thereby enlarging the lumen. In suprainguinal occlusions and complex disease metal stents may be deployed across the lesion to improve patency and reduce distal embolic complications. Endoluminal repair of the aortoiliac segment is routine practice in most vascular units because of its high patency rates and low morbidity compared to open surgery. Infrainguinal PTA is also widely used in the management of IC and CLI.

Intermittent claudication Claudicant patients should be chosen carefully for endoluminal repair because it is expensive and associated with a 1–2% morbidity rate. There

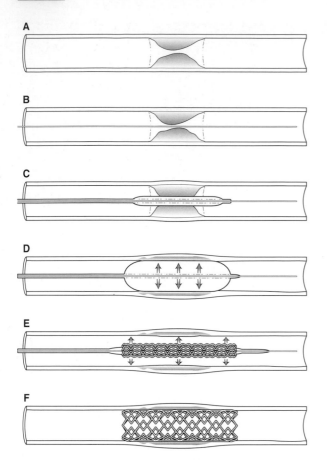

Fig. 27.8 Percutaneous transluminal angioplasty and stenting. **A** Critical arterial stenosis. **B** A guidewire is used to cross the lesion. **C** The guidewire is used to direct a balloon angioplasty catheter across the lesion. **D** The balloon is inflated. **E** A metal stent may be mounted on a catheter. The stent may be self-expanding or require expansion with a balloon. In many cases the first manoeuvre is to cross the lesion with a stent and in this circumstance steps C and D may be omitted. **F** Metal stent holding open the stenosis.

is controversy about its role in the femoropopliteal segment because two small trials have suggested a lack of durability of clinical benefit. However, PTA should be considered in patients with aortoiliac disease because they tend to be younger, may have normal infrainguinal arteries and tend to be more symptomatic (shorter walking distances and bilateral symptoms). Such patients may not achieve a satisfactory increase in walking distance with BMT alone, because the ability of the body to collateralize around aortoiliac disease is not as good as it is around femoro-popliteal disease. Furthermore, the long-term patency of PTA and stenting is optimal in high-flow large-calibre vessels.

Critical limb ischaemia Whereas the number of endoluminal repairs performed for IC is falling, the number performed for CLI is increasing. Endoluminal repair has a number of major theoretical advantages in this group of patients: it is safer, cheaper and quicker than surgery; it requires less hospitalization; it can be repeated; and, even if it is unsuccessful, does not appear to prejudice the chances of subsequently performing a successful arterial bypass. However, because patients with CLI tend to have complex multilevel disease, only a minority are suitable for conventional PTA. Studies comparing surgery and PTA in this patient group are currently underway.

Indications for arterial reconstruction

Intermittent claudication Most surgeons are reluctant to perform infrainguinal bypass surgery for IC because:

- The risk of limb loss is low with medical therapy
- Surgery is associated with a 1–2% risk of mortality and major morbidity
- Successful surgery on one side often reveals symptoms on the other, requiring a second operation
- Grafts have a finite patency.

As soon as a bypass graft is inserted, collaterals circumventing the original lesion involute. For this reason, when the graft occludes, usually suddenly, the patient is normally returned to a worse level of ischaemia than before the operation. A patient who was previously a claudicant may now have acute limb-threatening ischaemia, which then forces the surgeon or radiologist to reintervene. Secondary interventions such as thrombolysis or reoperation are technically more difficult, associated with higher risk and enjoy a lower patency rate. The patient must be fully apprised of

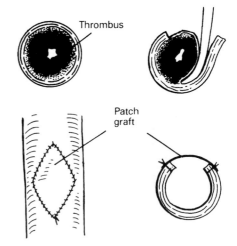

Fig. 27.9 Thromboendarterectomy and patch angioplasty.

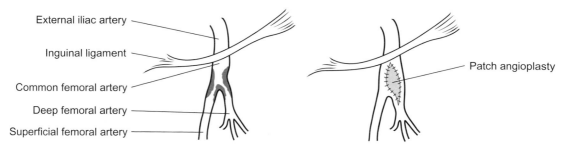

Fig. 27.10 Profundaplasty. Focal atherosclerotic disease of the left common femoral artery is causing severe ischaemia because it is obstructing flow down the superficial and deep femoral (profunda femoris) arteries. Local endarterectomy and closure of the profunda femoris using a patch (profundaplasty) restores normal flow to both vessels.

the risks and benefits so that they can make an informed decision.

As with PTA, the balance of risks and benefits is different in patients with aortoiliac disease because the long-term patency rates of such grafts is excellent, and one operation deals with both legs. However, the patient still needs to be aware that they are submitting to major surgery that carries a 30-day mortality of at least 5%.

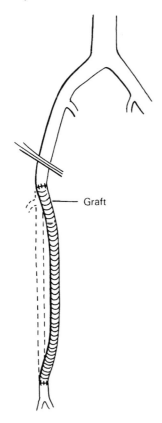

Fig. 27.11 Femorodistal bypass graft. Femoropopliteal graft inserted to bypass an occluded femoral artery.

Principles of arterial reconstruction

Endarterectomy This involves the direct removal of atherosclerotic plaque and thrombus (thromboendarterectomy) (Fig. 27.9). With the advent of prosthetic large-calibre grafts and the successful endovascular treatment of focal disease, endarterectomy is a relatively uncommon operation in modern surgical practice except at the carotid bifurcation (see below). In the lower limb common femoral endarterectomy, with or without a profundaplasty, is probably the commonest example (Fig. 27.10).

Bypass grafting For a femorodistal bypass (Fig. 27.11) to be successful in the long term, three conditions must be fulfilled:

1. There must be high-flow high-pressure blood entering the graft (inflow).
2. The conduit must be suitable.
3. The blood must have somewhere to go when it leaves the graft (outflow).

Two main types of conduit are available:

- Autogenous material, most commonly the ipsilateral long saphenous vein
- Prosthetic material, most commonly expanded polytetrafluoroethylene (ePTFE) or Dacron.

The main advantage of vein (Table 27.2) is that it is lined by endothelium that is actively antithrombotic and profibrinolytic, and therefore much less liable to induce coagulation than even the most inert of manmade materials. This translates into much better long-term graft patency. Vein is also much more resistant to infection (see below).

Reversed vs. in situ vein bypass It is generally agreed that, wherever possible, vein should be used for infrainguinal reconstruction. However, unless the long saphenous vein is reversed before being used as an arterial conduit its valves will prevent the flow of blood down the leg. Alternatively, the vein can be left as it is but the valves divided; this latter type of graft is called 'in situ'. There are

Table 27.2   Autogenous and prosthetic grafts

	Autogenous graft (vein)	Prosthetic graft (ePTFE, Dacron)
Advantages	No cost Superior long-term patency Resistant to infection	Easy to use Available 'off the shelf' in a variety of calibres and lengths
Disadvantages	Only available in small calibre Often diseased (varicose veins) or absent (previous bypass surgery, CABG, varicose vein surgery)	Expensive (£500–1000) per graft No resistance to infection Poor long-term patency below the knee

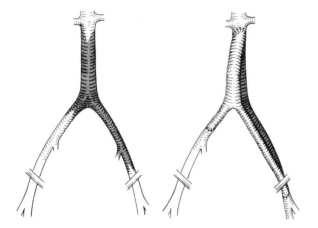

Fig. 27.12   Anatomic aortic bypass. Reconstruction of an occluded aortoiliac segment by a bifurcarian bypass graft.

pros and cons to each technique, but no difference in long-term patency between them has been demonstrated. The choice depends upon individual patient anatomy and surgeon preference.

Extra-anatomic bypass In most bypass operations the new conduit more or less follows the course of the original artery – so-called anatomic bypass (Fig. 27.12). Where this is not possible and/or desirable an extra-anatomic bypass can be inserted (Fig. 27.13). For example, if only one iliac artery is blocked, and the patient is unfit for abdominal surgery, a femorofemoral graft can be performed. If both iliac arteries are occluded then an axillobifemoral graft can be inserted. In general, these extra-anatomic grafts do not have as good long-term patency as anatomic aortoiliac reconstruction. However, they are much lesser procedures and the preferred option in high-risk patients or those that have a limited life expectancy.

Complications of arterial reconstruction In the early postoperative period (30 days) vascular patients are suscep-

tible to all the general complications of major surgery and anaesthesia. As such patients are usually elderly and unfit, the operations are lengthy and blood loss is often high, the morbidity of vascular surgery is considerably higher than for other types of major surgery, for example gastrointestinal surgery. Meticulous perioperative care is essential for optimal results, and close liaison between the surgeon, the anaesthetist and the intensivist is mandatory.

In the longer term the major complications are graft occlusion and infection. There are many reasons why a graft may occlude, and the correct management of this situation is a complex issue beyond the scope of this chapter. Suffice to say that the sooner a failed graft is identified and treated, the better, in general, the outcome. Many surgeons perform ultrasound scans of their grafts at regular intervals in the postoperative period – typically at 1, 3, 6, 12, 18 and 24 months. This so-called graft surveillance is designed to pick up technical problems with the graft that are likely to increase the risk of failure. It is generally better to correct a 'failing' graft before it has blocked than to try to resurrect one that has already failed.

Infection of prosthetic grafts is a serious and growing problem, largely due to the increasing prevalence of multiply resistant *Staphylococcus aureus* (MRSA). Once a prosthetic graft is infected it must be removed to rid the patient of sepsis and/or to prevent the anastomoses coming apart and causing life-threatening haemorrhage. Obviously this renders the distal part ischaemic and, where possible, a new graft is inserted through fresh uninfected tissue. This can be extremely challenging, and on occasions impossible. Measures to avoid graft infection include:

- Using autogenous material wherever possible
- Perioperative antibiotic prophylaxis
- Strict aseptic technique in the operating theatre and ward
- Washing hands between examining patients
- Prescribing antibiotics to patients with grafts in place whenever a bacteraemia might develop, for example dental extraction, cystoscopy, or any gastrointestinal intervention.

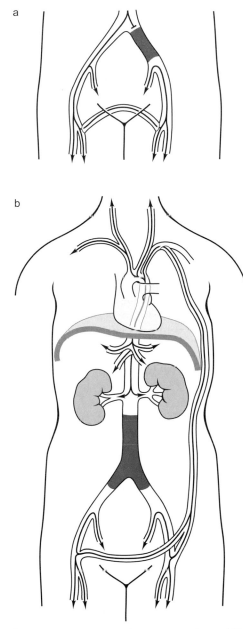

a

b

Fig. 27.13 Extra-anatomic bypass. **A** Unilateral iliac disease may be treated by femorofemoral cross-over graft. **B** Bilateral iliac disease may be treated with axillobifemoral bypass graft.

AMPUTATION

Indications

Amputation should only be considered where arterial reconstruction is considered by a vascular surgeon to be inappropriate or impossible.

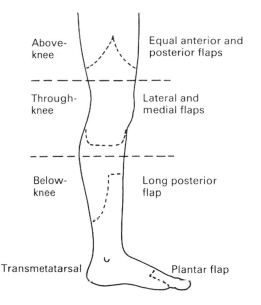

Fig. 27.14 Levels of amputation and types of flap used to close the residual defect.

In some cases patients are admitted profoundly unwell and septic from spreading gangrene and immediate amputation may be the only means of saving the patient's life.

Level of amputation

This is determined by local blood supply, the status of the joints, the patient's general health and their age. The broad principle is to amputate at the lowest level consistent with healing (Fig. 27.14). It is important to conserve the knee joint, as the energy required for walking with a below-knee prosthesis is only a fraction of that required with one above the knee. However, if the patient has other disabilities that make walking with a prosthesis impossible, there is no point in attempting to conserve the knee joint at the expense of healing. Most centres aim for a 2:1 ratio between below-knee (transtibial) and above-knee (transfemoral) amputations.

Surgical principles

A number of important principles must be observed if primary healing and satisfactory rehabilitation are to be achieved. The in-hospital mortality for major limb amputation is around 10–20%. The decision to amputate, the level of amputation and the procedure itself requires direct input from an experienced vascular surgeon.

Rehabilitation and limb fitting

At about 1 week the patient should begin to bear weight on the other limb between parallel bars, and at 10 days to walk with a pneumatic walking aid. If healing is progressing well, a temporary prosthesis can be fitted at about 3 weeks. Final fitting of the artificial limb must await shaping and firming of the stump. Approximately 70% of below-knee amputees and 30% of above-knee amputees eventually walk. It is important to appreciate that because of the prolonged hospital admission, rehabilitation, home modifications and, in some cases, long-term care, amputation is a much more expensive option than revascularization.

Patients need strong support and their care is a matter of teamwork, with the surgeon, nursing staff, physiotherapist, occupational therapist, prosthetist and social worker all playing vital roles. Amputation for vascular disease has high morbidity and mortality and only a few patients remain alive for 5 years.

Phantom pain

Phantom limb pain can be a late and troublesome complication, especially if pain has not been well controlled before and after the operation. With analgesia, reassurance and time it usually settles. There is some evidence that if the patient goes to theatre painfree, the risk of phantom pain is

much reduced. For this reason, many centres now commence epidural anaesthesia the night before surgery.

ARTERIAL DISEASE OF THE UPPER LIMB

Overview

Occlusive arterial disease is 10 times commoner in the leg than in the arm. Nevertheless, when the arm is affected treatment can be difficult, and the loss of an arm is more devastating for the patient than loss of a leg.

The subclavian artery just proximal to the origin of the vertebral artery is the commonest site of disease, especially on the left. This may lead to:

- *Arm claudication* This is relatively unusual, even when the subclavian artery is completely occluded, because of the very well developed collaterals.
- *Atheroembolism to the hand* Small emboli lodge in the vessels of the fingers and the hand and lead to symptoms that are often mistaken for Raynaud's phenomenon, except that in this case the symptoms are unilateral (see below). Failure to make the diagnosis may eventually lead to amputation.
- *Subclavian steal* In this circumstance, when the arm is used blood is stolen from the brain via the vertebral artery. This leads to vertebrobasilar ischaemia, characterized by dizziness, cortical blindness, and/or collapse when the arm is used (Fig. 27.15).

Management

Most subclavian artery disease should be treated by means of PTA and stenting, as the results are good and surgical access to the area is difficult. If surgery is required then the common operation is bypass from the common carotid artery to the subclavian or axillary artery distal to the lesion (carotid–subclavian bypass).

CEREBROVASCULAR DISEASE

Definitions

Stroke

Stroke may be defined as an episode of focal neurological dysfunction lasting more than 24 hours of presumed vascular aetiology.

Transient ischaemic attack

When such symptoms last for less than 24 hours the episode is described as a transient ischaemic attack (TIA).

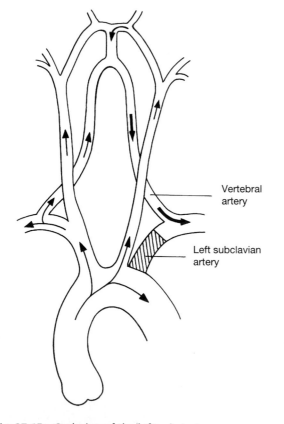

Vertebral artery

Left subclavian artery

Fig. 27.15 Occlusion of the left subclavian artery causing 'subclavian steal'.

Amaurosis fugax

This describes transient, usually incomplete, loss of vision in one eye owing to occlusion of a branch of the retinal artery by cholesterol emboli. The patient typically describes it as a veil or curtain coming across the eye, which remains for a few minutes and then disappears.

Carotid artery disease

Pathophysiology

Approximately 80% of strokes are ischaemic and about half of these are thought to be due to atheroembolism from the carotid bifurcation. The origin of the internal carotid artery is particularly prone to atheroma, which is often focal and therefore amenable to local carotid endarterectomy (CEA) (see below). In general, the tighter the degree of stenosis the more likely the plaque is to rupture and embolize. Atheroemboli entering the ophthalmic artery lead to amaurosis fugax or permanent monocular blindness on the same side (ipsilateral). If they enter the middle cerebral artery they may cause hemiparesis and hemisensory loss on the opposite side (con-

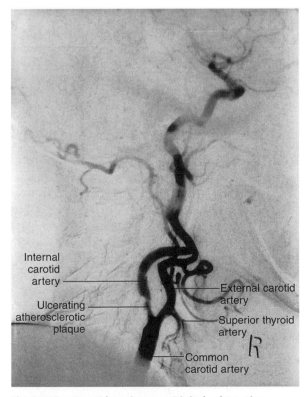

Fig. 27.16 Carotid angiogram. Digital subtraction carotid angiogram showing severe stenosis at the origin of the internal carotid artery.

tralateral). If the dominant hemisphere is affected there may also be dysphasia.

Assessment

The presence of a 'carotid' bruit bears no relationship to the severity of underlying internal carotid artery disease and thus the risk of stroke. Such a bruit may arise from the external carotid artery, and in the presence of a very tight internal carotid artery stenosis flow may be so slow that no audible turbulence is present. It is important to exclude other causes of cerebral ischaemia and haemorrhage.

Colour Doppler (duplex) ultrasound (CDU) is the initial investigation of choice for imaging the carotid arteries. However, CDU is limited by vessel calcification, and is very operator dependent. Magnetic resonance angiography (MRA) provides excellent images but is limited by availability. Angiography should be reserved for patients with unsuccessful or inconsistent non-invasive imaging (Fig. 27.16).

Treatment

Medical therapy

All patients should receive BMT.

Carotid endarterectomy (CEA)

Patients with completed major stroke are not candidates for surgical intervention; nor are those with an occluded internal carotid artery. However, CEA in addition to BMT is associated with a significant reduction in stroke compared with BMT alone in patients with amaurosis, TIA and stroke, with good recovery provided that:

- The degree of internal carotid artery stenosis exceeds 70%.
- The patient is expected to survive at least 2 years.
- The operation can be undertaken with a stroke and/or death rate of less than 5%.
- The operation can be performed soon after the index event, preferably within a month, but certainly within 6 months.

Patients who do not fulfil these criteria should, in most cases, be treated medically.

Carotid endarterectomy

The operation can be performed under general or local anaesthetic. The carotid bifurcation is dissected out, heparin is given and the arteries are clamped. If this leads to cerebral ischaemia then a shunt is inserted (Fig. 27.17). The plaque is shelled out and the artery repaired with direct suture or a patch graft.

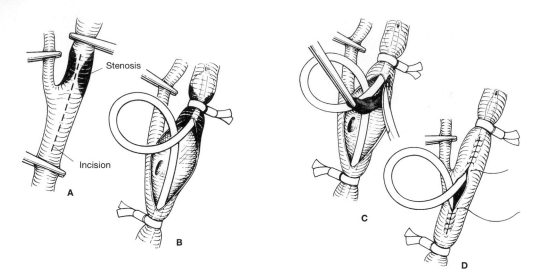

Fig. 27.17 Carotid endarterectomy using an internal shunt to maintain cerebral blood flow while the occluding plaque is removed.

Endovascular therapy

Although carotid stenting is still an experimental procedure, the initial results are encouraging and further trials are currently under way.

Asymptomatic carotid disease

Asymptomatic carotid artery stenosis is relatively common and is often picked up on a carotid duplex scan performed because a bruit has been detected in the neck. However, for the reasons outlined above, a bruit in isolation is not an indication for further carotid investigations. The risk of developing symptoms is quite low, and the role of CEA remains controversial. Such patients should be discussed with a vascular surgeon.

Vertebrobasilar disease

The vertebrobasilar system feeds the occipital cortex, cerebellum and brain stem. Patients with vertebrobasilar insufficiency (VBI) may complain of (bilateral) cortical blindness, vertigo and loss of balance. Only a minority of patients have focal, discrete disease amenable to vascular or endovascular intervention.

RENAL ARTERY DISEASE

Atherosclerosis

Critical stenoses impair the perfusion of the juxtaglomerular apparatus, which in turn leads to an increase in renin

---

SUMMARY BOX

Carotid artery disease

- Up to 50% of all ischaemic strokes may be caused by atheroembolism from the carotid bifurcation.

- Patients with carotid territory TIAs and amaurosis fugax should be assessed with a view to carotid endarterectomy.

- Carotid endarterectomy, in addition to best medical therapy, has been proved to significantly reduce the risk of further ipsilateral ischaemic stroke compared to best medical therapy alone in patients with symptomatic internal carotid artery stenosis exceeding 70%.

- Carotid endarterectomy for high-grade asymptomatic internal carotid artery stenosis is controversial; such patients should be discussed with a vascular surgeon.

- Angioplasty and stenting may be used to treat an increasing proportion of carotid artery disease in the future.

---

and angiotensin and hypertension. The disease may also lead to ischaemic necrosis of the renal parenchyma and progressive renal failure.

It is often difficult to determine whether renal artery disease is merely an incidental finding or is causally linked. Sometimes, the only way of clarifying the situation is to revascularize the kidney and observe what happens.

However, this means that a significant proportion of patients may be receiving unnecessary, potentially harmful, treatment.

Fibromuscular hyperplasia

This is a relatively uncommon and poorly understood stenosing condition that most commonly affects the renal arteries of young and middle-aged women. It may cause hypertension, but rarely renal failure.

Treatment

Indications

There are two indications for active intervention in cases of renal artery stenosis:

1. Control of hypertension that is refractory to medical therapy.
2. Preservation of renal function.

Endovascular therapy

Primary stenting is the treatment of choice for atherosclerotic renal artery disease. PTA is also very effective for FMD (fibromuscular dysplasia). Major complications (1–2%) include acute arterial occlusion, embolization and rupture.

Surgery

Renal artery reconstruction is a major undertaking with significant associated morbidity and mortality. It is largely reserved for patients who are not treatable by percutaneous means.

MESENTERIC ARTERY DISEASE

The coeliac axis and the superior and inferior mesenteric arteries supply the gastrointestinal tract. Owing to the rich collaterals it is usually necessary for two of the three vessels to be occluded or critically stenosed before patients develop symptoms and signs of mesenteric vascular insufficiency, often termed 'mesenteric angina'. Typically the patient develops severe central abdominal pain 15–30 minutes after eating, which may be associated with diarrhoea. Food avoidance leads to significant weight loss, which is universal. The condition can mimic many, much commoner intra-abdominal pathologies. Surgery is associated with significant morbidity and mortality (5–10%) but the long-term symptom relief is usually excellent; less commonly, angioplasty is used.

Acute embolic occlusion, of the superior mesenteric artery (SMA) presents with sudden onset of excruciating abdominal pain, collapse, bloody diarrhoea and peritonitis. Treatment comprises emergency SMA embolectomy and resection of non-viable bowel. Unfortunately, there is often extensive bowel necrosis by the time the patient is operated on and mortality exceeds 50%.

ACUTE LIMB ISCHAEMIA

Aetiology

Acute limb ischaemia is the most common vascular emergency. It is most frequently caused by acute thrombotic occlusion of a pre-existing stenotic arterial segment (60%), thromboembolism (30%) and trauma, which may be iatrogenic. Distinguishing between thrombosis and embolism is important because treatment and prognosis are different (Table 27.3). More than 70% of peripheral emboli are due to atrial fibrillation (AF). Thrombosis in situ may arise

Table 27.3 Embolus vs. thrombosis in situ		
Clinical features	Embolus	Thrombosis
Severity	Complete ischaemia (no collaterals)	Incomplete ischaemia (collaterals)
Onset	Seconds or minutes	Hours or days
Limb	Leg 3:1 arm	Leg 10:1 arm
Multiple sites	Up to 15%	Rare
Embolic source	Present (usually AF)	Absent
Previous claudication	Absent	Present
Palpation of artery	Soft; tender	Hard/calcified
Bruits	Absent	Present
Contralateral leg pulses	Present	Absent
Diagnosis	Clinical	Angiography
Treatment	Embolectomy, warfarin	Medical, bypass, thrombolysis
Prognosis	Loss of life > loss of limb	Loss of limb > loss of life

Table 27.4 Classification of limb ischaemia	
Terminology	Definition/comment
Onset	
Acute	Ischaemia < 14 days
Acute-on-chronic	Worsening symptoms and signs (< 14 days)
Chronic	Ischaemia stable for > 14 days
Severity (acute, acute-on-chronic)	
Incomplete	Limb not threatened
Complete	Limb threatened
Irreversible	Limb non-viable
Severity (chronic)	
Non-critical	Intermittent claudication
Subcritical	Night/rest pain
Critical	Tissue loss (ulceration +/– gangrene)

Table 27.5 Symptoms and signs of acute limb ischaemia	
Symptoms/signs	Comment
Pain	May be absent in complete acute ischaemia, also present in chronic ischaemia
Pallor	
Pulseless	Unreliable, as the ischaemic
Perishing cold	limb takes on the ambient temperature
Parasthesia	Important features of impending irreversible ischaemia
Paralysis	

from acute plaque rupture, hypovolaemia or 'pump failure' (see below).

Classification

Limb ischaemia is classified on the basis of onset and severity (Table 27.4). Incomplete acute ischaemia (e.g. thrombosis in situ) can usually be treated medically, at least in the first instance. Complete ischaemia (e.g. embolus) will normally result in extensive tissue necrosis within 6 hours unless the limb is revascularized. Irreversible ischaemia mandates early amputation or, if the patient is unfit, conservative therapy.

Clinical features

Apart from paralysis (inability to wiggle toes/fingers) and parasthesia (loss of light touch over the dorsum of the foot/hand), the so-called Ps of acute ischaemia (Table 27.5) are non-specific and/or inconsistently related to its completeness. Pain on squeezing the calf indicates muscle infarction and impending irreversible ischaemia.

At first, acute complete ischaemia is associated with intense distal arterial spasm and the limb is 'marble' white. As the spasm relaxes over the next few hours and the skin fills with deoxygenated blood, mottling appears which is light blue or purple, has a fine reticular pattern and blanches on pressure. At this stage the limb is still salvageable. As ischaemia progresses blood coagulates in the skin, leading to mottling that is darker in colour, coarser in pattern and does not blanch. Finally, large patches of fixed staining progress to blistering and liquefaction. Attempts at revascularization at this late stage are futile and will lead to life-threatening reperfusion injury (see below).

Management

All suspected acutely ischaemic limbs must be discussed immediately with a vascular surgeon – a few hours can make the difference between death/amputation and complete recovery of limb function. If there are no contraindications, administer an intravenous bolus of heparin to limit propagation of thrombus and protect the collateral circulation. If ischaemia is complete, proceed directly to the operating theatre because angiography will introduce delay, thrombolysis is not an option, and lack of collateral flow will prevent visualization of the distal vasculature. If ischaemia is incomplete obtain preoperative imaging wherever possible, as simple embolectomy or thrombectomy is unlikely to be successful, thrombolysis may be an option, and a 'road-map' for distal bypass is helpful.

Acute embolus

Embolic occlusion of the brachial artery is not usually limb-threatening and, in an elderly patient, non-operative treatment is reasonable. Younger patients should undergo embolectomy to prevent subsequent claudication, especially where the dominant arm is affected.

A leg affected by embolus is nearly always threatened and requires immediate surgical revascularization. Femoral embolus is associated with profound ischaemia to the level of the upper thigh because the deep femoral artery is also affected. Acute embolic occlusion of the aortic bifurcation (saddle embolus) leads to absent femoral pulses and a patient who is 'marble' white or mottled to the waist. Patients may also present with paraplegia due to ischaemia of the cauda equina, which may be irreversible. Embolectomy can be performed under local/regional or general anaesthetic (Fig. 27.18). Postoperatively, the patient should continue on heparin. Warfarin reduces the risk of recurrent embolism. The in-hospital mortality from cardiac death and/or recurrent embolism, particularly stroke, is 10–20%.

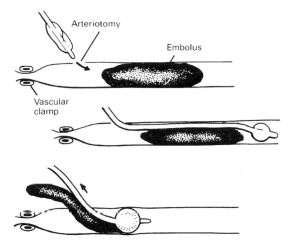

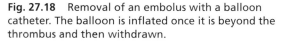

Fig. 27.18 Removal of an embolus with a balloon catheter. The balloon is inflated once it is beyond the thrombus and then withdrawn.

Thrombosis in situ

There is usually a reason why the limb affected by stable chronic ischaemia suddenly deteriorates, for example 'silent' MI or underlying, hitherto asymptomatic, malignancy. Septicaemia, particularly pneumococcal and meningococcal, may be associated with widespread thrombosis.

Popliteal aneurysm

Popliteal aneurysm can undergo thrombosis or act as a source of emboli. Catheter-directed intra-arterial thrombolysis of the crural vessels is often the treatment of choice, as simple thrombectomy usually leads to early rethrombosis and the distal run-off is often obliterated, precluding surgical bypass. Once the crural circulation is restored, a bypass should be performed to exclude the aneurysm (see below).

Trauma

In the UK acute traumatic limb ischaemia is frequently iatrogenic. The commonest causes of non-iatrogenic injury are limb fractures and dislocations, blunt injuries occurring in the course of road traffic accidents, and stab wounds. The presence of distal pulses does not exclude significant arterial injury. Where there is suspicion of major vascular injury, angiography should be performed.

Intra-arterial drug administration

This leads to intense spasm and microvascular thrombosis. The leg is mottled and digital gangrene is not uncommon, but pedal pulses are usually palpable. The mainstay of treatment is supportive care, hydration to minimize renal failure secondary to rhabdomyolysis, and full heparinization. Vascular reconstruction is almost never indicated, but fasciotomy may be required to prevent compartment syndrome (see below).

Thoracic outlet syndrome

Pressure on the subclavian artery from a cervical rib or abnormal soft tissue band may lead to a poststenotic dilatation lined with thrombosis, predisposing to occlusion or embolization. The distal circulation may be chronically obliterated and digital ischaemia advanced before the diagnosis is made. The diagnosis is made on duplex scan and/or angiography. Treatment options include thrombolysis, thrombectomy/embolectomy, excision of the cervical rib and repair of the aneurysmal segment.

Thrombolysis

This is performed percutaneously by interventional radiologists under local anaesthetic. A catheter is embedded into the distal extent of thrombus and recombinant tissue plasminogen activator (rTPA) is infused. TPA converts plasminogen to plasmin, which dissolves fibrin clot. The technique may be used in embolic occlusion but if the ischaemia is severe, lysis may be contraindicated because thrombus dissolution often takes several hours. Thrombolysis may dissolve the clot to reveal an underlying lesion amenable to endovascular therapy or surgery. Thrombolysis is associated with a significant major (5%) and minor (15%) complication rate, including stroke (2%).

Postischaemic syndromes
Reperfusion injury

Activated neutrophils, free radicals, enzymes, hydrogen ions, carbon dioxide, potassium and myoglobin released from reperfused tissue can lead to acute respiratory distress syndrome (ARDS), myocardial stunning, endotoxaemia and acute tubular necrosis, leading to multiple organ failure.

Compartment syndrome

Endothelial cell injury during ischaemia leads to increased capillary permeability and oedema on reperfusion. In the calf, where muscles are confined within tight facial boundaries, the increase in interstitial tissue pressure can lead to continuing muscle necrosis despite apparently adequate arterial inflow – the so-called compartment syndrome. There is swelling and pain on squeezing the calf muscle or moving the ankle. Palpable pedal pulses do not exclude the syndrome. The key to management is prevention through expeditious revascularization and a low threshold for fasciotomy (Fig. 27.19).

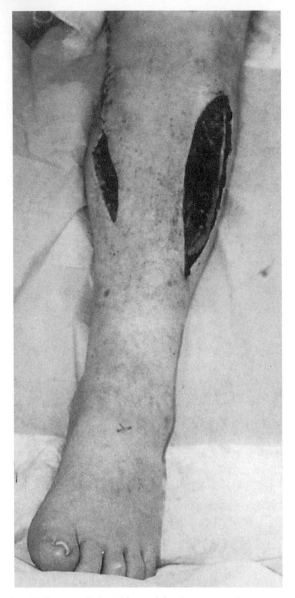

Fig. 27.19 Medial and lateral fasciotomy to decompress a compartment syndrome.

ANEURYSMAL DISEASE

Classification

An aneurysm may be defined as an abnormal focal dilatation of an endothelial-lined structure (artery, vein, heart chamber). Arterial aneurysms are by far the most common. Aneurysms may be classified according to their site, underlying aetiology and morphology.

Site

Any artery can be affected. The commonest site for aneurysmal disease presenting to the vascular surgeon is the infrarenal aorta; others include the popliteal, femoral and subclavian arteries.

Aetiology

Atherosclerotic Most aneurysms are 'non-specific' in aetiology; in the past they were termed 'atherosclerotic'. However, it is now clear that aneurysmal disease is a distinct pathological process from occlusive arterial disease, although they share some of the same risk factors (smoking and hypertension) and may coexist in the same patient.

Mycotic The term mycotic, meaning fungal, is a misnomer because fungi do not cause aneurysms. The term is used nowadays to include all aneurysms that are believed to be infected. The infection can be primary or secondary to other pathology. Arteries are generally resistant to infection, but two organisms, *Treponema pallidum* (syphilis) and salmonella, have a particular ability to produce primary mycotic aneurysms. Septic emboli from heart valves affected by subacute bacterial endocarditis may also lodge in the distal vasculature and produce secondary mycotic aneurysms. 'Non-specific' aneurysms and the layers of laminated thrombus within them may become infected in the course of a bacteraemia from another site. Lastly, infection of prosthetic grafts can lead to infected anastomotic aneurysms.

SUMMARY BOX

Acute limb ischaemia

- Acute limb ischaemia is the commonest vascular emergency.

- The most common causes are embolus from the left atrium in association with atrial fibrillation and acute thrombosis at a site of long-standing atherosclerotic narrowing.

- It is often possible to distinguish these two conditions on clinical grounds alone.

- The treatment of embolism is urgent embolectomy, usually without prior angiography.

- Patients with thrombosis in situ should undergo angiography, and treatment comprises a combination of medical therapy, thrombolysis, angioplasty and bypass.

- Paralysis, parasthesia and muscle tenderness are the cardinals signs of complete acute ischaemia; when present, the limb must be revascularized immediately if it is to be saved. Always consider a fasciotomy upon successful reperfusion in such cases to avoid compartment syndrome.

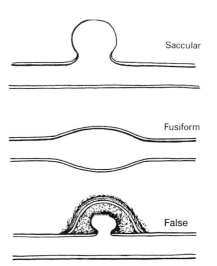

Fig. 27.20 True and false aneurysms.

True aneurysms

All three layers of the arterial wall enclose a true aneurysm (Fig. 27.20).

False aneurysms

If the wall of an artery is pierced, the resulting haematoma sometimes remains in continuity with the lumen. A pulsatile swelling then forms, whose wall consists of compacted thrombus and surrounding connective tissue. Small aneurysms (2–3 cm in diameter) often thrombose spontaneously. Larger aneurysms tend to expand, especially if the patient is on heparin or warfarin, and compress surrounding tissues. The commonest site is the groin after common femoral artery instrumentation, and this may cause femoral vein compression and DVT. Surgery is the traditional method of treatment, but ultrasound-guided compression repair and thrombin injection are increasingly used and successful.

ABDOMINAL AORTIC ANEURYSM (AAA)

Epidemiology

AAA is present in 5% of men aged over 60 years. In about 70% of cases only the infrarenal segment is involved. In the remainder the rest of the abdominal aorta, the thoracic aorta or a combination of both is involved. The incidence of AAA is increasing. They are three times more commoner in men than in women, and the median age at presentation is 65 years for elective and 75 years for emergency cases.

Clinical features

An abdominal aortic aneurysm may present in the following ways.

- *Asymptomatic (30%)* The AAA may be detected incidentally on routine physical examination, plain X-ray or, most commonly, abdominal ultrasound scan conducted for another reason. Even a large AAA can be difficult to feel, which explains why so many remain undetected until they rupture. Studies are currently under way to determine whether screening men over the age of 60 for AAA by means of ultrasound will result in a reduction in the number of deaths from rupture. All patients with an incidental finding of an AAA should be discussed with a vascular surgeon.
- *Symptomatic (20%)* AAA may cause pain in the central abdomen, back, loin, iliac fossa or groin. Thrombus within the aneurysm sac may be a source of emboli to the lower limbs. Less commonly the aneurysm may undergo thrombotic occlusion. AAA may also compress surrounding structures such as the duodenum, ureter, and the inferior vena cava.
- *Rupture (50%)* AAA may rupture into the retroperitoneum, the peritoneal cavity or surrounding structures, most commonly the inferior vena cava, leading to an aortocaval fistula.

Investigation

About two-thirds of AAAs are sufficiently calcified to show up on a plain abdominal X-ray (Fig. 27.21). Ultrasound (Fig. 27.22) is the best way of establishing the diagnosis, of obtaining an approximate size, and of following up patients with asymptomatic AAAs that are not yet large enough to warrant surgical repair. CT (Fig. 27.23) scanning will provide much more accurate information about the size and extent of the aneurysm, the surrounding structures, and whether there is any other intra-abdominal pathology. It is the standard preoperative investigation but is not suitable for surveillance. Arteriography is only indicated if there are concerns about associated lower limb, renal and/or visceral occlusive disease.

Asymptomatic AAA

Until an AAA has reached 5.5 cm in maximum diameter, the risks of surgery generally outweigh the risk of rupture. The best way of following up these patients is by ultrasound. However, ultrasound is only accurate to about 0.5 cm, and so when the AAA reaches 5.0 cm many surgeons would obtain a CT. Repair is considered when the AAA exceeds 5.5 cm.

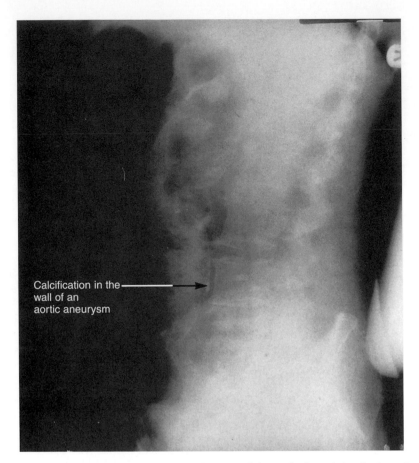

Calcification in the
wall of an
aortic aneurysm

Fig. 27.21 Plain lateral abdominal X-ray showing calcification of the wall of an abdominal aortic aneurysm (arrow).

Symptomatic

All symptomatic AAAs should be considered for repair, not only to rid the patient of their symptoms but also because pain often predates rupture. Distal embolization is a definite indication for repair, even if the AAA is small, as limb loss is common if left untreated.

Ruptured AAA

This is the commonest presentation of AAA to vascular surgeons in the UK. Patients survive rupture for the following reasons:

1. The rupture is usually into the retroperitoneum, which tamponades the leak.
2. There is intense vasoconstriction of non-essential circulatory beds.
3. The patient develops an intensely prothrombotic state.
4. The patient's blood pressure drops, which helps to seal the hole.

Any medical intervention that upsets this delicate balance will convert a relatively stable, salvageable patient into someone unlikely to reach the operating theatre, or to survive surgery. Specifically, large volumes of intravenous fluid (saline or plasma expander) increase the patient's blood pressure, impair haemostasis and abolish vasoconstriction, and must therefore not be given. The only way of saving the patient is to clamp the aorta, and there must be no delay in getting the patient to the operating theatre so that this can be done.

Open AAA repair

This entails replacing the aneurysmal segment with a prosthetic graft (Fig. 27.24). The 30-day mortality for this procedure is approximately 5–8% for elective asymptomatic, 10–20% for emergency symptomatic and about 50% for ruptured AAA. However, patients who leave hospital have a long-term survival that approaches that of the normal population.

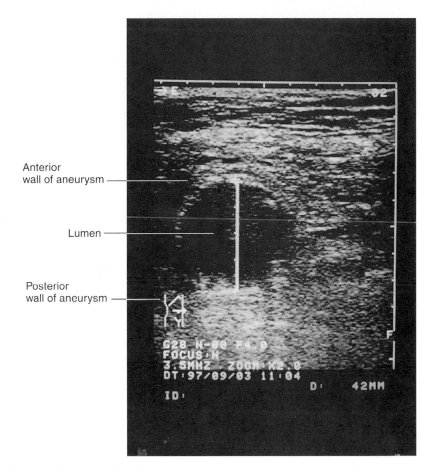

Anterior
wall of aneurysm

Lumen

Posterior
wall of aneurysm

Fig. 27.22   Abdominal ultrasound showing a transverse section through a large abdominal aortic aneurysm.

Endovascular AAA repair

Some AAAs may be treated with a covered stent placed via a femoral arteriotomy under radiological guidance (Fig. 27.25). Laparotomy and cross-clamping of the aorta are avoided. The procedure can be performed under regional anaesthesia. However, at present only a proportion of AAAs are suitable for this technique. In general, it is only suitable for the elective treatment of AAA, although devices have been placed successfully in patients with ruptured abdominal and thoracic aneurysms. The role of stenting is likely to increase in the future.

PERIPHERAL ANEURYSMS

Any peripheral artery, and very rarely vein, can be affected by aneurysmal dilatation. The aetiology, clinical features and treatment vary depending upon the site of disease.

Iliac aneurysms

Approximately 20% of AAA extend into one or both common iliac arteries and about a third of these extend into the internal iliac artery; for reasons unknown, the external iliac artery is rarely affected. Isolated iliac aneurysms can also occur. The bifurcation of the aorta is at the level of the umbilicus, so that a pulsatile mass below that level is likely to be iliac in origin. Iliac aneurysms are most often treated in the course of AAA repair. Isolated iliac aneurysms should be considered for endoluminal or surgical repair if they are causing symptoms or have reached twice the normal diameter of the native artery.

Femoral aneurysms

Three types of femoral aneurysm commonly present to the vascular surgeon: iatrogenic false aneurysm (see above), non-specific aneurysm and anastomotic aneurysm. 'Non-specific' aneurysms of the common femoral artery are

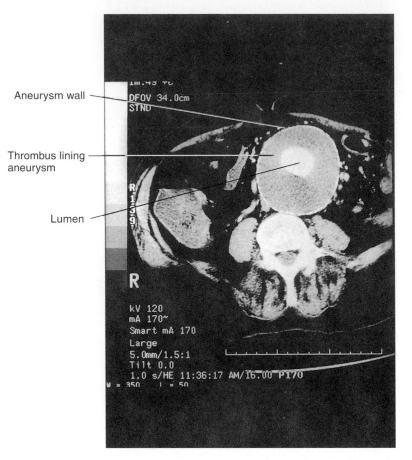

Aneurysm wall

Thrombus lining aneurysm

Lumen

Fig. 27.23 Computed tomography (CT) showing a transverse section through a large abdominal aortic aneurysm.

found in 10% of patients with AAA and as an isolated occurrence. Patients presenting with a femoral aneurysm should have an AAA excluded, if necessary, by ultrasound scan. In 50% of cases they are bilateral. They are frequently asymptomatic but may cause pain and compression of surrounding structures (femoral vein and nerve); rupture is uncommon. If large (>3 cm) or symptomatic they should be considered for surgical repair. Anastomotic false aneurysms are increasingly being seen in patients who have previously undergone aortobifemoral bypass grafting for occlusive or aneurysmal disease. They may not present until 10 years after the original surgery, but once present they, grow inexorably and require repair. They are usually due to mechanical disruption of the anastomosis as a result of late suture failure or progressive disease of the femoral artery; less commonly they are due to infection.

Popliteal aneurysms

These are present in 20% of patients with AAA and their presence must be sought, if necessary with ultrasound, in all

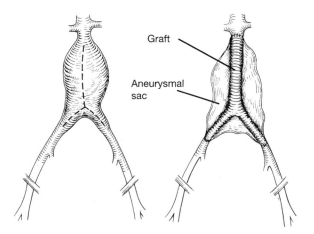

Graft

Aneurysmal sac

Fig. 27.24 Repair of an aortic aneurysm by insertion of a 'trouser' bifurcation graft within the opened aneurysmal sac.

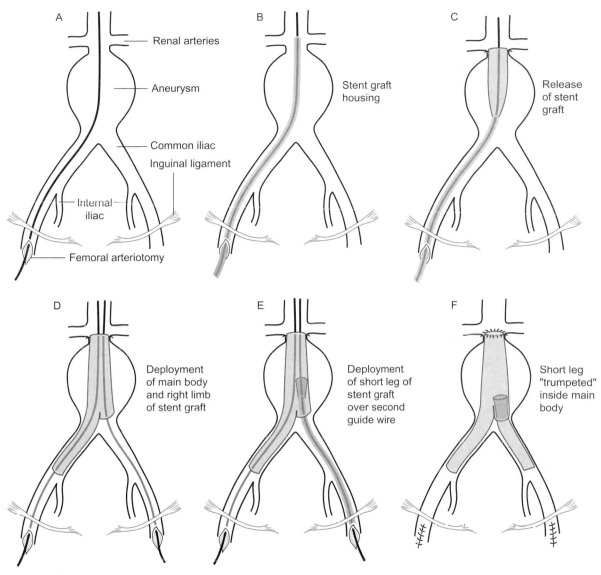

Fig. 27.25 Endovascular stent-graft repair of AAA. **A** A guidewire is passed through the aneurysm via an incision in the right common femoral artery. **B** A catheter containing the main body of the stent-graft is passed over the guidewire and into position within the aneurysm. **C** The outer cover of the catheter is removed, allowing the upper part of the stent-graft to spring open and become attached to the wall of the aorta just below the renal arteries by hooks. **D** The rest of the catheter is removed, allowing deployment of the main body of the graft and the right (long) limb within the common iliac artery. Note the short (left) limb of the graft. **E** Via an incision in the left common femoral artery a second guidewire is passed up though the short limb of the stent graft. A second catheter containing the rest of the stent-graft is passed over the guidewire and into the main body of the stent-graft. As before, retraction of the outer cover allows the top of the second limb of the stent-graft to open within the short limb of the main body. **F** Deployment is complete and the aneurysm sac completely excluded from the circulation. The femoral arteries are closed.

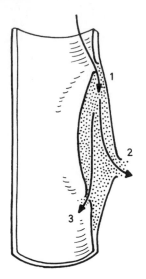

Fig. 27.26 Aortic dissection. (1) Initial intimal tear; (2) adventitial rupture; (3) intimal rupture.

such patients; 50% are bilateral. If a patient presents with a popliteal aneurysm there is a 50% chance that they also have an AAA, which again must be sought. The main complication of popliteal aneurysm is distal embolization and acute thrombosis; the latter is associated with limb loss in 50% of cases because the calf vessels are often chronically occluded, which makes surgical bypass difficult. As discussed above, the best treatment is usually thrombolysis followed by surgical bypass using the long saphenous vein (Fig. 27.27). Rupture of a popliteal aneurysm is extremely rare. Occasionally they can compress the popliteal vein and present as a DVT.

Subclavian aneurysms

This is usually associated with mechanical compression at the thoracic outlet from a cervical rib. Arterial stenosis causes a jet of high-velocity blood flow just distal to the narrowed area and, for reasons that are not entirely clear, this leads to post-stenotic dilatation (Fig. 27.28). This dilatation can become frankly aneurysmal and lined with thrombus which, as described above with regard to popliteal aneurysm, can lead to thrombotic occlusion and/or distal embolization. This presents as chronic or acute-on-chronic arm ischaemia; a pulsatile supraclavicular mass is often present.

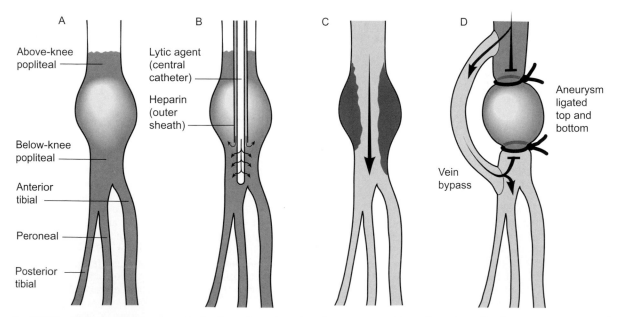

Fig. 27.27 Thrombolytic treatment of a thrombosed popliteal aneurysm. **A** Thrombosed popliteal aneurysm associated with complete thrombotic occlusion of the calf vessels. **B** The interventional radiologist has placed a catheter in the thrombosed aneurysm. The catheter has been introduced via the contralateral femoral artery, percutaneously under local anaesthesia. The outer part of the catheter is used to deliver heparin and the inner part to deliver lytic agent into the thrombus. **C** Lysis is complete and flow has been restored to the foot. The catheter has been removed. **D** The popliteal aneurysm has been bypassed and excluded from the circulation to prevent rethrombosis.

BUERGER'S DISEASE (THROMBOANGIITIS OBLITERANS)

This is an inflammatory obliterative arterial disease that is quite distinct from atherosclerosis. It is rare in the UK but common in Mediterraneans and North Africans; there is a strong genetic element. It usually presents in young (20–30 years) male smokers and characteristically affects the peripheral arteries, giving rise to claudication in the feet or rest pain in the fingers or toes. The condition also affects the veins and superficial thrombophlebitis is common. Wrist and ankle pulses are usually absent, but brachial and popliteal pulses are palpable. Arteriography shows narrowing or occlusion of arteries below the diseased segment, but relatively healthy vessels above that level. The condition often remits if the patient stops smoking; sympathectomy and prostaglandin infusions may be helpful. If amputation is required it can often be limited to the digits at first. However, if the patient continues to smoke then bilateral below-knee amputation is a frequent outcome.

RAYNAUD'S PHENOMENON

Raynaud's phenomenon describes digital pallor, due to vasospasm of the digital arteries, followed by cyanosis owing to the presence of deoxygenated blood, then rubor due to reactive hyperaemia upon restoration of flow, in response to cold and emotional stimuli.

> **SUMMARY BOX**
>
> *Aneurysmal disease*
>
> - AAAs are present in 5% of men aged over 60 and more than half are asymptomatic and undetected until they rupture.
>
> - Ruptured AAA is the 10th most common cause of death in men. Only a third of patients with ruptured AAA reach hospital alive and, of these, only about half survive surgery. The overall mortality for the condition is therefore in excess of 80%. Population screening of men over the age of 60 years with ultrasound may reduce this number.
>
> - Patients with asymptomatic AAA should be considered for repair if the maximum diameter reaches 5.5 cm and the surgeon believes the operation will be associated with a mortality of less than 5–7%.
>
> - An increasingly large number of AAAs may be repaired endoluminally using stent-grafts in the future.
>
> - Thrombosed popliteal aneurysm is a relatively common, but frequently overlooked, cause of acute and acute-on-chronic lower limb ischaemia.
>
> - Distal embolization from a subclavian aneurysm may be misdiagnosed as Raynaud's phenomenon, but Raynaud's is always bilateral.

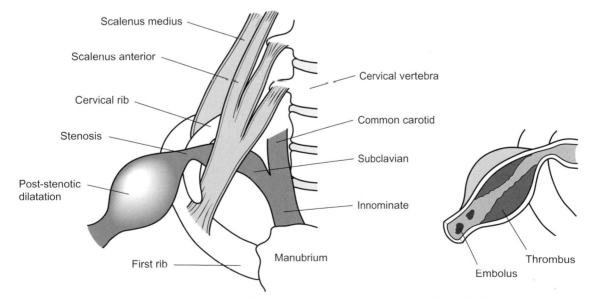

Fig. 27.28 Subclavian aneurysm. **A** Compression of the subclavian artery by a cervical rib has lead to poststenotic dilatation and aneurysm formation. **B** Thrombus within a subclavian aneurysm acting as a source of distal emboli.

Primary Raynaud's phenomenon

This is also called Raynaud's disease and affects 5–10% of young women in temperate climates. It usually appears between the ages of 15 and 30 years; a family history is common. It does not progress to ulceration or infarction. No investigation is necessary and the patient is given reassurance, advised to avoid exposure to cold, and treated in the first instance with nifedipine (a calcium channel blocker). The underlying cause is unclear.

Secondary Raynaud's phenomenon

This is also known as Raynaud's syndrome and tends to occur in older people in association with:

● Connective tissue disease, most commonly systemic sclerosis
● Vibration-induced injury, from the use of power tools
● Atherosclerosis, most commonly thoracic outlet obstruction from the cervical rib (see above).

Unlike primary disease that is due to reversible spasm, secondary disease is associated with fixed obstruction of the digital arteries. Fingertip ulceration and necrosis are often present. The fingers must be protected from cold and trauma, infection is treated with antibiotics, and surgery is avoided if possible. Vasoactive drugs have no clear benefit. Sympathectomy helps for a year or two. Prostacyclin infusions are sometimes beneficial.

PATHOPHYSIOLOGY OF VENOUS DISEASE

Anatomy

The long (LSV) and short (SSV) saphenous veins and their tributaries (Fig. 27.29) lie outside the deep fascia and carry only 10% of the venous return from the limb. The LSV begins at the medial end of the dorsal venous arch, crosses in front of the medial malleolus and ascends the medial side of the leg. It penetrates the deep (cribriform) fascia 2.5 cm below and lateral to the pubic tubercle, to enter the common

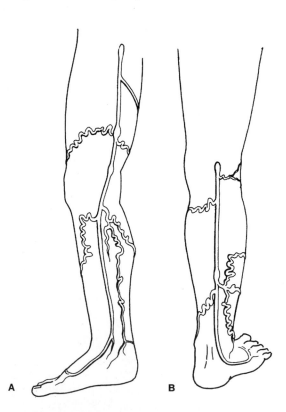

Fig. 27.29 Diagrammatic representation of varicose veins in the lower limb. **A** Long saphenous system. **B** Short saphenous system.

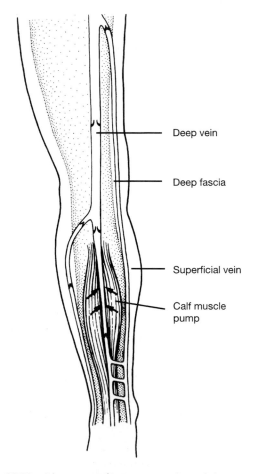

Fig. 27.30 Diagrammatic representation of the venous drainage of the lower limb.

femoral vein. The SSV starts at the lateral end of the dorsal venous arch, passes posterior to the lateral malleolus, then ascends the median line of the calf to join the popliteal vein usually just above the knee. Anatomical variations are common.

The deep venous system comprises intramuscular veins and axial veins, usually paired in the calf, that accompany the main arteries. Communicating veins perforate the deep fascia to connect the superficial and deep systems (Fig. 27.30).

Physiology

Weight bearing compresses the veins in the sole of the foot, which propels blood into the calf ('foot pump'). Pushing off is associated with calf muscle contraction and the compression of venous blood in the muscular sinuses and axial veins; this propels blood further up the leg ('calf pump'). When the leg is lifted off the floor and the muscles relax, blood is prevented from refluxing back down the leg by the closure of valves. During this relaxation phase blood passes from the superficial to the deep veins via perforators, ready to be expelled during the next step. In motionless standing the venous pressure at the ankle is approximately 100 mmHg; that is, the hydrostatic pressure exerted by the column of venous blood stretching from the ankle to the right atrium. However, upon walking the mechanisms described above reduce the ankle pressure to less than 25 mmHg (ambulatory venous pressure, AVP). The symptoms and signs of lower limb venous disease are largely due to failure of these protective mechanisms and the presence of a high AVP.

VARICOSE VEINS

Classification
Trunk varices

These involve the main stem and/or major tributaries of the LSV and SSV, are usually > 4 mm in diameter (and may be much larger), lie subcutaneously, are palpable, do not usually discolour the overlying skin, and are present in about a third of the adult population. Although five times more women than men present for treatment, the prevalence is roughly equal between the sexes. There appears to be a familial tendency and obesity, pregnancy, constipation and prolonged standing may be aggravating factors.

Reticular varices

These lie deep in the dermis, are < 4 mm in diameter, are impalpable, and render the overlying skin dark blue. They may or may not be associated with trunk varices and are present in about 80% of the adult population.

Telangectasia

These are also called spider and hyphen web veins. They lie superficially in the dermis, are usually 1 mm or less in diameter, are impalpable, and render the overlying skin purple or bright red. Again, they may be associated with trunk and reticular varices and are present in 90% of adults. Like reticular veins, they are slightly more common in women.

Epidemiology

Varicose veins (VV) are so prevalent that they could be considered a variant of normal. Their prevalence increases markedly with age and they are an almost universal finding in individuals over the age of 60.

Clinical features

The great majority of individuals with VV are asymptomatic, or at least they do not seek treatment. Those that do attend the surgical clinic do so because they are unhappy about the appearance of their leg(s), and/or they associate lower limb symptoms with their VV, and/or they are concerned about developing complications.

Cosmetic issues

Many patients, especially young women, seek treatment because they consider their veins to be unsightly. Possibly because they are embarrassed to admit that cosmesis is the main issue, they frequently complain of various lower limb symptoms as well.

Symptoms

A wide variety of lower limb symptoms have been attributed to VV. Lower limb symptoms are present in about a half the adult population, and there is a weak relationship between these symptoms and venous disease. Experience in the clinic confirms a poor relationship between the size and extent of VV on clinical examination and the presence and severity of symptoms claimed (see above).

Complications

Only a small proportion of patients with VV go on to develop the complications of chronic venous insufficiency (CVI); for example, leg ulcers, haemorrhage and thrombophlebitis. At present, it is difficult to predict which patients will progress and there is no evidence that early VV surgery will prevent these complications from developing.

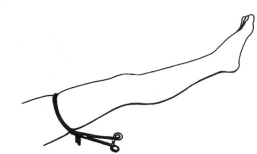

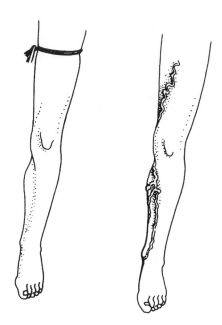

Fig. 27.31 Trendelenburg test to demonstrate saphenofemoral incompetence.

Indications for treatment

In correctly selected patients, VV surgery is associated with a marked improvement in quality of life and symptom relief. In patients with uncomplicated VV surgeons must use their own judgment to determine whether the patient truly does have symptoms; whether those symptoms are of venous aetiology, and, if so, whether they are likely to be relieved by surgery.

Aetiology

The aetiology of VV is unclear. The favoured hypothesis is that there is a structural defect in the vein wall, which may be at least in part inherited and which causes progressive dilatation in response to increased venous pressure consequent upon our bipedal posture and other factors. This leads to secondary incompetence of the valves, which in turn leads to more stress on the wall and more dilatation. Unlike the deep system, incompetence of superficial valves is only rarely due to post-thrombotic damage.

Examination

The patient should be examined standing in a warm room. The distribution of varices will usually, but not always, indicate whether they are long or short saphenous or both. Percussion over a varix while palpating with the other hand at a higher or lower level will help trace the pattern. The level at which deep-to-superficial reflux is occurring can be checked by the Trendelenburg test (Fig. 27.31). The leg is elevated and a rubber tourniquet applied just below the saphenofemoral junction. The patient is then asked to stand. Veins fill slowly from arterial inflow but quickly from venous reflux. If venous distension below the tourniquet is controlled, the site of reflux must be above it. By moving the tourniquet to different levels in the limb the pattern of incompetence can be mapped out. A more effective way to demonstrate reflux is to insonate over the site of incompetence and reflux with a portable continuous-wave Doppler ultrasound probe. This is particularly valuable in obese patients or those with recurrent VV, where the anatomy may be obscure.

Investigations

There is considerable debate as to which patients with VV should undergo further investigation. For all intents and purposes further investigation entails duplex ultrasound, as contrast venography is rarely performed nowadays. Imaging is particularly helpful in the following situations:

- Recurrent VV
- Short saphenous VV
- Where there is a suspicion of deep venous pathology, for example previous DVT or skin changes of CVI
- Atypical distribution.

Severe varicose veins, especially if in children, of atypical distribution or associated with cutaneous haemangioma, soft-tissue hypertrophy or limb overgrowth, should raise the suspicion of congenital arteriovenous malformations.

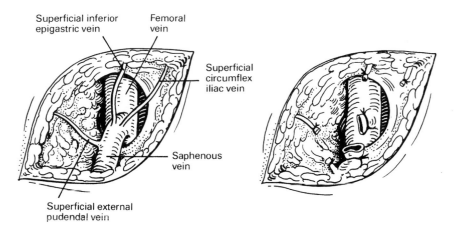

Fig. 27.32 Saphenofemoral disconnection with ligation of the tributaries of the long saphenous vein.

Management

Conservative treatment

Elderly patients or those with mild disease can be treated conservatively. Elastic support hose, weight reduction, regular exercise and the avoidance of constricting garments and prolonged standing all help to relieve tiredness and reduce swelling.

Sclerotherapy

Injection treatment is used for small varices below the knee which are due to incompetence of local perforators, or for recurrent varices after surgery. It is not satisfactory for varices associated with saphenofemoral or saphenopopliteal incompetence, as recurrence is inevitable. Sclerotherapy also makes subsequent surgery more difficult. The vein is injected with a sclerosant (for example sodium tetradecyl sulphate) and a compression bandage applied. This is left in place for 2 weeks.

Surgery

Varicose vein surgery aims to remove varices and intercept incompetent connections between deep and superficial veins so that further varices do not form. In patients with long saphenous disease the saphenofemoral junction is ligated flush with the femoral vein (Fig. 27.32). Recurrence is much less likely if the long saphenous vein is stripped out from knee to groin. Care must be taken not to damage the saphenous nerve. In patients with short saphenous disease the saphenopopliteal junction is dealt with in a similar fashion. However, the short saphenous vein is not normally stripped for fear of injuring the sural nerve. Remaining varices are then avulsed through multiple tiny incisions.

Superficial thrombophlebitis

Inflammation and thrombosis of a previously normal superficial vein may result from trauma, irritation from an intravenous infusion or from the injection of noxious agents. With the exception of septic puncture sites, it is usually non-bacterial. When superficial thrombophlebitis arises spontaneously, it almost invariably occurs in a varicose vein. Redness and tenderness follow the line of the vein.

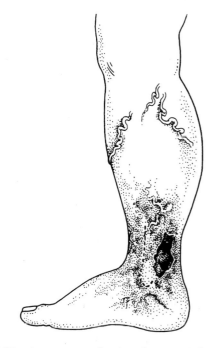

Fig. 27.33 Appearance of a chronic venous ulcer in the leg.

Thrombosis may spread through communicating channels into the deep veins and give rise to pulmonary embolism. Treatment comprises analgesia, anti-inflammatory drugs, support stockings and active exercise. Rapid propagation with deep vein involvement may require heparin therapy, and occasionally thrombectomy or vein ligation. Recurrent migrating superficial phlebitis is occasionally seen in malignant disease.

CHRONIC VENOUS INSUFFICIENCY

Pathophysiology

Chronic venous insufficiency (CVI) may be defined as the presence of irreversible skin damage in the lower leg as a result of sustained venous hypertension. This hypertension is due to failure of the mechanisms (see above) that normally lower venous pressure upon ambulation, namely:

- Venous reflux due to valvular incompetence (90%): this may affect the superficial veins, the deep veins or both, and may be due to primary valvular insufficiency (as in VV) or to postthrombotic damage (see below)
- Venous obstruction (10%): this is usually post-thrombotic in nature.

CVI affects 5–10% of the adult population. Chronic venous ulceration, the end result of CVI, affects 2–3% of people over the age of 65 and its treatment accounts for 1–2% of health care spending in developed countries (£400–600 million per annum in the UK). The female:male ratio is 3:1. Approximately 70% of all leg ulcers are venous in aetiology. Another 20% are due to mixed arterial and venous disease. In many cases the situation is aggravated by old age, poor social circumstances, obesity, trauma, immobility, osteoarthritis, rheumatoid arthritis, diabetes and neurological problems, for example stroke. It is usually possible to differentiate venous (Fig. 27.33) from arterial ulceration on clinical examination alone (Table 27.6).

Table 27.6 Differential diagnosis of leg ulceration

Clinical features	Arterial ulcer	Venous ulcer
Gender	Men > women	Women > men
Age	Usually presents > 60 years	Typically develops 40–60 years but patient may not present for medical attention until much older; multiple recurrences are the norm
Risk factors	Smoking, diabetes, hyperlipidaemia and hypertension	Previous DVT, thrombophilia, varicose veins
Past medical history	Most have a clear history of peripheral, coronary and cerebrovascular disease	More than 20% have a clear history of DVT, many more have a history suggestive of occult DVT, i.e. leg swelling after childbirth, hip/knee replacement or long bone fracture
Symptoms	Severe pain is present unless there is (diabetic) neuropathy; pain may be relieved by dependency	About a third have pain, but it is not usually severe and may be relieved on elevation
Site	Normal and abnormal (diabetics) pressure areas (malleoli, heel, metatarsal heads, 5th metatarsal base)	Medial (70%), lateral (20%) or both malleoli and gaiter area
Edge	Regular, 'punched-out', indolent	Irregular, with neo-epithelium (whiter than mature skin)
Base	Deep, green (sloughy) or black (necrotic) with no granulation tissue, may involve tendon, bone and joint	Pink and granulating but may be covered in yellow-green slough
Surrounding skin	Features of SLI	Lipodermato sclerosis, varicose eczema, atrophe blanche
Veins	Empty, 'guttering' on elevation	Full, usually varicose
Swelling	Usually absent	Often present

Assessment

History

This should include the history of the present and previous episodes of ulceration; previous thrombotic episodes; previous venous and non-venous surgery to the leg, pelvis and abdomen; arterial symptoms; diabetes; autoimmune disease; other medical conditions; locomotor problems; current medications, and allergies.

Examination

This should include a description of the ulcer, concentrating on the features outlined in Table 27.6. Pulse status and ABPI should be recorded. The pattern of venous disease should be determined as described above and gait, particularly ankle mobility assessed.

Investigations

Patients may require a full blood count, standard biochemistry, thyroid function tests, blood glucose determination,

15 mmHg

20 mmHg

25 mmHg

30 mmHg

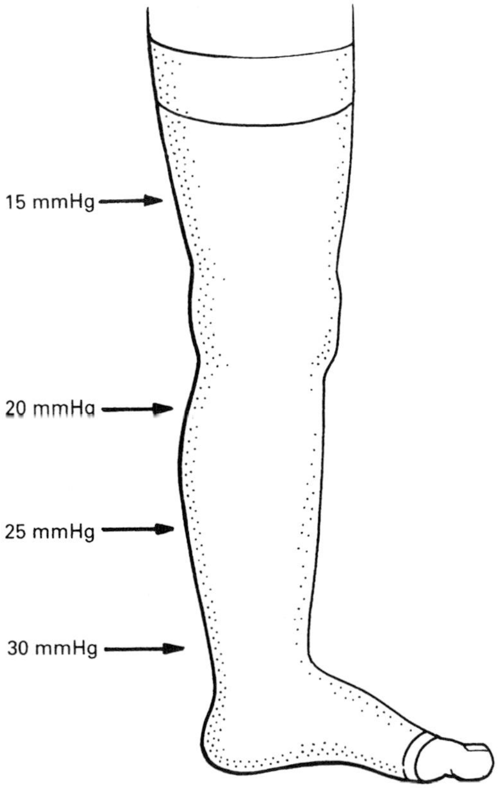

Fig. 27.34 Graduated elastic compression for venous ulcer. Compression from the base of the toes to the tibial tuberosity usually suffices.

lipid profile and rheumatoid serology. Duplex ultrasound can be performed to define the nature and distribution of superficial and deep venous disease, as this has a bearing on both treatment and prognosis. In patients with absent pulses and/or a low ABPI, it can also provide valuable information about the pattern of arterial disease.

Treatment

Medical therapy

Patients with leg ulcers often have multiple medical co-morbidity, the treatment of which must be optimal if the chances of ulcer healing are to be maximized. There are no drugs that have been proved to increase ulcer healing or reduce recurrence. Most ulcers are colonized with bacteria rather than infected, and antibiotics are not usually indicated.

Dressings

There are many different types of dressing on the market but none have been proved to increase ulcer healing. Leg ulcer patients are notorious for developing contact sensitivity to all manner of substances present in ointments and dressings. Thus, the least expensive, simplest and blandest forms of dressing are to be recommended. Topical antibiotics should never be applied.

Compression therapy

This continues to be the mainstay of treatment and, correctly applied, is highly effective in healing the majority of venous ulcers (Fig. 27.34). Compression should be:

- Elastic, as this achieves the best and most durable pressure profile
- Multilayer, as using many layers evens out the high- and low-pressure areas found under any bandage. The 'four-layer bandage' is a popular system
- Graduated: the pressure should be greatest at the ankle (c. 30–40 mmHg) and least at the knee (c. 15–20 mmHg).

It is still unclear how compression therapy works. It is vitally important to exclude arterial disease before compression is applied. If pulses are not easily palpable, the ABPI should be measured (see above). Any patient with an ABPI of < 0.8 should be referred to a vascular surgeon. Such patients will have to be treated with modified compression or undergo revascularization to allow compression to be applied. Oedema is frequently present and significantly reduces the chances of healing. Even expertly applied graduated compression may fail to control severe oedema while the patient is still ambulant, and a period of bed rest for leg elevation may be required.

Elastic compression

Once the ulcer has been healed with compression bandaging, compression stockings will reduce the chance of recurrence and should be prescribed to all patients for life (assuming the arterial circulation is adequate).

Surgical therapy

Many surgeons believe it is worth:

1. Correcting superficial venous reflux by means of short and long saphenous surgery, as described above for simple VV
2. Ligating medial calf perforating veins. This can be performed at open operation or endoscopically: so-called subfascial endoscopic perforator surgery (SEPS)
3. Performing split-skin grafting to speed up ulcer healing.

Patients with arterial disease may require angioplasty or bypass surgery.

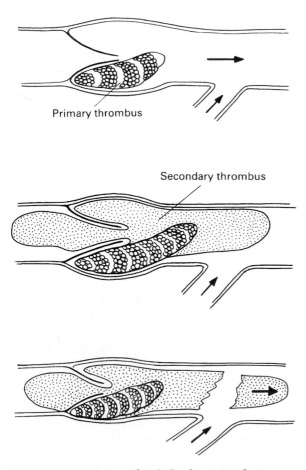

Fig. 27.35 Mechanism of embolus formation from thrombus in a deep vein.

VENOUS THROMBOEMBOLISM (VTE)

Epidemiology

DVT is a common condition in medical and surgical patients and pulmonary embolism (PE) is consistently cited as the commonest cause of potentially preventable death in the surgical patient. DVT also renders the leg prone to CVI and ulceration (the so-called postphlebitic limb).

Pathophysiology

DVT probably begins in the calf, in most cases (Fig. 27.35). Clot may extend into the popliteal, femoral or iliac veins, even the inferior vena cava. In some cases DVT originates in the pelvic veins.

At first the clot is free floating within a column of flowing blood. The risk of PE is highest at this point. Later, when thrombus has completely occluded the vein and incited an inflammatory reaction in the vein wall, the clot becomes densely adherent and unlikely to embolize. The classic features of the 'medical' DVT are due to this occlusion (leg swelling, dilated superficial veins) and thrombophlebitis (redness, pain and tenderness, heat). The important point is that most surgical patients developing a postoperative PE do so on about the 10th day and have clinically normal legs. By the time a clinically apparent DVT has developed the danger period for PE has largely passed.

Aetiology

Three factors are traditionally associated with thrombogenesis (Virchow's triad), namely, venous stasis, intimal damage and hypercoagulability of the blood. Many of the recognized clinical risk factors for DVT relate to venous stasis, for example immobility, obesity, pregnancy, paralysis, operation and trauma. In most instances of DVT no evidence of direct intimal damage can be detected. However, external trauma to a vein, for example during a hip replacement operation, can provide a starting point for thrombogenesis. There is increasing interest in hypercoagulable states, also known as thrombophilia, which can be congenital (primary) or acquired (secondary). These include antithrombin III, protein C, and protein S deficiency; as well as factor V Leiden (activated protein C resistance, APCR). These should be suspected if thrombosis occurs in a young patient (<45 years), if there is a family history, or if thrombosis is recurrent or at an unusual site. Secondary hypercoagulable states include pregnancy and the puerperium, and malignancy.

Diagnosis

Clinical examination alone is poor at confirming or excluding the presence of DVT. This means that the diagnosis of DVT cannot be made on clinical grounds alone, and that some form of investigation is required.

Ascending venography

This involves injecting contrast media into a pedal or a digital vein (Fig. 27.36) and directing flow into the deep veins by applying superficial tourniquets above the ankle. The aim is to delineate fully any thrombus in the deep veins of the calf, thigh and pelvis.

Colour flow duplex ultrasound

Colour duplex ultrasound imaging has largely replaced venography in the diagnosis of DVT. It is non-invasive, and avoids ionizing radiation and contrast, and is as accurate as venography in most cases.

Venous gangrene

In certain circumstances – notably where there is underlying malignancy – DVT may propagate to involve not only the main venous trunks, but also the venous collaterals and/or microcirculation. The former leads to an intensely swollen, cyanosed limb (caerula dolens), whereas the latter can lead to obstruction of the arterial inflow and the development of a swollen white leg (phlegmasia alba dolens). The patient may then go on to develop venous gangrene.

Prevention

Rationale

Because of our inability to diagnose DVT in its early and dangerous phase, prevention is very important. In this respect it is helpful to determine which patients are at the highest risk and thus have the most to gain from prophylactic measures. The most important risk factors are a history of previous DVT or embolism, advanced age, malignant disease, obesity, and con-

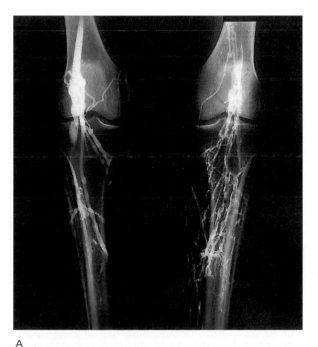

A   B

Fig. 27.36 Ascending phlebography showing **A** deep venous thrombosis in the left popliteal vein, and **B** thrombus in left iliac veins.

genital or acquired thrombophilia. However, even patients at apparently low risk do sometimes develop DVT and PE, and this fact, together with increasing concerns about litigation, has led many surgeons to institute active thromboembolic prophylaxis in almost all their patients.

General measures

Aspects of modern surgical care that help to reduce the likelihood of postoperative DVT include regional anaesthesia, accurate fluid replacement to avoid dehydration, and effective pain control to facilitate early ambulation.

Physical methods

Graduated compression (thromboembolic deterrent, TED) stockings, which exert a pressure of about 20 mmHg at the ankle, augment flow in the deep veins and reduce the risk of thrombosis.

Pharmacological methods

Low-dose subcutaneous unfractionated or low molecular weight heparin, protects against DVT and PE. The first dose may be given with the premedication (if an epidural is not being given) and treatment is continued until the patient is fully ambulant. In high-risk patients it can be continued following discharge.

Treatment

Overview

Before treatment is instituted, the diagnosis of DVT should normally have been established by means of ultrasound or venography. However, where the clinical suspicion of DVT and/or PE is high and there is no contraindication to heparin, then the potential benefits of 'blind' treatment may outweigh the risks. The aims of treatment are to relieve the acute symptoms, protect against PE, and minimize the risk of recurrent thrombosis and post-thrombotic sequelae to the limb.

Uncomplicated DVT

If thrombus is confined to the calf, the patient is fully mobile and other risk factors are reversible, then an elastic stocking and physical exercise may be all that is required. However, the 'surgical' patient does not usually fulfil these criteria and there is often thrombus extension into the femoropopliteal segment. In these cases, specific treatment is indicated. Traditionally:

- The patient was confined to bed.
- The foot of the bed was elevated to reduce swelling.
- The patient received a continuous intravenous infusion of heparin.

- Once the swelling had subsided the patient was mobilized, with graduated compression stockings.
- After 5 days of heparin the patient was changed to warfarin, which was continued for 3–6 months.

For most uncomplicated DVT it is now clear that:

- Bed rest is unnecessary: the patient can be mobilized almost immediately with a stocking.
- LMWH given by intermittent injection is just as effective.

DVT is thus increasingly treated entirely on an outpatient basis. Even some PEs are treated this way.

Complicated DVT

In a proportion of patients, however, treatment is more complicated because of one or more of the following:

1. The DVT is more extensive (iliofemoral, vena cava, phlegmasia).
2. The DVT is recurrent.
3. The patient has (probably) had a PE.
4. The patient has one or more major irreversible congenital and/or acquired thrombophilias.
5. Heparinization is contraindicated (heparin-induced thrombocytopenia, recent haemorrhage).

In these circumstances treatment must be tailored to the individual patient, and in selected cases it may be appropriate to use thrombolysis, insert a caval filter or consider thrombectomy.

Thrombolysis

Catheter-directed intraclot thrombolytic therapy has been advocated as a means of rapidly clearing the iliofemoral segment in patients with extensive proximal DVT. It is hoped that this will reduce the incidence of PE and post-phlebitic syndrome. Although the rate and extent of clot clearance is certainly greater than with heparin alone in the short term, it is not clear whether this results in improved patency and clinical outcome in the long term. The other potential role for thrombolysis is in phlegmasia with venous gangrene. In this situation, not only is the lytic agent given into the clot, it is also administered into the arterial circulation to try to clear the microcirculation. Again, although clot can be lysed in the short term, it is unclear whether this confers long-term benefit. Many of these patients have underlying malignancy and, unless the hypercoagulable state can be corrected, rethrombosis is likely. Furthermore, thrombolysis is associated with a significant incidence of serious haemorrhagic complications in these patients.

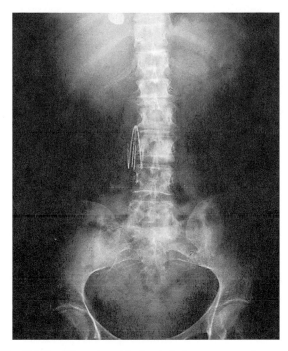

Fig. 27.37 Filter placed in the inferior vena cava to prevent pulmonary embolism.

Thrombectomy

Surgical thrombectomy to clear iliofemoral thrombus is rarely performed nowadays. Percutaneous mechanical venous thrombectomy is still under evaluation.

Caval filters

The rationale behind inserting a caval filter is that it will trap embolus that would otherwise have been destined for the lungs (Fig. 27.37). The most widely accepted indication for a filter is the patient in whom it can be proved that PE is still occurring despite adequate anticoagulation, or where anti-coagulation has been contra-indicated or has been discontinued owing to a complication of therapy. However, there are many other scenarios where their use has been advocated; for example, in a patient with severely impaired cardiorespiratory function in whom even a small embolus might be fatal, and in the patient who cannot be heparinized. Filters are usually inserted percutaneously under local anesthesia by interventional radiologists via the jugular or femoral veins. Some of the newer filters can also be removed percutaneously.

Other forms of venous thrombosis

Superior vena caval thrombosis

Mediastinal tumours or enlarged lymph nodes (e.g. from breast or bronchial carcinoma) may obstruct the superior vena cava and induce thrombosis. Central venous catheters for parenteral nutrition or pressure monitoring may cause thrombosis of the vena cava, or of the subclavian or axillary veins. The patient experiences an unpleasant bursting feeling in the head, neck and upper limbs. There is oedema, cyanosis and venous distension.

The obstruction is defined by bilateral upper limb venography. In occlusion secondary to malignancy, percutaneous stenting, radiotherapy or chemotherapy may relieve malignant obstruction, but the outlook is poor.

Subclavian and axillary vein thrombosis

Spontaneous axillary thrombosis is relatively common and usually occurs in otherwise healthy young adults following exercise, when it is termed 'effort thrombosis'. There may be a previous history of intermittent venous obstruction in the limb due to a mechanical cause at the thoracic outlet. A cervical rib, abnormal muscle or ligamentous band at the inner border of the first rib, or a narrow interval between the clavicle and the first rib, may constrict the vein and lead to thrombosis.

SUMMARY BOX

Venous disease

- Varicose veins are present in the majority of the adult population and chronic venous ulceration affects 5% patients over the age of 70.

- Compression therapy is the mainstay of treatment for chronic venous ulceration, but should never be implemented unless the arterial status of the leg is known to be satisfactory (palpable pedal pulses and/or an ABPI > 0.8).

- If patients with chronic venous ulceration are being considered for surgical treatment they should undergo duplex ultrasonography to delineate the pattern of superficial and deep venous disease.

- DVT in postoperative patients is often asymptomatic. Most postoperative patients developing (fatal) PE have normal legs on clinical examination. Duplex ultrasound or venography should be used to confirm the diagnosis of DVT; VQ scan or CT pulmonary angiography can be used to diagnose PE.

- All hospital patients, medical and surgical, should have their thromboembolic risk assessed and receive prophylaxis accordingly. PE is the commonest cause of potentially preventable death in hospital.

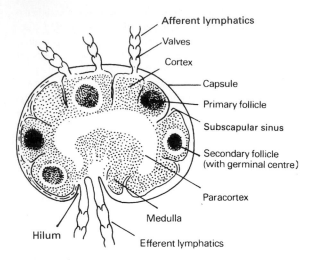

Fig. 27.38 Structure of a lymph node.

The patient complains of an uncomfortable, heavy, cyanosed arm with venous engorgement. Venous collaterals develop over the shoulder and anterior chest wall. Upper limb venous duplex scanning and/or venography defines the occlusion. The arm should be elevated, e.g. in a towel suspended from a drip stand. Heparin therapy followed by oral anticoagulants is standard treatment. Thrombolytic therapy can be very effective in early cases. Many surgeons believe that after the axillary thrombosis has been cleared the thoracic outlet should be explored and the first rib or other obstructing element removed. Stenting of any underlying venous-stenosis may be of value.

LYMPHOEDEMA

Pathophysiology

The lymphatic system removes excess water and protein from the interstitial space. Flow is directed centrally by intrinsic lymphatic contractions and endothelial valves, and is increased by muscle contraction. Lymph passes though lymph nodes (Fig. 27.38), before it re-enters the venous system, mainly through the thoracic duct. The total daily lymph flow is only 2–4 L. Failure of this mechanism leads to the accumulation of protein-rich oedema fluid in the tissues (lymphoedema) (Fig. 27.39). Lymphoedema may be primary or secondary, and must be differentiated from other causes of leg swelling (Table 27.7).

Primary lymphoedema

This often familial condition is caused by a developmental failure in which the lymphatics may be absent, hypoplastic, or varicose and dilated. It is defined by the age of onset:

● *Lymphoedema congenita* Swelling is present at birth or develops within the first year of life.
● *Lymphoedema praecox* Swelling develops between 1 and 35 years, usually during adolescence. It affects predominantly females, and may be unilateral or bilateral.
● *Lymphoedema tarda* In patients developing lymphoedema after the age of 35 an underlying pelvic tumour (benign or malignant) compressing the proximal lymphatic (and venous) systems must be excluded.

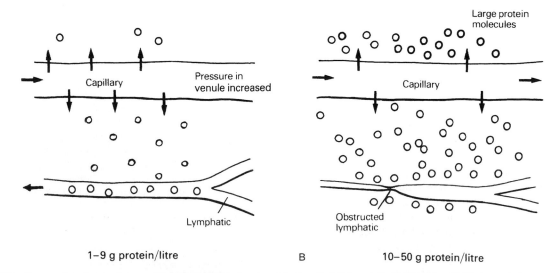

Fig. 27.39 Types of oedema. **A** Low-protein oedema due to abnormally high net fluid filtration. **B** High-protein oedema due to failure of lymphatics to remove interstitial protein.

Table 27.7 Differential diagnosis of the swollen limb

Non-vascular or lymphatic	General disease states	Cardiac, renal and liver failure. Hyperthyroidism (myxoedema). Allergic disorders. Immobility and lower limb dependency
	Local disease processes	Ruptured Baker's cyst. Myositis ossificans. Bony or soft tissue tumours. Arthritis. Haemarthrosis. Calf muscle haematoma. Achilles tendon rupture. Other trauma. Reflex sympathetic dystrophy
	Gigantism	Rare. All tissues are uniformly enlarged
	Drugs	Steroids
	Obesity	Lipodystrophy, lipoidosis
Venous	Deep venous thrombosis	The classic signs of pain and redness may be absent
	Post-thrombotic syndrome	Venous skin changes, secondary varicose veins on the leg and collateral veins on the lower abdominal wall. Venous claudication may be present
	Varicose veins	Do not usually cause significant swelling
	Venous malformations	Commonest is Klippel–Trenaunay syndrome. Abnormal lateral venous complex, capillary naevus, hypo(a)plasia of deep veins, and limb lengthening. Lymphatic abnormalities often coexist
	External venous compression	Pelvic or abdominal tumour including the gravid uterus. Retroperitoneal fibrosis
Arterial	Ischaemia – reperfusion	Following lower limb revascularization for chronic and particularly acute ischaemia
	Arteriovenous malformation	May be associated with local or generalized swelling
	Aneurysm	Popliteal. Femoral. False aneurysm following (iatrogenic) trauma

Secondary lymphoedema

This develops when the lymphatic system is obstructed by tumour, recurrent infection or infestation (filariasis), or obliterated by surgery or radiotherapy.

Clinical features

Symptoms

The patient usually complains of gradual painless swelling of one or both legs. At first, lymphoedema is like other forms of oedema in that it is present only upon dependency, that is, worse at the end of the day and absent in the morning. However, as the oedema fluid becomes more protein rich it is less and less affected by position. Lymphoedema nearly always commences distally on the foot and extends proximally, usually only to the knee.

Thus, there may be a complex interplay between nature and nurture: that is, many patients with apparently primary lymphoedema also have a secondary component. Some patients first present to medical attention because of acute cellulitis. Such patients are prone to recurrent episodes,

each one of which damages still further the lymphatic system, leading to a vicious spiral.

Signs

Unlike other types of oedema, lymphoedema characteristically involves the foot, as opposed to the lower calf and ankle. This is characterized by:

- Infilling of the submalleolar depressions
- A 'hump' on the dorsum of the foot
- 'Square' toes due to confinement by footwear; also, the skin on the dorsum of the toes cannot be pinched owing to subcutaneous fibrosis (Stemmer's sign).

Lymphoedema usually spreads proximally to knee level, and less commonly affects the whole leg. Lymphoedema will pit easily at first, but with time fibrosis and dermal thickening prevent pitting except following prolonged pressure. Chronic eczema, fungal infection of the skin (dermatophytosis) and nails (onychomycosis), fissuring, verrucae and papillae are frequently seen in advanced conditions. Frank ulceration is unusual.

Investigation

Lymphoedema is essentially a clinical diagnosis and most patients require no further investigation.

Treatment

Physical methods

The patient should elevate the foot above the level of the hip when sitting, elevate the foot of the bed when sleeping, and avoid prolonged standing. Various forms of massage are effective at reducing oedema. Intermittent pneumatic compression devices are also useful. The mainstay of therapy is graduated compression hosiery. Pressures exceeding 50 mmHg at the ankle may be required. Below-knee stockings are usually sufficient.

Drugs

Diuretics are of no value and are associated with side-effects, including electrolyte disturbance. No other drugs are of proven benefit.

Antibiotics

These should be prescribed promptly for cellulitis. Patients who suffer recurrent spontaneous episodes of cellulitis should be considered for long-term prophylactic antibiotic therapy. Fungal infection must also be treated aggressively. The feet must be dried after washing and the skin kept clean and supple with water-based emollients to prevent entry of bacteria.

Surgery

Only a small minority of patients will benefit from surgery. Operations fall into two categories: bypass procedures and reduction procedures; they are only rarely performed. The details of these procedures are beyond the scope of this book.

28 Cardiothoracic surgery

W.S. Walker

BASIC CONSIDERATIONS

Pathophysiological assessment

The history and examination suggest the presence of probable cardiac pathology. The initial clinical assessment is then refined and pathology quantified using specific investigations (Table 28.1).

Assessment of risk

The risks of perioperative mortality and stroke are significantly higher with cardiac than with other forms of surgery. A frank discussion of these risks is an essential element in the preoperative consultations between the surgeon and the patient.

Mortality

The risk of operative mortality is estimated by means of a scoring system (Parsonnet, Euroscore), where a variable number of points are given for specific clinical features. The sum of these, either directly or via a correction graph, indicates the percentage operative mortality, which ranges between 2% for routine and relatively straightforward procedures to over 50% for complex emergency procedures.

Stroke

Stroke risk varies from 1% to over 10%, and is associated with intracardiac thrombus and severe atheromatous disease of the proximal aorta and carotids. Patients with high-grade symptomatic carotid disease may benefit from carotid endarterectomy prior to cardiac surgery (see Chapter 27).

Specific aspects of surgical technique

Cardiopulmonary bypass

Modern cardiac and great vessel surgery became feasible with the development of cardiopulmonary bypass. Venous blood is extracted via cannulae inserted into the right atrium or vena cavae and drained to a reservoir. It is then pumped through an oxygenator, which adds O_2 and removes CO_2,

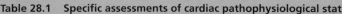

Table 28.1   Specific assessments of cardiac pathophysiological status

Investigation	Potential yield
ECG	
Resting	Rhythm; conduction abnormalities; atrial and ventricular hypertrophy; established ischaemic changes; evidence of previous myocardial infarction
Exercise	Exercise-induced ischaemic changes or arrhythmias
Chest X-ray	Cardiac enlargement; valvular calcification; evidence of pulmonary oedema: Kerley B lines, pleural effusion, interstitial marking, hilar flare; absent or enlarged cardiac or great vessel structures
Thallium isotope scan	Areas of low radiouptake indicative of impaired myocardial perfusion
Echocardiography	
Precordial	Ventricular contractility; valvular stenoses, regurgitation or leaflet abnormalities; intracardiac morphology, including septal defects and intracardiac masses; pericardial effusion.
Transoesophageal	Enhanced views of posterior cardiac structures: aortic and mitral valves, ascending aorta, great veins and posterior septae; posterior pericardial fluid collections
Cardiac catheterization	
Chamber pressures	Assess left and right ventricular function via determination of left ventricular end-diastolic pressure; atrial pressures in valve disease; transvalvular gradients (Fig. 28.1)
Angiography	Coronary arterial anatomy; intracardiac anatomy; trans-septal flow
O$_2$ saturations	Intracardiac shunts
Cardiac output	Cardiac function and determination of secondary derived parameters, including peripheral and pulmonary vascular resistance

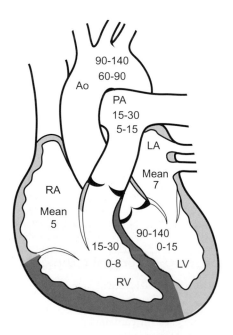

Fig. 28.1 Normal cardiac chamber pressures. AO = aorta, LA = left atrium, LV = left ventricle, RA = right atrium, RV = right ventricle, PA = pulmonary artery.

and through a heat exchanger coil so that its temperature can be varied. Finally, the blood is returned to the arterial circulation via a cannula in the ascending aorta or, occasionally, the femoral artery (Figs 28.2 and 28.3). Full anticoagulation with intravenous heparin is required to prevent blood clotting in the tubing, oxygenator and pump mechanisms. Roller or centrifugal pumps are used, as these minimize haemolysis related to red cell trauma. Semipermeable sheet membranes, or more commonly hollow fibres, form the blood–gas interfaces within the oxygenator. A trained perfusion technician (perfusionist) controls the bypass machine.

Cardiopulmonary bypass carries several risks. Cerebral damage occurs in about 1% of cases due to intracerebral bleeding, embolization of microbubbles or arterial debris, or inadequate cerebral perfusion. Subtle deterioration in cerebral function, as detected by psychological testing, is more frequent. There is also significant activation of systemic inflammatory mechanisms, with cytokine release, complement activation and white cell stimulation. These changes do not generally cause clinical problems but may occasionally be implicated in post-bypass pulmonary and renal dysfunction. Coagulopathy and haemolysis are associated with prolonged bypass.

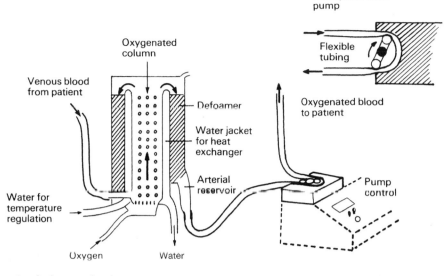

Fig. 28.2   Schematic of a bypass circuit.

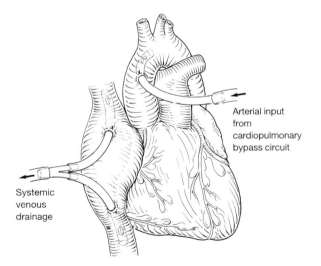

Fig. 28.3   Cannulation for cardiopulmonary bypass.

Myocardial preservation

Cardioplegia   Intracardiac surgery requires a still and bloodless heart. This is achieved by the use of cardioplegic arrest. A clamp is applied across the ascending aorta proximal to the point of insertion of the bypass arterial inflow cannula. This prevents blood flow into the coronary arteries. The heart is then arrested by perfusing the coronary circulation with a cardioplegic solution, either progradely via the aortic root or coronary artery ostia, or retrogradely via a catheter placed in the coronary sinus. The essential component of a cardioplegic solution is a high potassium concentration (circa 18 mmol/L), which causes the heart to arrest in diastole. Cardioplegia is typically delivered at a temperature of 4–6°C and via either a crystalloid solution or one derived from the patient's own blood. Blood-based solutions are believed to have buffering characteristics that are helpful in reducing the deleterious effects of ischaemic metabolites generated by the arrested myocardium. Local anaesthetic agents may be added to stabilize the myocardial cell membranes. In principle, therefore, cardioplegia solutions minimize myocardial energy requirements by abolishing energy expenditure on contraction and by reducing basal cellular metabolism by local tissue cooling. Reducing the core temperature to 26–34°C may enhance cardiac cooling. Cardioplegia combined with mild systemic hypothermia (32°C) will provide the surgeon with a safe period (90–120 minutes) within which to carry out surgery without the risk of myocardial damage.

In some circumstances the surgeon may elect to leave the coronary arteries perfused while on bypass and to operate on the beating heart. Alternatively, coronary bypass surgery can be performed using a technique in which an aortic clamp is intermittently applied to cut coronary flow while the heart is electrically fibrillated so as to reduce movement. The resulting ischaemic episodes are tolerated because they are brief and activate mechanisms within the myocardial cells that reduce damage caused by subsequent ischaemia – a phenomenon known as 'preconditioning'.

Recently, there has been considerable interest in the use of specific stabilizer instruments that allow the surgeon to perform coronary artery surgery on suitable patients without the use of cardiopulmonary bypass. Proponents of 'off-pump' surgery claim that the risks of artificial perfusion are avoided and that recovery may be quicker. Many surgeons, however, feel that the bloodless, still operative field provided by cardioplegic arrest may facilitate more accurate anastomoses.

Postoperative care

Intensive care

Postoperatively, patients are routinely ventilated for several hours until they are fully rewarmed and have satisfactory haemodynamics, pulmonary gas exchange and acid–base status. Urine output is copious and potassium levels are therefore checked frequently and potassium administered intravenously to correct urinary losses. Invasive measurement of arterial and central venous pressure is standard. Pulmonary artery catheters are frequently used to measure pulmonary artery pressure, pulmonary artery capillary wedge pressure and cardiac output.

Complications

Other than the catastrophes of death or stroke, established complications include:

- Low cardiac output
- Arrhythmias
- Fluid accumulation
- Short-term memory impairment
- Wound infection
- Pulmonary infection.

Recovery time

Patients undergoing routine elective coronary or valve surgery will usually leave acute hospital care within 1 week. Those requiring more extensive surgery or emergency procedures may take longer to recover. Most patients will have undergone a median sternotomy (Fig. 28.4). This wound heals quickly and well and, as the sternal edges are approximated securely by wire or heavy sutures, chest discomfort eases rapidly. Leg vein donor sites may take longer to heal, particularly around the knee. By 2 weeks the

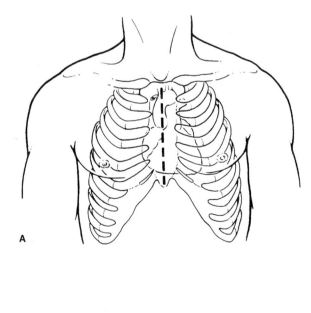

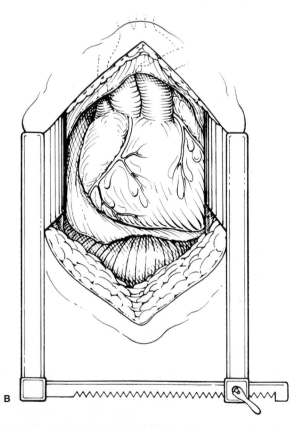

Fig. 28.4 Surgical approach to the heart. **A** Vertical sternotomy incision. **B** Right atrium and ascending aorta exposed.

patient should be able to walk a few hundred yards, and by 3 months they should have returned to full activity, including work.

ACQUIRED CARDIAC DISEASE

Surgical intervention may be required in the management of:

- Ischaemic heart disease
- Cardiac valvular disease
- Aortic aneurysm
- Pericardial pathology
- Cardiac trauma.

ISCHAEMIC HEART DISEASE

Ischaemic heart disease encompasses coronary artery disease and its complications, principally acute mitral regurgitation, ventricular septal defect and left ventricular aneurysm.

Coronary artery disease

This is caused by coronary artery atheroma (see Chapter 27). Most patients will present for surgery because of angina or previous myocardial infarction (MI).

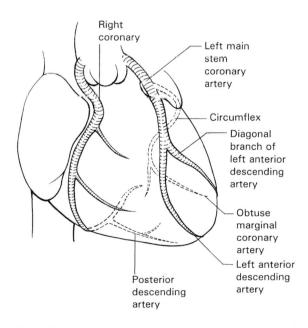

Fig. 28.5 Coronary circulation.

Evaluation

Exercise ECG is often used as an initial screening test for patients with suspected stable angina. Those with confirmed ischaemia then undergo coronary angiography and assessment of left ventricular function by means of angiography or echocardiography. Contrast medium is injected into the coronary circulation (Fig. 28.5) via a catheter which is usually inserted through the femoral artery (Fig. 28.6). Images are obtained in several different planes so as to minimize the risk of missing eccentric lesions. Bypass surgery is usually only advised for stenoses that exceed a 70% reduction in vessel diameter.

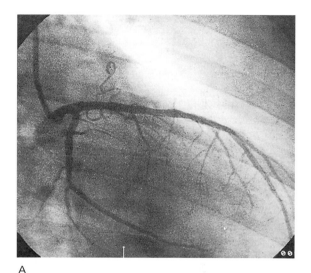

A

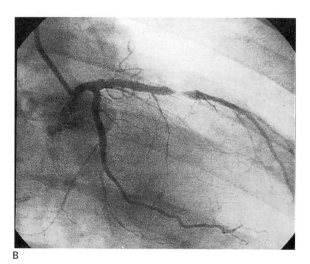

B

Fig. 28.6 **A** Selective left coronary angiogram showing appearances after balloon dilatation. **B** Selective left coronary angiogram, showing stenosis of descending artery.

> **SUMMARY BOX**
>
> *Coronary anatomy*
>
> - There are two coronary arteries.
>
> - The left coronary arises from the left posterior aspect of the aortic root and passes behind the pulmonary trunk before dividing into two large branches: the left anterior descending coronary which supplies the anterior left ventricle, and anterior two-thirds of the interventricular septum, and the circumflex coronary which supplies the posterior and lateral left ventricles.
>
> - The right coronary artery arises at the front of the aorta and passes down anteriorly between the right atrium and right ventricle, which it supplies via anterior right ventricle and acute marginal branches.
>
> - Either the right or circumflex may terminate as the posterior descending artery, which supplies the inferior surface of both ventricles and the lower septum.
>
> - The right, left anterior descending and circumflex are each considered to be a 'vessel system'. Disease within any one of these three vessels or its branches is termed single-vessel disease. Similarly, two- and three-vessel disease indicates involvement of two and three systems, respectively.

Indications

Elective surgery is indicated primarily for the control of angina that is refractory to medical treatment and which is caused by disease that is unsuitable for angioplasty and stent insertion. Historically, patients with three-vessel disease or left main stem disease have exhibited a high (*c.* 8%/year) risk of death from MI with medical therapy alone. Surgery may improve long-term survival for such patients, particularly when left ventricular function is also impaired. However, the data supporting this contention are derived from studies carried out over 15 years ago, long before modern 'best medical therapy' involving aspirin, statins and ACE inhibitors became available. Some patients requiring other cardiac procedures may be shown to have significant coronary disease during cardiological assessment. In these cases coronary surgery may be added to the primary procedure in order to improve perioperative survival and prevent future ischaemic problems. Emergency coronary surgery is rare. Patients with incipient or established MI usually fare better with supportive medical therapy, as the mortality of surgery in this setting is much increased. Emergency surgery is required mainly for failed interventional procedures that have caused coronary occlusion.

Coronary bypass

A coronary artery bypass graft (CABG) delivers blood to the distal coronary artery beyond a stenosis. If distal artery is obliterated by atheroma, an endarterectomy procedure may be performed to restore the lumen. Originally, nearly all grafts comprised reversed segments of the long saphenous vein anastomosed proximally to the anterior ascending aorta and distally to the coronary artery. Such grafts have patency rates of around 70% at 5 years and 40% at 10 years. Venous graft failure occurs as a result of intimal hyperplasia, which is thought to be, in part at least, a response to arterial pressure. The relatively high rate of vein graft failure stimulated interest in using the internal mammary artery (IMA). This is usually employed as a pedicled graft, when it is left attached to the subclavian artery proximally, but can also be used as a free graft in the same manner as vein. IMA graft patency exceeds 90% at 5 years and 70% at 10 years. The IMA's relatively short length restricts its use to the front of the heart. A common combination (Fig. 28.7) is to use the left IMA for the left anterior descending artery and vein grafts for the other vessels. The radial artery is currently enjoying a revival in popularity as a coronary graft and may be used as a free graft in place of saphenous vein, together with mammary grafts, to achieve 'total arterial revascularization'. Occasionally, the surgeon may consider using the inferior epigastric artery, the right gastroepiploic artery, the short saphenous vein and the cephalic vein. Prosthetic grafts occlude early and are not used.

Results

Angina is relieved completely in about 70% of cases, significantly improved in the remainder, and recurs with a frequency of about 10% per year. Successful revascularization may also improve breathlessness if it is related to myocardial ischaemia, and survival is probably enhanced in patients with three-vessel disease. Logically, increased use of arterial conduits should be associated with better graft patency and improved survival. There does appear to be a trend in that direction for patients with multiple arterial grafts followed up beyond 10 years, but the added benefit over one IMA graft placed to the left anterior descending coronary is small. This may reflect the progression of native coronary disease. Uncomplicated coronary surgery should carry a 2–3% risk of mortality and a 1–2% risk of stroke.

Surgery for the complications of coronary artery disease

Mitral valve reflux

Chronic Chronic ischaemia may cause reflux owing to papillary muscle fibrosis. Surgery may be indicated to replace the valve as an elective procedure, usually concur-

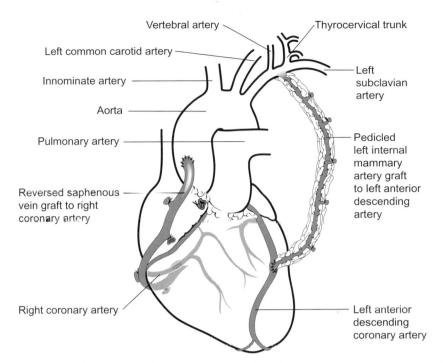

Fig. 28.7 Completed coronary bypass procedure with venous and left internal mammary artery grafts in situ.

rently with CABG. The operative mortality is around 8–11%.

Acute An infarcted papillary muscle may rupture, causing gross reflux. The patient is usually very ill, with pulmonary oedema and low cardiac output, and often requires emergency ventilation. Emergency mitral valve replacement and CABG is associated with a mortality of 15–40%, mainly because of poor myocardial function and secondary multiorgan failure.

Postmyocardial infarction ventricular septal defect

Necrosis of the intraventricular septum due to MI may lead to a ventricular septal defect. Blood flows from the high-pressure left to the low-pressure right ventricle (left-to-right 'shunt'). This increases right ventricular work and pulmonary blood flow and decreases cardiac output. Typically, the patient complains of sudden, severe breathlessness 3–8 days after an MI and is noted to have developed a pansystolic murmur. Cardiac chamber oximetry is used to calculate the shunt magnitude, which is expressed as the ratio between the pulmonary (Qp) and systemic (Qs) blood flows. Coronary arteriography and assessment of right and left ventricular function are also performed. In general, if the shunt is below 1.5:1 the patient will tolerate the defect reasonably well. A shunt ratio of 2 or more will usually cause death from right ventricular failure, pulmonary

oedema, renal failure and cardiogenic shock. Emergency repair is technically difficult because it can be impossible to find sound tissue to which a patch may be sutured. In addition, these patients are in the aftermath of an acute MI and consequently have impaired cardiac function. Surgical mortality ranges from 20 to 50%. Patients with lesser shunts are managed medically and considered for surgery some weeks later. By this stage cardiac function has stabilized and the margins of the defect have healed by fibrosis, making patch repair straightforward. Operative mortality is below 10%.

Left ventricular aneurysm

This occurs when a large left ventricular free wall MI scar becomes aneurysmal as a result of intraventricular pressure, and complicates about 8% of infarcts. A large aneurysm impairs cardiac contraction and increases myocardial work. Clot forms within the aneurysm and may embolize. Arrhythmias may be generated within the zone of ischaemic myocardium around the periphery of the aneurysm. The aneurysm is excised, the clot removed, and the resulting defect usually closed by direct suture, reinforced by buttressing strips of Teflon felt or vascular graft. Occasionally a small patch repair is performed to preserve the shape of the left ventricle. Surgery is performed electively, with a mortality of 6–10% and an increased risk of stroke.

CARDIAC VALVULAR DISEASE

Valve disease may obstruct forward flow (stenosis) or permit reverse flow (incompetence/reflux/regurgitation), or both. The aortic and/or mitral valves are primarily affected. Primary tricuspid pathology is rare and pulmonary valve disease is virtually unknown. Formerly, rheumatic fever following streptococcal infection was the commonest aetiological factor. This remains the case in many developing countries, but in the UK it is rare except in the elderly or in overseas patients.

Assessment

Precordial echocardiography provides useful data on forward gradients using Doppler techniques and can indicate regurgitation. Transoesophageal echocardiography can be particularly helpful, as this allows the valves and intracardiac anatomy to be imaged more effectively. Coronary arteriography is indicated in patients of middle age or older. Left ventricular angiography and aortic root angiography may allow the quantification of mitral and aortic reflux. A full catheterization study should include measurement of cardiac output and chamber and pulmonary artery pressures. Formulae exist which allow the effective orifice areas of stenotic mitral and aortic valves to be calculated.

Surgical management

Options include valve repair or replacement. Repair is relatively uncommon and is largely restricted to the mitral and tricuspid valves. Replacement may be achieved with mechanical or biological valves. Mechanical valves have developed from the original ball-in-cage design through single disc designs to the current range of bileaflet devices (Fig. 28.8). These devices should last indefinitely, but patients require lifelong warfarin to prevent thrombotic occlusion or embolism. Embolism risk is about 1–6% per year and is influenced by how accurately the INR is controlled. Mechanical valves produce audible clicks. Biological valves are derived from glutaraldehyde-preserved porcine aortic valves mounted on a frame or left within the porcine aortic root; glutaraldehyde-preserved bovine pericardium formed into a three-leaflet valve and mounted on a frame; and human homografts removed from cadaveric hearts and preserved in antibiotic solution (Fig. 28.9). Warfarin is not required and they are silent. However, such valves deteriorate over time and after 10–20 years will need to be replaced. Unless there is a contraindication to anticoagulation, mechanical valves are commonly used in those under the age of 70. In young women intending to have children it is usual to advise a biological valve, with the intention of replacing it with a mechanical device when the valve fails. This avoids problems with warfarin during pregnancy (placental separation and abortion and teratogenicity).

Endocarditis

Abnormal native heart valves and artificial valves are prone to subacute bacterial endocarditis and prosthetic valve endocarditis, respectively. Antibiotic prophylaxis is required to cover any surgical or dental procedure. If infection does develop, prolonged parenteral antibiotic therapy may be effective. However, surgery may be required if the infection does not respond or if the valve develops a large paravalvular leak or abscess. Surgery is a high-risk venture as the newly implanted prosthesis may itself become infected. Postoperative recovery is usually slow, with renal and ventilatory failure being common sequelae.

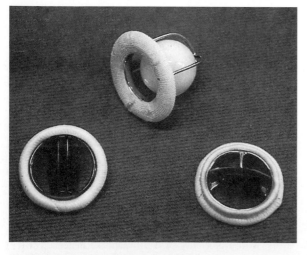

Fig. 28.8 Mechanical valve prosthesis.

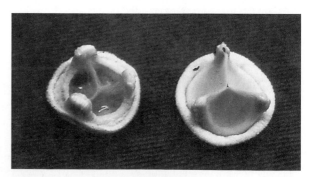

Fig. 28.9 Biological valve prosthesis.

Aortic valve disease

Stenosis

This is the most frequent indication for valve surgery in the UK. Although stenosis can be due to rheumatic disease, it usually results from a congenital bicuspid aortic valve. Such valves function normally in early adult life but develop progressive leaflet calcification from the sixth decade onwards (Fig. 28.10). Aortic stenosis causes left ventricular hypertrophy, effort angina, episodes of arrhythmia with syncope or even sudden death, and left ventricular failure. There is a slow rising pulse, a forceful apex beat and an ejection systolic murmur in the right upper parasternal area that may radiate to the root of the neck. Echocardiography and catheterization will confirm a valvular gradient, which is typically greater than 60 mmHg. If the patient is well an observational course is pursued; the onset of symptoms, however, should trigger referral for surgery. Patients with cardiac failure have a low output and consequently a low gradient. In these cases the decision to operate may be a difficult judgement, based on the absence of any other likely cause of poor left ventricular function and echocardiographic evidence of severe aortic valve disease.

Reflux

Native aortic reflux may be due to primary valve pathology (rheumatic fever, endocarditic valve destruction or, rarely, a bicuspid valve) or secondary to aortic root pathology (see below). Prosthetic valve reflux can occur as a result of deterioration of a biological prosthesis, partial obstruction of a mechanical device, or paraprosthetic leakage. Chronic aortic reflux causes progressive left ventricular dilatation and hypertrophy. There is a wide pulse pressure, lateral displacement of the apex beat and a diastolic murmur in the

left parasternal area. Chronic aortic reflux is well tolerated and often asymptomatic. In severe cases the patient may complain of dyspnoea and angina, and may exhibit features of congestive cardiac failure. Surgery is advised to forestall the onset of cardiac failure and irreversible myocardial damage when serial echocardiography indicates that the left ventricle is starting to dilate. Acute aortic reflux produces severe dyspnoea, with rapid onset of left ventricular failure and pulmonary oedema. The patient may require emergency ventilation and very urgent surgery.

Surgical outcomes

Elective aortic valve replacement is a relatively straightforward procedure with a mortality of about 3% and stroke rate of 1%. The risk is increased severalfold in cases which have progressed to cardiac failure, and in emergency cases with acute severe reflux.

Mitral valve disease

Stenosis

This is usually the end result of rheumatic disease and is becoming less common. Elderly women in their sixth or seventh decade are usually affected. Mitral stenosis restricts the flow of blood into the left ventricle, which is consequently small and thin-walled, and cardiac output is considerably reduced. The left atrium is dilated and left atrial and pulmonary artery pressures are raised. Chronic pulmonary hypertension causes right ventricular hypertrophy and dilatation, and in advanced cases tricuspid incompetence may develop (see below). Patients complain of shortness of breath on exertion and may experience palpitations. Most will have been on warfarin therapy for many years for chronic atrial fibrillation, and diuretic therapy for pulmonary congestion. Examination reveals atrial fibrillation, a left parasternal heave due to right ventricular enlargement, and a diastolic murmur best heard at the lower left sternal edge accompanied by a loud second heart sound. Chest X-ray shows right ventricular and atrial enlargement and the pulmonary artery is prominent. A progressive increase in heart size is often evident on serial yearly films. Renal function is frequently impaired.

The timing of surgery is a matter of judgement but an echocardiographic calculated mitral valve area below 1 cm^2 is indicative of severe stenosis and suggests that surgery should be advised. Very occasionally the patient may have echocardiographic evidence of leaflet fusion only, in which case percutaneous balloon valvuloplasty may be effective. Conservative surgery with separation of the fused leaflets and reconstruction of the valve is possible in some younger patients. Usually, however, there is extensive leaflet cal-

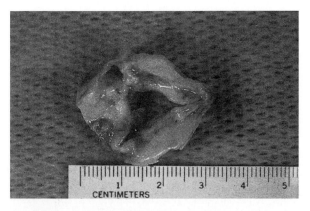

Fig. 28.10 Calcified aortic valve.

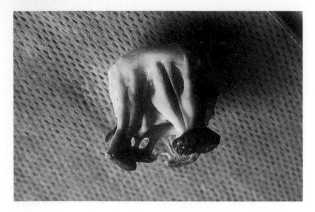

Fig. 28.11   Excised mitral valve showing the shortening and fusion of the papillary muscles and chordae tendinae in advanced mitral stenosis.

cification, with involvement of the papillary muscles and chordae tendinae, which become grossly thickened and shortened, tethering the leaflets to the tips of the papillary muscles (Fig. 28.11). Valve replacement is therefore the only practical option.

Rarely, patients with a mechanical mitral prosthesis may develop thrombotic occlusion of their valve secondary to inadequate control of anticoagulation or to fibrous tissue (pannus) ingrowth from the sewing ring. This acute emergency causes catastrophic pulmonary oedema and a severe reduction in cardiac output. Emergency salvage valve replacement or debridement is required.

Reflux

Chronic mitral reflux occurs with rheumatic disease, ischaemic papillary muscle dysfunction, myxomatous degeneration of the mitral valve, a variety of systemic connective tissue disorders and chronic paraprosthetic valvular leakage. Acute reflux is much less common and follows acute MI involving a papillary muscle, as noted above, but can also result from spontaneous rupture of a chorda tendina, sudden failure of a bioprosthetic valve leaflet or perforation of an infected native valve. Chronic mitral reflux presents a volume load to the left ventricle, which ejects blood preferentially backwards through the incompetent mitral valve. This situation is often well tolerated for years, with patients typically complaining of shortness of breath on exertion and of occasional episodes of palpitation. Clinical examination is often relatively unremarkable, apart from a pansystolic murmur radiating from the lower left sternal edge to the axilla and leftward displacement of the apex beat. Surgery is indicated where there is chest X-ray and echocardiographic evidence of left ventricular dilatation, as this process correlates with declining left ventricular function consequent upon the continued volume overload. Acute reflux causes pulmonary oedema and emergency surgery is necessary. Mitral valves that reflux are often replaced with a prosthesis, but some can be repaired.

Surgical outcomes

Elective mitral valve surgery for reflux is generally a low-risk procedure with a mortality rate of 4–6% and a stroke rate of about 2%. The risk is much greater (10–15%) for patients with ischaemic regurgitation, owing to the concomitant coronary disease and previous myocardial damage. Valve replacement for mitral stenosis also carries a significant mortality (8–12%) due to established pulmonary hypertension, right ventricular failure and poor renal function. The stroke rate is increased to 3–4%. Emergency valve replacement for acute obstruction or reflux carries a mortality of the order of 20%.

Tricuspid valve disease

Stenosis is very rare. Tricuspid endocarditis is occasionally encountered in i.v. drug abusers. Tricuspid incompetence secondary to enlargement of the tricuspid annulus is the commonest pathology and occurs when the right ventricle is dilated, as in advanced mitral valve disease. Typically, the patient will have the features of the underlying mitral valve disease, an elevated jugular venous pressure with 'v' waves, an enlarged pulsatile liver, peripheral oedema and, occasionally, ascites. Liver function tests are deranged and clotting is impaired. The preferred surgical option is to restore the normal dimensions of the valve through annuloplasty. It is uncommon to replace the tricuspid valve except in rare cases of organic stenosis. If replacement is performed a biological prosthesis may be preferable, as the risk of mechanical valve thrombosis is increased in this position.

Multiple and repeat valve procedures

Some patients require multiple valve procedures, typically aortic and mitral valve replacement, or mitral replacement and tricuspid annuloplasty. Such operations attract a higher operative mortality (10% and 35%) as the patient is often in poor condition. They may require prolonged periods of intensive care following surgery. Similarly, revisional valve surgery to re-replace a valve is technically more difficult and will involve a prolonged procedure against a background of impaired cardiac function or sepsis related to the defective prosthesis. Mortality is increased by two to three times the primary procedure risk, and the ICU stay is likely to be prolonged.

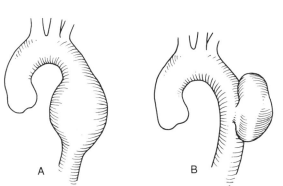

Fig. 28.12 Thoracic aortic aneurysm. **A** Tubular. **B** Saccular.

AORTIC ANEURYSM

Tubulosaccular aneurysm

These are 'true' aneurysms which form either a fusiform (tubular) or a focal (saccular) type of swelling (Fig. 28.12). They are lined by layered thrombus and most are due to medial degeneration secondary to smoking and hypertension (see Chapter 27).

False 'aneurysm'

This results when bleeding from an aortic injury is contained within the mediastinum so that the aneurysm wall is formed only by fibrous tissue and organized thrombus. There is usually a history of a road traffic accident or fall, which may have occurred many years previously.

Both true and false aneurysms may rupture and present as an acute emergency, with chest pain and catastrophic intrathoracic bleeding. However, they are often noted as incidental chest X-ray findings. Occasionally an aneurysm may present with symptoms due to secondary pressure effects, such as dysphagia (oesophagus), stridor (left bronchus), chest wall pain (erosion of ribs), back pain (erosion of the vertebrae) or hoarseness (stretching of the left recurrent laryngeal nerve).

Aortic dissection

This is caused when blood enters into the wall of the aorta through a split in the intima, creating a false lumen that spirals along the vessel within the medial layer. The entry point is usually either just above the aortic valve or immediately beyond the left subclavian artery. However, the dissection process may extend along the entire length of the aorta into the iliac vessels. The false lumen may rupture

through the adventitia into the mediastinum or pleural cavity, causing massive and frequently fatal haemorrhage, or into the pericardium causing fatal tamponade. The origins of aortic side branches, which are encountered by the false lumen, tend to be encircled and occluded. This process can lead to widespread ischaemic damage to the heart (coronaries), brain (branches of the aortic arch), spinal cord (spinal arteries), kidneys (renal arteries), abdominal viscera (coeliac and mesenteric arteries) and the limbs. A dissection that involves the aortic root tends to lift the aortic valve leaflets away from the wall, leading to reflux. Finally, a dissected aorta may dilate over months to years, causing a progressive aneurysmal process. Acute dis-

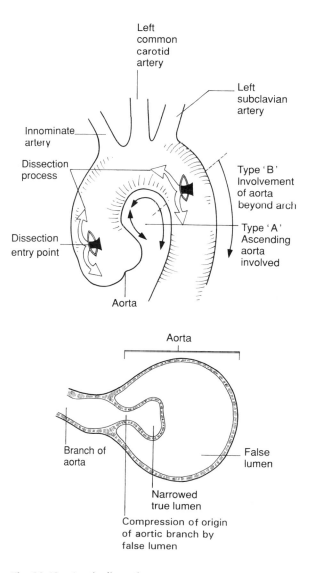

Fig. 28.13 Aortic dissection.

section is often fatal prior to arrival at hospital. There may be severe interscapular pain, collapse, shock aortic incompetence, unequal peripheral pulses, features of a left haemothorax, stroke, paraplegia and abdominal discomfort, and lower limb ischaemia. Dissections are classified using two systems (Fig. 28.13). Dissections which originate distal to the left subclavian and do not spread retrogradely to involve the aortic arch or ascending aorta, and are clinically stable, are usually managed conservatively by control of blood pressure, as the results of medical and surgical treatment are not different. The decision to operate on such patients is based on the development of rupture and organ/limb ischaemia. In contrast, most patients with dissections that involve the ascending aorta or arch are offered emergency surgery to prevent rupture, stroke, MI and aortic valve incompetence. Surgery involves excising and replacing the portion of the aorta containing the entry point. This prevents more blood entering the false lumen and reapposes the layers of the aortic wall. Additional surgery to repair the aortic valve or to replace the aortic arch or descending aorta will be determined by individual circumstances.

Aortoannulo ectasia

This is characterized by a flask-shaped aneurysmal dilatation of the aortic root and ascending aorta. This expanding aneurysm may rupture, initiate a dissection and lead to severe aortic reflux, with all the potential sequelae of these conditions. Aortoannulo ectasia is most frequently associated with Marfan's disease.

Assessment

A patient with an incidentally discovered aneurysm should be thoroughly investigated, including tests of respiratory function and coronary angiography and contrast CT to determine whether the magnitude of surgery required could be sustained. Aneurysms that extend from the chest into the abdomen (thoracoabdominal aneurysm) require further investigations to clarify the relationship of the aneurysm to the renal and visceral vessels. Larger aneurysms (6 cm or greater) are more likely to rupture, and several review appointments will confirm whether or not an aneurysm is enlarging. Based on these considerations, a decision can then be taken regarding the potential benefit of surgery. Patients presenting with acute rupture of an aneurysm may undergo emergency surgery if they are potentially salvageable and considered likely to benefit from operative intervention.

Surgery for aortic pathology

Lesions of the aortic root and ascending aorta are repaired on bypass via a median sternotomy. A woven nylon tube graft is used to replace an ascending aortic aneurysm, but in aortic annulo ectasia a graft containing an aortic valve prosthesis is used to replace the whole aortic root. The coronary artery ostia are then sewn into side holes cut in the graft. Aneurysms involving the aortic arch require complex surgery. The patient is cooled to 16°C on bypass, the circulation arrested and the patient exsanguinated. Profound hypothermia protects against cerebral damage while the surgeon operates in a bloodless field. The innominate, left carotid and left subclavian arteries are anastomosed to the arch graft. Descending aortic aneurysms can often be repaired using a local bypass system in order to deliver blood to the lower body. Clamps are applied to exclude the aneurysm, which is excised and replaced with a suitable length of graft. If a thoracoabdominal aneurysm is being repaired, the visceral arteries are also anastomosed to the graft.

All thoracic aortic aneurysm surgery is high risk. Elective procedures carry a 5–15% mortality risk and a risk of stroke of several percent. Procedures involving the descending aorta carry an additional 5–10% risk of paraplegia owing to interference with spinal arterial supply. Emergency thoracic aneurysm surgery is in most cases a desperate measure. Mortality rates vary between 10% and over 60%, depending upon the extent of surgery required and, very importantly, the degree of pre-existing and acquired morbidity the patient has prior to surgery. It is not uncommon for the primary repair procedure to proceed satisfactorily only for the patient to die later from multiorgan failure and/or stroke. In some instances it may be possible to manage a descending thoracic aneurysm or dissection by inserting an endoluminal stent under radiological guidance via the iliac artery (see Chapter 27).

Pericardial pathology

Pericardial effusion

In chronic pericardial effusion the pericardial sac will stretch and the clinical effects of the accumulated fluid may be modest. In contrast, a rapidly evolving effusion will prevent the heart from filling in diastole (tamponade) and lead to a low stroke volume. In order to maintain cardiac output and blood pressure there is a tachycardia and intense peripheral vasoconstriction. The raised intrapericardial pressure leads to elevation of atrial pressure, and hence the central venous pressure rises in order to maintain a filling gradient. A pericardial effusion can often be drained through a catheter placed under echocardiographic guidance. This may help clarify the diagnosis, but surgical drainage is likely to be required in infection, malignancy with reasonable life expectancy, and in chronic effusions. Chronic effusions are often drained into the left pleural cavity. This is achieved by creating a window in the left lateral pericardium via either an open left lateral thoracotomy or, more recently, as a minimal-access videothoracoscopic procedure. Acute and malignant effusions can be drained relatively simply into the peritoneal cavity via a short epigastric incision. Whichever approach is used, specimens of fluid and pericardium are sent for culture and histology.

Pericardial constriction

Chronic pericardial inflammation, often from tuberculosis, may heal by intense fibrosis and calcification (Fig. 28.14). This leads to chronic tamponade. Surgery is undertaken via a median sternotomy to remove the parietal pericardium and any fibrotic visceral pericardium. The results of surgery are frequently disappointing because the patient has developed irreversible hepatic cirrhosis and myocardial function is poor.

CONGENITAL CARDIAC DISEASE

This may be classified as cyanotic or acyanotic, depending on the presence of central cyanosis. Those with cyanosis will have a right-to-left shunt, preventing complete oxygenation of systemic arterial blood. Some patients with high-flow left-to-right shunts develop severe pulmonary

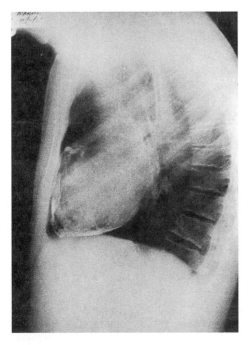

Fig. 28.14 Calcified constrictive pericardium.

hypertension as a consequence of the massive pulmonary blood flow. This can result in pressures in the right heart chambers which are greater than those in the left heart and, consequently, in reversal of the shunt direction to right to left, causing cyanosis. This situation is called Eisenmenger's syndrome. Primary repair is usually advised for congenital defects, but in some instances it may be helpful to delay definitive repair until the child is older, larger and fitter. In this situation a temporizing palliative procedure is performed. These are usually designed to augment or restrict pulmonary artery blood flow.

Atrial septal defect

This is the commonest abnormality, causing a left-to-right atrial shunt and hence an increase in right heart and pulmonary blood flow. Patients may be asymptomatic or present with frequent chest infections. There is a fixed split second heart sound and a pulmonary ejection systolic murmur. Small defects are of little haemodynamic significance, but if the pulmonary to systemic flow ratio exceeds 2:1 closure is necessary. ECG frequently demonstrates right ventricular hypertrophy and echocardiography is diagnostic. Three anatomical types exist, named after the developmental area giving rise to the defect:

- Sinus venosus defects arise in the upper atrium adjacent to the superior vena cava. They are repaired with a Dacron or pericardial patch, which must be placed with care as the right upper pulmonary vein can be abnormally located within the apparent right atrial area.
- Ostium secundum defects are the commonest lesions and are located at midatrial septal level. Closure by patch or simple suture is straightforward, but may also be achieved by an interventional cardiologist using a catheter-inserted closure device.
- Ostium primum defects are usually associated with clefts in the anterior mitral leaflet and septal tricuspid leaflet, which are repaired at the same time as closure of the atrial septal defect with a patch. Left axis deviation is common.

Surgical repair in children carries a low mortality (< 1%), but adults presenting with pulmonary hypertension are at greater risk (10%).

Ventricular septal defect

Many ventricular septal defects are small and close within the first year of life. Larger lesions cause a left-to-right shunt and pulmonary congestion. Defects may again be subdivided according to their embryological origins, but most (85%) occur in the membranous septum. Infants with large defects may present with frequent respiratory infections but patients are often asymptomatic. A pansystolic murmur is audible, maximal at the left sternal edge. The second heart sound may be loud. Biventricular hypertrophy is present on ECG and pulmonary plethora may be noted on chest X-ray. Echocardiography is diagnostic. Asymptomatic defects are observed, but early operation is preferred for larger defects to prevent irreversible pulmonary hypertension. Repair is undertaken using a patch, with an operative mortality of 3–5%.

Patent ductus arteriosus

If the ductus arteriosus fails to close after birth pulmonary blood flow is abnormally high, producing pulmonary congestion and hypertension. Infants have retarded growth and a continuous 'machinery' murmur is audible over the praecordium and back. The chest X-ray shows pulmonary congestion, and echocardiography can exclude concurrent intracardiac defect(s). In premature children the duct may close with an indomethacin infusion (prostaglandin E_1 inhibition), but clipping or division at left thoracotomy is likely to be needed. Endovascular closure is an option in older children. The operative mortality is low in older children (<1%) but high (25%) in preterm infants, who are generally very unwell.

Coarctation of the aorta

This condition is caused by a narrowing of the thoracic aorta, usually at the level of the ligamentum arteriosum. The lower body is perfused via extensive chest wall collaterals. Upper body hypertension develops, partly due to relative renal hypoperfusion, and may lead to heart failure in infancy. Untreated adults develop hypertensive cerebrovascular and renal problems and accelerated coronary atheroma. Most children and young adults are asymptomatic and present with high blood pressure or an abnormal chest X-ray. The femoral pulses may be impalpable or weak and delayed, and a systolic murmur may be audible over the back. Left ventricular hypertrophy is seen on the ECG and the chest X-ray shows an enlarged heart, reduced aortic knuckle and characteristic rib 'notching', caused by enlarged and tortuous intercostal arteries eroding the ribs near the posterior angles (Fig. 28.15). Balloon angioplasty has been used to dilate some coarctations in infants, but surgical correction is usually required. In infants an onlay patch graft created from the left subclavian artery is used. This has the advantage of growing with the child, although left arm growth is slightly decreased. Older children and adults are usually managed with a Dacron bypass graft. Surgical correction tends to reduce upper body hypertension in children. It is less effective in adults but pharmacological control of hypertension becomes more reliable. The operative risk is about 5%.

Tetralogy of Fallot

This is the commonest cause of cyanotic congenital heart disease and comprises a high ventricular septal defect, an aorta which tends to overlie the interventricular septum, pulmonary valvular and subvalvular stenosis, and right ventricular hypertrophy. Right ventricular outflow obstruction causes cyanosis as a result of right-to-left shunting across the ventricular septal defect. Clinical features depend upon the severity of the obstruction. This may not be significant when the child is at rest but it may be precipitated by adrenergic events, as these increase the subvalvular obstructive effect of hypertrophied right ventricular muscle. Consequently, the child may become blue and faint during feeding or crying. Right ventricular hypertrophy is found on ECG and the pulmonary artery shadow is small on chest X-ray. Echocardiography is diagnostic but complemented by right ventricular angiography, which demonstrates the pulmonary arterial tree. Correction entails closing the ventricular septal defect with a patch, resecting muscle bands contributing to right ventricular outflow obstruction, and enlarging the right ventricular outflow tract with a patch placed across the pulmonary valve annulus and along the pulmonary artery if necessary. In those not fit for this procedure, or with very small pulmonary vessels, a shunt (usually subclavian artery to pulmonary artery, Blalock–Taussig) is created in order to increase pulmonary blood flow and, hopefully, lead to further pulmonary arterial growth. Definitive correction may then be possible at a later stage. Operative mortality is about 10%.

THORACIC SURGERY

Assessment

This is concerned with confirming the diagnosis, determining in oncological cases whether resection is appropriate,

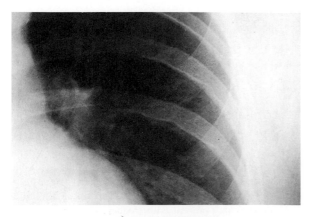

Fig. 28.15 Rib notching in coarctation.

Table 28.2   Common thoracic surgical investigations

Investigation	Yield
ECG	
Resting	Rhythm; conduction abnormalities; atrial and ventricular hypertrophy; established ischaemic changes; evidence of previous myocardial infarction
Chest X-ray	
PA & lateral	Preliminary assessment of location of lesion; malignant involvement of phrenic nerve or ribs; presence of additional lesions or effusion; presence of pneumothorax or mediastinal air
Thoracic CT scan	Further refine radiological assessment of mass lesions as above; review mediastinum for enlarged nodes in bronchogenic carcinoma; inspect bronchi for dilatations in suspected bronchiectasis, determine exact location of mediastinal mass lesions; determine areas of greatest disease in interstitial lung disease; locate intrathoracic collections; map out the distribution of bullous/emphysematous lung disease
Upper abdominal CT scan	Exclude or confirm liver abnormalities; identify adrenal metastases
Upper abdominal ultrasound	Determine probable nature of cystic hepatic lesions; provide guidance for biopsy of hepatic or adrenal lesions; review diaphragm motion in cases of suspected diaphragmatic rupture or phrenic nerve paralysis
MRI	Useful for detecting possible intraspinal extension of paravertebral neurogenic tumours
Isotope scans	
Bone	Search for skeletal metastases; review chest wall for possible direct invasion by carcinoma.
Lung	Identify areas of low uptake indicative of impaired perfusion (Q scan) or ventilation (V scan)
Pulmonary function tests	
FEV_1	Forced expiratory volume in 1 second provides a measure of airway obstruction
FVC	Forced vital capacity – indicates presence of restriction of ventilation
CO transfer	Measures the diffusion capacity of the patient's lungs
Walking test	Measures distance walked by the patient in a set time period (4 min) and the perceived exercise level achieved as assessed by the final heart rate – useful as an indicator of functional status in patients with poor FEV_1, as they may not comply well with the methodology of formal respiratory testing and hence underachieve
Arterial blood gas	Useful in demonstrating patients with CO_2 retention who should be excluded from surgical consideration

and establishing that the patient is fit for the intended surgical procedure. The principal investigations are summarized in Table 28.2. As noted below, history can be instructive in suggesting advanced malignant disease. It is also helpful in providing evidence of the patient's premorbid functional status.

Bronchogenic carcinoma

Aetiology, pathology and presentation

This usually presents from the fifth decade onwards and is now the leading cause of cancer death in the UK for both men and women. The principal risk factor is smoking, particularly cigarettes, but other rare causes include exposure to arsenic, radon gas, bichromates and nickel ore. The combination of asbestos exposure and cigarette smoking produces a many fold increase in risk. With the exception of alveolar cell carcinomas, which arise from cells lining the alveolae, primary lung cancers arise within the bronchial epithelium and are hence termed bronchogenic carcinoma. They are described as peripheral or central according to their location within the lung (Figs 28.16, 28.17). Peripheral lesions may grow to 8 cm or more before causing local symptoms such as chest wall pain. Many are detected as incidental findings on a chest film taken for unrelated reasons, or for

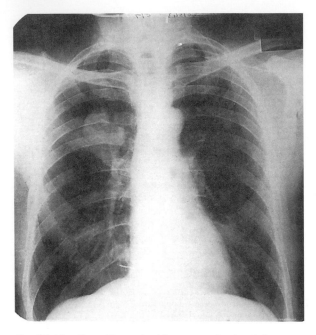

Fig. 28.16   Chest X-ray showing cancer in the right upper lobe.

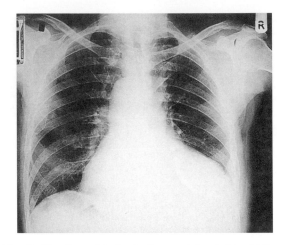

Fig. 28.18   Consolidation/collapse of the right middle and lower lobes associated with a bronchogenic carcinoma. Resection of these lobes would not alter respiratory function in the same way as resection of the tumour in Figure 28.16, as they are non-functional.

non-specific symptoms such as weight loss. Central lesions tend to occlude the airways, causing varying degrees of pulmonary collapse and consolidation (Fig. 28.18). Nodal spread occurs to the intralobar, hilar, mediastinal and thence to the scalene nodes. Metastases occur in bone, brain, liver, adrenals and lung. Local direct spread may involve the chest wall, vertebrae, trachea, oesophagus and great vessels.

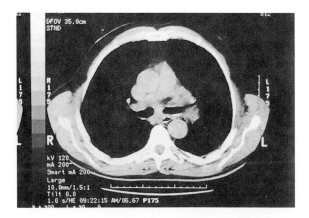

Fig. 28.17   Central bronchogenic carcinoma. This patient has an advanced carcinoma of the proximal left bronchus visible on this CT scan. There is extensive mediastinal lymphadenopathy visible in front of the bronchi and in the subcarinal area.

Cell types and approximate frequencies are: squamous 35%, adenocarcinoma 25%, undifferentiated 15%, small cell 20% and alveolar cell 5%. Patients with small cell lung cancer are not usually referred for surgery as this condition is regarded as a systemic disease at presentation and is therefore treated with chemotherapy. All other varieties are resected if possible, and bronchogenic carcinoma is therefore frequently split into two functional categories, small cell and non-small cell.

There may be no clinical features, but haemoptysis, pulmonary infection and weight loss are common presenting symptoms. Paraneoplastic syndromes are infrequent but well described, including ectopic hormone production (ACTH, PTH, ADH) and a painful periosteal reaction affecting the joints and long bones termed hypertrophic pulmonary osteoarthropathy (Fig. 28.19). Patients frequently have finger clubbing.

Assessment for pulmonary resection

Prior to referral to the surgeon, the diagnosis will often have been confirmed by sputum cytology, bronchoscopy or CT-guided needle biopsy, but approximately 30% of cases will be undiagnosed at this stage. Surgical assessment addresses two questions: Would the patient be fit for pulmonary resection and, if so, is the disease potentially curable?

Fitness for resection

Fitness is determined by cardiorespiratory investigations. A history of angina or myocardial infarction does not preclude

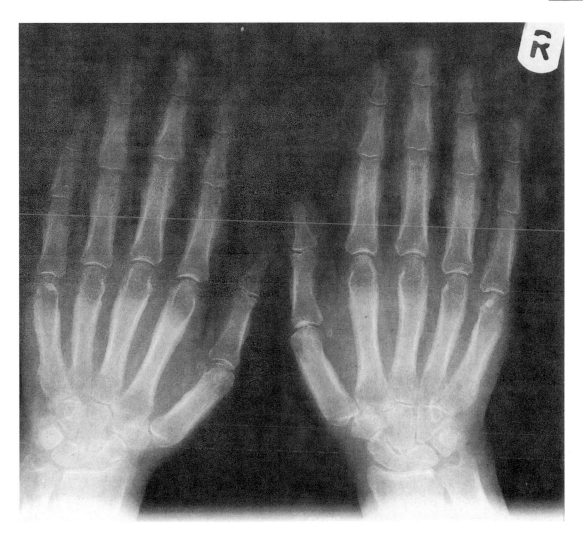

Fig. 28.19 Hypertrophic pulmonary osteoarthropathy.

surgery provided the symptoms are stable. However, patients with poor left ventricular function and/or unstable angina are not suitable for pulmonary resection. Respiratory investigations are orientated towards confirming that pulmonary reserve will be adequate following the intended resection. The forced expiratory volume in 1 second (FEV_1) and carbon monoxide (CO) transfer data are most helpful in this regard. Patients with an $FEV_1 < 50\%$ of predicted prior to resection are likely to be significantly breathless following surgery, and may not be suitable candidates for surgical management. If the CO transfer value is low, implying poor alveolar gas exchange, the minimum FEV_1 figure would have to be revised upwards. However, resection of consolidated or collapsed lung does not affect residual respiratory capability.

Staging

Assessment of the potential for curative resection is determined by staging. Initial clinical assessment will normally filter out advanced disease and provide evidence of incurability because of local irresectability or disseminated disease (Table 28.3). Simple chest X-ray may reveal an elevated diaphragm, indicating phrenic nerve involvement, bone metastases or direct invasion of the ribcage. If an effusion is present this should be aspirated, and if malignant cells are noted on cytology this would preclude resection. A contrast-enhanced thoracic and upper abdominal CT scan will clarify the nature and position of the pulmonary mass and should exclude other pulmonary lesions that might represent metastases or synchronous tumours. Mediastinal nodes <1 cm in

Table 28.3   Clinical indicators of locally irresectable or incurable lung cancer

Clinical finding	Pathological implication
Local inoperability	
Horner's syndrome	Involvement of upper sympathetic chain
Hoarseness	Involvement of left recurrent laryngeal nerve
Upper body venous congestion	Involvement of SVC
Severe shoulder/inner arm pain	Involvement of brachial plexus (Pancoast tumour)
Disseminated disease	
Scalene node enlargement	Nodal spread out of operative field
Hepatomegaly	Hepatic metastases
Focal bone pain	Bone metastases
Skin deposits	Cutaneous metastases
Behavioural/balance disturbance	Cerebral metastases
Headache	

long axis are generally considered to be benign, but surgical sampling is necessary to confirm this. The liver and adrenals are common sites for metastases. Suspicious areas can be sampled by means of ultrasound-guided biopsy. Further investigations, such as bone or brain scans, will depend upon the clinical suspicion.

Surgical staging is concerned with further refining the intrathoracic assessment so as to ensure that thoracotomy will be associated with a reasonable chance of cure. In practical terms this involves excluding those with involved mediastinal lymph nodes and, where possible, confirming the diagnosis and local operability. Three techniques are employed. Mediastinoscopy is used to sample the paratracheal and sub-carinal lymph nodes. A low anterior cervical incision is made just above the jugular notch and the mediastinoscope used to create a passage in the pretracheal region. The lymph nodes are dissected and biopsied. Mediastinotomy is used mainly to assess lymph nodes within the concavity of the aortic arch or anterior to the aorta, as these areas cannot be reached at mediastinoscopy. Access is gained via a short left anterior second interspace incision. Videothoracoscopy is a relatively new technique which allows the surgeon to inspect the pleural cavity, biopsy the primary lesion and sample the lower mediastinal and aortic arch lymph nodes. The extent of resection likely to be required can also be assessed in relation to the patient's lung function. Videothoracoscopy may also reveal unforeseen causes of irresectability, such as pleural seedlings.

Resection

Lung tumours are normally removed en bloc with the surrounding parenchyma and local draining lymphatics. This involves either lobectomy or pneumonectomy. Occasionally, in unfit patients small cancers are excised within a wedge or segment of lung. The risk of local recurrence is greater in these lung-sparing cases. An area of anterior chest wall directly invaded by tumour can be excised and replaced with

an acrylic patch, provided it is lateral to the posterior rib angles. Following assessment and surgical resection a final pathological TNM stage (Table 28.4) is allocated. This is

Table 28.4   Lung cancer staging

Stage Category	TNM Classification
0	Carcinoma in situ (Tis)
IA	T1 N0 M0
IB	T2 N0 M0
IIA	T1 N1 M0
IIB	T3 N0 M0
IIIA	T3 N1 M0
	T1/T2/T3 N2 M0
IIIB	Any T4, Any N3, M0
IV	Any M1

Abbreviated definitions:

T1 = peripheral tumour < 3 cm not involving pleura

T2 = tumour > 3 cm or involves: main bronchus beyond 2 cm from carina/parietal pleura

T3 = tumour involves: chest wall/mediastinal pleura/pericardium/diaphragm or main bronchus within 2 cm of carina

T4 = tumour involves: mediastinal structures/vertebral column/carina; tumour is associated with pericardial or pleural malignant effusion; satellite tumour deposits are present within lobe containing primary tumour

N0 = no lymph nodes involved by tumour

N1 = ipsilateral peribronchial or intrapulmonary nodes involved

N2 = ipsilateral mediastinal or subcarinal nodes involved

N3 = contralateral mediastinal nodes involved; involvement of scalene nodes on either side

M0 = no distant metastases

M1 = distant metastases present

helpful in indicating prognosis and determining whether a patient might benefit from adjuvant therapy or be suitable for inclusion in a trial. Patients who are found to have positive mediastinal nodes following resection are routinely referred for adjuvant radiotherapy to the mediastinum in view of the high risk of recurrence in that area. Operative mortality is about 2% for lobectomy and 6% for pneumonectomy.

Survival

Long-term survival depends on tumour stage at the time of resection. Reported 5-year survival data are of the order of 60% for stage I, 35% for stage II and < 20% for stage IIIa disease. Relatively few patients (< 20%) with non-small cell bronchogenic carcinoma are suitable for resection at presentation. One strategy to address this problem is the use of neoadjuvant preoperative induction chemotherapy to downstage tumours, although there are as yet no data to support the widespread use of this approach. The other obvious possibility for improving resection rates would be to detect lung cancers at an earlier stage. Previous mass chest X-ray screening studies did not appear to show an improvement in long-term survival, but there is currently renewed interest in screening using low-dose spiral CT as a more sensitive test.

Metastatic disease

Pulmonary metastases (Fig. 28.20) are the commonest form of intrathoracic malignancy. A confirmatory diagnostic lung biopsy may be helpful for patients with no evident primary. A palliative pleurodesis in patients with associated pleural effusion can be achieved by instilling an irritant such as

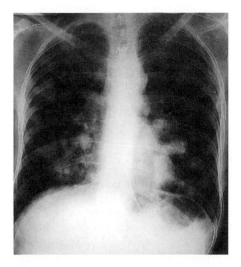

Fig. 28.20   Multiple pulmonary metastases.

aluminium silicate powder (kaolin) into the pleural cavity. Rarely, a solitary metastasis or limited pulmonary metastases (e.g. in osteogenic sarcoma) may be found in patients without any other evidence of disseminated disease. In these rare situations surgery may be advised to remove the metastatic lesion(s).

Other lung tumours

These tend to present either as an incidental chest X-ray finding, in which case the concern is that they may in fact be a malignant tumour, or as a cause of bronchial obstruction and infection. True benign lung tumours are rare and can arise from all tissue elements within the lung architecture. If the lesion can be shown to be benign by transthoracic biopsy no treatment is required. Where there is doubt, local excision will be required. If a main bronchus is obstructed lobectomy will be necessary to remove the tumour and the damaged portion of lung. Carcinoid tumours arise from argentaffin-containing cells within the bronchial epithelium. They are divided on histological grounds into 'typical' tumours, which grow slowly locally, and 'atypical' tumours which grow more quickly and can metastasize. Resection is by lobectomy. As local recurrence may occur up to 15 years following resection, good local clearance is essential. Unlike abdominal carcinoids, thoracic carcinoids do not secrete vasoactive substances.

An adenochondroma is a hamartoma, a tumour which develops from residual embryological tissue within the lung parenchyma. It presents as an incidental chest X-ray finding and is typically partly calcified and with a very smooth outline. CT-guided needle biopsy should provide the diagnosis, and surgery is only undertaken when the diagnosis is in doubt.

Mesothelioma

This causes progressive thickening of the parietal and visceral pleura, with subsequent encasement of the lung and the formation of a large pleural effusion. In the later stages the growth penetrates the chest wall, causing pain, and involves the mediastinal structures and abdominal cavity. Metastatic spread is rare until an advanced stage is reached. Mesothelioma is strongly related to a history of asbestos exposure, but there is usually a latent period of 20–40 years before the onset of symptoms. The patient commonly presents with shortness of breath owing to a large pleural effusion. In many cases the diagnosis is made by a percutaneous pleural biopsy, but if this is not successful thoracoscopy or open pleural biopsy will provide the diagnosis. The main differential diagnosis is disseminated adenocarcinoma involving the pleural cavity. It can be difficult to distinguish these two pathologies on light microscopy, and diagnosis may be delayed while immunohistochemistry and electron microscopy studies are performed. Surgical resection by excision of the parietal pleura and lung (pleuropneumonectomy) is not generally reported to offer a survival benefit, except possibly in very early lesions. Radiotherapy and chemotherapy have no curative value. Therapy is therefore usually directed towards controlling symptoms as they occur. If the lung re-expands after drainage of the effusion, kaolin may be instilled in order to promote pleurodesis and so prevent recurrence. Life expectancy varies between 1 and 4 years from initial presentation, depending on age, the rate of tumour growth and the stage at presentation.

Mediastinum

Mass lesions

Benign and malignant masses may arise in the mediastinum. Some clue to the likely diagnosis is provided by the location of the lesion (Fig. 28.21) within the mediastinum. Where the diagnosis is in doubt, tissue may be obtained by CT-guided needle biopsy. If this is either not feasible or is unsuccessful, a surgical biopsy can be obtained using mediastinotomy,

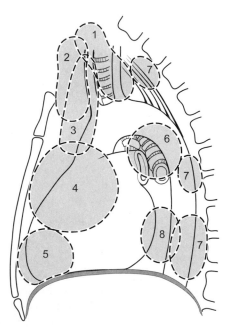

1 Goitre
2 Lymph node tumours, primary and metastases
3 Thymoma
4 Dermoid/teratoma
5 Pleuropericardial cyst
6 Bronchogenic cyst
7 Neurogenic tumour
8 Enterogenous cyst

Fig. 28.21 Topography of mediastinal lesions.

mediastinoscopy or videothoracoscopy. The clinical features vary considerably, with some quite large masses being asymptomatic and identified on routine chest films. Non-specific symptoms include vague chest pain, cough, weight loss, fever and general malaise. Other lesions may cause direct pressure effects, such as tracheal compression by a retrosternal thyroid goitre or oesophageal compression by malignant lymphadenopathy. Small thymic tumours may be identified during the evaluation of patients with myasthenia gravis.

Wherever possible primary mediastinal tumours are resected, although in many cases this is precluded because the growth encircles or invades the great vessels and mediastinal viscera. Benign cysts are usually resected or, less commonly, marsupialized in order to prevent pressure effects or the development of infection. Surgery is generally undertaken via a median sternotomy for anterior lesions and via a thoracotomy for mid and posterior lesions.

Infection

Mediastinal infection is an uncommon but serious condition that is associated with a rapid onset of septicaemia and septic shock. It is almost always a consequence of oesophageal or pharyngeal leakage, which may follow perforation or breakdown of an oesophageal anastomosis. Perforation usually occurs after attempted dilatation of a stricture but can result from swallowing sharp objects or caustic substances, and rarely with external trauma. The diagnosis may be suggested by the history. A chest film will usually show mediastinal widening, gas streaks from mediastinal emphysema together with pleural fluid, and possibly a hydropneumothorax. Surgical management requires broad-spectrum parenteral antibiotics, adequate mechanical drainage, and correction of the cause if possible. Mechanical drainage may be achieved by pleural drainage alone if the lesion is low in the mediastinum and has burst directly into the pleural cavity, as may be the situation with a leaking oesophagogastric anastomosis. It is often necessary to perform a thoracotomy so that the pleura can be widely opened and the mediastinum fully drained and debrided. Further surgery to attend to the underlying cause, for example by repairing the oesophagus, may be necessary either immediately or subsequently when the patient is more stable.

Pneumothorax

Pneumothorax occurs when air enters the potential space between the visceral and parietal pleura through either an external chest wound or an internal air leak. External air entry occurs with a traumatic chest wall defect, and the resulting open pneumothorax is often associated with a 'sucking wound', where air moves in and out of a chest wound with respiration. Internal air leakage may follow oesophageal perforation or anastomotic breakdown, as air can enter the pleural cavity via the mouth.

However, by far the most common cause of pneumothorax is leakage of air from the lung, due either to a traumatic puncture wound or to spontaneous leakage from a large (bulla) or small (<1 cm, 'bleb') air sac on the lung surface. Occasionally, the pulmonary leak point may have a flap valve mechanism which allows air out of but not back into the lung, causing a rapid build-up of pressure within the pleural cavity and 'tension' pneumothorax (Fig. 28.22). This can be fatal, as the high intrapleural pressure completely flattens the ipsilateral lung while deviating the mediastinum to the opposite side, impeding venous return. Spontaneous pneumothorax is described as primary or secondary. Primary pneumothorax typically occurs in young (15–35 years) individuals with essentially normal lungs apart from a few apical bullae or blebs. Secondary pneumothorax develops in elderly patients (55–75 years) with a background of emphysema and chronic obstructive pulmonary disease. It is caused by rupture of a large bulla.

Treatment

Initial management involves inserting a chest drain connected to an underwater seal drain into the pleural space (Fig. 28.23). This allows the lung to re-expand. In most cases of primary pneumothorax air leakage stops within 48 hours or so, after which the drain can be removed. If the

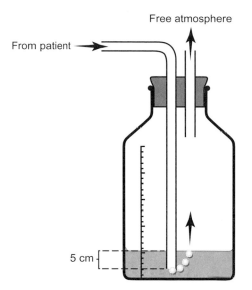

Fig. 28.23 Underwater seal drain. The water acts as an hydraulic valve. This allows air to escape from the pleural cavity with ease but the pressure required to cause reverse air flow is much greater, being increased by the ratio of the surface areas inside and outside the tube which enter the water.

pneumothorax recurs, or the air leakage does not stop, surgery is indicated. This is now undertaken as a thoracoscopic procedure. The lung is inspected and any blebs or bullae are stapled. These are usually found at the apices of the upper or lower lobes. Pleurodesis is then performed using either an abrasion technique to scarify the parietal pleura, a pleural strip (pleurectomy), or by insufflation of kaolin. Bullectomy and abrasion or pleurectomy has about an 8% risk of further recurrent pneumothorax. This is reduced to 1–2% with kaolin insufflation, but as this technique involves leaving foreign material in the chest of a young person it is usually kept in reserve for recurrent pneumothorax, or for patients with no obvious culprit bulla or bleb.

Secondary pneumothorax may not settle rapidly owing to the poor quality of the underlying lung tissue. However, it occurs in individuals who are clearly poor candidates for general anaesthesia and major thoracic surgery. It is customary, therefore, to wait for 1–2 weeks to see if the air leak will stop spontaneously. If not, videothoracoscopy is undertaken in better-risk patients to inspect the lung for a leaking bulla, which can be closed by stapling. Alternatively, kaolin mixed with local anaesthetic can be inserted as a slurry up the drain. This option avoids general anaesthesia but results in significant pain. Either treatment is associated with an appreciable mortality of 5–10% owing to respiratory and cardiovascular complications.

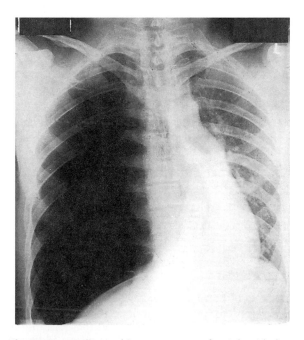

Fig. 28.22 Radiographic appearance of a right-sided tension pneumothorax (note the mediastinal shift to opposite side).

Emphysema

Emphysema causes progressive loss of respiratory function, culminating in respiratory failure and death. Recurrent infection and pneumothorax are common. It is characterized by progressive loss of interalveolar septae. Large air spaces form throughout the lung which become grossly enlarged, and areas of severely diseased lung develop which are neither ventilated nor perfused. This is a typically a smoking-related disease affecting patients from the fourth or fifth decade onwards, with a tendency towards an upper lobar distribution. In less than 10% of cases, however, it can also result from a deficiency of α_1-antitrypsin, affecting younger patients from the third decade and having a lower lobar distribution. Medical treatment with bronchodilators and steroids may improve symptoms but transplantation is the only definitive cure. This is only an option for younger patients, and even in these it should be put off as long as possible. Recently, a new surgical procedure called lung volume reduction has been developed which aims to improve lung function by excising the worst-affected areas. This removes the space-occupying effect of these non-functional areas and allows the overall lung volume to return towards normal, thereby improving diaphragmatic and chest wall function. The improvement in respiratory function is modest in absolute terms, being in the order of 0.5 L for FEV_1. However, patients eligible for this surgery typically have FEV_1 values less than 1 L, so that the percentage improvement and hence the perceived benefit can be significant. The procedure may be performed as either a videothoracoscopic operation or through a median sternotomy. The operative mortality is high (6–12%), reflecting the generally very poor condition of these patients.

Interstitial lung disease

This can arise from many causes and correct treatment depends on an accurate diagnosis. Transbronchial biopsy can be undertaken but provides only a small tissue sample, which is often not diagnostic. It is usually preferable to use videothoracoscopic techniques to excise a wedge of affected lung. The patient is typically allowed home on the first postoperative day.

Pleuropulmonary infection

Empyema

This is a collection of pus within the pleural cavity and commonly follows a pneumonia due to secondary infection of a reactive parapneumonic effusion. In the initial phase the infected fluid is thin and may be completely evacuated by a low intercostal drain. The empyema quickly becomes

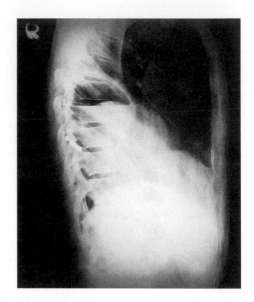

Fig. 28.24 Lateral X-ray of empyema. This film shows the D-shaped outline of a typical empyema. Infected fluid collections can, however, occur anywhere within the chest.

thick and loculated as a result of the deposition of fibrin, and at this stage formal surgical drainage is required. The collection is typically placed posteriorly towards the base of the pleural cavity and causes a D-shaped shadow on the chest film (Fig. 28.24). Drainage is achieved by excising a 2 cm segment of rib over the lowest part of the empyema and suctioning and curetting the cavity clean. Dense fibrosis surrounds an empyema, so that drainage creates a fixed cavity. In elderly or unfit patients a simple open tube drain is left in situ for many months, during which the cavity gradually shrinks and finally obliterates. In younger patients open thoracotomy allows the fibrous cavity to be excised and any cortex over the lung removed. This returns more lung function to the patient and avoids open drainage, so that recovery is more rapid.

Other causes of empyema include postsurgical bronchial or oesophageal suture line leakage, oesophageal rupture or perforation, repeat aspiration of pleural effusion, secondary infection of a clotted haemothorax and, rarely, a subphrenic abscess.

Bronchiectasis

Dilatation of bronchi and bronchioles can follow childhood infections. The stagnant pools of secretions that collect are subject to continued infection, resulting in episodes of acute pulmonary infection or pneumonia and, more rarely, in haemoptysis. Management is by antibiotic therapy, physiotherapy and daily postural drainage.

Evaluation by CT scan usually demonstrates that the condition is fairly widespread throughout the lungs, but occasionally one lobe may be particularly badly affected. This is more likely when the bronchiectasis is secondary to chronic bronchial obstruction by an inhaled object or, more rarely, from external glandular compression. In this relatively uncommon situation lobectomy may result in a gratifying decrease in chronic sputum production and in the frequency of recurrent infection. Resection can be technically difficult, as dense vascular adhesions surround the affected lobe.

Chest wall deformities

Sternal protuberance (pectus carinatum) or retraction (pectus excavatum) may be detected and corrected in early childhood. Pectus excavatum can be associated with connective tissue disorders such as Marfan's syndrome, and with unilateral breast hypoplasia. There is often a mild degree of scoliosis present and patients characteristically stand with a hunched posture. Often, however, patients with these deformities present in their early teenage years. At this time the deformity is exacerbated by accelerated growth and the individual becomes extremely sensitive about their appearance. Neither deformity is of physiological significance, and correction is only indicated when the patient's quality of life is clearly impaired because of their appearance. Correction involves major surgery, with resection of the costal cartilages from the third rib downwards bilaterally in order to mobilize the sternum so that it can be repositioned. In addition, a steel bar is implanted behind the elevated sternum for excavatum cases so as to maintain the new sternal position. The patient and their family must be advised that, as with all major thoracic surgery, this procedure can be associated with serious postoperative complications, including death. Also, the sternum must be given time to fuse in the corrected position, and so contact or vigorous sports are not permitted for about 9 months after surgery. In general, if repair is to be undertaken it is best delayed until the patient is at least 17 years old, as major growth has stopped by this time, thereby reducing the chance that further deformation could follow repair.

Postoperative care

The majority of major thoracic surgery is performed through a lateral thoracotomy incision, which is inherently much more painful than a median sternotomy. However, patients are not usually electively ventilated, as this is not helpful to healing lung or to lung function. Patients undergoing major thoracic surgery are therefore usually cared for in a high-dependency unit for the first 24–48 hours follow-

ing surgery. The key objectives are to enable the patient to breathe effectively and to clear secretions properly.

Pain control

Pain management during the HDU phase is achieved in two ways An epidural catheter can be placed prior to surgery. This provides very effective pain control in the immediate postoperative period but can have disadvantages related to increased fluid requirement, nursing care, and marked pain appreciation when the epidural infusion is stopped. Many units prefer not to place an epidural catheter and to rely instead on a combination of patient-controlled morphine infusion supplemented by parenteral non-steroidal analgesics and local intercostal nerve blocks. These can be conveniently given via a paravertebral catheter inserted at surgery.

Management of secretions

It is vital that patients cough and clear secretions. This requires humidification of oxygen to prevent the secretions becoming excessively viscous, effective pain control, and considerable input from physiotherapy. Many patients undergoing thoracic surgery have been chronic heavy smokers and have impaired lung function. They have heavy production of secretions and in some cases these accumulate, threatening to cause pneumonia and respiratory failure. In this situation a suction bronchoscopy is performed under light general anaesthesia to remove the secretions, and a minitracheostomy tube may be inserted via the cricothyroid membrane so that secretions can be aspirated. In severe cases ventilation and formal tracheostomy may be required.

Fluid management

Following major thoracic surgery the pulmonary alveolar–capillary membrane becomes relatively leaky, so that fluid tends to accumulate within the pulmonary interstitial spaces. This decreases lung compliance and increases the work of breathing. A degree of postoperative fluid restriction for the first 48 hours ensures that the left atrial pressure is kept low, thereby decreasing pulmonary venous pressure and the transcapillary gradient.

Late management

All patients receive subcutaneous heparin as DVT prophylaxis until fully mobile, because the risk of thrombosis is high in thoracic surgery and the consequences of pulmonary embolism are that much worse when lung has been resected. Drains are withdrawn when air leakage stops, and patients are mobilized as rapidly as possible. In an uneventful recovery, discharge home should occur about

6–9 days after major open resection, and after 1–5 days following a videothoracoscopic minimal-access procedure. The patient's age, general health and social circumstances will influence these estimates.

Cardiac and pulmonary transplantation

Transplantation for end-stage cardiac and pulmonary disease is discussed in Chapter 31.

29 Urological surgery

L.H. Stewart

ASSESSMENT

General points

Many patients who present to a urological clinic have symptoms and/or signs suggestive of an abnormality in the urinary tract worthy of investigation. Importantly, any patient with blood in the urine (haematuria), irrespective of other symptoms, requires a full urological assessment. Patients also present to a variety of other clinics complaining of symptoms which may be urological, for example backache from metastatic prostatic carcinoma; fever of unknown origin from renal carcinoma; lethargy and anaemia due to obstructive renal failure; or headaches from renal hypertension. Common things are common, and an elderly male complaining of difficulty in passing urine *probably* has outflow tract obstruction due to benign prostatic enlargement. Alternatively, he may have been recently prescribed a diuretic leading to a change in his urinary habit, withdrawal of which may solve the problem. Environmental and geographic factors must not be ignored. In some parts of the world bilharziasis is a common cause of haematuria. In the developed world, exposure to certain carcinogens may lead to bladder cancer many years later.

Urinary tract symptoms

Pain

Any pain must be precisely described. Pain 'in the side' could originate from the chest, loin or spinal column. Renal pain occurs in the angle between the 12th rib and the sacrospinalis muscles. Ureteric pain (or colic) may start in the renal angle but typically radiates forwards and down-

515

wards into the groin, testes or labia. Acute bladder obstruction usually causes severe central lower abdominal pain. By contrast, chronic bladder obstruction may be virtually asymptomatic even though the bladder is grossly distended. Disease of the bladder and prostate cause ill-defined perineal or penile pains. A prostate that is grossly enlarged can cause rectal symptoms, including tenesmus. Recognition of penile and testicular pain is usually easy.

Disorders of micturition

Patients may use a wide range of phrases to describe alterations in their urinary habit. The principal aim of the history is to determine whether they are describing obstruction (e.g. poor stream), detrusor contraction (e.g. urgency), infection (e.g. frequency, dysuria) or a more sinister sign of malignancy (e.g. dark, discoloured or brown urine). Frequency is recorded numerically: D/N 6/3 indicates that the frequency by day is six times and by night three. Poor stream and dribbling are characteristic of mechanical obstruction of the urinary outflow tract. Urgency describes the sudden uncontrollable urge to empty the bladder. This may be associated with incontinence (urge incontinence). Stress incontinence indicates the involuntary loss of urine due to stress, such as straining, lifting, running or even laughing. Dysuria describes painful micturition that is often burning or scalding.

Examination

Examination should not be confined to the urinary system, as cardiological, neurological and gynaecological problems may be associated with urological symptoms and signs. Many urological patients are elderly and require their fitness for further investigations and operative treatment to be assessed. Furthermore, the patient's cardiovascular status may be relevant to subsequent treatment, for example administration of oestrogens for carcinoma of the prostate.

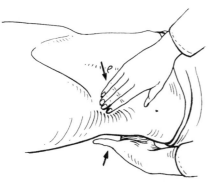

Fig. 29.1 Bimanual palpation of the right kidney.

Physical examination of the kidneys is difficult. The patient must relax the abdominal muscles so that the kidney can be lifted with one hand placed behind the loin and compressed by the other hand pressing downwards (Fig. 29.1). The ureter cannot be palpated even though it passes close to the posterior fornix of the vagina. An enlarged bladder rises centrally out of the pelvis is dull to percussion and may even be visible. Abnormalities of adjacent abdominal organs should also be considered: for example, a mass in the iliac fossa could be ovarian in origin. In a man, the hernial orifices, cords, testes and epididymes are examined with the patient standing and lying. The penis should always be examined. If it is uncircumcised it must be confirmed that the foreskin retracts and that the glans and meatus are normal. In the female patient the vulva, urethra and vagina must also be examined. A speculum examination should be carried out if there is any suspicion of vaginal or cervical abnormality. A full pelvic bimanual examination, whether in males or females, is best carried out under general anaesthesia with a muscle relaxant. A rectal examination is mandatory, not only to examine the prostate but also to detect abnormalities of the anal margin (haemorrhoids, fissures) and lower rectum (carcinoma).

Investigations

Urine

The urine must be tested for protein (proteinuria) and sugar (glycosuria) using proprietary test papers. In the absence of infection, urine is normally almost protein free. Proteinuria of more than 150 mg/24 h mandates further investigation. Glycosuria suggests the presence of diabetes. Screening for urinary tract infection may also be done by dipstix. Microscopic examination is only carried out to detect casts or tubular epithelial cells associated with renal parenchymal disease, to detect the crystals that are often present in patients with renal calculi, or to detect ova in a patient suspected of having bilharziasis. Urine cytology for malignant cells is a useful examination both in the diagnosis and in the follow-up of bladder (urothelial) cancers. For microbiological examination a fresh sample of urine must be collected in a sterile container. In order to avoid contamination by normal urethral flora, the patient is asked to pass some urine into the toilet; then, without interrupting the flow, the next part is directed into a special container, and the remainder into the toilet – hence the term *midstream specimen* of urine (MSU). If it is necessary to store the specimen, it should be kept at 4°C. To rule out possible contamination, fine-needle suprapubic aspiration of a full bladder may be required in difficult cases. The microbiologist cultures the urine on a suitable medium, and then determines the sensitivity of any organism identified to antimicrobial agents.

Blood

Blood creatinine provides an overall measure of renal function. However, creatinine does not begin to rise until the glomerular filtration rate (GFR) is halved. Creatinine clearance can be used to estimate GFR. Blood chemistry may also be examined to exclude a metabolic disorder (see below). Patients with chronic renal disease often have a normocytic, normochromic anaemia. The erythrocyte sedimentation rate (ESR) can be markedly raised in idiopathic retroperitoneal fibrosis, a cause of ureteric obstruction. Human chorionic gonadotrophin (HCG), α-fetoprotein (AFP) and prostate-specific antigen (PSA) are useful tumour markers

Intravenous urography (IVU)

A plain X-ray of the abdomen and pelvis is obtained to outline the kidneys, ureters and bladder (KUB film). The lumbar spine and pelvis, as well as stones in the region of the urinary tract, will be shown. An iodine-containing contrast material is then injected intravenously and serial X-rays are taken as the contrast is excreted (Fig. 29.2). The concentration of contrast is influenced by the urine flow, which in turn depends on the hydration state of the patient. Routine preparation for an IVU should include fluid restriction for 12 hours. As faeces within the large bowel will obscure the radiographic outline of the urinary tract, an aperient may be given on the day before the X-ray. An IVU demonstrates the renal pelvis and calyces and the rate of emptying from the kidneys. The calibre of the ureters is seen as contrast passes down to the bladder. Once the bladder has filled with contrast, the patient empties the bladder and a 'postmicturition' film is taken to show the efficiency of bladder emptying and to indicate the amount of residual urine. Delayed excretion of the contrast is a sign of obstruction somewhere in the urinary tract. Delayed films, taken up to 24 hours after contrast injection, may then give added detail of the affected kidney and ureter.

Ultrasonography

The quality of ultrasonography has improved so dramatically in recent years that it now rivals IVU as a means of first-line imaging (Fig. 29.3). It tends to give superior information about the renal parenchyma but less about the collecting system. It also allows visualization of other related organs, such as the liver, spleen and gynaecological organs.

Special radiological investigations

To define the ureter, pelvis and calyces more clearly, a retrograde ureteropyelogram may be necessary. This involves retrograde injection of contrast material through a catheter placed in the lower ureter (Fig. 29.4). A ureteroscope can also be used to directly examine the ureter. Abnormalities of the renal vessels can be demonstrated by renal angiography. CT is now the preferred method for imaging renal tumours (Fig. 29.5). A micturating cystourethrogram (MCU) is required to outline the bladder, detect ureterovesical reflux and examine the bladder neck and urethra. The bladder is filled with contrast material (via a catheter) and emptying is then studied by X-ray screening. An *ascending urethrogram*, in which contrast medium is injected into the urethra, can be used to define strictures, but is less useful than an MCU which provides a descending urethrogram.

Nuclear imaging

Radiolabelled substances are used for two main purposes:

1. Detection of metastases in bones. ^{99m}Tc-labelled methylene diphosphonate (MDP) is the most reliable marker for detecting metastases from carcinoma of the prostate.
2. Measurement of renal function. MAG3 is now used extensively as it is excreted by the proximal tubules

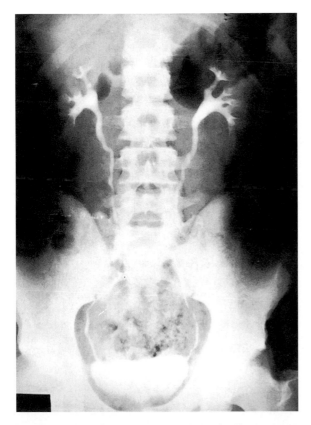

Fig. 29.2 Normal intravenous urogram (IVU).

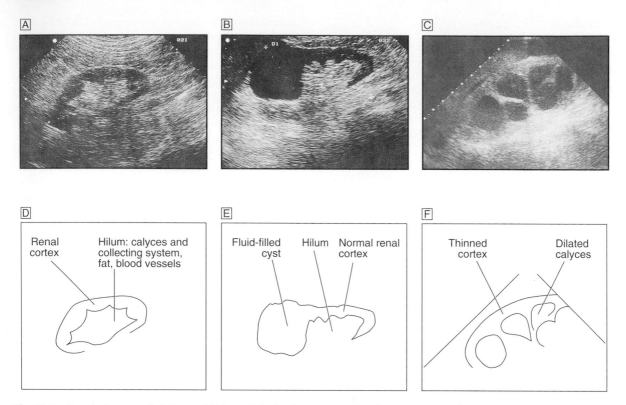

Fig. 29.3   Renal ultrasound. A Normal kidney. **B** A simple cyst occupies the upper pole of an otherwise normal kidney. **C** The renal pelvis and calyces are dilated by a chronic obstruction to urinary outflow. The thinness of the remaining renal cortex indicates chronicity. **D, E** and **F** The diagrams beneath show the anatomical features.

rather than by glomerular filtration. Diethylenetetramine penta-acetic acid (DTPA) is reserved for patients in whom there is renal failure. Dimercaptosuccinic acid (DMSA) is concentrated in the renal tubule. As only 5% is excreted, static imaging can be carried out some 2–3 hours after injection. Parenchymal defects such as scars, haematomas, lacerations or ischaemia may be demonstrated. Differential renal function can be quantified from measuring the DMSA concentration in each kidney.

Urodynamic studies

The maximum urinary flow rate during micturition can be measured using a flowmeter. The normal in males is 15–30 ml/s and in females 20–40 ml/s. It is important to measure flow rate when the voided volume is at least 150 ml, otherwise the values may be misleading and reflect bladder dysfunction rather than outflow obstruction. A flow rate of less than 6 ml/s is abnormal. The urinary stream may be so poor that quantification is unnecessary. However, in a proportion of patients with equivocal symptoms, the flow rate can help to determine the degree of obstruction (Fig. 29.6). Measurements of flow rate can be combined with cystometry to provide a measure of residual urine, bladder capacity, the capacity at which a desire to void occurs, and the detrusor pressures when the bladder is full and during maximum flow. Spontaneous detrusor contractions during bladder filling may indicate an unstable bladder, a cause of urgency and urge incontinence. Pressures along the urethra may also be measured (urethral pressure profile). These measurements are of particular value in distinguishing between bladder and urethral abnormalities in an incontinent patient. They also help to distinguish between neurological, pharmacological and mechanical causes of outflow tract symptoms.

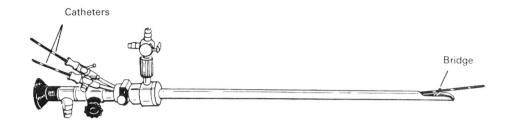

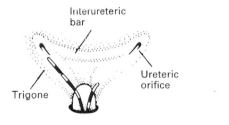

A

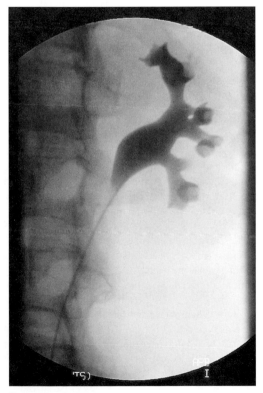

B

Fig. 29.4 Retrograde ureteropyelography. **A** Cystoscope and ureteric catheterization. **B** The best views of the normal collecting system are shown by pyelography. A catheter has been passed into the left renal pelvis at cystoscopy. The anemone-like calyces are sharp-edged and normal.

Semen analysis

Microscopic examination of the semen is a basic investigation in infertile males. The specimen is collected 3 days after the last ejaculation and is examined within 2 hours. Normal semen has a volume of 2–6 mL and a sperm concentration of $20–120 \times 10^6$/mL. More than 60% of the sperm should be motile at 2 hours. The morphology, biochemistry and viability of the sperm may also be studied. In selected cases immunological tests may help to determine the cause of infertility.

Biochemical screening for stones

All patients with urinary tract calculi should be screened for hyperparathyroidism, idiopathic hypercalciuria, hyperoxaluria and cystinuria. Serum calcium, phosphate, oxalate

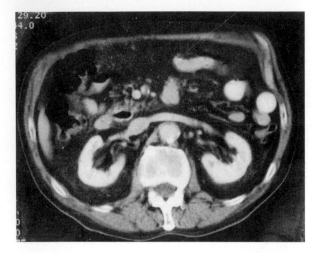

Fig. 29.5   Normal renal CT scan.

and uric acid are measured. More detailed investigation requires 24-hour collection of urine for determination of calcium, phosphate, oxalate and uric acid excretion. The composition of passed or removed stones should be analysed to determine their metabolic type.

UPPER URINARY TRACT (KIDNEY AND URETER)

Anatomy

The two kidneys lie retroperitoneally on the posterior abdominal wall. Each is approximately 12 cm long, 6 cm wide and 3 cm thick. The upper pole of the kidney lies on the diaphragm, which separates it from the pleura and the

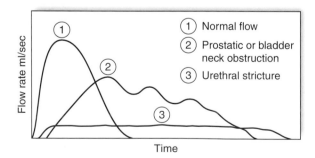

Fig. 29.6   Urinary flow rates. 1. Normal, rapid rise to maximum high peak flow. 2. Typical bladder outflow obstruction due to BPH. Slow rise to poor maximum flow rate, prolonged variable flow. 3. Typical urethral stricture, prolonged flow with little variability giving plateau or box-shaped curve.

> **SUMMARY BOX**
>
> *Urinary tract obstruction*
>
> Common causes of obstruction of the *lower* outflow tract are:
> - Benign prostatic hyperplasia
> - Prostatic cancer
> - Bladder cancer involving the bladder neck
> - Bladder-neck obstruction (dyssynergia, infection, neurological disorders)
> - Urethral obstruction (congenital posterior urethral valves, blocked urinary catheter, trauma, infection, stricture)
>
> Common causes of obstruction of the *upper* urinary tract are:
> - Renal and ureteric calculi (80% are calcium oxalate/phosphate stones)
> - Pelviureteric junction obstruction (idiopathic hydronephrosis)
> - Retroperitoneal fibrosis (idiopathic/malignant infiltration/radiotherapy)
> - Transitional cell carcinoma (with or without bleeding and clot)
> - Congenital abnormalities (e.g. ectopic ureter, ureterocele)
> - Infections (notably bilharziasis and tuberculosis)

11th and 12th ribs. Below this it lies on the psoas, quadratus lumborum and transversus abdominis muscles from medial to lateral (Fig. 29.7). Anteriorly, the right kidney is covered by the liver, the second part of the duodenum and the ascending colon. The spleen, stomach, tail of pancreas, left colon and small bowel overlie the left kidney. The renal hilum lies medially and transmits from front to back the renal vein, renal artery and renal pelvis. The ureter begins at the renal pelvis and runs for 25 cm to the bladder. The abdominal ureter lies on the medial edge of the psoas muscle, which separates it from the tips of the transverse processes. It then crosses the bifurcation of the common iliac artery, which separates it from the sacroiliac joint, to enter the pelvis. The pelvic ureter runs on the lateral pelvic wall to just in front of the ischial spine, when it then turns medially and forward to enter the bladder. In the male it is crossed by the vas deferens. In the female it lies close to the lateral fornix of the vagina and is crossed by the uterine vessels, where it is vulnerable to damage during hysterectomy. The section of ureter that lies within the bladder wall functions as a flap valve to prevent reflux. Stones tend to impact at the three points where the ureter narrows, namely, the pelviureteric junction, the pelvic brim and the ureteric orifice.

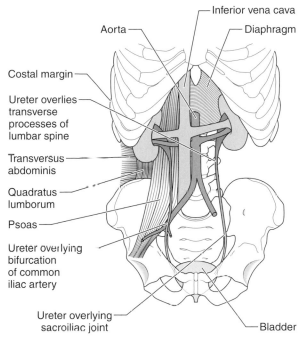

Fig. 29.7 Anatomy of kidneys and ureters.

Labels in figure:
- Aorta
- Inferior vena cava
- Diaphragm
- Costal margin
- Ureter overlies transverse processes of lumbar spine
- Transversus abdominis
- Quadratus lumborum
- Psoas
- Ureter overlying bifurcation of common iliac artery
- Ureter overlying sacroiliac joint
- Bladder

Physiology

The kidney produces on average 1 ml of urine per minute. This is transported down the ureter by four to five peristaltic waves per minute to reach the bladder, where it is stored without reflux up the ureters. For details of physiology of the nephron see *Davidson's principles and practice of Medicine* p. 418.

Trauma

Kidney and renal pedicle

Penetrating injuries Gunshot or stab wounds may injure the kidney and renal pedicle. Inadvertent damage during percutaneous access surgery or needle biopsy can cause severe bleeding and, rarely, an arteriovenous fistula. Open lacerations of the parenchyma, collecting system or pedicle are usually associated with other injuries within the abdomen.

Blunt injury This may be caused by a fall against a hard object or by a blow to the loin. These injuries are commonly associated with fractured ribs and occasionally damage to the spleen (left) or liver (right).

Deceleration injury Rapid deceleration, for example during a road traffic accident, tends to damage the renal pedicle rather than the parenchyma, often through the development of intimal tears, resulting in thrombosis of the major vessels.

Late effects These include perirenal collection of urine (urinoma), scarring of the kidney, or renal artery stenosis (hypertension). Hydronephrosis may be an early or a late complication.

Clinical features Whereas a gunshot wound is obvious, a penetrating knife wound may appear trivial even if it involves several important deep structures. Commonly, the patient presents with a history of injury to the loin followed by haematuria. Usually, the worse the haematuria the worse the renal damage. Thus, a bruise or contusion of the kidney causes mild haematuria, a laceration moderate haematuria, and a fragmented kidney causes gross haematuria. Severe injuries are characterized by a mass in the loin that is increasing in size, and signs of shock. These patients often have other serious injuries. Damage to the renal pedicle may cause few signs, or the patient may be severely shocked.

Investigation Urgent intravenous urography is indicated to determine the extent of renal damage. Urographic information about the other kidney must be obtained prior to emergency surgery. With mild contusion the urogram may be normal. With increasing damage there is distortion of the renal outline and calyces, and extravasation of contrast. A CT scan will more accurately determine the extent of the injury. Non-visualization of the kidney implies serious damage to the pedicle and is an indication for angiography. Angiography is also helpful in assessing parenchymal/ vascular damage in patients who are likely to need surgical exploration. Ultrasonography and isotope scanning are of more help in the follow-up of an injured kidney than in immediate care.

Treatment A shocked patient must be resuscitated. Renal contusion is managed conservatively by bed rest and observation. Lacerations that are part of an open injury are explored to determine the extent of the damage. Those due to closed injury may be treated conservatively at first, but should be explored if haematuria persists or loin swelling increases. Severe lacerations with fragmentation of the kidney must be explored if the patient is shocked. The extent of operation depends on the severity of the laceration. Whenever possible, partial rather than total nephrectomy is carried out.

Ureter

Mechanism of injury The ureter is occasionally damaged by a knife or a bullet, but always in association with other injuries. The principal cause of open injury to a ureter is inadvertent damage during an operation involving the colon, rectum, bladder, major abdominal blood vessels and, most commonly of all, the uterus. The proximity of the ureter to these organs means that it is frequently affected by direct spread of a variety of pathological conditions. Surgical damage may lead to complete or partial obstruction, with subsequent hydronephrosis, or to a urinary fistula. A fistula may occur immediately (if the damage is not recognized at operation) or later (if the injury to the ureter causes late necrosis). Urine may leak to the skin (cutaneous fistula), form a 'urinoma' or, after a gynaecological operation, leak through the vagina (ureterovaginal fistula). The ureter is occasionally damaged in major road traffic accidents and during endoscopic procedures to treat stones.

Clinical features The patient may complain of renal pain, but even a completely obstructed kidney may cause few symptoms. If there is infection in the obstructed kidney the patient may be extremely ill, with pain, fever and rigors. Any excessive 'watery' discharge from a wound is suspicious.

Investigation A rapid way to determine whether a watery discharge is urine or serum is to measure its concentration of urea. Alternatively, intravenous methylene blue quickly appears in a urinary leak. An IVU will show the site of the damage, and after ureteric injury there is always some hold-up in the contrast on the affected side. If there is still uncertainty as to whether a vaginal leak is from the ureter or bladder, discoloration of a vaginal swab after intravesical instillation of methylene blue will confirm that the leak is from the bladder. Occasionally, cystoscopy and ureteric catheterization are indicated.

Treatment A percutaneous nephrostomy tube should be placed to drain the kidney on the affected side. This should minimize further leakage from the distal ureter. It may now be possible to pass a stent up or down the ureter if there is only a partial injury; this may lead to complete recovery. If conservative management fails surgical exploration is required. Provided it has sufficient length, a damaged lower ureter can be reimplanted directly into the bladder. If the ureter is short, the gap may be bridged by a tube of bladder (Boari flap) (Fig. 29.8) or by drawing up the bladder and fixing it to the psoas muscle (psoas hitch). If the ureter is too short for these procedures, it may be joined to the other ureter (uretero-ureterostomy) or a segment of small bowel used to bridge the gap (ileal interposition).

Renal cysts

Simple cysts

These are usually single, almost always asymptomatic, and are often found incidentally on IVU or ultrasound. A cyst is easily differentiated from carcinoma by ultrasound. Malignant change in a cyst can occur but is very rare.

Polycystic kidney disease

This is an autosomal-dominant congenital anomaly that affects both kidneys and often leads to chronic renal failure in middle life. Despite their very large size the cystic kidneys cause few symptoms. Infection or bleeding into a cyst can occur and may require exploration to relieve symptoms. The condition may cause haematuria.

Benign tumours

Renal adenomas are small and usually an incidental finding. Haemangiomas are a rare cause of dramatic haematuria.

Nephroblastomas

Epidemiology

This tumour usually occurs in children under 4 years of age, and is the commonest childhood urological malignancy, with an incidence of 7 per million children per year. The tumour is probably derived from embryonic

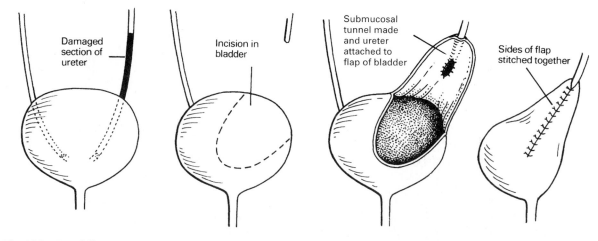

Fig. 29.8 Boari flap.

Damaged section of ureter

Incision in bladder

Submucosal tunnel made and ureter attached to flap of bladder

Sides of flap stitched together

mesodermal tissue, and microscopically has a mixed appearance of spindle cells, epithelial cells and muscle fibres. Growth is rapid and there is early local spread, including invasion of the renal vein. Invasion of the renal pelvis occurs late, and so haematuria is seen in only 15% of cases. Distant metastases most commonly appear in the lungs, liver and bones. Tumours presenting in the first year of life have a better prognosis.

Clinical features

The cardinal sign is a large abdominal mass. Some of the unusual clinical features associated with a renal carcinoma in adults, such as fever or hypertension, may be present.

Investigation

A CT scan of the abdomen and chest is essential for diagnosis and staging. The main differential diagnosis is from neuroblastoma affecting the adrenal, but other causes of a large kidney, such as hydronephrosis and cystic disease, must also be considered. The tumour is bilateral in 5–10% of cases.

Treatment

Transabdominal nephrectomy with wide excision of the mass is carried out after preliminary ligation of the renal pedicle. This is followed by chemotherapy using actinomycin D and vincristine. Radiotherapy is reserved for residual disease. In some centres, pre-operative radiotherapy is used to downsize the tumour prior to resection. As a result of this treatment, the 5-year survival rate has improved from 10% to 80%.

Renal adenocarcinoma

Epidemiology

This is the commonest malignant tumour of the kidney. The incidence is 16 cases per 100 000 and it is twice as common in males. It is uncommon before the age of 40 years and has a peak incidence between 65 and 75 years of age. The tumour arises from renal tubules. Haemorrhage and necrosis give a characteristic mixed golden-yellow and red appearance to the cut surface. Microscopically there are clear and granular cell types; the former are more common. There is early spread into the renal pelvis, causing haematuria. Invasion of the renal vein, often extending into the inferior vena cava, also occurs early. Direct spread into perinephric tissues is common, so that the whole fascial envelope and kidney should be removed *en bloc*. Lymphatic spread occurs to para-aortic nodes, but bloodborne metas-

tases (which may be solitary) may develop almost anywhere in the body.

Clinical features

The triad of pain, haematuria and a mass is an important but late feature, occurring only in 15% of cases; 60% present with haematuria, 40% with loin pain and only 25% with a mass. A remarkable range of systemic effects may occur early on. These include fever, a raised ESR, polycythaemia, disorders of coagulation, and abnormalities of plasma proteins and liver function tests. The patient may present with pyrexia of unknown origin (PUO) or, rarely, with neuromyopathy. Systemic effects may be due to tumour secretion of products such as renin, erythropoietin, parathormone and gonadotrophins. The effects disappear when the tumour is removed but may reappear when metastases develop, and so can be used as markers of tumour activity.

Investigation

The initial investigation is ultrasound. Thereafter, a contrast CT scan of the abdomen and chest should be performed for staging (Fig. 29.9).

Treatment

Radical nephrectomy, including the perirenal fascial envelope and ipsilateral para-aortic lymph nodes, is performed whenever possible. Renal adenocarcinoma is resistant to

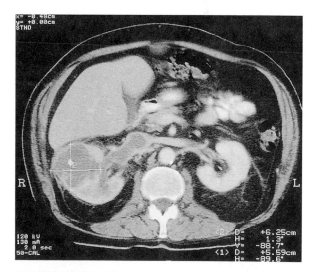

Fig. 29.9 Contrast-enhanced CT scan of renal cancer. The right kidney is expanded by a low-density cancer which fails to take up the contrast. Tumour is seen extending into the renal vein and IVC (arrow).

radiotherapy and chemotherapy, but some benefit has been seen with immunotherapy using interferon and interleukin-2. Because of the unusual features associated with renal carcinomas, nephrectomy should always be considered. Not only may systemic effects disappear, but also there may even be regression of a solitary metastasis. Solitary metastases tend to remain single for long periods and excision is often worthwhile.

SUMMARY BOX

Renal carcinoma

- Renal carcinoma is much the commonest malignant renal tumour and is twice as common in males.

- The carcinoma arises in the renal tubules and spreads early to the renal pelvis, producing haematuria. Later spread involves the renal vein (with bloodstream dissemination), perinephric invasion and lymphatic spread.

- The clinical presentation is very varied. The triad of pain, haematuria and a mass may be late features, and early systemic effects include fever, polycythaemia, disordered coagulation and PUO.

- The key investigations are ultrasonography, chest X-ray and contrast CT scanning.

- Treatment consists of radical nephrectomy; the tumour is not radiosensitive. The natural history of renal carcinoma is very variable and excision of solitary metastases may be worthwhile.

Transitional cell carcinoma of the upper tracts

Transitional cell carcinoma (TCC) arises from the urothelium that lines the whole of the urinary tract from collecting system to urethra. They are common in the bladder (see below) but uncommon in the upper tracts. They tend to present with haematuria and/or obstruction of the upper tract. They are diagnosed on IVU. Treatment is by nephroureterectomy and regular surveillance of the bladder. If the tumour is solitary and low grade it may be treated endoscopically; however, surveillance remains problematic.

Renal and ureteric calculi

Types of stone

Stones that form in the kidney are of two main types, infective and metabolic. An infective stone is whitish and chalky and crumbles or breaks easily. It is composed mainly of calcium, ammonia and magnesium phosphates. Such stones

develop wherever drainage is impaired, and are usually associated with an anatomical abnormality such as a diverticulum or with long-term recumbency or paraplegia. Their formation indicates an established infection that cannot be eradicated by antibiotics alone. As the stone enlarges drainage is further impaired and there is progressive damage to the kidney. A metabolic stone, commonly of calcium oxalate, is usually hard and dark with an irregular sharp surface. It develops as a result of an abnormality of the composition of the urine. There may be abnormal concentration of normal constituents (e.g. due to dehydration); excess excretion of normal constituents (e.g. calcium in hyperparathyroidism, or uric acid in gout); or the urine may contain abnormal constituents (as in cystinuria). It is likely that several aetiological factors must occur together or in sequence for a stone to form. As indicated above, all patients with recurrent urinary calculi should be screened for metabolic abnormalities. Up to 80% of the stones seen in the UK are mixed calcium oxalate/phosphate stones. Some 10% are magnesium ammonium phosphate stones with a variable proportion of calcium. Most of the remainder are uric acid stones. Cystine and xanthine stones are rare.

Clinical features

Renal pain, renal colic or ureteric colic are characteristically unilateral. Renal pain is dull and aching, whereas ureteric colic is acute and severe and occurs in waves that pass down the line of the ureter. A stone may cause bleeding or there may be symptoms of urinary tract infection. However, a stone in the kidney may remain silent, even one large enough to fill the pelvis and calyces (a 'staghorn' calculus).

Investigation

An IVU usually provides all the necessary information on the position of the stone (Fig. 29.10). Routine haematological and biochemical tests are needed to assess renal function and to exclude metabolic causes of stones. A urine sample is cultured to determine whether there is infection. If obstruction is acute, its relief is the prime clinical need; if it is chronic and has caused renal damage, the surgical approach depends on the function of the affected kidney. This is best determined by radioisotope methods.

Treatment

Symptomatic treatment should be instituted as soon as the diagnosis is confirmed. Intramuscular diclofenac, a non-steroidal anti-inflammatory, is the most effective analgesic; pethidine is an alternative. The likelihood of spontaneous passage depends on the size of the stone and on its

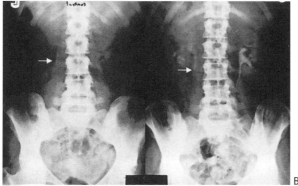

Fig. 29.10 IVU showing ureteric stone. **A** Eighty per cent of stones are visible on a plain X-ray (arrow). **B** The contrast excreted by the kidney in an IVU clearly shows the obstruction caused by the stone in the ureter (arrow).

smoothness. A stone less than 0.5 cm in diameter should pass down the ureter. If it becomes fixed (causing increasing hydroureter and hydronephrosis), if the urine is infected or the patient has increasing pain and fever, treatment is necessary. Extracorporeal shockwave lithotripsy (ESWL), the technique of focusing external shock waves to break up stones, has revolutionized the treatment of renal and ureteric stones (Fig. 29.11). If a stone can be visualized on X-ray or ultrasound then it can be treated by ESWL. Other stones can be visualized directly by passing a fine telescope up the ureter (ureteroscope) and the stones either broken up or removed intact. Some stones in the kidney that are unlikely to pass even if broken up are best treated by direct puncture of the kidney, insertion of a sheath and removal under vision with a nephroscope (percutaneous nephrolithotomy, PCNL). Stones within a kidney can be the cause of renal destruction, especially if

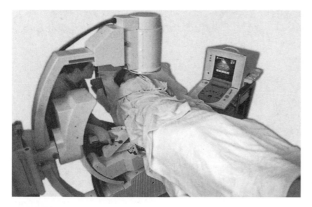

Fig. 29.11 Extracorporeal shockwave lithotripter.

Table 29.1 Causes of urinary tract obstruction

Extrinsic
Retroperitoneal fibrosis
External pressure (e.g. carcinoma of the cervix, prostate)

Intrinsic
Transitional cell tumours
Tuberculosis/bilharziasis
Ureterocele
Ectopic ureter

Intraluminal
Calculi

the urine is infected. If the damage is severe so that the kidney contributes less than 10% of total renal function, then a nephrectomy is recommended. It is now very rare to need to remove stones from the renal tract at open operation.

Upper tract obstruction

The upper urinary tract includes the pelvicaliceal system and ureters. As with any tubular structure, obstruction may be due to extrinsic, intrinsic or intraluminal causes (Table 29.1). In the kidney, stones within the pelvicaliceal system and a congenital abnormality of the pelviureteric junction (PUJ) (see below) are the main causes of obstruction leading to hydronephrosis. More rarely, a sloughed renal papilla, blood clot or a tumour may be the cause. During pregnancy there is a physiological dilatation of the ureters due to progesterone, which reduces smooth muscle tone.

Pelviureteric junction obstruction (idiopathic hydronephrosis)

Narrowing of the junction between the renal pelvis and the ureter is a common cause of hydronephrosis. As the aetiology is obscure, the term 'idiopathic' hydronephrosis is appropriate. Electron microscopy shows normal muscle cells with normal innervation, but the muscle bundles are separated by an excess of collagen fibres which may prevent relaxation of the segment.

Pelviureteric junction obstruction This condition is seen in very young children. It is likely to be congenital and is often bilateral, but gross hydronephrosis may present at any age.

Clinical features

Idiopathic hydronephrosis may produce a large painless mass in the loin; in its grossest form the volume of urine in the hydronephrotic sac may simulate free fluid in the peritoneal cavity. The more usual moderate hydronephrosis causes ill-defined renal pain or ache that may be exacerbated by drinking large volumes of liquid. The patient may regard these symptoms as 'indigestion'. Rarely, there may be no symptoms.

Investigation

An IVU, with or without delayed films, provides sufficient information in many cases. The calibre of the ureter is normal. There are a few patients in whom there is doubt as to whether the dilatation of the pelvis and calyces is truly obstructive in nature. Methods to resolve this include urography and renography during induced diuresis, and antegrade pressure–flow measurements.

Treatment

Operation (pyeloplasty) is designed to remove the obstructing tissue and refashion the pelviureteric junction (PUJ) so that the lower part of the renal pelvis drains freely into the ureter (Fig. 29.12). Occasionally, an aberrant vessel to the lower pole of the kidney crosses the PUJ and gives the appearance of having caused the obstruction (though this is unlikely); in this situation, the PUJ is reconstructed in front of the vessels. Endoscopic alternatives to pyeloplasty have been developed and give as good results in most cases.

Outcome

It is not possible to predict the degree of recovery of renal function after the relief of obstruction, but it is generally felt that a kidney contributing less than 10% of total renal function should be removed.

Retroperitoneal fibrosis

Pathology

Fibrosis of the retroperitoneal connective tissues may encircle and compress the ureter(s), causing hydroureter and hydronephrosis. Fibrosis occurs in three groups of conditions:

- *Idiopathic* In this, the largest group, the fibrosis extends across the pelvic brim to involve the ureters, the vena cava and even the aorta. The aetiology is unknown, although it may be associated with methysergide or analgesic abuse. Mediastinal fibrosis and Dupuytren's contracture may coexist.
- *Malignant infiltration* The fibrosis contains malignant cells that have metastasized from primary sites such as the breast, stomach, pancreas and colon.
- *Reactive fibrosis* Radiotherapy to the pelvic organs, resolving blood clot after major vascular or other surgical procedures, or extravasation of sclerosants (e.g. phenol for a nerve block) can lead to fibrotic change in the retroperitoneum.

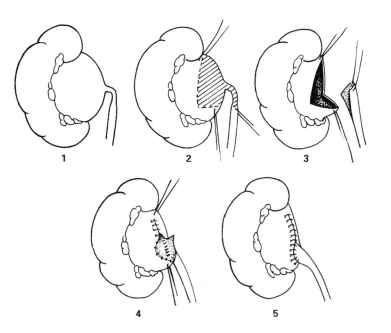

Fig. 29.12 Anderson-Hynes pyeloplasty.

As the gross appearance of fibrosis in all three groups may be similar, biopsy of the tissue is essential for diagnosis.

Clinical features

Ureteric obstruction may cause symptoms similar to idiopathic hydronephrosis, namely, ill-defined renal pain or ache. Some patients complain of low backache.

Investigation

An IVU shows hydronephrosis and usually hydroureter down to the level of the obstruction. The anatomy of the ureter is often difficult to define, but it is usually pulled medially. It is rarely necessary to pass a ureteric catheter up to the kidney, although it is characteristic of retroperitoneal fibrosis that a ureteric catheter will pass easily through what appears to be a severe obstruction. A markedly raised ESR is found in more than 50% of cases with idiopathic fibrosis.

Treatment

Relief of obstruction may be difficult. The ureter is dissected out of the fibrous sheet of tissue (ureterolysis) and wrapped in omentum to prevent further involvement. Although obstruction may regress with steroids, these agents are reserved for recurrent obstruction.

Miscellaneous causes of obstruction

Congenital abnormalities

A ureterocele develops behind a pinhole ureteric orifice. The intramural part of the ureter then undergoes dilatation, bulges into the bladder, and can become very large. Incision of the pinhole opening relieves the obstruction. An ectopic ureter occurs with congenital duplication of one or both kidneys (duplex kidneys). Developmentally, the ureter has two main branches and, if this arrangement persists, the two ureters of the duplex kidneys may drain separately into the bladder (Fig. 29.13). One ureter enters normally on the trigone, and the ectopic ureter (from the upper renal moiety) enters the bladder or, more rarely, the vagina or seminal vesicle. A ureter that is ectopic and drains into the bladder is liable to have an ineffective valve mechanism, so that urine passes *up* the ureter on voiding (vesicoureteric reflux). Reflux can occur in normally sited ureters if the normal intramural ureter fails to act as a valve. The pressure of refluxing urine behaves as an intermittent obstruction which in children may lead to serious renal damage. Vesico ureteric reflux is treated by reimplantation of the ureter with the formation of an effective valve, or by a subureteric injection of inert material to endoscopically recreate a flap valve. In primary obstructive megaureter

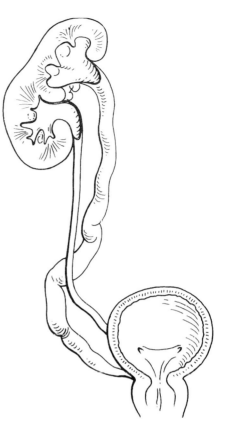

Fig. 29.13   Duplex kidney.

there is dilatation of the ureter in all but its terminal segment, without obvious cause and without vesicoureteric reflux. There are normally no ganglionic cells in the ureter, so that megaureter cannot be due to neuromuscular incoordination. Radiographic and pressure–flow studies may be needed to determine whether there is obstruction to urine flow. Narrowing of the ureter and reimplantation may be necessary.

Urinary tract infections (UTIs) are common in children. All microbiologically proven UTIs in boys and recurrent proven UTIs in girls should be investigated for evidence of underlying structural urinary tract abnormalities including vesicoureteric reflux (VUR), pelviureteric junction obstruction causing hydronephrosis and ureterocele causing vesicoureteric junction obstruction. Initial imaging investigations should include a urinary tract ultrasound scan and a DMSA radioisotope study. Where reflux is suspected on the basis of these two initial investigations, a micturating cystogram or a DTPA reflux study (in toilet-trained children) should be undertaken. VUR is graded from I (mild reflux into lower ureter) to V (severe reflux with dilatation of the ureter, renal pelvis and calyces). The milder grades (I and II) of reflux are managed with prophylactic antibiotics to prevent renal injury and scarring. More severe grades require a surgical procedure to abolish or reduce the grade of reflux. Cystoscopic sub-ureteric injection of an inert material or formal reimplantation of the ureter are the operative procedures of choice.

Infections

Tuberculosis of the urinary tract is a rare cause of stricture of the ureter and even complete obstruction. This process may be silent and 'autonephrectomy' may be detected at a later date. Bilharziasis affecting the urinary tract is common in parts of Africa and the Middle East. Ureteric fibrosis and obstruction are part of the process that can affect the whole of the urinary tract. Many patients present in such an advanced state of the disease that surgical treatment is not feasible. Both infections require specific drug treatment. When the ureters are involved and obstructed, a variety of reconstructive surgical procedures may be used to conserve renal function and correct obstruction and/or reflux.

SUMMARY BOX

Micturition

- Micturition requires para-sympathetic (S2–S4) innervation of the detrusor, sympathetic innervation (T10–L2) of the bladder neck and proximal urethra, and somatic innervation (S2–S4) of the bladder, pelvic floor and urethra.

- Structural causes of disordered micturition in the male include prostatic enlargement, prostatectomy (dribble, stress and urge incontinence) and chronic illness/debility.

- Structural causes of disordered micturition in the female include childbirth, surgery, radiotherapy and cystitis (infection, chronic interstitial cystitis and urethral syndrome).

- Neurogenic causes of disordered micturition are:
  - Impaired cortical control
  - Alcohol abuse and drugs
  - Spinal cord damage (at/below T12–L1 – flaccid bladder with overflow; above T12–L1 – reflex bladder with reduced cortical control which fails to empty completely)
  - Pelvic nerve damage (surgery, diabetic autonomic neuropathy)
  - Atonic myogenic bladder (prolonged outlet obstruction).

LOWER URINARY TRACT (BLADDER, PROSTATE AND URETHRA)

Anatomy

The bladder is a muscular reservoir that receives urine via the ureters and expels it via the urethra. In children up to 4 years it lies predominately in the abdomen, in the adult it is a pelvic organ, well protected in the bony pelvis. Superiorly the bladder is covered with peritoneum, which separates it from coils of small bowel and the sigmoid colon and, in the female, the body of the uterus. Posteriorly lie the rectum, the vas deferens and seminal vesicles in the male, and the vagina and supravaginal cervix in the female. Inferiorly the neck of the bladder transmits the urethra and fuses with the prostate in the male and with the pelvic fascia in the female. The bladder is composed of whorls of detrusor muscle, which in the male become circular at the bladder neck. They are richly supplied with sympathetic nerves that cause contraction during ejaculation, thereby preventing semen from entering the bladder (retrograde ejaculation). There is no such sphincter in the female. The bladder is lined with specialized waterproof epithelium, the urothelium. This is thrown into folds over most of the bladder, except the trigone where it is smooth. The male urethra is 20 cm long, the prostatic urethra descends for 3 cm though the prostate gland, and the membranous urethra is 1–2 cm long and intimately associated with the main urethral sphincter, the rhabdosphincter. The spongy urethra is 15 cm long and is surrounded by the corpus spongiosus throughout its complete length, opening on the tip of the glans penis as the external meatus. The spongy urethra is further subdivided into the proximal bulbar urethra and the distal penile urethra. The female urethra is 3–4 cm long, descends through the pelvic floor surrounded by the urethral sphincter and embedded in the anterior vaginal wall to open between the clitoris and the vagina. In the male the prostate is pyramidal, with its base uppermost. It resembles the size and shape of a chestnut and surrounds the prostatic urethra. Traditionally described as having a median and two lateral lobes, it is better considered as being composed of a small central and a larger peripheral zone (Fig. 29.14).

Physiology

Neurological control of micturition

Parasympathetic fibres arising as preganglionic axons from S2 to S4 relay through ganglia, mostly within the detrusor muscle. Postganglionic nerves supply the detrusor muscle. These (cholinergic) nerves stimulate detrusor contraction.

Sympathetic nerves arise from T10 to L2 and relay in the pelvic ganglia. Their exact role in the control of micturition

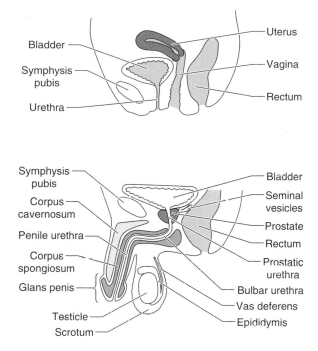

Fig. 29.14 Anatomy of the male and female lower urinary tracts.

is unclear. It is known that α-adrenergic receptors and their nerve terminals are found mainly in the smooth muscle of the bladder neck and proximal urethra, whereas β-receptors are found in the fundus of the bladder. The α-receptors respond to noradrenaline by stimulating contraction, whereas the β-receptors relax the smooth muscle. It is possible that the sympathetic neurons play a role in both urethral closure and detrusor relaxation during the filling phase of the micturition cycle.

The distal sphincter mechanism is innervated from the sacral segments S2–S4 by somatic motor fibres that reach the sphincter either by the pelvic plexus or via the pudendal nerves. Afferent nerves are carried in both the parasympathetic and pudendal pathways and transmit sensory impulses from the bladder, urethra and pelvic floor. These sensory impulses pass to the cerebral cortex and the micturition centre, where they produce reflex bladder relaxation and increased tone in the distal sphincter, so helping maintain continence. Cortical control is a basic part of the micturition cycle described below. The higher centres suppress detrusor contractions and their main function is to inhibit micturition until an appropriate time. Afferent impulses pass to the brain via the posterior columns. The higher centres are situated in the pons, the periaqueductal grey, the anterior cingulate gyrus and the preoptic area of the hypothalamus.

The micturition cycle

The micturition cycle has two phases.

Storage (or filling) phase Because of the high compliance (elasticity) of the detrusor muscle the bladder fills steadily without a rise in intravesical pressure. As the volume of urine increases stretch receptors in the bladder wall are stimulated resulting in reflex bladder relaxation and reflex increased sphincter tone. At approximately three-quarters of bladder capacity, sensation produces a desire to void. Voluntary control is now exerted over the desire to void, which temporarily disappears. Compliance of the detrusor allows further increase in capacity until the next desire to void. Just how often this desire needs to be inhibited depends on many factors, not the least of which is finding a suitable place in which to void.

Emptying (or micturition) phase The act of micturition is initiated first by voluntary and then by reflex relaxation of the pelvic floor and distal sphincter mechanisms, followed by reflex detrusor contraction. These actions are coordinated by the pontine micturition centre in the pons. Intravesical pressure remains greater than urethral pressure until the bladder is empty.

The normal control of micturition requires coordinated reflex activity of autonomic and somatic nerves, as described above. These responses depend on normal anatomical structures and normal innervation. There are thus two main types of disorders of micturition: structural and neurogenic. Examples are extensive carcinoma of the prostate that has damaged the sphincter mechanism (structural), and spinal cord injury that has damaged the innervation (neurogenic).

Trauma

Bladder

Open injuries The bladder may rupture as a result of a penetrating injury to the lower abdomen, in which case the bladder, urethra and rectum are all likely to be damaged. The bladder may also be injured in the course of extensive cancer surgery in the pelvis. Occasionally, a large inguinal or femoral hernia may include the bladder in the medial wall of the sac and it may be damaged during repair of the hernia. Unrecognized damage during surgical procedures may lead to a wound fistula, a vesicovaginal fistula or a vesicocolic fistula.

Closed injuries Intraperitoneal rupture typically occurs in a patient who has been drinking alcohol, has a full bladder and is assaulted and kicked in the abdomen. The dome of the bladder ruptures and urine extravasates into the peritoneum (Fig. 29.15A), causing intestinal ileus and abdominal distension.

Extraperitoneal rupture is usually due to a major road traffic accident in which the pelvis has also been fractured when the bladder is not full (Fig. 29.15), but may follow endoscopic resection of the prostate or a bladder tumour.

Clinical features The ileus and distension that occur with intraperitoneal rupture of the bladder are often detected late because of the circumstances surrounding the injury. However, the patient will soon note that he is not passing urine and seek advice. Extraperitoneal extravasation of urine, if part of a major accident, adds to what already are severe pelvic injuries. When the leak occurs during an endoscopic procedure, the patient later complains of suprapubic pain with varying degrees of lower abdominal tenderness.

Investigation Generally, the circumstances of the bladder injury establish the diagnosis. If confirmation of injury is required, water-soluble contrast is injected via a urethral catheter and the bladder examined on the X-ray screen (cystogram).

Treatment Intraperitoneal rupture demands laparotomy. The bladder rupture is oversewn, the viscera are examined for other injuries, and drainage by a suprapubic catheter is established. Extraperitoneal rupture of the bladder may require surgical exploration to remove blood and serum, correct bony injuries, close the tear and establish bladder drainage. However, if a small extraperitoneal rupture is recognized during any pelvic operation, a urethral catheter to keep the bladder empty is usually all that is needed. Very rarely a suprapubic drain is required.

Urethra

Open injuries Penetrating injuries resulting in damage to the anterior or posterior urethra are rare.

Closed injuries Damage to the anterior urethra is typically due to falling astride a hard object, although a kick can cause a similar injury. There may be contusion or lacer-

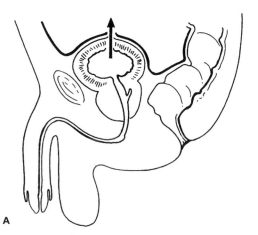
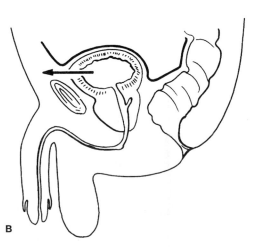

Fig. 29.15   Rupture of the bladder: **A** intraperitoneal; **B** extraperitoneal.

ation, and a laceration may be partial or complete. The mechanism of injury to the posterior urethra is similar to that of extraperitoneal rupture of the bladder, for example a road traffic accident. For such an injury to damage the urethra, a fracture of the pubis or fracture-dislocation of the pelvis must occur. Both the posterior urethra and bladder are damaged in 10% of cases. The urethral rupture may be partial or complete.

Injury to the posterior urethra may also be iatrogenic. Inexpert instrumentation can tear the mucosa and cause a false passage, with subsequent stricture formation.

Clinical features Anterior urethral injuries are usually located at the bulb, so that the patient presents with a perineal haematoma. If this becomes infected, there may be sloughing of the skin, urethra, and even the scrotal tissues. Because of the mechanism of injury, patients with posterior urethral tears are usually shocked and require resuscitation before a detailed assessment can be made. If the patient has passed clear urine, the bladder and urethra are probably intact. If there is blood at the external meatus, urethral injury must be suspected. A distended bladder can occur because of spasm of the urethral sphincter or because of a torn posterior urethra.

Investigation If the physical signs suggest an anterior urethral injury and the patient has passed clear urine, no further steps need be taken. If there is blood at the external meatus or the urine is bloodstained, a urethrogram using water-soluble contrast material may demonstrate the extravasation (Fig. 29.16). Any investigative procedure of the posterior urethra is potentially dangerous and may worsen the injury. A catheter should never be passed in the emergency room 'just to see'. If the patient passes clear urine, nothing further should be done. If the urine is blood-stained, retrograde urethrography may be carried out. The radiological distinction between a rupture of the membranous urethra and an extraperitoneal bladder rupture may be difficult.

Treatment All patients with an injury to the bulb of the urethra have a perineal haematoma. If the injury is only a contusion this will resolve, but prophylactic antibiotics are indicated. A large haematoma may need to be drained if the urethra has been lacerated. The extent of injury should be defined and the urethra repaired if possible. A urethral or suprapubic catheter drains the bladder. Treatment of a posterior urethral injury depends on the expertise available. It is quite acceptable to perform a suprapubic cystostomy and deal with the injury to the urethra at a later date. If laparotomy is necessary for other reasons, this may give an opportunity to pass a catheter. If the rupture is incomplete, the catheter will act as a splint. If the rupture is complete the ends of the urethra can be approximated and splinted by the catheter. The late complication of these injuries is stricture and impotence.

Bladder tumours

Pathology

The vast majority of bladder tumours arise from the urothelium or transitional cell lining, which it shares in continuum with the renal pelvis and the proximal urethra. The urothelium is exposed to chemical carcinogens excreted in the urine, such as naphthylamines and benzidine, which were extensively used in the chemical and dyes industries until their carcinogenic properties were recognized. The bladder is more susceptible to urinary carcinogens as urine is stored in the bladder for relatively long periods of time.

Almost all tumours are transitional cell carcinomas. Squamous carcinoma may occur in urothelium that has undergone metaplasia, usually due to chronic inflammation or irritation due to a stone or bilharziasis. An adenocarcinoma is a rarity but may occur in a urachal remnant in the dome of the bladder, or from local infiltration, e.g. bowel cancer. The incidence of transitional cell carcinoma in the bladder is 45 cases per 100 000, and it is three times more common in men than women. The appearance of a transitional cell tumour ranges from a delicate papillary structure to a solid ulcerating mass. The appearance correlates well with subsequent behaviour, in that papillary tumours are relatively benign cancers, whereas those that ulcerate are much more aggressive.

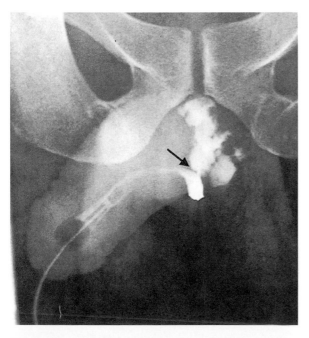

Fig. 29.16 Ascending ureterogram in urethral rupture. Contrast is seen extravasating at the site of the disrupted urethra.

Staging

A biopsy is essential to confirm the diagnosis and to determine the degree of cell differentiation (i.e. the grade) and the depth to which the tumour has penetrated the bladder wall (i.e the stage). The TNM system of tumour classification is also applicable to bladder tumours. Assessment of the primary tumour (T) is of prime clinical importance and requires bimanual examination under anaesthesia to judge the degree of penetration through the bladder wall. This is especially important for T2 and T3 tumours (Fig. 29.17). Clinical examination, urography and CT are used to assess the involvement of regional and juxtaregional lymph nodes (N). Assessment of distant metastases (M) requires clinical examination and radiography. Histopathological examination allows a much more accurate assessment of the tumour and guides the choice of treatment. Biopsy gives accurate information on superficial tumours, but invasive tumours cannot be assessed precisely without examining the full thickness of the bladder wall.

Clinical features

More than 80% of patients have haematuria, which is usually painless (Fig. 29.18). It should be assumed that such bleeding is from a tumour until proved otherwise. In women, symptoms of cystitis are so common that occasional bleeding may be thought to be part of an infective problem. In men, symptoms of bladder outflow obstruction are common and may include bleeding. Bleeding at the end of micturition, and especially the passage of pink/red urine, suggests that the bladder is the site of bleeding. Uniformly dark-coloured urine suggests that the source is in the upper tract. A tumour at the lower end of a ureter or a bladder tumour involving the ureteric orifice may cause obstructive

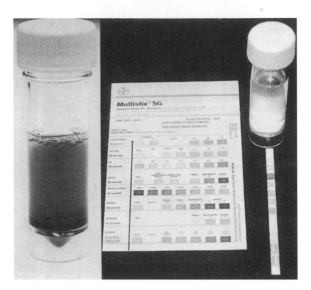

Fig. 29.18 Macroscopic (frank) and microscopic haematuria. The presence of microscopic amounts of blood in the urine is now more commonly detected by dipstick testing than by microscopy.

symptoms, but there are often few symptoms apart from discolouration of the urine. Examination is usually unhelpful. Rectal examination detects only advanced tumours.

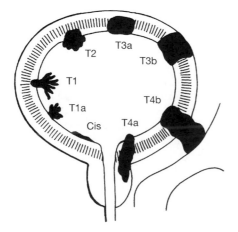

Fig. 29.17 T categories of bladder tumour. Cis = carcinoma-in-situ.

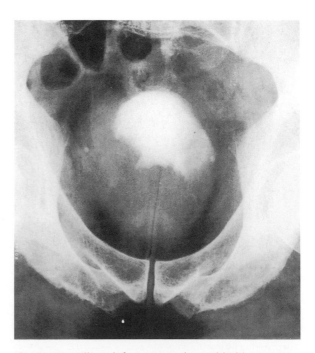

Fig. 29.19 Filling defect on IVU due to bladder tumour.

Investigation

Because upper tract tumours are much less common, they may be overlooked in the presence of an obvious bladder tumour. Both may occur together, and the whole of the urothelium must be examined on the IVU (Fig. 29.19). If there is any suspicious filling defect in the ureter, a retro-grade ureteropyelogram is necessary. Cystourethroscopy and examination under anaesthesia are the basic investigations for all suspected bladder tumours (Fig. 29.20). With the patient relaxed under general anaesthesia, the bladder and tumour are examined bimanually to determine the depth of spread. The physical features of the tumour(s) are noted, the normal bladder mucosa is inspected and the tumour is fully resected if possible. If not, biopsies are taken from the tumour and any other suspicious areas.

Treatment

Superficial bladder tumours (Ta, T1) Small superficial tumours can be treated by endoscopic diathermy alone, but whenever possible a biopsy followed by formal transurethral resection of the tumour (TURT) is recommended. Larger, even multiple, superficial tumours can also be treated effectively by TURT. Intravesical chemotherapy (epirubicin, mitomycin C) is useful to treat multiple low-grade bladder tumours and to reduce the recurrence rate. Regular check cystoscopies are required; recurrences are treated either by extensive diathermy or by cystectomy. Carcinoma in situ (Cis) may be present in normal-appearing mucosa or in association with a proliferative tumour. Cis can also exist as a separate entity, when there may be only a generalized redness (malignant cystitis). Untreated patients with Cis have a high risk of progression to invasive cancer. The tumour responds well to intravesical Bacille Calmette–

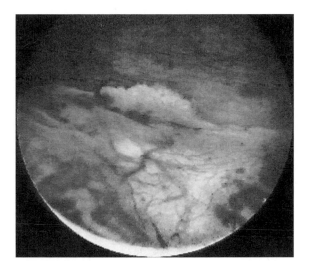

Fig. 29.20 Typical endoscopic appearance of papillary bladder tumour.

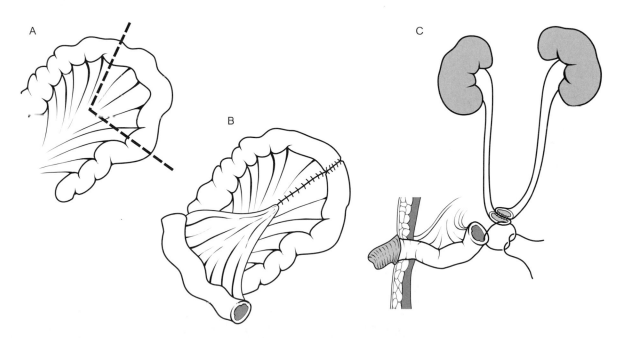

Fig. 29.21 Ileal conduit urinary diversion. **A** and **B** Isolation of segment of terminal ileum; **C** fashioning of ureteroileal anastomosis. The stoma is made to protrude from the skin to minimize skin contact with urine and so reduce irritation.

Guérin (BCG) treatment. However, if there is any doubt about the response, and especially if there is any pathological evidence of progression, more aggressive treatment is warranted.

Invasive bladder tumours The management of invasive (T2–T3) tumours is controversial. For patients under 70 years of age radical cystectomy is recommended, the morbidity and mortality associated with such a radical procedure suggests that in older patients radiotherapy may be a better option. Unfortunately this may not always cure the tumour, and 'salvage' cystectomy may be needed for recurrence or for symptoms such as intractable bleeding. Cystectomy always necessitates urinary diversion. In favourable cases, where the urethra can be retained, it may be possible to construct a new bladder from colon or small bowel (orthotopic bladder replacement). In such cases the patient may retain normal continence. Alternatively a continent urinary diversion can be constructed. The urine is collected in an internal reservoir which is connected to the body surface via a continent conduit (ileum or appendix), through which the patient drains the urine at regular intervals with a catheter. In less favourable circumstances an ileal conduit should be performed. The principle here is to implant the ureters into a short segment of ileum, which then opens on to the abdominal wall as a urinary stoma (Fig. 29.21). In some countries where an 'ostomy' is not acceptable, the ureters can be implanted into the sigmoid colon (ureterosigmoidostomy). However, renal infection and metabolic disturbances are potentially serious complications of this procedure. An invasive T4 tumour, fixed to the pelvis or surrounding organs, is inoperable and only palliative treatment can be given. The place of adjuvant chemotherapy is not yet established.

Both cisplatin and methotrexate have an effect on transitional cell cancer, but response rates in the treatment of metastatic disease are modest (about 20%).

Prognosis

The prognosis of bladder tumours depends on tumour stage and grade. The 5-year survival rate varies, from 20 to 30% in those with deep muscle invasion, to 50–60% in those with mucosal tumours. Overall, about one-third of patients survive for 5 years.

Carcinoma of the prostate
Epidemiology

In the UK this is the third most common malignancy in males, with an incidence of 50 cases per 100 000 population, and is increasing in frequency. It is the second commonest cause of cancer death in men in the UK. The tumour is common in northern Europe and the USA (particularly in the

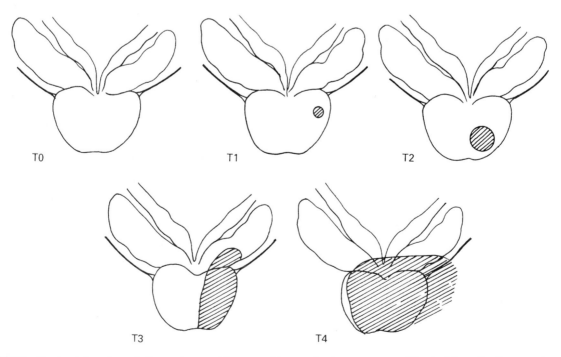

Fig. 29.22 T categories of prostatic carcinoma. T0 = no evidence of primary tumour; T1 = incidentally diagnosed, not palpable; T2 = palpable tumour confined within prostate; T3 = extending beyond prostate capsule; T4 = fixed – or invades adjacent structures.

black population), but rare in China and Japan. It rarely occurs before the age of 50 and is uncommon before the age of 60. The mean age at presentation is approximately 70 years. The aetiology is unknown, but hormonal and possibly viral factors are implicated.

Pathology

Almost all malignant tumours of the prostate are carcinomas. If a prostate is examined by serial section, a small malignant focus is detected in almost all men over the age of 80. Thus, there is a very high incidence of histological prostate cancer and many men will die with a cancer of the prostate – but not *from* that cancer. It is estimated that the incidence of focal histological cancer in men aged 50–75 is approximately 40%, whereas the incidence of clinical prostate cancer is approximately 8%, one-quarter of whom will die from that cancer. The TNM system is used in classification (Fig. 29.22). Metastatic spread to pelvic lymph nodes occurs early. One-third of clinically localized tumours at the time of presentation will have spread to regional nodes. Metastases to bone, mainly the lumbar spine and pelvis, are common; more than half of all new cases have such metastases.

Clinical features

Most patients with prostatic carcinoma present with frequency, urgency and dysuria; a quarter present with acute retention. Occasionally, the tumour extends posteriorly around the rectum and causes alteration in bowel habit. Presenting symptoms and signs due to metastases are much less common, but include back pain, weight loss, anaemia and ureteric obstruction. On rectal examination the prostate feels nodular and stony hard. The diagnosis must never be made on clinical grounds alone: many irregular prostates, even those with nodules, are not malignant. Conversely, 10–15% of malignant prostates are not palpably abnormal on rectal examination.

Investigation

As most patients present with outflow tract obstruction, ultrasound and serum creatinine determinations are performed to assess the urinary tract. An X-ray of the pelvis or lumbar spine (to investigate backache) may show osteosclerotic metastases as the first evidence of prostatic malignancy. Whenever possible the diagnosis is confirmed by needle biopsy, usually performed under transrectal ultrasound (TRUS) guidance (Fig. 29.23), or by histological examination of tissue removed at endoscopic resection if this is needed to relieve outflow obstruction. The patient is assessed for distant metastases by a radioisotope scan. Prostate-specific antigen (PSA) is now the main serum

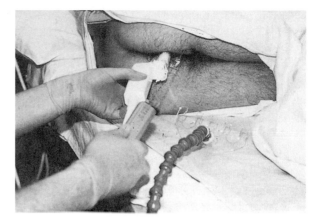

Fig. 29.23   Transrectal ultrasound of the prostate (TRUS) and needle biopsy. Scanning alone will miss 40% of cancers and biopsy is mandatory.

marker for the detection of prostate cancer. High levels (>100 ng/mL) almost always indicate distant bone metastases. PSA is also the main test for monitoring response to treatment and disease progression. A bone scan may be carried out at follow-up to localize and define the extent of metastases.

Treatment

Prostatic cancer, like breast cancer, is sensitive to endocrine influences. Management is best considered in four clinical groups, as follows.

Incidental or focal cancer Such patients will usually have had a prostatectomy and the diagnosis of cancer is made incidentally on histological examination. With increasing use of PSA, a raised value may be the only abnormality that leads to the diagnosis of cancer confirmed by a needle biopsy. A patient with a small focus of well-differentiated carcinoma may be managed by a watch and wait policy, because treatment is rarely required for these tumours and the patient has a normal life expectancy. A large tumour with a less well-differentiated cell pattern may progress; either radical surgery or radiotherapy is recommended for a man with a life expectancy of more than 10 years.

Organ-confined cancer; no evidence of bone metastases If the general health of the patient is good then either radical surgery or radiotherapy should be considered. Endocrine treatment is kept in reserve until there is evidence of tumour progression.

Metastatic prostate cancer Approximately half of the men diagnosed with prostate cancer will have metastatic disease. The basis of treatment is androgen depletion (orchiectomy) or androgen suppression (gonadotrophin-releasing hormone analogues with or without an antiandrogen). A small number of patients fail to respond to endocrine treatment; a larger number respond for a year or two, but then suffer disease progression. Other oestrogens or progestogens are of limited value, but chemotherapy with 5-fluorouracil, cyclophosphamide or nitrogen mustard may be effective. Radiotherapy is an effective treatment for localized bone pain. For severe generalized bone pain, hemibody radiotherapy or strontium-89 may give effective palliation, but the basis of treatment remains pain control by analgesia.

Prognosis

The life expectancy of a patient with an incidental finding of focal carcinoma of the prostate is that of the normal population. With tumours localized to the prostate, a 10-year survival rate of 50% can be expected; but if metastases are present this falls to 10%.

SUMMARY BOX

Prostatic cancer

- In the UK this is the third most common cancer in men, presents at a mean age of 70, and is increasing in incidence.

- The carcinoma may be incidental (i.e. found incidentally on histological examination), clinically apparent (bladder outflow obstruction and a hard craggy prostate) or occult (metastatic disease).

- Metastatic spread may occur early; one-third of clinically confined cancers have spread to lymph nodes, and more than half of all new cases have bony spread (to lumbar spine and pelvis).

- Treatment of prostatic cancer varies:

  - *Incidental or focal cancer.* If well differentiated, then life expectancy can be normal with a watch-and-wait policy. If the cancer contains undifferentiated cells then either radical surgery or radiotherapy is considered.

  - *Localized cancer with no evidence of bony metastases* is treated by either radical surgery or radiotherapy, keeping endocrine therapy in reserve.

  - *Metastatic cancer* is treated by androgen depletion (orchiectomy) or androgen suppression (gonadotrophin-releasing hormone analogues).

- The overall 5-year survival rate is 25%, but tumours localized to the prostate carry a 10-year survival rate of 50%.

Urethral cancer

Transitional cell tumours, which may be associated with bladder tumour, and squamous carcinoma of the distal urethra are uncommon. They may cause obstructive symptoms, urethral bleeding, or haematuria confined to the initial stream. The external meatus must always be examined and, if present, the foreskin retracted for full inspection. The urethra should be palpated, but usually the diagnosis can only be made at cystoscopy and biopsy. As the urothelium of the urethra is attached directly to vascular corpus spongiosum these tumours spread early, and should be treated aggressively by cystourethrectomy.

Benign prostatic hyperplasia

Pathology

From about the age of 40 years the prostate undergoes progressive change in size and consistency. Gland enlargement results from the hyperplasia of periurethral tissues, which forms adenomas in the central zone of the prostate. These characteristically form lateral 'lobes', and often a 'middle lobe'. The normal prostatic tissue is gradually compressed to form a shell or capsule around these adenomas. There is considerable variation in the growth rates of the adenomas and in the proportions of stromal and epithelial tissue. A prostate that has been previously infected or has a preponderance of stromal tissue is firm and fibrous on rectal examination. Adenomas with an epithelial preponderance can grow to form large discrete masses weighing more than 100 g, and on examination have a characteristic rubbery consistency. These changes are generally referred to as benign prostatic hyperplasia (BPH).

Enlarging adenomas lengthen and obstruct the prostatic urethra, and lead to the signs and symptoms of outflow obstruction. The increased work of the detrusor muscle in overcoming this obstruction results in detrusor muscle hypertrophy. The muscle bands form trabeculae, between which saccules form diverticula (Fig. 29.24). Occasionally a diverticulum may become quite large, even larger than the bladder. Bladder diverticula empty poorly and are liable to the three main complications of urinary stasis: infection, stones and tumour.

With progressive inability to empty the bladder completely (chronic retention), the risk of urinary infection and stone formation increases.

Bladder stones have become rare in western countries but are often seen in areas of poor nutrition, especially in children.

Eventually the residual urine volume may exceed 1 L, leading to progressive obstruction and dilatation of the ureters (hydroureter) and pelvicaliceal system (hydronephrosis). This ultimately leads to obstructive renal failure.

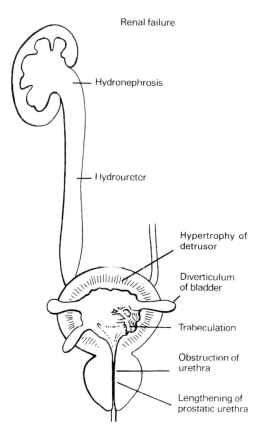

Renal failure

Hydronephrosis

Hydroureter

Hypertrophy of detrusor

Diverticulum of bladder

Trabeculation

Obstruction of urethra

Lengthening of prostatic urethra

Fig. 29.24 Late sequelae of prostatic obstruction.

Clinical features

The pathological changes at the bladder neck produce signs and symptoms that correlate poorly with the size of the prostate. Frequency, urgency and dysuria are common. Nocturia may become increasingly troublesome. The force of the stream is noticeably weaker and, with straining in an attempt to empty the bladder, vessels at the bladder neck may bleed. These clinical features may be separated into two main groups: those that are due to obstruction (slow stream and hesitancy) and those that are due to detrusor instability (urgency and urge incontinence). The presence of the latter in isolation is not an indication for prostatectomy.

Increasing frequency may deceive the patient into thinking that he is passing an adequate amount of urine, whereas the bladder may be almost full all of the time (chronic retention), that is, it has a small functional capacity. Frequency may progress to continual dribbling incontinence. Such patients are liable to develop the signs and symptoms of obstructive uraemia, including drowsiness, anorexia and personality changes. Urinary infection, cold weather, anticholinergic drugs or excessive alcohol intake can cause sufficient congestion of the bladder neck to tip the balance from difficult micturition to acute painful retention. If obstruction has already led to chronic retention, acute-on-chronic obstruction may occur. If the patient has a bladder stone he may have obstructive symptoms during micturition, and there may also be bladder pain at the end of micturition. Examination of a patient with symptoms of bladder outflow obstruction reveals little except enlargement of the gland on rectal examination. The enlargement is symmetrical and smooth, with a median groove between the two lateral 'lobes'. The consistency of an adenoma is described as rubbery. Asymmetry or a hard consistency raises the suspicion of malignancy. In a patient with acute painful retention of urine, the size of the prostate is more difficult to determine. This is due partly to the pelvic discomfort, but also to the fullness of the bladder, which changes the normal relationship of the prostate to the lower rectum so that the gland appears to be larger than it is. In patients with chronic retention the painless, enlarged bladder rises out of the pelvis, almost to the umbilicus. Even if it is not visible, the overlying area will be dull on percussion. In addition, the patient with chronic retention may be ill from obstructive uraemia.

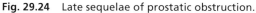

Table 29.2 Factors affecting level of PSA	
Causes of increase in PSA	Cause of decrease in PSA
Increase in age Acute retention of urine Urethral catheterization TURP Prostatitis Prostate cancer Large benign prostatic hyperplasia Prostatic biopsy	Patient taking a 5-α reductase inhibitor (finasteride)

Investigation

All patients must have an assessment of renal function, and haemoglobin and serum electrolyte estimations. The urine must be cultured in all cases. PSA is measured as a routine. Although the normal range is given as 0–4 ng/ml, prostatic cancer can occur with values within this range, and BPH can cause elevated values. Interpretation of a raised PSA therefore depends on many factors, including the age of the patient and the size of the prostate (Table 29.2). If the digital rectal examination is suspicious of malignancy then a needle biopsy of the prostate is always indicated. An ultrasound is necessary to detect the secondary effects of obstruction on the bladder (diverticula, stones) and upper urinary tract, and especially to assess the volume of residual urine after micturition. A urine flow rate measurement is essential to quantify a reduction in the urinary stream. The patient may also complete a symptom score sheet to quantify the degree of inconvenience and bother. In some patients, especially the elderly, neurological or pharmacological causes for the changes in micturition must be considered. A pressure–flow urodynamic assessment may be necessary.

Treatment

Patients can be divided into three clinical groups, each requring a different approach to management.

Symptomatic only The patient's assessment of the severity of symptoms is influenced by his age, the social inconvenience caused, and their frequency and progression. A young man may be greatly inconvenienced by symptoms that are quite acceptable to one who is elderly. If the exact role of the prostate in causing symptoms is difficult to determine, urodynamic studies may be helpful, especially if the symptoms appear to be irritative rather than obstructive. Once sinister pathology has been excluded (prostate carcinoma, renal failure) and it is established that the prostate is the principal problem, initial management should be medical. α-blockers can relax the smooth muscle of the bladder neck and prostatic capsule, and are useful in small prostates. 5-α-reductase inhibitors block the intraprostatic conversion of testosterone to dihydrotestosterone, resulting in shrinking of the prostate, and are useful in large glands. Prostatectomy (transurethral or open) is reserved for medical failures. Few patients are unfit for this operation; only if there is a history of myocardial infarction within the last 3 months should operation be delayed.

Acute retention This is an emergency that usually requires admission to hospital. If there is a history of bladder outflow obstruction, conservative measures aimed at encouraging micturition (sedation, a warm bath) only delay the inevitable requirement for catheterization. A self-retaining Foley catheter (size 16 Fr) is passed using strict asepsis and connected to a closed drainage system. If it is not possible to pass a urethral catheter, the bladder is entered directly by puncture with a trocar/cannula (suprapubic cystostomy). A specimen of urine is cultured and if there is microbiological evidence of an infection antibiotics are given. If the history of urinary symptoms is short the catheter can be removed after 12 hours (trial without catheter), following which normal voiding may occur. This is more likely if the patient is also given α-blockers. If retention recurs then definitive treatment is carried out.

Chronic retention It is essential to determine whether the patient has any complications of obstruction, especially renal damage. Although the upper urinary tracts may be dilated, renal function is not necessarily impaired. If the patient is well, with no haematological or biochemical disturbance, there is no indication for preliminary bladder drainage and prostatectomy may be planned in the usual way. If the patient is uraemic, his general fitness for operation must be assessed. Uraemia alone is not a contraindication, but hyperkalaemia, dehydration or other evidence of fluid and electrolyte disturbance must be corrected. The bladder is catheterized and prostatectomy is carried out as soon as the patient is fit. Relief of chronic obstruction is almost always followed by a diuresis, due partly to an osmotic (urea) diuresis and partly to renal tubular changes resulting from back pressure. Accurate intake/output fluid charts can detect these losses. The blood pressure should be monitored and intravenous fluid replacement may be necessary.

Open prostatectomy

Earlier open procedures used a transvesical approach, during which the bladder was opened and the adenomatous obstruction enucleated from the capsule. Later, a retropubic approach was used in which the adenoma was enucleated through a transverse incision in the prostatic capsule (Fig. 29.25). These open procedures are now reserved for very large adenomas. Apart from the length of hospitalization (7–10 days) and the presence of an abdominal wound, enucleation of smaller adenomas may damage the external sphincter and cause incontinence. This is a particular problem with more fibrous glands and those that contain a focus of cancer.

Closed (endoscopic) prostatectomy

During transurethral resection of the prostate (TURP) the prostate is removed piecemeal by electroresection using a resectoscope (Fig. 29.26). The advantages of this approach are patient acceptance, short hospitalization (3–5 days), and the precision of removal of the obstructing tissue. However, serious damage can be inflicted on the prostatic sphincter mechanism by inexpert use of the resectoscope. Also, a

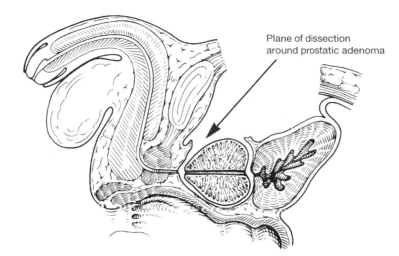

Fig. 29.25 Retropubic prostatectomy.

prolonged resection can result in excessive absorption of irrigating fluid and electrolyte imbalance (TURP syndrome). Retrograde ejaculation is a common sequel to any operative procedure on the prostate (and bladder neck), and all patients should be advised preoperatively of this effect. If the patient has a bladder stone, this may be crushed with a lithotrite or removed by suprapubic lithotomy.

After either form of prostatectomy the bladder must be allowed to drain freely via a urethral catheter while the prostatic bed heals and bleeding stops. After TURP the catheter is normally removed on the second postoperative day. After an open procedure, because of the bladder or prostatic incision, it is usually left in place until the fifth postoperative day. The main postoperative hazard is bleeding. In an open procedure blood vessels at the bladder neck are sutured, but bleeding within the capsule is less easy to control. With TURP, coagulation of the blood vessels is more precise but not always complete. If postoperative bleeding is excessive, clot may lead to obstruction (clot retention). This hazard can be minimized by continuous irrigation through a three-way urethral catheter. The results of all forms of prostatectomy continue to improve, but TURP has the lowest morbidity and mortality (<1%) and requires a shorter hospital stay (50% less) than other procedures.

Bladder neck obstruction

Occasionally the obstruction to the outflow tract appears to be at the bladder neck. The prostate is often quite small. The cause may be an infective condition such as prostatitis

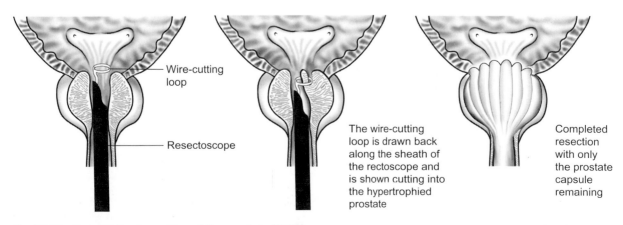

Wire-cutting loop

Resectoscope

The wire-cutting loop is drawn back along the sheath of the rectoscope and is shown cutting into the hypertrophied prostate

Completed resection with only the prostate capsule remaining

Fig. 29.26 Transurethral resection of the prostate (TURP).

or schistosomiasis, or a neurological disorder such as diabetes or a prolapsed intervertebral disc. More commonly, the obstruction is due to failure of the bladder neck to open when the detrusor contracts (dyssynergia). Characteristically, bladder neck dyssynergia is found in younger middle-aged men, that is, at an age when benign prostatic hyperplasia is not expected. The urinary stream is poor, although the patient may have thought it normal, and there may be frequency and urgency. α-Adrenergic blocking drugs may improve the muscular dysfunction that causes dyssynergia. Endoscopic incision or excision of the bladder neck is preferable to long-term drug treatment, but surgery is contraindicated if the risk of retrograde ejaculation and hence infertility is of concern to the patient.

External sphincter obstruction

In cases of spinal injury, spina bifida and multiple sclerosis the external sphincter may have high resting tone (isolated distal sphincter obstruction) or lose its normal coordination with the detrusor muscle. This results in the sphincter closing when the detrusor contracts (detrusosphincter dyssynergia). In both cases the result is a functional obstruction. Specialized urodynamics is required to make the diagnosis accurately and treatment may require endoscopic sphincterotomy.

Urethral obstruction

Pathology

Obstruction of the urethra may be congenital, due to a stricture, or due to malignancy (Fig. 29.27). Foreign bodies, including urinary stones, may also be responsible. The complications include infection with periurethral abscess,

fistulation and stone formation. Congenital valves in the posterior urethra occur only in boys. They lie at the level of the verumontanum and may cause gross obstructive changes in the bladder and upper urinary tracts at birth. Increasingly, this diagnosis is being established during pregnancy by ultrasound examination. If the diagnosis is established after birth, it is confirmed by micturating cysto-urethrography. Treatment consists of endoscopic incision of the valves. Urethral diverticulum is a rare cause of obstruction. More commonly, it is secondary to obstruction and infection in women. An important late sequel of urethral trauma or infection is a stricture, the severity of which is related to both the site and the extent of the insult. Thus, a posterior urethral stricture that follows major trauma to the pelvis may be surrounded by dense fibrous tissue, whereas healthy tissues may surround a stricture of the bulb of the urethra. The former requires major reconstructive surgery; urethral dilation or incision can readily manage the latter. It must be remembered that rough inexpert use of any instrument (including a catheter) in the urethra can be followed by stricture formation. The principal organism responsible for inflammatory scarring and stricture of the urethra is *Neisseria gonorrhoeae*. Long-term use of a self-retaining catheter, although not necessarily associated with infection, can also cause an inflammatory reaction in the urethra. This may result in a stricture, most commonly at the external meatus.

Clinical features

A change in micturition due to urethral narrowing may be indistinguishable from that which occurs with BPH and bladder neck obstruction. However, the diagnosis should be considered if there is a history of urethral infection, instru-

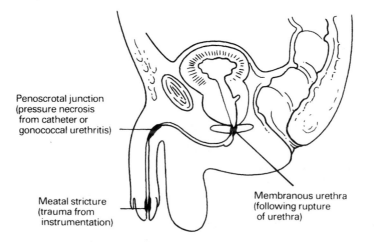

Penoscrotal junction
(pressure necrosis
from catheter or
gonococcal urethritis)

Meatal stricture
(trauma from
instrumentation)

Membranous urethra
(following rupture
of urethra)

Fig. 29.27 Common sites and causes of urethral stricture.

mentation or trauma. The external meatus must always be examined and, if present, the foreskin retracted for full inspection. The urethra is palpated. It is still possible for a patient to pass urine, albeit with difficulty, in the presence of a urethral stone.

Investigation

Urinary flow rate will help differentiate urethral strictures from bladder neck and prostatic obstruction, the former giving a uniformly low and prolonged (box-like) pattern (Fig. 29.6). Postmicturition ultrasound is more useful than an IVU in assessing bladder emptying and residual volume. An ascending and descending urethrogram will adequately demonstrate the urethral anatomy. Urodynamic assessment of the urethra and bladder may be helpful, especially when neurological and mechanical problems coexist. The final investigation to assess a urethral lesion is cystourethroscopy.

Treatment

Many simple strictures are easily treated by repeated dilatation with metal bougies, or may be incised under direct vision using a urethrotome. Most simple short strictures in the region of the bulb respond well, but recurrence is common (50%) and may require operative reconstruction (urethroplasty). Short strictures can be excised and the healthy urethra reanastomosed. Longer strictures can be patched with full-thickness skin flaps, or buccal mucosal grafts, to restore normal calibre.

DISORDERS OF MICTURITION – INCONTINENCE

Overview

Incontinence may be due to problems in storage, resulting in urge and stress incontinence or continual incontinence with fistulae, or to problems in emptying, resulting in chronic retention with overflow incontinence. In stress incontinence, leakage occurs because passive bladder pressure exceeds normal urethral pressure. This may be because of poor pelvic floor support or because of a weak urethral sphincter; most often there is an element of both. In urge incontinence, leakage usually occurs because detrusor overactivity produces an increase in bladder pressure that overcomes the urethral sphincter (motor urgency). A hypersensitive bladder (sensory urgency) resulting from UTI (urinary tract infection) or bladder stone may also drive urgency. Incontinence in these circumstances is less common. Stress incontinence and urge incontinence may coexist (mixed incontinence). All of the above terms, with the exception of a fistula, are descriptive only and do not accurately diagnose the underlying pathophysiology, which can only be determined by urodynamic testing.

Structural disorders

Assessment

Abnormalities of function of the lower urinary tract are notoriously difficult to assess because there is frequently dual underlying pathology. For example, incontinence in an elderly man may be due to cerebral cortical degeneration, but could also be due to chronic outflow tract obstruction resulting from prostatic hyperplasia. The history is important but may be deceptive, mainly because different abnormalities can produce similar symptoms. The exact character of the urinary abnormality must be determined so that structural causes can be separated from neurological ones. Details of drug treatment are noted. Diuretics and drugs with anticholinergic side-effects may tip the balance when there is already dysfunction. Urine is tested for glycosuria and infection. In addition to intravenous urography there is now a range of more specific methods for assessing micturition, but not all are required for a diagnosis. Their value lies in resolving specific clinical questions relating to management. They include radiology (cystourethrography), urodynamic studies (uroflowmetry, cystometrography and urethral pressure measurement) and direct inspection (cystourethroscopy and pelvic examination under anaesthesia). A full history and physical examination, with cystourethroscopy and bimanual examination, remain the basic initial investigation of structural disorders.

Structural causes of incontinence in males

Post prostatectomy Disordered control of micturition occurs in 3–5% patients after prostatectomy. In this operation the bladder neck sphincter is deliberately excised posteriorly but the external sphincter is carefully preserved. However, any inadvertent damage to the external sphincter can lead to difficulties with continence. Stress incontinence may occur, but as the damage to the sphincter is usually incomplete it usually responds to physiotherapy.

Chronic outflow obstruction Chronic obstruction commonly leads to involuntary contractions or unstable bladder. Relief of obstruction alone is usually sufficient to correct the associated urgency and urge incontinence, but in about 10% of cases the instability is primary and antispasmodics may be necessary. Chronic retention may also lead to overflow or dribbling incontinence. It must be emphasized that continence requires normal cortical control, and in an elderly patient this may be impaired. Possible abnormalities of both structure and innervation need to be considered in these patients.

Carcinoma of the prostate This may involve the external sphincter, preventing it from closing. Repeated transurethral resections for recurring obstruction may convert the posterior urethra into a rigid tube so that dribbling incontinence occurs, that is, there is leakage of urine during the storage phase. An indwelling catheter or condom incontinence appliance may be necessary.

Postmicturition dribble incontinence This is very common, even in relatively young men, and is caused by a small amount of urine becoming trapped in the 'U-bend' of the bulbar urethra. This then leaks out passively when the patient moves. The condition is more pronounced if associated with a urethral diverticulum or urethral stricture.

Chronic illness and debility Especially in the elderly, this may lead to incontinence because of poor tone in the periurethral striated muscle of the pelvic floor and difficulty in getting to the toilet. This may be worsened by loss of cortical inhibition of micturition.

Structural causes of incontinence in females

Incontinence is more prevalent than generally suspected: approximately 14% of all women have been incontinent at some time, half of them within the last 2 months. This figure rises rapidly in older patients, and reaches 50–70% in geriatric units. Only a proportion of younger women seeks advice, either because of embarrassment or because of stoical acceptance of some incontinence as being normal.

Childbirth and operations Multiparous women commonly lose some of the tone in the pelvic floor muscles with each pregnancy. Symptoms may range from occasional stress incontinence to almost continual dribbling incontinence. Examination shows weakening of the pelvic floor muscles and anterior vaginal wall (cystocele). It is important to distinguish stress incontinence from urge incontinence. The former responds well to pelvic floor exercises and to surgical procedures designed to support the bladder neck, but the latter should be treated by bladder retraining and drug therapy. Stress incontinence is characterized by an involuntary loss of urine during coughing, laughing, sneezing or any other activity that suddenly raises the intra-abdominal pressure. A cough, however, may stimulate involuntary detrusor contractions (cough-induced detrusor instability), which cause motor urge incontinence. This differential diagnosis can be made only by urodynamic assessment. In parts of the world where obstetric services are poor, prolonged labour may lead to a vesicovaginal fistula, which presents as continuous dribbling incontinence. The association with delivery is usually clear, but a small fistula may be missed. Investigation of dribbling incontinence must distinguish between urethral damage and a fistula. Treatment consists of closing the fistula through a vaginal or suprapubic approach.

Hysterectomy may also be followed by urinary incontinence, suggesting either vesicovaginal fistula or damage to the ureter(s) at operation, resulting in ureterovaginal fistula. Investigations are directed at establishing whether the bladder or the ureters are involved, and which ureter has been damaged. Treatment consists of reimplanting the ureter into the bladder.

Cystitis Cystitis is common in women and, in addition to causing frequency, urgency and dysuria, sometimes causes sensory urge incontinence. Treatment of both the infection and the bladder spasm is required. Chronic interstitial cystitis (Hunner's ulcer) is a chronic inflammatory condition which, in addition to causing frequency and dysuria, may also cause urgency and urge incontinence. Treatment is often unsatisfactory. Hydrostatic dilatation may be effective. The urethral syndrome is characterized by symptoms of cystitis in the absence of infection. There may be some incontinence. The urethral syndrome usually responds to regulation of micturition habits and careful perineal hygiene. Resistant cases may benefit from urethral dilatation, although they are seldom, if ever, strictured.

Ectopic ureter Dribbling incontinence in a child should raise the suspicion of an ectopic ureter, in which the lower of the two ureters opens outside the control of the urethral mechanism. The abnormal ureter must be relocated in the bladder.

Cervical cancer Carcinoma of the cervix or its treatment by radiotherapy may cause vesicovaginal fistula and incontinence.

Neurogenic disorders

Assessment

A full history, including an interview with relatives, is required. Examination must include assessment of the plantar reflexes and the sensation and tone of the anal canal. Glycosuria and urinary infection should be excluded. Urodynamic, radiological and electromyographic studies may all be required.

Aetiology of abnormal micturition

Impaired cortical control Diseases affecting the frontal lobe can alter the pattern of micturition by increasing or decreasing its frequency, or by affecting the social awareness of incontinence. There may also be failure to inhibit initiation of micturition. The paracentral lobule controls the activity of skeletal muscle, so that lesions in this area may cause sustained pelvic and perineal muscular contraction. It must be remembered that a disorder of micturition may be accentuated by, or even due to, the physical inability to prepare for micturition.

Emotional state This may affect the postponement of micturition, giving rise to 'giggle' incontinence and possibly to enuresis in some patients. Incontinence with epilepsy is also due to a loss of inhibitory control. Excessive sensory stimuli, as with the pain of cystourethritis in women, may cause 'sensory urge incontinence'.

Drugs Drugs, including alcohol, may alter cortical control of micturition. Sedatives can affect the postponement phase and precipitate incontinence, especially at night. The intoxicated patient may lack the mental alertness to maintain continence, or may continually suppress the desire to void, leading to prostatic congestion and retention.

Damage to the spinal cord Two aspects of disease or injury to the spinal cord influence disordered micturition, namely the level of the disease and the completeness of the damage.

Injury at or below the sacral outflow (S2, 3, 4) may be due to a fracture of the spine at the level of T12 and L1, which damages the conus medullaris, a central prolapsed intervertebral disc, leading to cauda equina injury, or to spinal stenosis. The bladder distends without sensation, the external sphincter is weak and the cystometrogram is flat. The patient develops retention with overflow, but emptying is possible with abdominal straining or hand pressure.

Injury between the sacral segment and the pontine micturition centres (upper motor neuron lesions) may be due to fractures of the spine; tumours that compress the cord; surgical removal of such a tumour; and diseases of the cord itself, such as multiple sclerosis, transverse myelitis and cervical cord stenosis. If these central connections are disrupted, the patient develops a reflex bladder with impaired or absent cortical control, that is, the bladder loses the coordination imposed by the pontine micturition centre. The detrusor becomes overactive (hyperreflexic) and attempted voiding results in detrusor contraction occurring synchronously with that of the external sphincter (detrusor– sphincter dyssernegia). The net result is poor bladder emptying and the development of a thick, trabeculated bladder wall. The resultant high-pressure bladder will, over time, lead to renal impairment. Usually the central connections are not completely disrupted and there may be some sensation and some cortical inhibition.

Damage to pelvic nerves may occur in the course of surgery, especially when dissection involves the side walls of the pelvis, as in radical dissection of the rectum or the uterus. Similarly, aneurysm surgery may disrupt neural pathways in the pelvis. Diseases affecting the autonomic system, principally diabetes mellitus, also affect the control of micturition. With the loss of sensation and contraction the bladder becomes an atonic sac, prone to the complication of stasis infection. The external sphincter remains closed by uninhibited tonic contractions, but the internal sphincter is partly open as it partly depends on detrusor activity.

Abnormalities within the bladder itself may also be responsible. Primary failure of the detrusor has been described, but is usually secondary to chronic overdistension. Atonic myogenic bladder is caused by prolonged outlet obstruction and is found in the late stages of bladder decompensation. The commonest cause is silent prostatic obstruction, where progressive loss of the desire to void results in overflow incontinence. In women, conscious postponement can lead to a large, atonic bladder.

Principles of management

The diagnosis must be as complete as possible. More than one mechanism may account for disordered micturition. A urodynamic assessment is mandatory in all patients with a suspected or proven neuropathic bladder.

Neurologically intact patients

Patients with congenital defects or fistulae should have these repaired surgically if possible. If the fistula is malignant or the surrounding tissues poor because of radiation, urinary diversion is preferable. Stress incontinence in both males and females should be treated initially with pelvic floor exercises. If it persists in males it is best treated by the insertion of an artificial urinary sphincter. In females the urethra and bladder neck should be returned to their natural positions and supported by means of colposuspension or a pubovaginal sling. The injection of bulking agents at the bladder neck can improve continence, but remains under evaluation. Urge incontinence should be treated initially by bladder retraining, supplemented by anticholinergic drugs. If this fails good results can be obtained by surgery, either by stripping off a substantial proportion of the detrusor muscle (myectomy) or by splitting the bladder in half and suturing a strip of small bowel to augment the bladder (clam ileocystoplasty). Patients with atonic bladders are best managed by regular intermittent self-catheterization (ISC).

Neuropathic patients

These patients are prone to urinary infection and renal impairment, and the preservation of renal function takes priority. Management depends as much on the patient's overall condition as on their specific urological problem. Regardless of pathology, poorly motivated immobile patients with poor cognition and hand function are best managed by suprapubic catheterization or urinary diversion. Highly motivated intelligent patients should be treated in much the same way as the neurologically intact, although the results are often less good.

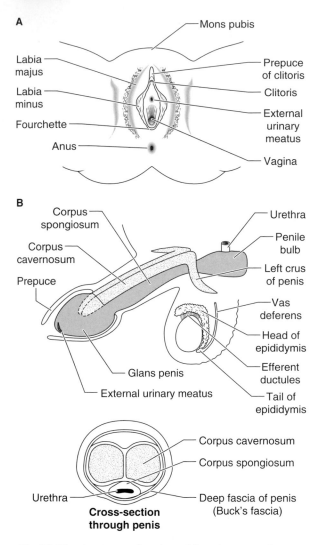

A

- Mons pubis
- Labia majus
- Labia minus
- Fourchette
- Anus
- Prepuce of clitoris
- Clitoris
- External urinary meatus
- Vagina

B

- Corpus spongiosum
- Corpus cavernosum
- Prepuce
- Glans penis
- External urinary meatus
- Urethra
- Penile bulb
- Left crus of penis
- Vas deferens
- Head of epididymis
- Efferent ductules
- Tail of epididymis

- Urethra
- Corpus cavernosum
- Corpus spongiosum
- Deep fascia of penis (Buck's fascia)

Cross-section through penis

Fig. 29.28 Anatomy of male and female external genitalia.

EXTERNAL GENITALIA

Anatomy

In the male this comprises the penis, testicles and scrotum; in the female the mons pubis, labia majora, labia minora and the clitoris (Figs 29.14 and 29.28). The penis comprises three cylinders of erectile tissue. The ventral corpora spongiosum is expanded proximally as the bulb and distally as the glans penis, and transmits the urethra. Two dorsolateral corpora cavernosa attach to each side of the inferior pubic arch as the crura. They form the body of the penis and become embedded in the glans. The penile skin is hairless, free of fat, and extends over the glans as the prepuce or foreskin. Blood is supplied from the internal pudendal

arteries. The scrotum is a thin rugose pouch of skin containing the two testicles. Each testicle is contained within a tough capsule (tunica albuginea) and has the epididymis attached to it posteriorly. This highly coiled tubular structure arises from the rete testis, where some 20 small tubules enter it. This head of epididymis is considerably larger than the lower tail, from which the vas deferens arises to traverse the spermatic cord and finally to open into the prostatic urethra as the ejaculatory duct. The testicle and epididymis are invaginated into the tunica vaginalis, which lies anteriorly, so providing a potential space where a hydrocele may form. The testicular arteries supply the testes. Venous blood drains along the spermatic cord as the pampiniform plexus. The scrotum drains lymph to the inguinal lymph nodes, and the contents of the scrotum drain along the spermatic cord to nodes in the pelvis and abdomen. In the female the mons pubis is the fatty elevation over the pubis from which the labia run backwards, enclosing between them the vestibule into which open the vagina and urethra. The clitoris lies above the urethral opening and is a smaller replica of the penis, with the same erectile tissues.

Physiology

Parasympathetic stimulation leads to erection through the release of nitric oxide, with resultant vasodilatation of the arterioles, increased penile blood flow and passive closure of the venules. After sufficient stimulation, sperm from the epididymis and seminal fluid from the seminal vesicles are emptied into the prostatic urethra. Sympathetic stimulation is responsible for this emission, and also closes the bladder neck to prevent leakage of semen into the bladder. Ejaculation proper is due to rhythmic contraction of the bulbospongiosus muscles expelling the semen out through the urethra.

Circumcision

The foreskin is normally non-retractile for the first few months of life. By the end of the first year half will retract, but it may be 3–4 years before all do so. Provided the parents are reassured, there is no reason, apart from religious grounds, to remove the foreskin within the first few years of life. In some children the foreskin remains non-retractile and has to be treated by division of preputial adhesions or by circumcision. Otherwise, secretions collect under the foreskin, leading to infection (balanitis) and narrowing of the orifice (phimosis).

Severe phimosis may obstruct urinary flow. In those whose foreskin retracts only with difficulty, pain during intercourse may be a problem. Keeping the glans and coronal sulcus clean can also be difficult; accumulated secretions may predispose to carcinoma of the penis. If a poorly retracting foreskin remains retracted, it can act as a tight band and cause engorgement and oedema of the glans (paraphimosis). This demands urgent treatment. It may be possible to compress the glans and draw the foreskin forwards, but if this fails the tight band must be incised under general anaesthesia. Later elective circumcision is advocated.

Congenital abnormalities of the penis

Hypospadias

Failure of the embryonic folds to fuse results in abnormal placing of the external urinary meatus on the ventral surface of the penis. The opening may be coronal, penile, scrotal or even perineal. The corpus spongiosum may be scarred and fibrosed, leading to a ventral curvature or chordee of the penis. The aim of treatment is to correct the chordee by excising the fibrosis, and then to construct a new urethral opening in the normal position on the glans. This procedure should be completed before the boy goes to school.

Epispadias

In this condition the external urinary meatus opens on the dorsal surface of the penis. The extent of the malformation varies from an isolated penile abnormality to gross malformation of the bladder and urethra. The mucosa of the bladder and the ureteric orifices may be exposed and form the infraumbilical part of the abdominal wall (exstrophy). The urethra then lies opened out and the testes are undescended. Other abnormalities include separation of the symphysis pubis and rectal prolapse. Reconstruction of these deformities is not always successful, and urinary incontinence may remain a major problem and require urinary diversion.

Disorders of erection (impotence)

Impotence may be psychogenic, organic or drug induced. Psychogenic problems, the commonest cause, can usually be established from a careful history that includes details of sexual habits. Organic impotence is associated with diabetes mellitus, neurogenic disorders, major pelvic injury or operations, vascular disease of the pelvic vessels (Leriche's syndrome), priapism and Peyronie's disease. Most of these conditions cause irreversible impotence, but angiography may help to define a treatable abnormality in the arterial inflow to the penis. Drug-induced causes occur in patients receiving hormonal manipulation for prostatic cancer. In addition, some antihypertensive drugs may cause loss of erection or inability to ejaculate. Drugs such as barbiturates, benzodiazepines, corticosteroids, phenothiazines and spironolactone may all affect libido. Medical treatment is by oral sildenafil (Viagra), intracavernosal injection of papaverine, or prostaglandin E. Vacuum suction devices or a prosthesis implantated into the corpora cavernosa are effective alternatives to self-injection.

Priapism

In this condition there is a painful maintained erection unassociated with sexual desire. It is associated with leukaemia, disorders of coagulation, renal dialysis and sickle-cell trait, and is believed to be due to sludging of venous blood in the sinuses of the corpora cavernosa. Thus, the painful erection affects the corpora cavernosa but not the corpus spongiosum or glans. The commonest cause now seen is due to intracavernosal self-injection for impotence. Non-operative methods to relieve the congestion, such as aspiration of the thickened blood and intracavernosal injections of vasoconstrictors (phenylephrine), may be effective, especially in self-injection treatment. However, if these fail the creation of a venous shunt (e.g. saphenous vein to corpus cavernosum or corpora cavernosa to corpus spongiosum) within 6–12 hours gives satisfactory results, and the patient can achieve normal erections subsequently. If treatment is delayed or incomplete, the erectile tissue is damaged and the patient will be impotent.

Peyronie's disease

This is the occurrence of a hard fibrous plaque (or plaques) in the wall of a corpus cavernosum, causing lateral curvature of the penis. The cause is obscure but is possibly related to trauma, leading to the formation of hard scar tissue. In addition to the deformity, the patient complains of pain during intercourse. Various treatments, including cortisone injections, vitamins and radiotherapy, have met with little success. Excision of the plaque and replacement by a dermal patch graft, or excision of a wedge of tissue on the convex (opposite) border of the penis, may be effective.

Carcinoma of the penis

This uncommon tumour has an incidence of 1.5 cases per 100 000 and is generally attributed to poor hygiene associated with a non-retractile foreskin. It is very rare in circumcised men and almost always occurs in the elderly. The cancer may be a papillary or an ulcerating squamous cell carcinoma. Local spread occurs early and the tumour may ulcerate and fungate. Lymphatic spread to inguinal lymph nodes is common; associated infection may also lead to lymphadenopathy. The patient may present with a purulent or bloodstained discharge. Unfortunately, many patients do not seek help until the lesion is advanced – some only when much of the penis is already destroyed and the inguinal lymph nodes are involved. The diagnosis must be confirmed by biopsy. Circumcision may cure early tumours confined to the prepuce. Early tumours confined to the glans may be treated by excision of the glans and skin grafting. Advanced tumours will require partial or total penile amputation, and often bilateral block dissection of the inguinal lymph nodes. Inoperable tumours are treated by radiotherapy.

Inflammation of the penis

Inflammation of the glans penis (balanitis) usually also involves the prepuce (posthitis) and is common in children with poorly retractile foreskins. Specific infections are beyond the scope of this chapter (see *Davidson's principles and practice of medicine*, p. 184). Circumcision usually cures recurrent non-specific balanitis. Balanitis xerotica obliterans (BXO) is the local manifestation of lichen sclerosis et atrophicus of the glans and prepuce. It causes typical white scarring of the prepuce and glans, and may involve the urethral meatus and distal urethra. Meatal stenosis occurs as a result of either recurrent infection, trauma or BXO. It may respond to removal of the inflammation (by circumcision) and meatal dilation; alternatively, it may require meatotomy or meatoplasty.

Undescended testes (cryptorchidism)

Retractile testis

Normally, both testes are in the scrotum by 6 months of age. However, they may be excessively mobile and readily retract towards the external inguinal ring, even into the inguinal canal, especially when the patient is examined in a cold room. Such retractile testes may easily be misdiagnosed as being incompletely descended. Care must be taken to examine the baby in a warm room or after a bath. True undescended testes are of two types:

1. *Incomplete* Such a testis is arrested in its normal pathway to the scrotum. Usually this is within the inguinal canal, more rarely within the abdomen. The testis is smaller than normal and cannot be palpated. Its ability to produce sperm is doubtful. As the spermatic cord is short, such testes are difficult to bring down into the scrotum by operation (orchidopexy). If this can be carried out before the age of 2–4 years, the testis may be of some use; otherwise it should be removed. Occasionally, an incompletely descended testis is situated just inside the external inguinal ring, through which it can be coaxed (emergent testis). Testes that remain incompletely descended have a 1 in 80 chance of becoming malignant; the risk is greater if the testis is retained in the abdomen. Laparoscopy is increasingly used to locate and remove an intra-abdominal testis.

2. *Ectopic* An ectopic testis has developed normally, but after passing through the external inguinal ring its further descent is impeded. It either remains in the superficial inguinal pouch (common) or is transposed to perineal, femoral or prepubic sites (rare). Because an ectopic testis is normal in size, it is palpable and its cord is normal. Orchidopexy is achieved without difficulty. Provided this is done early, preferably before the age of 6 years, spermatogenesis is believed to occur normally. However, even if the diagnosis is not made until later (frequently just before puberty), orchidopexy should still be performed. This consists of mobilizing the testis and its cord and placing the testis in the scrotum. Various methods are used to stop the testis from retracting towards the inguinal canal. The simplest is to place the testis in a pouch between the dartos muscle and the scrotal skin.

Torsion of the testis

Torsion of the cord can occur where the visceral layer of the tunica vaginalis completely covers the testis so that it lies suspended within the parietal layer. The patient, usually a teenager, presents with sudden onset of testicular pain and swelling. There may be a history of minor trauma, or previous episodes of pain due to partial torsion. On examination there is a red, swollen hemiscrotum that is usually too tender to palpate. Misdiagnosis of the swelling as epididymo-orchitis, which is rare in teenagers, is a serious error. This a surgical emergency: if the blood supply is not restored within 12 hours, the testis infarcts and must then be excised. If at operation the testis is viable, it is sutured to the parietal tunica to prevent recurrence. As the underlying abnormality of the tunica is bilateral, the other testis must be fixed at the same time.

Testicular tumours

Pathology

Tumours of the testes are uncommon, with an incidence of 5 cases per 100 000. They most commonly affect men between 20 and 40 years of age. Seminoma and teratoma account for 85%; malignant lymphoma, yolk-sac tumours, interstitial cell tumours and Sertoli cell/mesenchyme tumours make up the remainder. Seminomas arise from seminiferous tubules and are of relatively low-grade malignancy. Metastases occur mainly via the lymphatics and may involve the lungs. Teratoma (non-seminomatous tumour) arises from primitive germinal cells. It may contain cartilage, bone, muscle, fat and a variety of other tissues, and is classified according to the degree of differentiation. Well-differentiated tumours are the least aggressive; at the other extreme, trophoblastic teratoma is highly malignant. Occasionally, teratoma and seminoma occur in the same testis.

Clinical features

The commonest presentation is the incidental discovery of a painless testicular lump. The history is often vague, however, and symptoms may be attributed to an injury, or there may be pain and swelling suggesting inflammation. The patient may wrongly have received treatment for 'acute epididymitis'. Very rarely, patients with teratoma may complain of gynaecomastia. Irrespective of the history, any new painless testicular lump in a young man must be regarded with suspicion. A hydrocele in a young man also demands investigation, as testicular tumours may be accompanied by bloodstained effusion in the tunica vaginalis.

Investigation

All suspicious scrotal lumps should be imaged by ultrasound, which provides a high degree of accuracy. As soon as a tumour is suspected, and before orchiectomy, serum levels of α-fetoprotein (AFP) and the β-subunit of human chorionic gonadotropain (HCG) should be determined. The levels of these 'tumour markers' are increased in extensive disease. Accurate staging is based on CT scans of the lungs, liver and retroperitoneal area, and an assessment of renal and pulmonary function (Table 29.3).

Treatment

Through an inguinal incision the spermatic cord is divided at the internal ring; only then is the testis removed. Radiotherapy is the treatment of choice for early-stage seminoma, as this tumour is very radiosensitive. The management of a teratoma depends on the stage of the disease. Early disease confined to the testes may be managed without further treatment, provided that there is close surveillance for at least 2 years; tumour progression is treated by chemotherapy. More advanced cancers are managed initially by chemotherapy, usually with a combination of bleomycin, etoposide and cisplatin. Retroperitoneal lymph node dissection is now only performed for residual or recurrent nodal masses. AFP and β-HCG each offer a valuable means of monitoring response to treatment and detecting recurrent disease. Both markers should be monitored in all patients with testicular tumours for at least 2 years after they are considered to be tumour-free. CT is used to follow the response of enlarged lymph nodes to treatment.

Table 29.3 Royal Marsden classification for testicular cancer	
Stage 1	Tumour confined to testis
Stage 2	Tumour spread only to lymph nodes below diaphragm
Stage 3	Tumour spread only to lymph nodes above and below diaphragm
Stage 4	Tumour spread to inguinal lymph nodes or distant metastases

SUMMARY BOX

Testicular tumours

- In the UK there are about 1000 new cases of testicular tumour per year and the age group 20–40 years is predominantly affected.

- Seminomas and teratomas account for 85% of all testicular tumours.

- Seminomas arise from the seminiferous tubules, are of relatively low-grade malignancy, spread predominantly via the lymphatic system and are very sensitive to radiotherapy.

- Teratomas arise from germinal cells, their differentiation reflects their aggressiveness (well-differentiated tumours are the least aggressive), and they are not radiosensitive.

- Treatment consists of radical orchiectomy (with division of the spermatic cord at the level of the deep inguinal ring). Radiotherapy is used if the tumour proves to be a seminoma, whereas chemotherapy (bleomycin, etoposide and cisplantin) is used for teratomas that are advanced or recurrent.

- Seminomas have a 5-year survival rate of 90–95%, whereas teratomas have a more varied prognosis (60–95% 5-year survival rate).

Prognosis

The 5-year survival rate for patients with seminoma is 90–95%. The more variable prognosis of teratomas depends on tumour type, stage and volume. With more favourable tumours the 5-year survival rate may be as high as 95%, but in more advanced cases 60–70% is more usual.

Epididymo-orchitis

Acute epididymo-orchitis is usually the appropriate term, as both testis and epididymides are involved in the acute inflammatory reaction. The spermatic cord is also often thickened (funiculitis). After infection has subsided the epididymis alone may remain thickened and irregular, so that chronic epididymitis may be diagnosed. Thus a late effect of tuberculosis is an irregularly hard (craggy) epididymis. Apparent involvement of the testis alone may be a feature of viral infections such as mumps orchitis. The usual cause of epididymo-orchitis is bacterial spread, either from infected urine or from gonococcal urethritis. The affected side of the scrotum is swollen, inflamed and very tender. In all cases the urine or urethral discharge must be cultured. Sometimes there is no evidence of a bacterial cause and a viral aetiology is then likely. Treatment consists of antibiotics, bed rest and a scrotal support. The choice of antibiotic depends on the results of culture and sensitivity determination of the organism responsible. If there is any doubt about the diagnosis, the testis should be explored. Abscess formation is now rare, but if signs of localization or fluctuation develop the pus should be drained. Infertility is an important late complication of epididymo-orchitis.

Hydrocele

This is a common condition, especially in older men, in which fluid collects in the tunica vaginalis, resulting in an enlarged but painless scrotum. The inconvenience of its size usually leads the patient to seek advice. The cause of most hydrocoeles is unknown (idiopathic). The fluid is straw coloured and protein rich. In some patients it develops as a reaction to epididymo-orchitis. Rarely, it may develop with a malignant testis (secondary hydrocele) and the fluid may then be bloodstained. On examination of the scrotum a normal spermatic cord can be palpated above a smooth oval swelling. Typically a hydrocele transilluminates, but where it is long-standing this may be difficult to elicit owing to fibrosis and thickening of its wall. It is important always to seek this physical sign and also to examine the neck of the scrotum carefully to exclude an inguinal hernia as the cause of the swelling. It may be possible to palpate the testis and confirm that it is normal, but this is unusual as it lies behind and is enveloped by the hydrocele. If there is any doubt about the diagnosis then an ultrasound should be done. If ultrasound is not available, then the fluid is aspirated and the testes re-examined to exclude a tumour. Injury to the scrotum may result in a swelling that resembles a hydrocele but does not transilluminate because the tunica has filled with blood (haematocele). Aspiration alone does not cure an idiopathic hydrocele and the tunica soon refills. It is possible to obliterate the sac by injecting a sclerosant after aspiration, but surgical excision and eversion is associated with a much lower recurrence rate. If the hydrocele fluid becomes infected, incision and drainage of the pus are necessary. Similarly, a haematocele may require treatment by incision and drainage.

Hydrocele is a common abnormality in children. It is due to failure of closure of the processus vaginalis after descent of the testis. This patent processus vaginalis allows fluid to drain into the scrotum around the testis. Most congenital hydroceles of this sort resolve before the first birthday. Those that persist require surgical treatment comprising ligation of the PPV through a small groin incision.

Cyst of the epididymis

Cysts in the epididymis arise from diverticula of the vasa efferentia. The distinction between a cyst of the epididymis and a hydrocele is easy. Epididymal cysts are almost always multiple and therefore nodular on palpation; are located above and behind the testis, which is palpably separate from the cysts; and always transilluminate brightly. A solitary epididymal cyst may even resemble a testis, so giving rise to fables of three testes and the term 'pawnbroker's sign'. Sometimes the fluid within an epididymal cyst is opalescent and contains sperm (spermatocele). Usually the fluid is clear. It is best to leave these cysts alone unless increasing size warrants excision. Careful dissection is needed to remove the cyst completely. Often several other little cysts are present which, if not removed, will eventually increase in size and produce a so-called recurrence. If all the cysts are removed, the pathway for sperm will almost certainly be damaged. Bilateral operations can result in sterility.

Varicocele

The veins of the pampiniform plexus are dilated and tortuous, producing a swelling in the line of the spermatic cord that resembles a 'bag of worms'. It is more common on the left side, possibly because of the right-angled drainage of the left testicular vein into the renal vein rendering it more liable to stasis. In some men varicocele is associated with infertility. A dragging sensation in the scrotum may cause concern. Treatment is by ligation of the spermatic vein, which may be done surgically (laparoscopically) at the internal inguinal ring or radiologically by embolization.

Infertility

Assessment

Although only the causes of male infertility are discussed here, the investigation and management of infertility does, of course, require the assessment of both partners. A detailed history is essential, particularly with regard to factors that may contribute to an abnormal sperm count. These include operations (e.g. for hernia), infections (mumps, tuberculosis and gonorrhoea) and certain drugs (nitrofurazone, cyclophosphamides and possibly some tranquillizers). Excessive smoking, alcohol intake, obesity and working in a hot environment may all suppress spermatogenesis. The patient should be asked about any psychosexual problems, including impotence or premature ejaculation. Physical examination may be entirely normal. Physical build and hair distribution are noted. Testicular size is a crude but useful guide to spermatogenic potential. For example, a tall male with female hair distribution and pea-sized testes almost certainly has Klinefelter's syndrome. Examination of the scrotum may reveal dilated spermatic veins (varicocele).

Investigation

The principal investigation is the analysis of seminal fluid. Values given as 'normal' are only a guide, as pregnancy can occur even with low sperm concentrations (oligozoospermia). However, the lower the concentration of sperm the less the chance of pregnancy. If a patient has no sperm (azoospermia) it is necessary to distinguish between obstruction and primary failure of spermatogenesis. This may be possible by measuring plasma gonadotrophins (FSH, follicle-stimulating hormone). A normal value indicates obstruction, which is usually in the epididymis. In these patients the testes are also normal in size. More detailed tests such as immunological compatibility and chromosome analysis may be necessary.

Management

There is no treatment for a patient with azoospermia due to primary spermatogenic failure. Testicular biopsy to confirm the diagnosis is all that is possible. Azoospermia due to obstruction may be treated by bypass (epididymovasostomy). This may be successful if the obstruction is in the tail of the epididymis. However, if it is elsewhere in the epididymis or the vasa efferentia, the results are generally poor. In these circumstances aspiration or biopsy can usually recover sperm. The introduction of intracytoplasmic sperm injection (ICSI), which requires only a single sperm for fertilization, has greatly increased the pregnancy rate in those circumstances. Patients with oligozoospermia are initially advised to reduce their weight, improve dietary and smoking habits, and (if possible) adjust their occupation or working environment. It is important to ensure that the patient understands the basis of reproductive biology, especially the timing of intercourse in relation to the menstrual cycle. These measures alone often lead to a successful pregnancy. The role of a varicocele as a cause of infertility remains controversial. There is evidence that some varicoceles affect testicular temperature and, therefore, spermatogenesis. Most series have shown improvements in seminal quality following the ligation, but none of these studies is controlled. Drug treatment for oligozoospermia is disappointing; clinical trials are in progress but no one treatment can at present be recommended. If infertility is due to antisperm antibodies, courses of high-dose steroids may be of use.

Vasectomy and vasectomy reversal

Bilateral ligation of the vasa deferentia, in the neck of the scrotum, is now widely practised as a form of permanent contraception. This is usually done as an outpatient procedure under local anaesthesia. Each vas is divided and ligated, and the ends are separated in order to avoid recanalization. It is essential to repeat the semen analysis 6–8 weeks postoperatively to confirm azoospermia. Two negative tests are required for assurance that fertilization cannot occur, but the patient is still warned of the very rare chance of recanalization. Reversal of a vasectomy may be requested, usually because of remarriage. Reported pregnancy rates vary from 50% to 80% following microsurgical repair.

30 Neurosurgery
I.R. Whittle, L. Myles

INTRODUCTION

Although surgery has been performed on the brain since antiquity, neurosurgery as we would recognize it today dates back no more than 120 years. Over the last 50 years there have been major advances in neuroimaging, neuro-anaesthesia, surgical instrumentation, neuropharmacology, microsurgery and, most recently, computer-assisted surgery.

SURGICAL ANATOMY AND PHYSIOLOGY

The skull

The skull is made up of the skull base and the calvarial skeleton, which comprises the frontal bone, the paired parietal and temporal bones and the occipital bone. The frontal and parietal bones are joined by the coronal suture, the parietal bones by the sagittal (midline) suture, and the parietal and occipital bones by the squamosal sutures. These sutures close at about 18 months, and thereafter the brain is enclosed in a rigid container. The skull base comprises the orbital roof, cribiform plates and sphenoid bones (anterior cranial fossa); sphenoid wings and petrous temporal bone (middle cranial fossa); and the squamous occipital bones, the clivus and petrous temporal regions (posterior cranial fossa). The cranial cavity is subdivided by thick folds of dura. The falx separates the two cerebral hemispheres and the tentorium separates the middle from the posterior cranial fossa. At the base of the posterior cranial fossa is the foramen magnum, through which the medulla projects inferiorly towards the spinal cord.

The spine

The bony axial spinal skeleton comprises seven cervical, 12 thoracic and five lumbar vertebrae, as well as the sacrum and coccyx. Although vertebral structure varies between regions, they are basically comprised of a body, pedicles, lamina and a posterior spine. The bony spinal canal is formed by the body (anteriorly), the pedicles (laterally) and the lamina (posteriorly). The canal contains the spinal dura, the spinal cord and, inferiorly, the cauda equina. The vertebral bodies are joined by fibroelastic discs and articulate via facet joints.

The brain

The brain is a gelatinous structure which in adults weighs about 1.4 kg. It comprises the paired cerebral hemispheres, the brain stem and the cerebellum. Primary fissures divide the brain into lobes (frontal, parietal, occipital, temporal and limbic). The temporal lobe is separated from the frontal and parietal lobes by the sylvian fissure and the rolandic (central) sulcus separates the frontal from the parietal lobes. Commissural fibres, the largest of which is the corpus callosum, connect the cerebral hemispheres. Cortical grey matter lies on the surface of the brain and comprises laminae of neurons which project into the white matter (tracts). Important deep cortical nuclear regions include the basal ganglia, thalamus and hypothalamus. The brain stem comprises the midbrain, pons and medulla. The cerebellum attaches to the back of the pons and is responsible for movement, coordination, balance and posture.

The coverings

The brain and spinal cord are encased by the meninges. The outer layer is like leather and is called the dura. The two inner layers are much finer: a spider's web-like tissue, the arachnoid, and a very thin layer over the surface of the brain called the pia. Between arachnoid and pia lies the cerebrospinal fluid (CSF) space. The CSF is secreted from the choroid plexus. Paired lateral ventricles communicate via the foramina of Munro with the third ventricle, which communicates via the aqueduct with the fourth ventricle in the pons and medulla. Outflow foramina connect with the spinal subarachnoid space.

Cranial nerves

The 12 paired cranial nuclei arise from the base of the brain. The optic nerves connect through the optic tracts to the lateral geniculate body of the thalamus. The olfactory nerve tracts connect the olfactory bulbs to the rhinencephalon ('old smell brain'). The third (oculomotor) and fourth (trochlear) cranial nerves project from the midbrain and control ocular motility. The fifth (trigeminal) nerve provides sensation to the face, as well as innervating the muscles of mastication. The sixth (abducens) nerve controls abduction of the eye. The seventh (facial) nerve rises from the pontomedullary junction and controls the facial musculature. The eighth (vesibulocochlear nerve) conveys hearing from the cochlea and balance from the labyrinth. The ninth (glossopharyngeal), tenth (vagus), 11th (accessory) and 12th (hypoglossal) nerves project from the medulla to innervate the tongue, pharynx, bronchus and intestines.

The spinal cord

The spinal cord consists of grey (neurons) and white (tracts) matter and gives off eight cervical, 12 thoracic, five lumbar and four sacral paired spinal roots. Each root comprises a ventral and a dorsal rootlet. The spinal cord is enlarged in the lower cervical region and at the L1–2 region (conus). The lower part of the spinal canal contains the nerve roots that innervate the lower limbs, bladder and genitalia (cauda equina).

BLOOD SUPPLY

The brain requires a large blood flow (800 mL/min, 16% of cardiac output) to satisfy its oxygen and glucose requirements. The anterior and posterior circulations of the brain communicate with each other and across the midline through the circle of Willis (Fig. 30.1). In some circumstances occlusion of a major artery can be compensated for by collateral flow.

Anterior circulation

The major vessels supplying the anterior circulation of the brain are the paired internal carotid arteries. These arise from the common carotid artery, pass through the skull base and cavernous sinus, and then divide into the anterior and middle cerebral arteries. Smaller but important branches include the posterior communicating artery, which interconnects the anterior and posterior circulations, the anterior choroidal arteries, and fine perforating vessels to the inferior part of the brain. The anterior cerebral arteries supply large parts of the frontal and medial parts of the parietal lobes. The middle cerebral artery supplies the posterior frontal and most of the temporal and parietal regions.

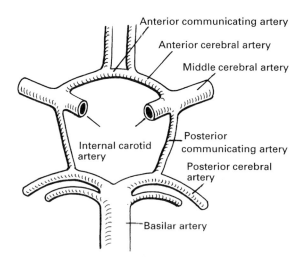

Fig. 30.1 Circle of Willis.

Posterior circulation

The posterior cerebral circulation arises from paired vertebral arteries that pass through the cervical foramina, enter
the skull and join to form a single midline basilar artery.
This divides terminally into the paired posterior cerebral
arteries. The posterior cerebral arteries communicate with
the anterior circulation through the posterior communicating arteries. The posterior circulation supplies the brain
stem, cerebellum, occipital lobes and inferior parts of the
temporal lobes. Because many of these are 'end-arteries',
occlusion often leads to a well-defined stroke syndrome.

INTRACRANIAL PRESSURE

The brain is enclosed within a rigid bony container.
Intracranial pressure (ICP) therefore depends on the relative
volumes of intracranial blood, CSF and brain parenchyma.
ICP also fluctuates throughout life in response to changes in
intrathoracic pressure (coughing, defaecation) and cardiac
pulsation. These transient increases do no harm. In a normal
supine adult ICP is the same as the CSF pressure obtained at
lumbar puncture ($5–15$ cmH$_2$O, $4–10$ mmHg). In patients
with intracranial mass lesions (tumour, haemorrhage),
oedema or CSF obstruction the extra volume is at first compensated for by a reduction in blood and CSF volume.
However, a critical point is soon reached where no further
compensation is possible, and any additional volume will
lead to exponential rises in intracranial pressure.

The rate of growth of the intracranial mass is crucial to
the shape of the ICP pressure–volume curve. With more
chronic, slow-growing lesions such as brain tumours,
abscesses or congenital abnormalities, extraordinary
degrees of compensation can occur. In some situations even
massive lesions can lead to minimal symptoms and signs.

The cerebral perfusion pressure (CPP) equals mean arterial
pressure (MAP) less the ICP (CPP = MAP–ICP). Initially,
raised ICP leads to dilation of intracranial vessels (autoregulation), a reduction in peripheral resistance and maintenance of
an effective perfusion pressure. However, if there is a severe
and sustained elevation of ICP autoregulation will be ineffective and cerebral perfusion may be focally or general compromised, leading to cerebral ischaemia and infarction. A
CPP of > 60 mmHg is generally required to sustain adequate
cerebral perfusion. Although children and young adults can
tolerate lower levels, the consequences of a profound prolonged lowering of CPP are often devastating (e.g. following
severe head injury with raised ICP, or after cardiac arrest).

Herniation

Generalized or localized increases in ICP may lead to
marked displacement of intracranial structures (herniation)

Transfalcine herniation

The cingulate gyrus may herniate beneath the free edge of
the falx. The anterior cerebral artery may be compressed
sufficiently to cause medial hemispheric infarction, but
otherwise there are no obvious clinical signs except deteriorating conscious level.

Transtentorial herniation

The medial part of the temporal lobe is pushed down
through the tentorial notch to become wedged between the
tentorial edge and the midbrain (Fig. 30.2). The opposite
cerebral peduncle is pushed against the sharp tentorial
edge, and the midbrain and uncus become wedged at
the tentorium. The aqueduct is compressed, obstructing
CSF flow, and venous obstruction leads to midbrain
haemorrhage.

Foraminal herniation

The cerebellar tonsils and medulla are displaced downwards through the foramen magnum (Fig. 30.3). Cerebellar
impaction leads to medullary compression. This may
happen following the removal of CSF at lumbar puncture in
patients with raised ICP, and is also known as 'coning'.
There is a rapid deterioration in conscious level, with
decerebration. Lumbar puncture must not be performed in
patients suspected of having raised ICP.

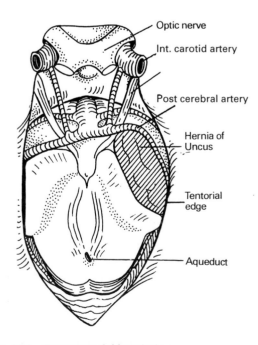

Fig. 30.2 Transtentorial herniation.

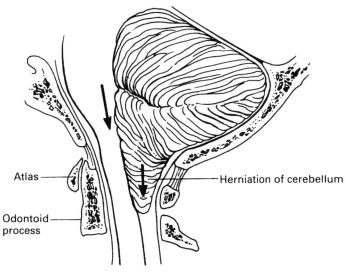

Fig. 30.3 Foraminal herniation.

Clinical features

The clinical features of acute ICP decompensation are classically seen as a result of traumatic extradural haematoma:

1. The Glasgow Coma Score (GCS) falls (Table 30.1)
2. The motor component of the GCS becomes asymmetrical.
3. The ipsilateral pupil dilates and becomes unreactive to light.
4. The blood pressure rises.
5. The pulse slows.
6. The respiratory rate falls and the patient become apnoeic.

This combination of signs denotes acute uncal herniation syndrome and is a medicosurgical emergency. Without intervention death is inevitable.

Generalized or localized increases in ICP may lead to marked displacement of intracranial structures (herniation)

Table 30.1	Glasgow Coma Scale	
Eyes open	Spontaneously	4
	To verbal command	3
	To pain	2
	No response	1
Best motor response to verbal command	Obeys verbal command	6
	Localizes pain	5
	Flexion withdrawal	4
to painful stimulus	Abnormal flexion (decorticate rigidity)	3
	Extension (decerebrate rigidity)	2
	No responses	1
Best verbal response	Orientated and converses	5
	Disorientated and converses	4
	Inappropriate words	3
	Incomprehensible sounds	2
	No response	1
Total number of points (minimum 3, maximum 15)		–

INVESTIGATIONS

Plain X-ray

Plain X-rays of the skull and spine may reveal evidence of metastatic tumour spread, narrowing of the intervertebral discs, congenital abnormalities, bony erosion due to tumour, or abnormal vascular markings. Calcification of the pineal gland or choroid plexus may allow displacement to be detected, and abnormal calcification can develop in certain cysts and tumours.

Computed tomography

Although computed tomography (CT) does not image brain tissue as well as magnetic resonance imaging (MRI), it is particularly good for imaging bony tissue and has the advantage that images can be acquired more simply and rapidly. Spiral CT allows the skull base and blood vessels to be reconstructed in remarkable detail.

Magnetic resonance imaging

MR images can be reconstructed in axial, coronal or sagittal planes. Because the water in bony tissue is tightly bound, the cranium is not as well visualized as it is with CT. However, as the cortical grey matter comprises approximately 78% water and white matter approximately 68% water, these two areas, as well as subnuclei within the brain, can be clearly distinguished. CSF is also well imaged. By using different sequencing techniques not only can the anatomy of the normal and abnormal brain be imaged in millimetre detail,

but so too can the function of brain tissues. MRI is limited by certain conditions (cardiac pacemakers, early pregnancy, certain metallic aneurysm clips). By employing certain contrast agents MRI (and CT) can be used to perform angiography (MRA, CTA). In some circumstances these non-invasive techniques are replacing conventional intra-arterial digital subtraction angiography (IA-DSA)

CEREBROVASCULAR DISEASE

Brain injury can be caused by vascular disease through either occlusion or haemorrhage. Occlusive disease predominantly affects the extracranial vessels and is a common cause of stroke and transient ischaemic attack, usually managed by vascular surgeons (see Chapter 27). In contrast, intracranial haemorrhage is managed by neurosurgeons and may be extradural, subdural, subarachnoid or intracerebral.

Subarachnoid haemorrhage

Spontaneous subarachnoid haemorrhage (SAH) affects 100 persons per million per year and most frequently (70%) results from the rupture of an intracranial 'berry' aneurysm. Other causes include arteriovenous malformation (AVM), cavernoma, tumour, infection and trauma.

Intracranial aneurysm

Risk factors include smoking, hypertension and female gender. The median age of affected patients is 47 years, although familial aneurysms may rupture earlier. Most aneurysms (85%) affect the anterior circulation and 15% of patients have more than one. The great majority have no symptoms until rupture occurs, although a few may suffer compressive symptoms, for example an oculomotor nerve palsy due to an aneurysm of the posterior communicating artery.

Clinical features

Typically the patient complains of a sudden onset of severe headache that peaks in intensity within 1 minute. Patients often describe it like being 'hit on the head with a hammer', or as 'the worst headache they have ever had'. There is usually associated neck stiffness and photophobia. A positive Kernig's sign denotes meningism. In some cases a small 'herald' bleed may go unnoticed, or only be remembered when a major bleed occurs. Nausea and vomiting are common. The patient's conscious level is variably affected (Table 30.2), ranging from mild disorientation to coma to rapid death. Sudden death is not uncommon when an aneurysm ruptures into the brain substance rather than the

WFNS grade	Glasgow Coma Score	Focal neurological deficits
Table 30.2 World Federation of Neurosurgical Societies' (WFNS) grading system for subarachnoid haemorrhage		
WFNS grade	Glasgow Coma Score	Focal neurological deficits
1	15	No
2	13–14	No
3	13–14	Yes
4	7–12	Yes/no
5	3–6	Yes/no

subarachnoid space. The focal signs depend upon the vessel affected. When symptoms and signs are mild the differential diagnosis is quite extensive, and diagnosis depends on having a high index of suspicion.

Investigation

The standard investigation is a CT scan, which characteristically shows blood in the CSF basal cisterns in the acute phase (Fig. 30.4). As CSF blood is broken down, the CT detection rate falls after the first 72 hours. If the diagnosis is in doubt then a lumbar puncture should be performed, but only in patients whose clinical condition is good and in whom CT has excluded an intracranial mass lesion or midline shift. If performed early, the CSF will be uniformly bloodstained; later it will contain haem pigments that will be apparent on naked-eye inspection (xanthochromia) or can be detected by spectrophotometry.

Next, a search must be made for the site of the bleeding. About 80% of aneurysms involve the anterior circulation. Conventionally, carotid or vertebral angiography has been performed (Fig. 30.5). However, CT and MR angiography are equally good at revealing aneurysms greater than 5 mm, and are non-invasive and so associated with less morbidity. As the consequences of missing a diagnosis of SAH are serious, there is a tendency to perform angiography in patients in whom the diagnosis is equivocal. For that reason, a source of bleeding will be identified in only 70% of angiograms. This is usually an aneurysm, less commonly an arteriovenous malformation or cavernoma. In 30% of cases no source is found. In the majority this is a 'true' negative, and many of these patients will have a condition called perimesencephalic SAH, which is of unknown aetiology.

Management

The medical management of SAH includes intravenous fluids, nimodipine, analgesia and antiemetics. Patients in coma will usually be intubated and managed in a

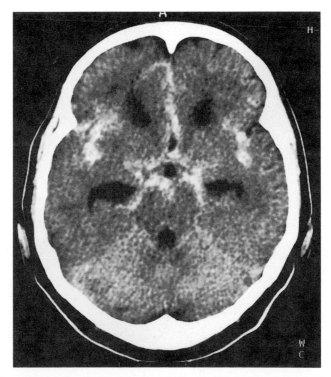

Fig. 30.4 Axial CT scan of a patient following subarachnoid haemorrhage. Blood is seen in the basal cisterns. There is also hydrocephalus.

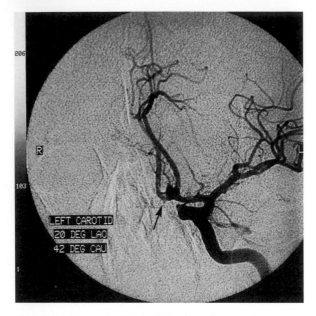

Fig. 30.5 Intra-arterial digital subtraction angiogram outlining the cerebral vasculature and showing an aneurysm of the anterior communicating artery (arrow).

neurointensive care unit. Having initially been quite well, many patients begin to exhibit signs of focal cerebral ischaemia 4–10 days following a SAH. This has been attributed primarily to vasospasm and can be ameliorated by the prophylactic use of the calcium antagonist nimodipine.

Rebleeding is a major cause of morbidity and mortality following aneurysm rupture. Standard surgical treatment entails occluding the aneurysm from the cerebral circulation by clipping its neck (Fig. 30.6) at operation. It has recently become possible to place detachable coils within the aneurysm via a catheter passed into the cerebral circulation (Fig. 30.7). The coils unwind in the aneurysm and induce thrombosis. Although coiling is a much less invasive procedure, only a proportion of aneurysms are suitable. A randomized control trial is currently comparing the clinical and cost effectiveness of surgery and coiling.

Even when an aneurysm has been successfully excluded by means of coiling or surgery, the patient can still suffer stroke. Although nimodipine has significantly decreased the risk of stroke and death there is still no effective treatment for delayed cerebral ischaemia following SAH. Clinical practice has included the induction of hypertension and volume loading (to keep up CPP), as well as haemodilution (to reduce blood viscosity in the hope of increasing flow), but this triple therapy has its own problems, such as heart failure.

The outcome following aneurysmal SAH is heavily dependent upon the condition of the patient on admission. Patients admitted in good condition (grade 1) enjoy a complete recovery in about 90% of cases. By contrast, about 50% of those admitted in coma (grade 5) die or are severely disabled. The outcome of intermediate patients is unpredictable and not necessarily dependent on the clinical excellence of either the attending surgeon or interventional neuroradiologists.

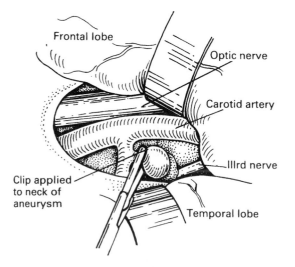

Fig. 30.6 Treatment of an intracranial aneurysm by clipping of the neck.

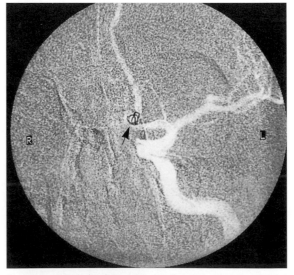

Fig. 30.7 Digital subtraction angiogram showing initial coil placement in an anterior communicating artery aneurysm (arrow).

Primary intracerebral haemorrhage

Primary intracerebral haemorrhage (PICH) is four times commoner than SAH. It increases with age and is particularly common in hypertensive patients and those with amyloid angiopathy. In hypertension, the perforating arteries of the middle cerebral arteries develop microaneurysms that rupture and tear open the internal capsule. Many such haemorrhages are small and deep; others may be very large and cause death by raising ICP and causing herniation. Other causes include the rupture of a 'berry' aneurysm or arteriovenous malformation (AVM). The onset is usually abrupt, with most patients entering coma and developing a flaccid hemiparesis. One-third of patients die within a few days and most of those who survive are permanently disabled. Emergency removal of the haematoma is not usually successful if it is deep and large. If patients survive the initial bleed then haematoma evacuation may be of value. The role of surgery in PICH is being evaluated in a multinational randomized controlled trial.

Arteriovenous malformations

Cerebral arteriovenous malformations are congenital abnormalities of the capillary system that lead to a direct arteriovenous communication (fistula). This leads to gross dilatation of the draining cerebral veins, as well as ectasia and occasionally aneurysmal dilatation of the feeding artery. AVMs can lead to cerebral ischaemia (because blood preferentially enters the venous system, bypassing the tissues), focal seizures and haemorrhage. Rupture of an AVM typically causes an intracerebral haemorrhage rather than a SAH. As the haematoma is under less pressure the overall prognosis is better than for aneurysmal SAH. The diagnosis is confirmed on CT and angiography. If the AVM can be excised then the risk of further haemorrhage is removed and the incidence and frequency of seizures is considerably reduced. Sometimes, however, the AVM is large and in an important or inaccessible location. In this case endovascular 'glueing' or stereotactic radiosurgical treatment is appropriate. The latter is a focused form of X-ray therapy that leads to fibrosis over a 2-year period. AVMs may also affect the spine and lead to cord ischaemia. Symptoms are often progressive and include pain, weakness and, ultimately, paraplegia. The treatment is excision.

Cavernomas

These are well-circumscribed collections of small vascular channels (usually capillaries). They typically present as headaches, focal neurological deficits or even epilepsy, owing to small, recurrent focal haemorrhages. CT and angiography often miss these lesions, but they have a characteristic appearance on MRI and may be much more common than was previously appreciated. Those causing epilepsy or haemorrhage are usually excised, unless they are in a vital and/or inaccessible place (e.g. brain stem). The risk of rebleeding from cavernomas and AVMs is poorly documented and prospective natural history studies are under way so that the risks and benefits of intervention can be better defined.

SUMMARY BOX

Vascular disorders and the central nervous system

- Symptoms due to occlusive vascular disease most often originate from blockage of extracranial vessels by atherosclerosis. Intracranial occlusion can be thrombotic or embolic.

- Transient ischaemic attacks are associated with a high risk of major stroke within 5 years unless treatment is instituted (e.g. by carotid endarterectomy or aspirin therapy).

- Intracranial haemorrhage may be extradural, subdural, subarachnoid or intracerebral. Extradural and subdural haemorrhage are usually the result of trauma; subarachnoid bleeding is due to rupture of an aneurysm in around 70% of cases, and intracerebral bleeding is frequently associated with hypertension and amyloid angiopathy.

- Surgical treatment of spontaneous intracerebral bleeding is currently being evaluated in a trial.

- Patients with subarachnoid haemorrhage from an aneurysm should be considered for either clipping or coiling of the aneurysm to avoid recurrent bleeding.

NEUROTRAUMA

Head injury comprises a large proportion of emergency neurosurgical practice. Primary brain injury occurs as a direct result of trauma. It may be diffuse or focal, of varying severity, and is essentially irreversible. Secondary brain injury occurs after the primary trauma as a result of hypotension, hypoxia, pyrexia, infection and raised ICP. Secondary brain damage can have a devastating effect on what may initially have been a relatively minor injury and amenable to prevention and treatment.

Assessment

Glasgow Coma Score

The Glasgow Coma Score (GCS) is a measure of conscious level and has greatly facilitated the classification and objective management of head-injured patients. It is used internationally and records the best verbal response, best motor response and eye opening. The maximum score is 15 and the minimum is 3. Change in GCS over time is much more informative than an absolute reading at any one point in time.

The Glasgow Coma Scale can be used in children of all ages. The *best verbal* component of the scale needs to be modified to take into account the age of the child, particularly in children under the age of four years.

Neurological examination

This should routinely include an assessment of pupillary size and reaction; a search for CSF leaks from nose, mouth and ears; a survey of the scalp for penetrating injuries; and an assessment of the maxillofacial skeleton.

Other systems

Patients with head injury often have extracranial injury. It is important to remember that head injury alone *never* causes hypovolaemic shock.

Management

As with all injured patients, management commences with airway, breathing and circulation. The neck should be immobilized until a cervical spine injury has been excluded. The GCS should be documented on arrival and following resuscitation, and the findings of a neurological survey recorded. Many patients with head injury are under the effects of alcohol and other drugs that affect conscious level. If in doubt, assume that depressed consciousness is due to brain injury. Continued monitoring of conscious level over time by means of GCS is a key aspect of management, and sedatives must be avoided.

In general, patients with a GCS of 8 or less are intubated and ventilated. This is to prevent hypoxia and aspiration pneumonitis, and to allow hyperventilation, which reduces the partial pressure of carbon dioxide in the blood and so lowers ICP through cerebral vasoconstriction.

Following resuscitation, stabilization and prioritization of injuries, a CT scan is performed. This will visualize intracranial haematoma, brain contusions (bruises), depressed bone fragments, intracranial air and associated maxillofacial fractures (Fig. 30.8). Mass lesions such as extradural haematoma, subdural haematoma and haemorrhagic contusions may cause brain swelling and shift and are often surgically evacuated.

Brain injury evolves over several days and the principal aim of management is to limit secondary damage due to ischaemia and brain herniation caused by raised intracranial

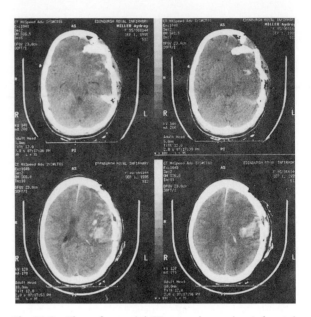

Fig. 30.8 These four axial CT scans show a large frontal depressed fracture, multiple left-sided brain contusions, effacement of the lateral ventricle and midline shift. This patient had been assaulted with a hammer.

pressure (ICP), hypoxia and hypotension. ICP is often severely elevated following neurotrauma, because of oedema, haematoma, contusions, engorgement of the brain vasculature, hydrocephalus or even infection. A sustained pressure that exceeds 25 mmHg is associated with a poorer outcome. Severely brain-injured patients are kept sedated and ventilated and an ICP monitor is inserted so that cerebral perfusion pressure (CPP) can be calculated. Hyperventilation, mannitol and barbiturates are used to reduce ICP, and the systemic blood pressure may be raised using fluids and inotropes. A common misconception is that brain-injured patients should be fluid restricted to avoid brain oedema. On the contrary, hypotension must be avoided at all costs.

Skull fracture

The presence of a skull fracture is an important pointer to the likelihood of significant primary and/or secondary brain injury, especially if accompanied by a depressed GCS. However, the absence of a fracture does not exclude life-threatening brain injury, particularly in young children. A patient without a fracture and a GCS of 15 has a risk of intracranial haematoma of 1:6000. If a fracture is present this rises to 1:30, and if the GCS is 14 or less this is 1:4. Plain X-ray will miss many fractures, particularly of the skull base.

Extradural haematoma

This is usually due to disruption of the middle meningeal vessels as a result of fracture of the temporal bone. The primary brain injury is often minimal, there is a typical 'lucid' interval and then rapid deterioration. In the past, haematomas used to be evacuated through burr holes. However, the use of CT scanning to locate the haematoma precisely has made burr holes redundant, and nowadays craniotomy is performed over the site of bleeding.

Subdural haematoma

This is more common than extradural haematoma and is due to laceration of vessels (especially small cerebral veins) on the brain surface. CT shows a haematoma that is concave on its inner surface. Craniotomy is performed to remove the haematoma and arrest the bleeding.

> **SUMMARY BOX**
>
> *Head Injury*
>
> Minor, GCS   13–15
> Moderate, GCS   8–12
> Severe, GCS   < 8
> May cause:
>
>   Extradural haematoma
>   Subdural haematoma
>   Intracerebral haematoma
>   Cerebral contusions
>   Diffuse axonal Injury
>
> Avoidance of hypotension, hypoxia, hypercapnia, pyrexia and ICP > 25 mmHg minimizes secondary brain damage.

INTRACRANIAL INFECTIONS

Infection of the central nervous system and its meninges acquires surgical importance if it produces a mass (abscess or oedema), hydrocephalus or osteomyelitis, or if it occurs as a result of a breach in or absence of the coverings of the brain. In developed countries intracranial infections are relatively uncommon in immunocompetent patients. However, immunocompromised patients, particularly those affected with HIV, frequently suffer from a range of opportunistic organisms, for example toxoplasmosis and tuberculosis. Infection may affect the scalp, cranium and meninges, as well as the brain itself (Fig. 30.9).

Bacterial infections

Brain abscess and subdural and epidural empyema usually present in a subacute manner with headache, seizures and

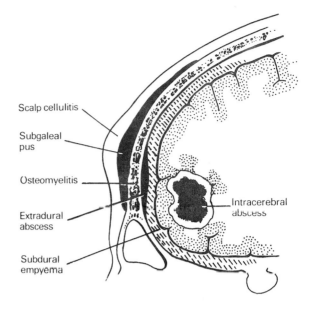

Fig. 30.9 Types of bacterial cranial infection.

focal neurological deficit. There may be an obvious source of concurrent infection, but in the majority of younger patients the infection appears to arise de novo. Treatment is a medicosurgical emergency. As well as loculations of pus, the other major problems are severe perilesional brain oedema and venous sinus thrombophlebitis. CT permits the rapid diagnosis and localization of pus and greatly facilitates surgical drainage, often through multiple burr holes. High-dose intravenous antibiotics should be prescribed and pus should be sent for Gram staining, culture and sensitivity. Anaerobic streptococci are the most common agents, although infections are often mixed. Dexamethasone can be used to reduce the brain oedema. Although the mortality from brain abscess and subdural empyema has fallen considerably owing to earlier diagnosis, patients frequently have significant neurological sequelae and there is a high incidence (50–60%) of postinfective seizures. Anticonvulsants are prescribed routinely and are often required indefinitely.

Osteomyelitis of the skull

Bone may become infected via penetrating wounds, during surgery, by local extension (from sinuses, middle ear or mastoid), or through bloodborne infection. Pus may track into the subgaleal space or involve the overlying scalp, or form a small extradural abscess. The infection is difficult to eradicate and may require the removal of large portions of calvarium and later replacement with acrylic plate.

Extradural abscess

This usually arises secondary to osteomyelitis and most often occurs close to the middle ear, mastoid air cells or paranasal sinuses. It may spread out through the skull or inwards through the dura to produce meningitis, subdural empyema or cerebral abscess. Systemic upset is usually severe. There is local tenderness, and focal neurological signs may result from thrombophlebitis and oedema. Facial nerve palsy may complicate mastoiditis.

Subdural abscess (empyema)

Pus may spread over the whole hemisphere and beneath the falx to involve the opposite hemisphere. It may accumulate in multiple sites, making treatment difficult.

Cerebral abscess

The brain is relatively resistant to infection but abscesses may form, particularly if there has been previous penetrating neurotrauma or immunocompromise. Initially there is cerebritis (encephalitis), following which the brain necroses to form pus surrounded by a tough glial capsule that is resistant to the passage of antibiotics. Abscess may form as a result of direct extension of infection or via haematogenous spread, for example in patients with bronchiectasis. The presentation may be acute, with high fever, seizures, reduced consciousness and evidence of raised ICP. If the infection is walled off it may simply present as a space-occupying lesion with little systemic upset. Surgical drainage is the mainstay of treatment. Sometimes, the abscess is excised, but most commonly drainage is performed by image-guided stereotactic aspiration.

Postsurgical infection

Postcraniotomy wound infections occur in less than 1% of procedures and are generally due to staphylococcus. Once the flap is colonized and a nidus of osteomyelitis has developed, the infection will not usually be eradicated by antibiotic therapy. Quite frequently, a sinus will develop along the line of the craniotomy scar and intermittently discharge pus. In most cases the flap needs to be removed and some form of cranioplastic procedure performed 9–12 months later. Fortunately, infection of the brain itself following surgery is extremely rare, even following the implantation of prosthetic material.

Meningitis

Although most forms of meningitis are treated by physicians, some involve neurosurgeons. For example, a dural tear following a skull base fracture leads to the egress of CSF into the paranasal sinuses or mastoid air cells. From there the CSF can pass through the Eustachian tube into the nasopharynx. Under these circumstances, pneumococcal infection can occur either early or extremely late following injury. Early treatment of post-CSF fistula meningitis is important, as this generally leads to a very satisfactory outcome. Conversely, failure to recognize the disorder can result in death. With post-traumatic CSF fistula there is no evidence that prophylactic antibiotics reduce the incidence of meningitis. If the CSF leak continues then the site of leakage needs to be surgically repaired.

INTRACRANIAL TUMOURS

Tumours of the skull

Osteoma

This is a relatively common, usually solitary, benign tumour that most frequently arises in a paranasal sinus or the orbit. It typically grows outwards to form a hard mass, but may grow inwards to compress the brain. It is excised if symptomatic.

Glomus jugulare tumours

These tumours arise in the middle ear and invade the posterior fossa. They often present with bleeding from the ear and may be seen as a soft fleshy red mass protruding through the eardrum. Deafness, tinnitus and facial paresis are common. Treatment is often by embolization, radical excision and radiotherapy.

Multiple myeloma

This usually affects patient over the age of 50 and is twice as common in men as in women. The tumour is multicentric and may involve bones outside the skull. It may be confused with metastatic disease. The treatment is cytotoxic chemotherapy.

Paget's disease

This condition of unknown aetiology leads to thickening, softening and deformity of the skull. Men and women are equally affected and it usually begins between the four and sixth decades. The disease process encroaches on the optic and auditory foramina, leading to visual and auditory disturbance. In 10% of cases it may undergo sarcomatous change. Surgical decompression of entrapped cranial nerves may be required.

Metastatic disease

The skull is a common site for metastases. The majority are osteolytic; those from the prostate and breast may be sclerotic.

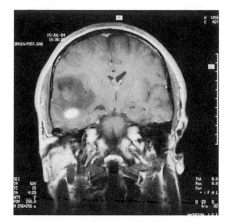

Fig. 30.10 This coronal MRI scan shows a right temporal mass lesion of low signal intensity, with an oval-shaped region of gadolinium enhancement. The latter suggests malignancy. This tumour was an anaplastic astrocytoma.

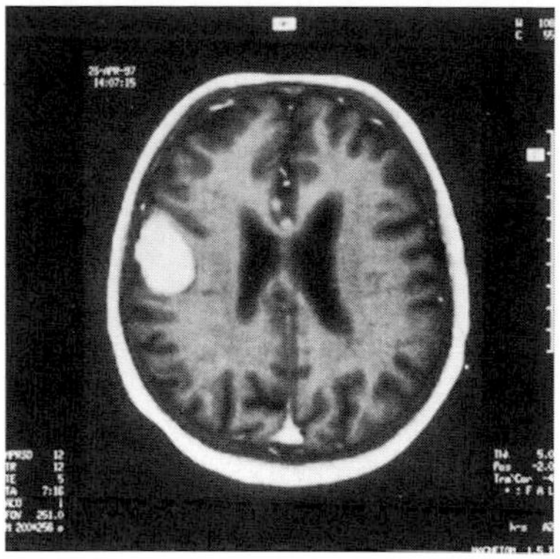

Fig. 30.11 Axial MRI showing a gadolinium-enhancing meningioma attached to the dura. There is no associated brain oedema. This was an asymptomatic tumour in an elderly patient.

Intracranial tumours

Glioma

Gliomas arise from the supporting cells of the brain (Fig. 30.10) are the most common brain primary tumour, and account for more than 50% of all primary intracranial tumours. Astrocytomas are often slow growing initially but may then become rapidly invasive (glioblastoma multiforme). The less common oligodendrogliomas are slow-growing, sometimes calcified, and have less tendency to infiltrate the brain. Complete removal of gliomas is often difficult owing to infiltration. Tumours in a single lobe may be treated by lobectomy. Recurrence is common despite postoperative radiotherapy

Ependymoma

These tumours arise from cells lining the ventricles. They most commonly occur in the fourth ventricle and cause hydrocephalus. They may emerge from the ventricle into the cisterna, spread over the brain stem and cause multiple cranial nerve palsies.

Meningiomas

These arise from the dura (Fig. 30.11) and account for 20% of all primary intracranial tumours. They usually arise from the skull convexity, skull base or sagittal sinus region. They may compress the motor cortex or temporal lobe and cause seizures. They are generally slow-growing but may spread widely over the dura, and may invade the skull to form a palpable mass. The treatment is excision.

Neurinomas

Cranial nerve tumours account for 5% of intracranial tumours and virtually all of them affect the vestibulocochlear nerves (acoustic neuroma or vestibular schwanoma) (Fig. 30.12). The tumour grows within, expands and erodes the internal auditory meatus. The seventh and eighth nerves become stretched over its surface as it grows in to the cerebellopontine angle. Early eighth-nerve symptoms include progressive nerve deafness, tinnitus and vertigo. Later seventh-nerve involvement leads to facial weakness. Larger tumours may involve the trigeminal nerve, leading to diminished facial sensation, as well as the pons and cerebellum leading to ataxia and nystagmus. Displacement of the fourth ventricle and aqueduct may lead to hydrocephalus.

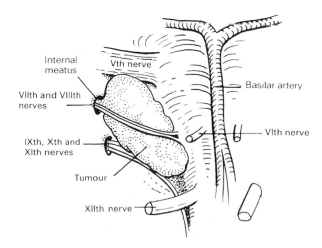

Fig. 30.12 Right acoustic neuroma.

Patients are often misdiagnosed as having Ménière's disease and the tumour may reach a large size before it is discovered. Treatment is excision, stereotactic radiosurgery or observation.

Pituitary tumours

These account for 15% of all intracranial tumours and produce symptoms through pressure and endocrine effects (pituitary adenomas). Typically pressure on the optic chiasma leads to bitemporal hemianopia.

Brain metastasis

Metastatic tumours are present at postmortem in 20% of patients dying of cancer, and in 50% they are multiple (Fig. 30.13). They most commonly arise from the lung, breast, kidney, melanoma and colon. Such metastases may be the presenting feature or appear only late in the course of a previously diagnosed primary cancer. Prostate cancer classically spreads to the cranium and never involves the brain parenchyma.

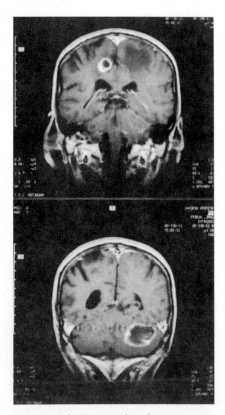

Fig. 30.13   Coronal MRI scan showing two gadolinium-enhancing lesions in the brain. The larger is in the cerebellum and the smaller in the cingulate region of the cerebral hemisphere. Both have low signal intensity centres, suggesting necrosis. The multiplicity of the lesions is highly suggestive of metastatic neoplasia. This patient has lung cancer.

Clinical features

Symptoms of raised ICP Intracranial tumours commonly present as an intracranial mass lesion, either from tumour volume itself or from surrounding oedema. This classically leads to morning headache that is aggravated by bending or straining. If the lesion is large there may be psychomotor slowing, that is, the patient does everything normally but does it slowly and apathetically. This is a generalized sign of brain hypofunction.

Focal neurological deficit This refers to any sign or symptoms that indicates focal neuronal hypofunction. The commonest is hemiparesis due to dysfunction of the motor cortex. Dysphasia occurs in about 50% of dominant hemispheric brain tumours and may be receptive, expressive or mixed. Visual field defects, dyslexia, dysgraphia and dyspraxia are also common.

Seizures These represent local neuronal hyperfunction. The disorder may be generalized, partial or focal, and their precise nature will reflect the anatomical position of the lesion. Seizures are more common with lower-grade tumours and may respond well to anticonvulsant therapy.

Personality disintegration There may behavioural disturbances and problems with judgement, memory and planning abilities. The patient usually has no insight into their progressive decline and may be referred initially to a psychiatrist.

Endocrinopathy Secondary amenorrhoea, galactorrhoea or (in men) loss of libido caused by a prolactin-secreting pituitary adenoma is the commonest example. Acromegaly, Cushing's syndrome, diabetes insipidus and precocious puberty may also occur.

Diagnosis

MRI and/or CT usually reveals the locality and pathology of the lesion and often shows the disease to be multifocal. The next step is to obtain a biopsy. Stereotactic biopsy involves a 2.5 cm incision, a burr hole and the insertion of a biopsy needle under CT/MRI guidance. The procedure is accurate to within 1 mm and diagnostic tissue is obtained in 98% of cases. The morbidity and 30-day mortality are low (< 5% and < 2%, respectively) and generally related to the disease rather than to the procedure.

Management

Tumours are often surrounded by oedema and the administration of dexamethasone can lead to a dramatic reduction in symptoms and signs over a 12–24-hour period. How steroids work in brain tumours is not well understood, but their use has led to a major reduction in morbidity and mortality. Excision of the lesion is warranted to reduce mass effect, control seizures and restore lost brain function. If the preoperative neuroradiology suggests a malignant glioma then extensive resection may provide optimal symptomatic control, a smoother course during radiotherapy and a reduction in steroid requirement. If the lesion is a meningioma then a total excision is generally planned, as this is a benign lesion. Similarly, if a posterior fossa lesion looks like a vestibular schwannoma, complete excision would be the treatment of choice. During excisional surgery a whole variety of adjunctive techniques can be used, ranging from the use of surgical ultrasonic aspirators to the use of intraoperative localization techniques, as well as cortical stimulation of the brain of the awake patient with neurophysiological assessment. The latter technique is extremely useful in operating in areas of eloquent brain, such as the language cortex and motor region.

Outcome after surgical resection is influenced by many factors, but for malignant gliomas the 30-day mortality is around 5% and neurological morbidity around 10%. Common complications include iatrogenic neurological deficits, cavity and extradural haematomas, and superficial wound infections. Patients with glioblastoma who have biopsy, or excision, and external beam radiotherapy survive a median of 9–10 months. Patients with anaplastic gliomas have a median survival of around 2 years. Meningioma cure and recurrence rates depend primarily on the extent of excision, but vary between 9 and 18% at 5 years. Except for anaplastic oligodendroglioma, there is no convincing role for chemotherapy in any primary brain neoplasm. Outcome following surgical excision of brain metastases depends on the state of the primary disease as well as the locality and multiplicity of intracranial disease. Excision plus radiotherapy of a solitary metastasis is typically associated with a median survival of 7 months.

Paediatric neuro-oncology

Tumours of the central nervous system are the second most common tumours of childhood after leukaemia. The incidence of paediatric central nervous system tumours in the UK is 15 per million of the paediatric population. In children under the age of 2 years the commonest tumours are teratomas, astrocytomas or primitive neuroectodermal tumours (PNET). These may occur anywhere in the central nervous system. Between the ages of 2 and 15 years the commonest site for tumours is in the posterior fossa, the most common being PNET (also known as medulloblastoma when found in the posterior fossa), astrocytoma and ependymoma (Fig. 30.14).

There may be an insidious onset of symptoms, such as lethargy, nausea and vomiting, with progressive ataxia in posterior fossa tumours. The symptoms of raised intracranial pressure (headache, drowsiness, nausea and vomiting) due to hydrocephalus or to the mass effect of the tumour itself may be the factors precipitating admission. Not infrequently children with posterior fossa tumours present with a torticollis, which is persistent and not related to trauma. General surgeons may be asked to see a child because of persistent vomiting and weight loss, with no other symptoms or signs. Suprasellar tumours such as craniopharyngioma may present with visual failure, hydrocephalus or endocrine dysfunction. Brain-stem gliomas may present with cranial nerve deficits.

One should take seriously the information that a previously well child has lost ground or fallen behind its peers. A clumsy child may have ataxia. Endocrine dysfunction may show as short stature, obesity or cachexia. Optic atrophy or papilloedema should always be looked for, as visual problems are difficult to diagnose in small children and visual failure may be profound at the time of presentation. Hemiparesis is occasionally the presenting feature of a hemispheric neoplasm. Spinal cord tumours, although rare in children, may present with back pain, scoliosis, limb weakness or bladder dysfunction. Occasionally children will present in coma because of a catastrophic bleed into a tumour, or the rapid onset of obstructive hydrocephalus.

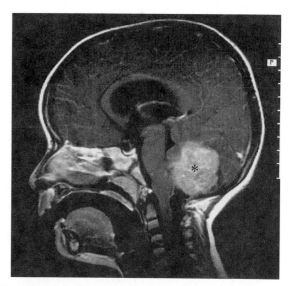

Fig. 30.14 Sagittal MRI of a medulloblastoma. The tumour (*) can be seen filling the fourth ventricle between the pons anteriorly and the cerebellum posteriorly. There is associated obstructive hydrocephalus due to blockage of CSF flow through the fourth ventricle.

If in doubt the investigation of choice is MRI, but a CT scan with contrast will often make the diagnosis. MRI should image the spine in order to exclude spinal metastases. The child should be referred to a paediatric neurosurgeon as a matter of urgency. Treatment consists of a combination of surgery, chemotherapy and radiotherapy. Surgical excision remains the mainstay of treatment in most cases, but is usually not curative by itself in malignant tumours, e.g. PNET, ependymoma, malignant astrocytoma. Surgery alone may be curative in the benign tumours, e.g. pilocytic astrocytoma, low-grade glioma, pineocytoma. Radiotherapy cannot be used in children under the age of 3 because of the risk of damaging the developing brain. Between 3 and 8 years of age radiotherapy may cause loss of IQ and other neurodevelopmental delays, but to a lesser extent. Some tumours are chemosensitive, e.g. germinomas, but most of the childhood brain tumours have had a disappointing response to chemotherapy, although it has a role as adjunctive treatment and as a treatment for recurrent disease. The prognosis for PNET is poor, with only 50% of children surviving for 5 years. In those children who are older than 3 years at the time of presentation, with no CSF seeding or metastatic disease and with a gross total excision of tumour at the time of surgery, the prognosis is better, with 5-year survival as high as 70%. Benign astrocytomas of the posterior fossa in children do well with complete surgical excision alone, and 90% 5-year survival is the norm.

SPINAL DYSRAPHISM

This is a congenital abnormality of the spine and underlying spinal cord, meninges and nerves owing to failure of the neural tube to close. Closure usually begins in the mid-dorsal region and extends cranially and caudally. Thus, thoracic defects are rare, cervical defects uncommon, and

> ### SUMMARY BOX
>
> *Tumours affecting the skull and its contents*
>
> - Common tumours involving the skull are osteomas and metastatic deposits. Less common tumours include deposits of multiple myeloma, histiocytosis, glomus jugulare tumours and chordomas.
>
> - Intracranial tumours have a bimodal age distribution (peaks at 6–7 years and fifth decade). Almost 50% of intracranial tumours are metastatic (most common primary sources are lung and breast).
>
> - Primary cerebral tumours arise from the supporting cells of the brain (gliomas), from the walls of ventricles (ependymomas) and from the roof of the fourth ventricle (medulloblastomas). They constitute about 60% of intracranial tumours
>
> - Meningiomas account for 20% of intracranial tumours (90% of meningiomas are supratentorial), grow slowly, can cause focal seizures, and are treated by excision.
>
> - Pituitary and parapituitary (craniopharyngioma and cholesteatoma) account for 15% of all intracranial tumours. Pituitary tumours may be functional, both types can cause pressure effects and both types are best removed surgically.
>
> - Neurinomas of the cranial nerves account for 5% of all intracranial tumours, Acoustic neurinomas develop in the internal auditory meatus and involve the seventh and eighth cranial nerves, to cause deafness, tinnitus, vertigo and facial weakness. Involvement of the fifth nerve may cause loss of facial sensation.

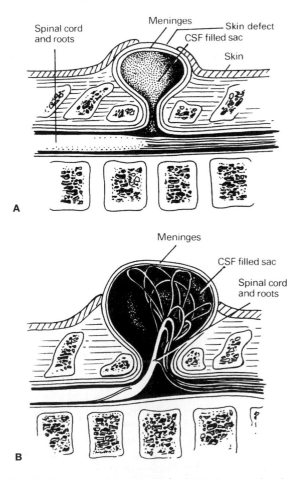

Fig. 30.15 A Simple meningocele. B Meningomyelocele.

most affect the lumbar/lumbosacral region. Fortunately, maternal folate supplementation and prenatal screening for raised serum α-fetoprotein at 16 weeks' gestation have reduced the incidence of this condition.

Open spinal dysraphism

This is also known as classic spina bifida aperta (Fig. 30.15). Simple meningocele is usually lumbar and results from a failure of the lamina to fuse. The subarachnoid space is distended and protrudes through the defect. The arachnoid fuses with the skin, forming a membrane to which the nerve roots can adhere. The cord, however, is normal and the child neurologically intact.

In meningomyelocele spinal nerve roots and the cord adhere to the membrane because of distension of the central canal, and may be exposed to the surface. The child usually has lower motor neuron signs below the level of the

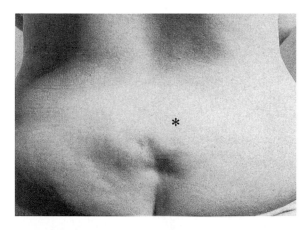

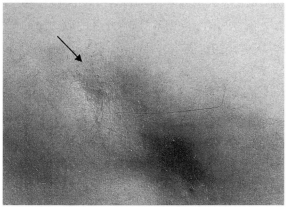

Fig. 30.16 The skin 'signatures' of closed spinal dysraphism. Note the fatty lump over the spine (*) with hairy patch (arrow) and angioma. Each of these abnormalities may be seen in isolation.

lesion and a neurogenic bladder (paralysis of the detrusor and pelvic floor muscles). Affected children often develop hydrocephalus following surgical closure of the spinal lesion, and require ventriculoperitoneal shunting. They usually have an associated abnormality of the hindbrain known as a Chiari II malformation, which may cause respiratory or feeding difficulties. These children require lifelong follow-up in a multidisciplinary clinic where the renal tract, neurological status and orthopaedic deformities can be regularly reviewed.

Closed spinal dysraphism

This is also known as spina bifida occulta. The condition may be apparent at birth owing to the characteristic overlying skin lesions, which include midline lumbar lipomas, hairy patches, dimples and sinuses (Fig. 30.16). However, the diagnosis may not be noted until later in childhood, when the child develops neurological symptoms (often following minor trauma or a growth spurt) and/or recurrent urinary tract infections. Late neurological deterioration and/or bladder dysfunction are due to tethering of the developing spinal cord at the level of the lesion. The treatment is surgical untethering. Other causes include splitting of the cord by a bony projection from the posterior surface of the vertebral body (diastematomyelia) (which can be removed), and the presence of intracord lipomata, which are often diffuse and multiple and whose removal is difficult and hazardous. Dural sinus tracts may lead to meningitis. In general, affected individuals do not develop hydrocephalus and there is no association with the Chiari malformation.

HYDROCEPHALUS

CSF is produced by the interventricular choroid plexus and passes from the lateral ventricles via the narrow foramen of Munro into the slit-like third ventricle, and then through the aqueduct of the upper brain stem to the fourth ventricle. From here the fluid passes via exit foramina into the cisterna magna and then flows over the surface of the brain and spinal cord to be absorbed by cerebral veins and arachnoid granulations. Hydrocephalus is the accumulation of CSF within the ventricles or over the surface of the brain. This may be due to overproduction of CSF (because of a choroid plexus papilloma), but the vast majority are due to reduced drainage secondary to obstruction of normal CSF flow (Fig. 30.17). Obstruction may be congenital such as in aqueduct stenosis (Fig. 30.18) or acquired as a result of tumour or fibrosis after infection or haemorrhage. Hydrocephalus due to obstruction to flow within the ventricular system, leading to dilatation of the ventricles, is

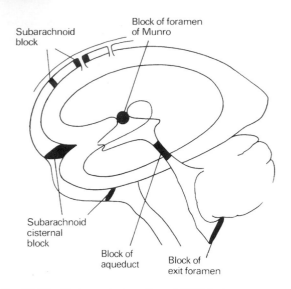

Fig. 30.17 Hydrocephalus: sites of CSF blockage.

termed 'internal', 'non-communicating' or 'obstructive'. In 'external' or 'communicating' hydrocephalus the ventricular system is patent but there is reduced absorption of CSF in the basal cisterns by the arachnoid granulations in the basal cisterns. This is commonly due to fibrosis following meningitis or subarachnoid haemorrhage, or to sagittal sinus thrombosis. In this type the ventricles and the CSF spaces around the surface of the brain will be enlarged.

Congenital hydrocephalus usually presents at birth or in early infancy. The cranial sutures may start to open and the fontanelle will be tense and bulging. The veins of the scalp and the bridge of the nose will be dilated. As the hydrocephalus worsens the eyes may become downcast (sunsetting). The child may be floppy and develop apnoeic spells and episodes of bradycardia.

In older children and children with closed fontanelles the symptoms are those of raised ICP (headache, vomiting and drowsiness). Bradycardia may also be present. The eyes may develop a squint owing to cranial nerve palsies. Papilloedema may be present and, if severe or chronic, may lead to blindness. Growth may be retarded.

Treatment consists of relieving the pressure by bypassing the block to CSF drainage. In some cases of aqueduct stenosis this can be done in a minimally invasive way by endoscopic third ventriculostomy. In this procedure a small hole is formed in the floor of the third ventricle, allowing CSF to flow into the basal cisterns. In most cases, however, a ventriculoperitoneal (VP) shunt will have to be inserted (Fig. 30.19). This consists of a catheter in the lateral ventricle which drains CSF through a valve (which sits on the skull under the scalp) into the peritoneal cavity. The risk of bleeding into the ventricular system or brain during the insertion or removal of a VP shunt is of the order of 1–2%. There is also a risk of early infection, usually with skin commensal organisms such as *Staphylococcus albus* or

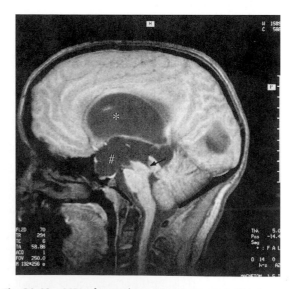

Fig. 30.18 MRI of aqueduct stenosis (arrow). This is an example of an obstructive hydrocephalus. There is gross ventricular enlargement (*) and herniation of the floor of the third ventricle into the interpeduncular cistern (#).

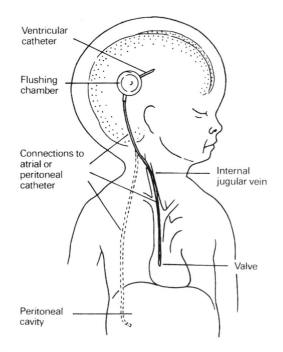

Fig. 30.19 Ventriculoatrial and ventriculoperitoneal shunt for hydrocephalus.

aureus. Shunts can become blocked or malfunction, causing a rapid return of symptoms, and this is a medical emergency. Prompt referral to a neurosurgeon is required. Shunts can also become infected many months or years after insertion, in which case the shunt has to be removed and reinserted once the infection has cleared. Occasionally a shunt will overdrain the ventricles, leading to premature closure of the cranial sutures and microcephaly. Overdrainage may be symptomatic, with headache and vomiting. It also predisposes to blockage of the ventricular catheter.

The long-term prognosis depends very much on the underlying cause of the hydrocephalus. In cases of simple aqueduct stenosis treated early, the prognosis for normal IQ and normal neurological function is good. Repeated episodes of raised intracranial pressure or ventriculitis can lead to loss of IQ and neurological deficit.

MALFORMATIONS OF THE SKULL

Abnormalities of the scalp and skull are often a source of worry for parents. The common problems are moulding at the time of birth, which is self-limiting, and scalp haematomas caused by ventouse extractions. These usually resolve spontaneously. Subgaleal haematomas in infants, often related to underlying skull fractures, can be extensive and can cause the haemoglobin to drop significantly.

Growing skull fractures are peculiar to infancy and are caused when a fracture is associated with an underlying dural tear. The CSF pulsations cause the edges of the bone at the fracture site to absorb, and the child may present some months later with a palpable skull defect in the line of the fracture. The treatment is to repair the dura. The defect can be repaired with bone, but this is not always required.

Craniosynostosis

This refers to the premature closure (before 4 years) or absence of a cranial suture (Fig. 30.20) and leads to asymmetrical skull growth. Fusion of a single suture is associated with certain typical head shapes. Sometimes more than one suture can be affected. Craniosynostosis may lead to a reduction in cranial volume and raised ICP. Surgery can be undertaken to remodel the skull into a more acceptable shape if necessary, or to increase the cranial volume.

Cranial dermal sinuses and angular dermoids

Dermal sinuses are midline tracts lined with squamous epithelium that may communicate with the intracranial

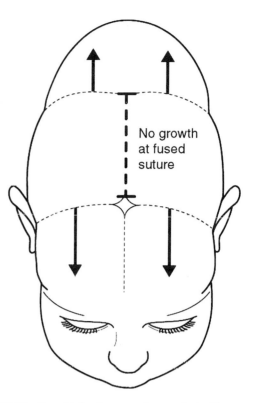

Fig. 30.20 Saggittal suture craniosynostosis. The sagittal suture is prematurely fused (dashed line). Growth normally occurs perpendicular to the suture line. In this case the skull cannot widen as there is no growth at the fused suture, which may be palpable as a ridge in the midline. There is compensatory growth at the coronal and lambdoid sutures, leading to an elongated head shape (scaphocephaly), with bulging of the forehead (frontal bossing) in severe cases.

cavity and may predispose to meningitis. They are also found in the spine. In the head most are found in the occipital region; 70–80% are associated with inclusion dermoids and 80% extend subdurally. In the face, because of the complex embryology dermoids can be found at the tip of the nose and the lateral aspect of the eye.

FUNCTIONAL NEUROSURGERY

A relatively small but highly specialized branch of neurosurgical practice involves the treatment of movement disorder, intractable epilepsy, and even certain cases of psychiatric disorders.

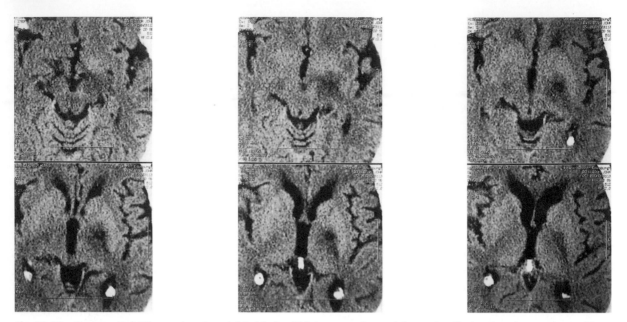

Fig. 30.21 Postsurgical CT scan showing right-sided pallidotomy performed for motor fluctuations in a patient with Parkinson's disease.

Movement disorders

Surgery for movement disorders such as tremor (Parkinson's disease), dystonia, chorea and tics involves selecting a target within the central nervous system for either ablation (Fig. 30.21) or stimulation (Fig. 30.22). The latter is thought safer and is thus preferred. Neural transplantation is still

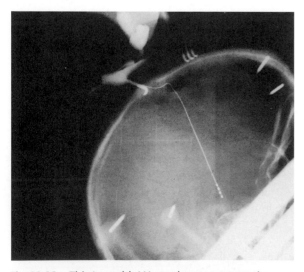

Fig. 30.22 This 'on-table' X-ray shows stereotactic placement of a deep brain electrode into the thalamus of a patient with intractable movement disorder.

being evaluated and involves the implantation of functional tissues into the target brain areas in the hope that they will produce missing neurosecretory products. These various techniques are currently the subject of ongoing trials.

Epilepsy

Neurosurgical intervention for epilepsy is appropriate where medical treatment has failed, and the seizure has a focal onset and a structural disorder of the brain associated with the disorder that relates to the seizure focus. The commonest indication for surgery is in complex partial seizures, usually known as temporal lobe epilepsy. Many of these patients will either have a hamartoma or a low-grade neoplasm that is causing the seizure disorder or, alternatively, have a condition termed hippocampal sclerosis which leads to chronic seizures. Resection of the involved temporal tissues and hippocampus leads to the cessation of seizure disorder in about 80% of cases. The success rates for surgery in non-temporal epilepsy are lower.

VERTEBRAL COLUMN

Degenerative disease

Each intervertebral disc comprises two cartilage end-plates that adhere to the vertebral bodies, a central semifluid

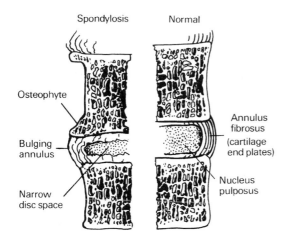

Spondylosis   Normal

Osteophyte

Annulus
fibrosus
(cartilage
end plates)

Bulging
annulus

Narrow
disc space

Nucleus
pulposus

Fig. 30.23   Intervertebral disc.

nucleus pulposus, and the slightly elastic annulus fibrosus that surrounds and retains it. Degenerative changes in the intervertebral discs are common at all levels. In response to acute or chronic trauma the nucleus pulposus may protrude (herniate) through either the annulus or the end-plate (Fig. 30.23). Horizontal protrusion usually occurs postero-laterally and may compress the cord or nerve roots. Such herniation is usually gradual and intermittent, so that symptoms remit between exacerbations. Acute herniation due to severe trauma or flexion injury may lead to (central) posterior herniation, with sudden neurological deficit. Disc degeneration is associated with loss of 'disc space' height. This throws abnormal strain on the intervertebral (apophyseal) joints, leading to osteophyte formation and narrowing of the intervertebral foramina. This condition is known as spondylosis and may lead to nerve root – even cord – compression. Spinal osteoarthritis may also affect the posterior apophyseal joints, leading to back pain. However, unlike with spondylosis, there is no nerve root compression and so no radiation of pain.

Degenerative changes in the cervical spine are common (especially at C5/6) and may lead to neck pain that radiates to the shoulder and arm and which is exacerbated by rotation. Plain X-ray will show narrowing of one or more disc spaces and osteophyte formation. If there is concern about compressive neurological symptoms then MRI can be used to image the bony and soft tissues precisely. Treatment is usually conservative, with physiotherapy, traction and a collar. Nerve or cord compression may require surgical decompression. Thoracic disc degeneration is also common but seldom requires surgery. Lumbar spine problems are extremely common. Low back pain (lumbago) with pain radiating down one or both legs (sciatica) may be due to a wide range of pathologies. Although most affected patients have degenerative disease (spondylosis), it is important not to overlook

metastatic deposits. Acute central, lumbar disc prolapse may result in compression of the cauda equina, leading to severe back pain, urinary retention and weakness below the knee. More commonly, posterolateral protrusion leads to nerve root compression, with back pain radiating down the leg that is exacerbated by coughing and sneezing. Tendon jerks and muscle power are diminished according to the site of the lesion. Straight leg raising pulls on the sciatic nerve and stretches the nerve roots over the protruding disc, and may be limited to 30° or less. There is usually loss of normal lumbar lordosis, and a scoliosis often develops that is concave to the affected side.

L5/S1 prolapse affects the S1 nerve root and produces pain down the back of the thigh, the lateral side of the calf and the lateral border of the foot. There is sensory loss in this distribution. The ankle jerk is diminished or absent and, as plantar flexion of the ankle is weak, the patient may have difficulty standing on tiptoe.

L4/L5 prolapse compresses the L5 root. Pain radiates down the back of the thigh, the lateral aspect of the calf and the dorsum of the foot in to the great toe. There may be accompanying sensory loss, the ankle jerk is normal but ankle dorsiflexion is weak.

SUMMARY BOX

Acute lumbar disc prolapse

- The condition is most common in the fourth and fifth decades, and men are most often affected.

- The annulus fibrosus ruptures, allowing protrusion of the central nucleus pulposus. The prolapse most commonly occurs posterolaterally and compresses and angulates the spinal nerve(s) it as leaves the spinal canal. Less commonly the disc ruptures posteriorly, with compression of the cauda equina.

- The commonest levels for disc prolapse are L4–5 and L5–S1.

- Pain is the predominant symptom and is exacerbated by coughing and sneezing. Tendon jerks and muscle power are diminished, straight leg raising is restricted (e.g. from 80–90° to 30°) and lumbar lordosis is flattened, with scoliosis concave to the side of the lesion.

- Most cases settle on conservative therapy but those with major protrusions or persistence of symptoms beyond 6 weeks should be considered for removal of the prolapsed material.

- The cauda equina syndrome (severe back pain, urinary retention and weakness bilaterally below the knees) requires urgent surgical relief.

L3/L4 prolapse compresses the L4 root and leads to pain down the front of the thigh and the medial aspect of the calf to the medial malleolus. The knee jerk is affected and there may be quadriceps weakness.

Full examination of the abdomen is mandatory to exclude retroperitoneal and pelvic pathology. A rectal examination should be performed to assess anal tone and sensation. The diagnosis can often be made on clinical examination, and plain X-rays may show degenerative changes in the relevant disc space. Most patients are treated conservatively at first with analgesia and bed rest. Failure to improve and neurological deficit are indication for surgical removal of the protruding disc material.

PERIPHERAL NERVE LESIONS

Lesions of the peripheral nerves can be classified as: traumatic, compressive, metabolic, inflammatory, autoimmune, neoplastic and genetic. The neurosurgeon will see many compressive lesions, a small amount of trauma and the occasional nerve tumour. The common compressive neuropathies are carpal tunnel syndrome, ulnar nerve compression at the elbow, meralgia paraesthetica, and posterior interosseous nerve entrapment syndrome.

Carpal tunnel syndrome

The syndrome consists of symptoms of pain and numbness in the distribution of the median nerve in the hand. This may be intermittent and may be relieved by shaking the hand while holding it in a dependent position. The symptoms are often provoked by wrist flexion. On examination there may be wasting of the thenar eminence and weakness of the abductor pollicis brevis. There may be loss of sensation in the median nerve distribution. The skin of the palm is usually spared. Tapping over the nerve in the carpal tunnel may elicit paraesthesia in the median nerve distribution (Tinel's sign). Phalen's test involves acutely flexing the wrist and holding it in this position. This may precipitate paraesthesia or numbness, and this is abnormal if it occurs within 1 minute. The diagnosis can be confirmed using electrophysiology to measure nerve conduction velocity and distal motor latency. Treatment should be conservative in the first instance, especially if there are no clinical findings of wasting or numbness. Splinting the wrist or injections of steroid into the carpal tunnel provide relief in a third of cases. If this fails the transverse carpal ligament can be divided surgically, and in many cases this can be performed as a day case under local anaesthetic.

Ulnar nerve compression at the elbow

This is usually due to acute and chronic trauma, osteo- or rheumatoid arthritis. There is pain in the forearm and wasting of the small muscles of the hand, leading in the worst cases to an ulnar 'claw' hand. There may be reduced sensation in the ulnar distribution of the hand. The diagnosis may be made clinically, but electrophysiology is recommended to confirm the diagnosis. Treatment consists of surgically releasing and decompressing the nerve.

Meralgia paraesthetica

This is numbness and painful paraesthesia in the lateral thigh caused by compression or injury of the L2/3 sensory lateral cutaneous nerve. The nerve emerges from the lateral border of the psoas muscle just above the iliac crest and crosses the iliacus to pass beneath or through the inguinal ligament, 1 cm medial to the anterior superior iliac spine, to pass into the thigh. Seat belts, pregnancy, trauma, and post-surgical scar tissue, to name but a few, can cause mechanical compression. Diabetes is present in up to 10% of cases. The clinical diagnosis can be confirmed by injecting local anaesthetic into the inguinal region 1 cm medial to the anterior superior iliac spine. Treatment includes weight loss, the removal of constricting clothes and belts, non-steroidal anti-inflammatory drugs, ice packs and injections of corticosteroid. Most cases will settle within 2 years. Surgical decompression is reserved for those that do not.

EVIDENCE-BASED NEUROSURGERY

Much of neurosurgery lacks an evidence base but is performed because the results are considered generally satisfactory. There are, however, many areas of controversy and there is an increasing demand for evidence-based practice. Where randomized controlled trials (RCTs) have been performed the results have usually led to significant improvements in practice and a softening of entrenched opinion. One study showed quite clearly that the prescription of nimodipine, a calcium channel antagonist, significantly reduces both death and delayed ischaemic neurological deficit following SAH. Another RCT showed that the timing of aneurysm clipping after SAH made little difference to outcome, and another that most unruptured aneurysms should probably be treated conservatively. There are many other areas, such as the management of malignant gliomas, where evidence from RCTs is urgently required in order to optimize patient treatments.

31 Transplantation

H. Pleass, J. Forsythe

The surgical techniques necessary for the transplantation of tissues or organs were described in the early part of the 20th century. However, as the immunology of these procedures was not understood, they were destined to fail. In 1937 a skin graft was performed from one identical twin to another, which survived permanently. Yet it was not until 1954 that kidney transplantation succeeded, again between identical twins. The first immunosuppressant drug was 6-mercaptopurine, introduced in 1959 and subsequently modified to azathioprine, which is still in use today.

Liver transplants have been carried out since 1963 and the world's first heart transplant was performed 4 years later. The early results were dismal, and it has only been with the greater understanding of transplant immunology, and an increasing armamentarium of immunosuppressant drugs, that solid organ transplantation has become the accepted and successful form of treatment that we know today. For example, the 1-year graft survival rate for both kidney and liver transplantation has been reported at over 90%.

IMMUNOLOGY

Terminology

Allograft Transplantation between individuals of the same species who are not genetically identical.

Autograft An organ or tissue moved from one part of the body to another within the same person.

Isograft A transplant performed between genetically identical individuals.

Xenograft A transplant performed between one animal species and another.

Rejection

The bulk of clinical transplantation involves allografting and, because individuals are not genetically identical, the recipient's immune system acts to reject the foreign allograft. Rejection is a complex, multifaceted process, but it can be broken down into three main steps:

1. Antigen presentation
2. Immune system activation
3. Effector action.

Antigen presentation

What defines self? On the surface of most cells there are antigens which have a particular importance to transplantation. These are called human leukocyte antigens (HLA) and are encoded by genetic loci of the major histocompatibility complex (MHC) found on chromosome 6 in humans. There are three main loci within this complex, namely A, B and DR. In transplantation DR is more important than B, which in turn is more important than A in terms of graft rejection. This genetic 'blueprint' provides each individual with a specific group of alloantigens – or tissue type – that will be recognized as foreign by another individual from within the same species.

The variation in HLA is enormous and the chance of two unrelated individuals having an identical tissue type is, therefore, very small. For example, with the HLA-A locus, 99 different haplotypes have been identified. This variation is advantageous to the individual, as it provides resistance to infective organisms and thus protects the species as a whole. The disadvantage is that transplantation between genetically dissimilar individuals results in rejection of the transplanted organ.

Acute allograft rejection involves antigen presentation by macrophages and dendritic cells of the recipient. These highly specialized cells phagocytose foreign alloantigen from the transplanted organ, and then process and present this antigen in combination with self HLA (Fig. 31.1). Recipient T cells (termed CD4 cells) recognize alloantigen seen with class II HLA coded for by the DR locus of the HLA complex. Class II HLA are found on only a few specific cell types, which are designated antigen-presenting cells. CD4 cells activated in such a manner lead to an inflammatory response, with the production of cytokines (including interleukin-2), cytotoxic T-cell activation (CD8), and antibody production by the activation of B lymphocytes.

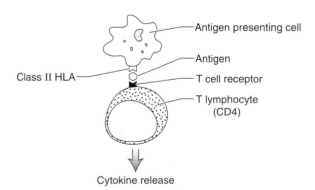

Fig. 31.1 An antigen-presenting cell interacting with a CD4 (T-helper) cell, leading to lymphocyte activation and cytokine release.

Immune system activation

Although the immune system is complex, the cell central to the coordination of allograft rejection is the T-helper or CD4 lymphocyte. Activation of this cell leads to clonal expansion and cytokine production, resulting in the activation of both T-cytotoxic cells and B lymphocytes. This immune system activation directs effector cells to attack and reject the transplanted organ, and leads to the production of an acute inflammatory response.

Effector action

Cytotoxic T cells within the recipient recognize foreign antigen in association with class I HLA, which are found on almost all cells within the body. Following such an interaction, activated cytotoxic T cells kill the cells displaying such antigen by cytolysis. This is termed cell-mediated rejection, and tends to occur 5 days after engraftment; it takes this long for the processing and presentation of alloantigen. In addition, antibody production from activated B lymphocytes can lead to antibody-dependent cell-mediated cytotoxicity through the activation of complement, resulting in cell lysis and vascular occlusion.

Clinical rejection

These immunological processes lead to clinical reactions within the transplanted patient. In truth, the total reaction may be a combination of each immunological step described.

Hyperacute rejection

Fortunately this is rarely seen in the modern transplant setting, but used to occur because circulating antibodies within the recipient could recognize and bind with antigens within the allograft to activate both the complement and the coagulation cascades. As a result, the allograft would be rejected within minutes of being revascularized with the recipient's blood. These antibodies can now be detected, and combinations of donor and recipient that would lead to hyperacute rejection are now avoided.

Acute rejection

This can occur at any time but is most common 5–7 days after the transplantation. Foreign antigen from the allograft is processed by antigen-presenting cells, which in turn recruit and activate cytotoxic T lymphocytes. If left unchecked, this acute inflammatory response will destroy the allograft. Increased numbers of T lymphocytes and macrophages within a transplant biopsy can confirm acute rejection.

Chronic rejection

This tends to occur after a minimum of 6 months post transplantation, but can be seen up to years later. It is thought to be caused by a complex interaction of the immune system, leading to chronic graft dysfunction and subsequent failure. Treatment of chronic rejection has largely been unsuccessful and remains a major hurdle for both transplant team and immunologist.

Immunosuppression

Without immunosuppression all transplant recipients, except identical twins, will reject the new organ. A variety of drugs are available, with different mechanisms of action. The aim of their usage is to prevent both acute and chronic rejection in solid organ transplantation. However, because they suppress the immune system in a non-specific way they increase the patient's susceptibility to both infection and malignancy.

Azathioprine

This was the first widely used immunosuppressant and is still in use today. It is metabolized to 6-mercaptopurine and inhibits DNA and RNA synthesis by interfering with purine metabolism. It reduces the number of lymphocytes, phagocytes and natural killer cells, thereby reducing the incidence of rejection. The main side effects are leukopenia and thrombocytopenia secondary to marrow suppression.

Corticosteroids

Corticosteroids have a general anti-inflammatory action, but suppress the immune system by inhibiting cytokine production. Although they can prevent and reverse rejection, they have a variety of unwanted metabolic effects, causing diabetes, osteoporosis, skin changes, and increasing the risk of infection. They are still used as the main agent, in bolus doses, to treat an acute rejection episode.

Cyclosporin

This drug was revolutionary to transplantation during the 1980s. It acts as a calcineurin antagonist and thereby prevents the production of IL-2. It has significantly improved graft survival, but the side-effects of renal toxicity, hypertrichosis, hypertension and hyperlipidaemia are a significant disadvantage. A new formulation of the drug, known as Neoral, was introduced in 1994 and has a better absorption profile, but with identical side-effects. It is often used as part of a triple-therapy regimen with azathioprine and prednisolone.

Tacrolimus

This agent acts in a similar way to cyclosporin but binds to a different cytosolic protein. Like its competitor it has marked renal toxicity, but it can also induce neurotoxicity and has a higher incidence of diabetes. It is probably a more powerful agent than cyclosporin, although trials are not conclusive. It is also used in combination with azathioprine and prednisolone.

Other agents

Antibody preparations directed at single (monoclonal) and multiple (polyclonal) cell surface molecules are used to target the cells of the immune system. However, anaphylaxis and pulmonary oedema due to cytokine release remain major complications with such biological agents. They are frequently used as rescue therapy in patients with steroid-resistant rejection, and who are already on a triple-drug regimen. Newer agents are also available against the receptor for IL-2, which appears on activated T cells. These appear to have a lower side-effect profile, although clinical usage is limited.

SUMMARY BOX

Clinical rejection

- Hyperacute rejection is now rarely seen
- Acute rejection is seen in up to 40% of organ transplants
- Chronic rejection is the commonest cause of late allograft loss

---

CADAVERIC ORGAN DONATION

Organ shortage

At present the major obstacle to solid organ transplantation is the shortage of suitable organ donors. This has resulted in part from the reduced incidence of subarachnoid haemorrhage, but also better resuscitation techniques and seatbelt legislation have reduced the number of donors available following major trauma. Although this is good news for the population in general, it results in a large number of patients with organ failure dying while on the transplant waiting list. This organ shortage cannot be overemphasized.

The multiorgan donor

With the definition of brain-stem death becoming more widely accepted after 1969, it has been possible to retrieve organs from heart-beating, ventilated donors. For such a diagnosis to be made, three conditions have to be met:

1. A diagnosis compatible with brain-stem death
2. Irreversible structural brain damage
3. Apnoeic coma.

If these are met, specific causes of reversible coma must then be excluded, for example sedative drugs, hypothermia, metabolic and endocrine abnormalities. Clinical tests to confirm the absence of brain-stem reflexes and the presence of persistent apnoea can then be performed, as long as the conditions and exclusions have been met. In the UK, two physicians not connected with the transplant unit perform these tests on two separate occasions.

Clinical tests for absent brain-stem reflexes

1. No pupillary response to bright light
2. No corneal reflex in response to light touch stimulation
3. No vestibulo-ocular reflex using ice-cold water (free access to tympanic membrane must be visualized)
4. No motor response within the cranial nerve distribution.

Clinical test for persistent apnoea

1. Preoxygenate with 100% oxygen for 10 minutes.
2. Disconnect from ventilator while providing diffusion oxygenation via a catheter placed in the endotracheal tube.
3. Allow Paco$_2$ to rise above 6.65 kPa and confirm no spontaneous respiration, before reconnecting the patient to the ventilator.

Contraindications to organ donation

There are several absolute contraindications to organ donation, irrespective of whether the potential donor is alive or dead.

Contraindications to cadaveric organ donation

1. A history of malignancy, except primary brain tumour and basal cell carcinoma of the skin
2. Hepatitis B carrier
3. Hepatitis C carrier
4. HIV positive
5. Major systemic sepsis.

These factors hold true for all solid organ donation. In addition, established organ failure will prevent donation of the failed organ, but may not preclude the patient becoming a donor for other organs that have retained their function. For example, a patient dying from liver failure could theoretically become a kidney donor, although systemic sepsis often prevents this.

Multiorgan retrieval procedure

Cadaveric organs are usually retrieved as part of a multi-organ donor procedure (Fig. 31.2). The donor, having been confirmed brain-stem dead and never having expressed a wish against organ donation, can then be referred to the transplant team. Normally, a transplant coordinator will speak with the grieving family and, with their agreement, obtain consent for organ donation. This is a very difficult time for the patient's relatives: usually after a sudden event their loved one appears 'alive', pink and breathing on a ventilator, although to the physician they are brain-stem dead. Tact, diplomacy and experience are required, organ donation being promoted as the only positive thing to come out of such a tragic circumstance.

Normally, the heart, lungs, liver, kidneys, pancreas, eyes, bone, skin and other tissues can all be retrieved from the same donor, and so the coordination of a number of different surgical teams is required. The abdomen is opened longitudinally and the sternum split to expose the heart. A thorough laparotomy is carried out to exclude any possible contraindication to organ donation, such as a previously undiagnosed bowel cancer. The intra-abdominal viscera to be retrieved are mobilized and the major vessels dissected out and slung with vessel loops. In a similar way the tho-

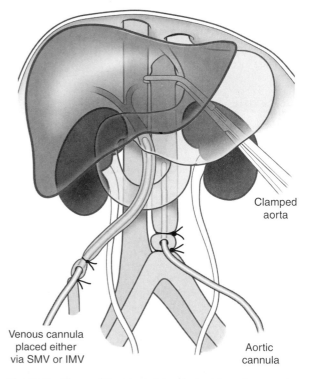

Clamped aorta

Venous cannula placed either via SMV or IMV

Aortic cannula

Fig. 31.2 The multiorgan retrieval, showing placement of intra-abdominal cannulae.

racic surgeons will inspect and palpate the heart to exclude macroscopic coronary artery disease. The lungs are fully inflated, often by hand ventilation, to assess suitability. When all teams have completed their mobilization the patient is heparinized and a cannula placed in the lower aorta. A further cannula is often placed via the inferior mesenteric vein to perfuse the portal venous supply of the liver. At this stage the thoracic team places a cannula in the ascending aorta and, if the lungs are to be retrieved, a further cannula is placed in the main pulmonary artery. With close cooperation between abdominal and thoracic surgical teams the aorta is cross-clamped at the level of the diaphragm, with simultaneous perfusion of viscera both above and below the diaphragm. Using this technique, the organs can be cooled and flushed without any period of warm ischaemia. Venous blood and perfusate are vented by either transecting or placing a cannula within the inferior vena cava.

The heart–lung bloc can be removed together after fully inflating the lungs and stapling the trachea to maintain inflation during transport. A cardioplegic solution is used to cool and stop the heart: University of Wisconsin (UW) solution is infused via the portal cannula for liver retrieval and storage. UW can also be used for renal perfusion via the aortic cannula, and is the perfusate of choice if the pancreas is also to be harvested. However, if the pancreas is not suitable then a less expensive kidney perfusion solution can be used via the aortic cannula.

After retrieval of the heart–lung bloc the intra-abdominal viscera are normally well perfused, and are then removed from the cadaver and placed in ice-cold saline in sterile bowls. The liver is normally the first to be removed and can be taken en bloc with the pancreas. Finally, the kidneys are removed. All organs retrieved from such a multiorgan donor are carefully inspected for injury and suboptimal perfusion prior to transportation.

Each organ is flushed again with perfusate, placed submerged in fresh perfusion solution and carried in two sterile plastic bags (Fig. 31.3). These are then placed in a further bag containing crushed ice, within an insulated box for transport. Samples of spleen and lymph nodes from the donor are placed in sterile containers and transported with each kidney, as shown. Donor iliac artery and vein are similarly transported with the liver and pancreas, as they are often required to facilitate the implantation procedure.

Non-heart-beating donors

Owing to the increasing numbers of patients on transplant waiting lists, attempts have been made to increase the donor pool. One such method is to use non-heart-beating donors who die following failed resuscitation. Units in Maastricht and Leicester have pioneered this development with considerable success. Following confirmation of death a double-balloon catheter is placed within the femoral artery to perfuse the kidneys; the femoral vein is used to drain out effluent blood. A period of 10 minutes must elapse after confirmation of death before cannulation commences. Such a non-heart-beating donor is not suitable for multiorgan retrieval, but it may well reduce the organ shortage in the field of renal transplantation.

> **SUMMARY BOX**
>
> *Organ shortage*
>
> - Insufficient numbers of cadaveric organs available
> - Patient deaths on transplant waiting lists are increasing
> - Greater need to promote organ donation
> - Greater need for live donation in renal transplantation

RENAL TRANSPLANTATION

Epidemiology

In the UK, end-stage renal failure affects approximately 80 per million each year. Renal failure may be classified as acute or chronic, the latter being the commonest category for transplantation referral. Glomerular disease, diabetes mellitus and interstitial disease account for more than half the cases. Currently, there are almost 6000 patients on the renal transplant waiting list, with only 1500 transplants

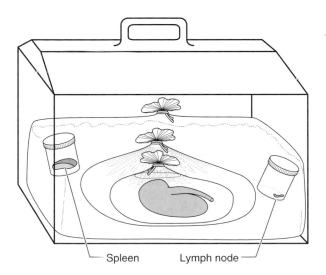

Spleen   Lymph node

Fig. 31.3 The kidney is double-wrapped in two sterile plastic bags and then placed in a third bag containing crushed ice.

being performed each year. It is clear that the demand outstrips the supply.

Source of organs

Cadaveric

In the UK most kidneys are obtained from multiorgan brainstem-dead donors. Kidneys retrieved in such a way may be stored for up to 48 hours prior to implantation, although their long-term survival has been shown to benefit if the cold ischaemic time is kept below 24 hours. Non-heart-beating donors are also providing a significant source of donor kidneys at certain centres. Although questions as to the viability of such kidneys remain, this source should be increasingly utilized.

Live related and live unrelated donors

Live donors provide almost 40% of kidneys available for transplantation in Scandinavia, compared to 10–15% in the UK. The advantages are a planned operation for the recipient and a significantly improved graft survival compared to a cadaveric organ. The improved survival holds true for both matched and totally mismatched kidneys, as is the case with live unrelated donors such as spouse-to-spouse transplantation. It is thought that the benefit is due to the significantly shorter cold ischaemic time, as the kidney is removed from the healthy living donor and transplanted within a matter of minutes. This is because both donor and recipient can be operated on simultaneously, ideally in adjacent theatres. The major disadvantage is the risk of morbidity and even mortality to the donor – someone who is undergoing surgery for no personal direct benefit. Worldwide, the risk of death from a live donor procedure has been estimated at 1 in 1600 to 1 in 3300 procedures, pulmonary embolus and occult coronary artery disease being the most common causes.

Because of these risks it is vitally important that a potential live donor makes the decision to donate without coercion, threat or bribery. In the UK, the Human Organ Transplant Act of 1989 specifically forbids the purchase of kidneys and outlaws commerce in transplantation. In addition, all cases of unrelated live donation in the UK must receive the approval of the Unrelated Live Donor Transplant Regulatory Authority (ULTRA).

Great care must be taken in both the physical and the psychological preparation of the live donor. Obviously they must have no evidence of renal disease, and an ultrasound scan, isotope glomerular filtration rate assessment and renal angiography are usually carried out prior to surgery. Normally the left kidney is taken, because the renal vein is longer on this side, but multiple renal vessels on one side would transfer attention to the opposite kidney.

The live donor nephrectomy is usually performed with the patient positioned on their side, using a loin incision centred over the twelfth rib. A more recent innovation has been laparoscopic donor nephrectomy, with a small suprapubic incision being made at the end of the procedure to aid removal of the kidney. This technique appears to be less painful in the postoperative period, although there is an increase in the warm ischaemic time prior to kidney flushing with cold preservation fluid. This relatively new technique has helped to increase public awareness of live donation, and in some countries it is claimed to have led to an increase in both related and unrelated live renal transplantation.

Recipient assessment

Potential recipients are usually seen in the transplant assessment clinic prior to being placed on the active cadaveric renal transplant waiting list. Age is a factor in patient selection, but the presence of comorbidity is more influential on selection and each patient is assessed individually. A recent history of cancer is an exclusion criterion because of the postoperative immunosuppression required, but the patient may still receive a transplant in the future if follow-up demonstrates no recurrence.

Persistent sepsis, such as recurrent pyelonephritis, is a contraindication to transplantation and the patient may require native nephrectomy before being placed on the list. Bladder function is also assessed at this time and may require further investigation, even surgery, before transplantation can be considered.

Patients with a history of peripheral vascular disease may require duplex ultrasonography and angiography to investigate the severity of the problem. It is important to inform a potential recipient that a renal transplant may worsen the distal circulation on the same side, especially if there is no vascular lesion amenable to angioplasty or surgery.

Likewise, a history of cardiovascular disease needs to be thoroughly investigated and the patient's cardiological status optimized. Myocardial infarction is one of the major causes of graft loss beyond 5 years post transplant, and also accounts for the 5% perioperative mortality seen with renal transplant recipients.

If the patient is deemed suitable for inclusion on the active list, then blood group, tissue type and up-to-date virology are checked, including HIV status. Positive serology for HIV or hepatitis B is a contraindication to transplantation. The advantages and disadvantages of transplantation are discussed with particular reference to complications, drug treatment, rejection and graft failure. Only patients who are fully informed should be put forward for transplantation.

Recipient procedure

Ideally a cadaveric kidney is matched to a potential recipient in terms of age, blood group and tissue type, but a final compatibility test is performed prior to surgery. This is

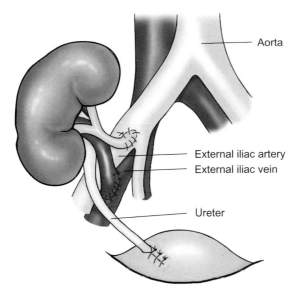

Fig. 31.4 The renal transplant is placed retroperitoneally on to the iliac vessels with the ureteric anastomosis as shown.

Labels: Aorta, External iliac artery, External iliac vein, Ureter

termed a cytotoxic cross-match and involves the incubation of donor lymphocytes with the potential recipient's serum. With the subsequent addition of complement, cell lysis indicates the presence of IgG antibodies, thereby predicting hyperacute rejection of the graft. In such a case a 'positive' cross-match will prevent the transplant procedure from going ahead, and an alternative recipient is sought.

If the immediate preoperative work-up is satisfactory the patient is taken to theatre and, following catheterization, a renal transplant performed. Normally, the iliac vessels are used, with the ureter being anastomosed on to the dome of the bladder (Fig. 31.4). Most units routinely place a ureteric stent across the vesicoureteric anastomosis, which can be removed by flexible cystoscopy between 6 weeks and 3 months postoperatively. The procedure is performed under antibiotic cover.

Complications

Vascular complications tend to occur in the early postoperative period and are largely technical, although they may be related to graft rejection. Haemorrhage, renal artery and vein thrombosis can all occur, the latter two almost always leading to graft loss, with a reported incidence of 4%. Late renal artery stenosis can also occur because of poor surgical technique or accelerated atherosclerosis during the follow-up period. This complication tends to cause hypertension and a decline in renal function, correction being attempted by either radiological or surgical means. Such correctional procedures pose a significant risk of graft loss, although

this has to be weighed against the dangers of uncontrolled hypertension.

Urological complications are notoriously difficult to diagnose, as a urine leak in an immunosuppressed patient may produce little in the way of symptoms or signs. Urine leaks can occur in the immediate postoperative period owing to poor surgical technique, but may also present later as a result of ischaemic necrosis of the distal ureter. A high index of suspicion is required and surgical exploration may be required to make the diagnosis. Ureteric obstruction is the other major urological complication. Both leak and obstruction tend to occur in about 5% of most series, but have been reported in up to 16% of renal transplants. Such problems are managed by the radiologist, urologist and transplant surgeon, and may require percutaneous nephrostomy, ureteric stenting and revisional surgery. They are most common within the first 3 months, their incidence being significantly reduced by the routine use of ureteric stents.

Lymphoceles occur in approximately 2% of renal transplants because of the disruption of lymphatic channels within the retroperitoneal space, giving rise to a lymph leak. Fluid aspirated from a lymphocele has a characteristically high lymphocyte count, which can help to differentiate the collection from a simple seroma. Lymphoceles can obstruct the transplant ureter and require drainage, either by an open procedure or by a laparoscopic fenestration into the peritoneal cavity.

LIVER TRANSPLANTATION

Epidemiology

Like renal transplantation, the demand for liver transplantation has outstripped the supply of suitable donor organs over the last 30 years. Approximately 90% of liver transplants are performed for an underlying chronic liver disease. They are usually carried out to prolong life, but in certain cases an improvement in quality of life may be the predominant indication. The remaining 10% are performed for fulminant hepatic failure and, as such, their assessment is quite different.

Source of organs

Cadaveric

The majority of donor livers are obtained from brain-stem-dead multiorgan retrieval procedures. The liver is perfused with University of Wisconsin (UW) solution, which can preserve a liver satisfactorily for up to 16 hours. Longer cold ischaemic times lead to a higher incidence of primary non-function (PNF) and the need for emergency retransplantation. At present there is no artificial liver available, and without retransplantation a patient with PNF will die within 48–72 hours. Livers are stored in a manner similar to kidneys. Donor iliac arteries and veins are also retrieved, as they may be required for the vascular reconstruction of the graft.

Reduced liver transplantation

A variety of techniques have been developed to combat the natural shortage of suitable donor livers for children. This shortage has been most severe in paediatric practice and has led to the use of a reduced liver graft. A cadaveric liver is retrieved in the standard fashion and then cut down to size. The unwanted portion is discarded and the reduced liver is transplanted into the child. Although this technique has been successful in reducing the paediatric waiting list, it has led to increasing competition between adult and paediatric centres.

Live related and split-liver transplantation

Live related liver transplantation was first carried out successfully in 1989. The main advantages are a planned elective operation for the recipient and a short cold ischaemic time. The major disadvantage is the risk of significant morbidity and mortality to the live donor. Because of these risks, split-liver transplantation (SLT) using a cadaveric donor organ has been developed. Two SLT techniques have been described. The ex vivo technique involves retrieving the whole liver in the standard fashion and then splitting it in theatre at the recipient centre. The split liver is usually then placed in one adult and one child. The in situ technique involves splitting the cadaveric donor liver prior to cross-clamping, perfusion and subsequent retrieval. This provides a shorter cold ischaemic time, meticulous haemostasis and a better assessment of the viability of the divided liver parenchyma. Compared to the ex vivo technique, the in situ technique is associated with a decrease in the inci-

dence of biliary complications and primary non-function, and an increase in patient and graft survival.

Recipient assessment

The requirement for transplantation in patients with chronic liver disease is less clear cut than the decision to transplant patients with chronic renal failure. Spontaneous bacterial peritonitis and variceal haemorrhage are both predictors of mortality without a liver transplant. In addition, the prolongation of prothrombin time, deranged liver function tests, low albumin and the presence of ascites are all used to assess the need for transplantation. The patient's quality of life is also regarded as an important factor in determining the need for transplantation. Chronic itch and fatigue are often the main indications for transplantation, irrespective of the synthetic liver function tests. In the UK, hepatitis C, alcoholic liver disease and primary biliary cirrhosis account for the majority of cases. A thorough assessment of the patient's cardiovascular status is made, as well as routine ultrasound Doppler examination of the diseased liver and its blood supply. The patient needs to be able to tolerate a major procedure and investigations are aimed at detecting comorbidity such as ischaemic heart disease and respiratory compromise. If no contraindication is found, patients with chronic liver disease can be placed on the active cadaveric transplant waiting list.

Fulminant hepatic failure

Patients with fulminant hepatic failure (FHF) carry a high risk of mortality without a liver transplant. In the UK, paracetamol overdose is the commonest cause. In such cases there is a 90% mortality if the King's College Hospital criteria are met. If a patient reaches the criteria listed below and there are no contraindications, then they are listed for a super-urgent liver transplant.

Criteria for paracetamol-induced FHF

1. Arterial pH < 7.3 on admission after full rehydration or all of the following:
2. Prothrombin time > 100 s
3. Creatinine > 300 μmol/L
4. Encephalopathy.

Criteria for non-paracetamol induced FHF

1. Prothrombin time > 100 s or three of the following, irrespective of the grade of encephalopathy:
2. Age < 10 or > 40 years
3. Cause being non-A non-B hepatitis, halothane hepatitis or idiosyncratic drug reaction

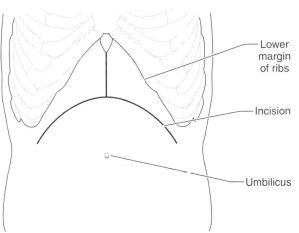

Fig. 31.5 The Mercedes incision for orthotopic liver transplantation.

4. Duration of jaundice before encephalopathy > 1 week
5. Prothrombin time > 50 s
6. Serum bilirubin > 300 μmol/L

Recipient procedure

The donor liver must be blood group compatible, ideally blood group identical, and of a similar size to that of the recipient. A difference in body weight between the cadaveric donor and the recipient of up to 10% is usually acceptable. Unlike renal transplantation no attempt is made to match the patient's tissue type, as no increase in rejection has been seen with mismatch.

A bilateral subcostal incision with xiphisternal extension (Mercedes incision) is generally used (Fig. 31.5). An orthotopic transplant is usually performed, that is, removal of the diseased liver and replacement with the donor liver at the same site. The classical orthotopic liver transplant (OLT) includes removal of the retrohepatic vena cava with the

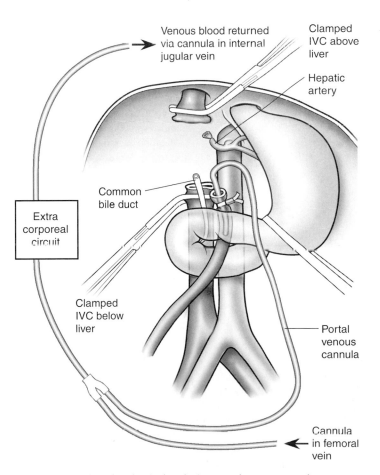

Fig. 31.6 Recipient hepatectomy using the classical technique and venovenous bypass.

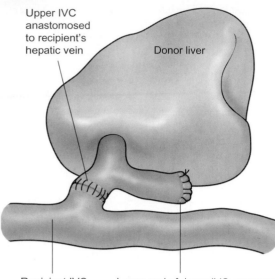

Upper IVC anastomosed to recipient's hepatic vein

Donor liver

Recipient IVC   Lower end of donor IVC oversewn

Fig. 31.7 Side view of the caval preservation (piggyback) technique of OLT.

diseased liver (Fig. 31.6). To improve haemodynamic stability, venovenous bypass, which recirculates portal and caval blood flow to the superior vena cava via an extracorporeal circuit, has been introduced. Caval preservation is an alternative technique that is widely practised in both adult and paediatric OLT (Fig. 31.7). In this technique the diseased liver is dissected off the vena cava, maintaining venous return throughout and obviating the need for veno-

venous bypass. Whichever technique is employed, the vascular anastomoses are similar for the implant procedure. The vena cava is joined first, followed by the portal venous anastomosis, then the hepatic artery and finally the bile duct. The whole procedure usually takes about 6 hours (Fig. 31.8).

Complications

Primary non-function (PNF) occurs in 2–5% of patients and is an absolute indication for emergency retransplantation. Haemodynamic instability and persistent acidosis, hypoglycaemia, coagulopathy and coma are all indicators of PNF. Fatty livers and livers from older, more unstable cadaveric donors have a higher incidence of PNF. However, there is no preoperative test that will reliably predict this often fatal complication.

Hepatic artery thrombosis (HAT) complicates 5% of all adult OLT procedures and in the early post-transplant period usually mandates retransplantation. Later on, HAT leads to biliary ischaemia, with stricturing and abscess formation. Retransplantation to prevent recurrent sepsis is often the end result, and is associated with significant morbidity and mortality. Biliary complications occur in 5–15% of cases and are frequently associated with HAT. However, an early biliary leak may simply denote a technical anastomotic error, which may require endoscopic placement of a stent and percutaneous drainage of the bile collection. Such complications may ultimately require revisional surgery, particularly if a biliary stricture ensues.

Haemorrhage in the postoperative period is common and due to the large raw area created by the removal of the

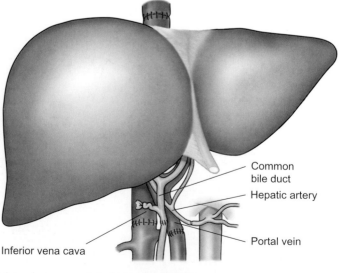

Common bile duct
Hepatic artery
Portal vein
Inferior vena cava

Fig. 31.8 All anastomoses have been completed in a classic OLT.

diseased liver, coagulopathy secondary to liver failure, and thrombocytopenia secondary to portal hypertension and hypersplenism. Bleeding may necessitate a return to theatre, although correction of platelet and coagulation factor deficiencies may alleviate the problem.

PANCREAS TRANSPLANTATION

Epidemiology

Pancreas transplantation is now an accepted form of treatment for type I diabetes mellitus. Most commonly a combined pancreas and kidney transplant from the same donor is transplanted into a type I diabetic with renal failure. Since it was first reported in 1966, the technique has evolved largely to cope with the unwanted exocrine secretions. Such evolution has not been without a price, and a high morbidity and mortality have been associated with the procedure in the past. Better patient selection, correction of coronary artery disease and technological and immunological advances have all led to a significant improvement in survival.

Source of organs

The pancreas is retrieved from a heart-beating cadaveric donor, ideally under 40 years of age. The pancreas and liver can be retrieved *en bloc* after perfusion with UW solution, the two organs then being separated in theatre. A handful of live related pancreas transplants have been performed, but donor morbidity and mortality currently prevent this from becoming accepted clinical practice.

Recipient assessment

Recipients are type I diabetics, under 50 years of age, with absent or corrected coronary artery disease. The majority have renal failure secondary to diabetic nephropathy, although pancreas transplants alone are performed for brittle diabetes and hypoglycaemic unawareness. Patients are selected according to blood group compatibility, and a cytotoxic cross-match is always performed prior to implantation.

Recipient procedure

The implant procedure commences with a thorough preparation of the pancreas. A Y-shaped segment of donor iliac artery is used to anastomose the splenic and superior mesenteric arteries of the pancreas (Fig. 31.9). Venous drainage is via the portal vein, which often requires an extension graft using donor iliac vein. With the gland fully prepared, the arterial and venous conduits are anastomosed

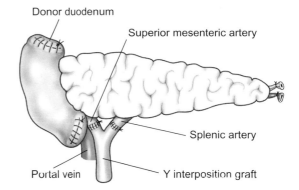

Fig. 31.9 Pancreas graft showing interposition Y graft prior to implantation.

to the recipient's common iliac vessels. Controversy still exists as to how best to deal with the exocrine secretions. Many units still favour drainage into the bladder, although enteric drainage is currently the technique of choice.

Complications

Vascular thrombosis occurs in 10% of cases and almost invariably leads to graft loss. Postoperative haemorrhage can also occur, but is less frequent than in liver transplantation. Pancreatic fistulae were common in the early years, but better patient preparation and meticulous technique have significantly reduced this problem. If a bladder drainage technique is employed, 40% develop severe cystitis and urethritis owing to the chemical action of pancreatic secretions on urothelium. These patients require an enteric conversion at a later date – a further operation with its own morbidity.

HEART AND LUNG TRANSPLANTATION

Epidemiology

Ischaemic heart disease and cardiomyopathy account for more than 80% of the heart transplants performed today. Children can be treated as successfully as adults, although the shortage of suitable paediatric donors is limiting. A bilateral lung and heart bloc is often advocated for the treatment of patients with congenital heart disease, pulmonary hypertension and secondary respiratory failure. However, frequently the heart may be healthy, as in cystic fibrosis, and in such cases bilateral lung transplantation is carried out, to remove all potential sources of sepsis. It is also possible to perform single lung transplants in selected patients with emphysema or fibrosing lung disease.

Source of organs

Hearts are retrieved as part of a cadaveric multiorgan retrieval procedure and are generally from donors under the age of 55. Through a midline sternotomy the heart is inspected and palpated to exclude macroscopic coronary artery disease. A perfusion cannula is placed in the ascending aorta following anticoagulation, and the heart is perfused with cool cardioplegic solution. If the lungs are also retrieved, a second cannula is placed in the main pulmonary artery for perfusion. The heart–lung bloc can be removed after fully inflating the lungs and stapling the trachea to maintain inflation during transport. Living related lung transplantation has been performed, although it is unclear whether the results justify the significant risks to the donor.

Recipient assessment

The assessment of patients for heart and lung transplantation involves an intensive assessment of cardiac function, including exercise testing with monitoring for arterial gas desaturation. Similar contraindications exist as for any form of solid organ transplantation.

Recipient procedure

With cardiac transplantation the cold ischaemic time is kept to a minimum, and certainly under 6 hours. To facilitate this, the recipient procedure is normally well under way before the heart reaches the recipient centre. The recipient is fully heparinized and placed on cardiopulmonary bypass with systemic cooling to 28°C. Following removal of the diseased heart through a midline sternotomy, implantation commences by suturing the atrial remnants to the donor heart as well as performing aortic and pulmonary artery anastomoses. The patient is rewarmed and then the heart is reperfused. Cardioversion may be required to establish sinus rhythm, and temporary pacing may also be needed. Patients are transferred to the cardiac intensive care unit and, following extubation, are rapidly mobilized back to the ward.

Lung transplantation similarly requires a short cold ischaemic time. A lateral thoracotomy is used for single lung transplants, and cardiopulmonary bypass may be required if the patient becomes unstable. With a bilateral procedure a median sternotomy can be used, although improved access is gained by using a submammary incision.

Complications

A complication common to all types of lung transplantation is dehiscence of the tracheal or bronchial anastomosis, which is life-threatening, with prolonged air leak and mediastinitis. This is thought to result from ischaemia, and can be reduced by careful surgical technique and gentle tissue handling.

Routine endocardial biopsies are taken from the right ventricle of heart transplant recipients using X-ray screening and right internal jugular venous access. If rejection is confirmed, augmentation of immunosuppression is carried out. Rejection can also cause rapidly progressive coronary artery disease, with thickening and narrowing of the coronary arteries. Because the donor heart is denervated the patient will not experience angina, and therefore coronary angiography is performed annually from 2 years onwards.

SMALL BOWEL TRANSPLANTATION

The technique of intestinal transplantation is not new but is still rarely performed. One of the major obstacles has been the amount of lymphoid tissue transplanted with the gut and which can give rise to graft-versus-host disease. The other difficulty has been the bacterial load, coupled with the heavy immunosuppression that is required postoperatively. The indications for small bowel transplantation are intestinal failure where nutrition cannot be maintained by total parenteral nutrition. Contraindications are active sepsis, malignancy, or eventual adaptation and a return to an enteral diet.

COMPLICATIONS COMMON TO ALL TRANSPLANTS

The medical complications of renal transplantation are related to the use of immunosuppression and are therefore common to all solid organ transplant procedures. *Pneumocystis, Candida* and viral infections can all cause serious morbidity and mortality. Transplant recipients receive prophylaxis in the form of co-trimoxazole for *Pneumocystis* and nystatin for fungal infection as routine for the first 3 months. Antiviral treatment is also given if the patient is at risk from cytomegalovirus (CMV).

CMV is commonly an asymptomatic viral infection in normal healthy adults, with more than 50% of the adult population being CMV positive. This prevalence increases with age, and has been reported as high as 85% in the elderly. Following transplantation, an immunosuppressed patient who has not had CMV (CMV negative) is at risk of being infected by the organ from a donor who has (CMV positive). This may manifest itself 6–12 weeks post transplant, with fever, malaise, thrombocytopenia, diarrhoea, pneumonitis or hepatitis. There is a wide spectrum of disease severity, but recurrence following intravenous antiviral therapy is common and immunosuppression may have to be reduced for full patient recovery.

Another complication common to all immunosuppressed patients is the increased incidence of cancer, particularly skin cancer and lymphoma. In the former, squamous cell cancers outweigh the normal preponderance of basal cell cancers: they tend to occur at an earlier age and are often multiple. The lymphoproliferative disorders are often associated with Epstein–Barr virus infection and may respond to a reduction in immunosuppression, although the long-term survival of such patients is disappointing.

SUMMARY BOX

Complications common to all transplants

- Increased risk of malignancy, especially skin cancer and lymphoproliferative disease
- Increased risk of *Pneumocystis* and fungal infections
- Increased risk of CMV disease

RESULTS OF ORGAN TRANSPLANTATION

Renal

Almost 40% of renal transplant patients experience an early rejection episode, which is normally reversible with augmentation of the immunosuppression. Such episodes are usually easy to recognize, and treatment can be prompt and effective. Rejection occurring later, when the patient has been discharged from hospital, is often not identified as quickly and carries a poorer prognosis. The 1-year renal allograft survival rate is now 90%, and patient survival exceeds this. However, there remains a 2–5% perioperative mortality, as many renal patients have severe comorbidity which is a relative but not an absolute contraindication to transplantation. The 5-year graft survival is around 70%, and at this time graft losses are commonly due to chronic rejection or to cardiovascular death in a patient with a functioning graft.

Liver

Immunosuppression of the liver transplant recipient is vital, but acute rejection is less of a problem than in the kidney recipient. One-year survival after an elective OLT for chronic liver disease is consistently 90%, although the results for fulminant hepatic failure are closer to 70%. Chronic rejection, disease recurrence, cardiovascular complications and the development of malignancy all account for graft failure and patient deaths.

In the long term the liver does appear to be an immunologically privileged organ, with late graft loss being uncommon compared to other solid organ transplants. The 5-year survival for OLT recipients is in excess of 70%, although multiple regrafts as a group have a significantly poorer survival. Some individuals develop tolerance of their graft and fail to reject despite stopping all immunosuppression, although as yet it has not been possible to safely predict this patient group.

Pancreas

Rejection of a pancreas transplant alone has been notoriously difficult to diagnose, whereas renal function and renal biopsy can be usefully employed as a surrogate marker of pancreas rejection if a combined kidney–pancreas procedure has been carried out. This, coupled with better immunosuppression, has enabled 5-year combined kidney–pancreas graft survival to exceed 70%. In addition, some recent evidence has indicated that diabetics who receive a renal transplant alone have a worse patient and graft survival than those who receive a combined kidney and pancreas.

Heart

The results of cardiac transplantation are similar, with 85% of recipients being alive and well at 1 year, and a 75% 5-year survival having been reported. These recipients are able to lead a very normal life although, like other transplant patients, they do require lifelong immunosuppression, with its attendant complications. Sadly, demand outstrips organ supply and the death rate on the cardiac transplant waiting list is high.

Lung

The 5-year survival of lung transplant recipients is close to 50% or better in some series, with chronic rejection causing obliterative bronchiolitis being quoted as a major cause of both graft and patient loss.

Small bowel

Small bowel transplantation is still in its infancy and remains a major technical and immunological challenge. Graft survival is only 30% at 3 years, although graft loss does not inevitably result in patient death. Patient survival is currently better with total parenteral nutrition if this is technically possible, although complications from this may prompt transplant referral.

CONCLUSION

Solid organ transplantation has progressed dramatically over the last 30 years to become a successful and accepted form of treatment for end-stage organ failure. Transplantation has been shown to improve the quality of life, as well as saving life in many instances, and is often more cost-effective than continued treatment of a chronic disease, such as dialysis. The targets for the new millennium must be improved rates of organ donation, increasing usage of live donors and the induction of immunological tolerance.

32 Ear, nose and throat surgery

R.P. Mills

EAR

Anatomy

External ear

The pinna (Fig. 32.1) is made of fibroelastic cartilage. Postauricular muscles are attached posteriorly and allow limited movement in some individuals. The external auditory meatus consists of an outer portion made of cartilage and inner part formed by the tympanic bone (Fig. 32.2). It is lined by squamous epithelium and contains ceruminous glands that produce wax. As there is very little subcutaneous tissue, soft tissue swelling is very painful.

Middle ear

The tympanic membrane is a conical vibrating membrane which is attached to the margin of the bony ear canal

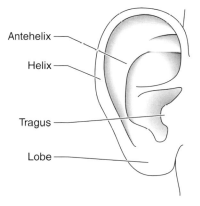

Fig. 32.1   Anatomy of the pinna.

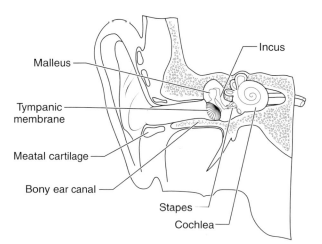

Fig. 32.2   Anatomy of the ear.

585

peripherally and the handle of the malleus, the first of the three ossicles, centrally (Fig. 32.2). The head of the malleus is attached to the body of the incus in the space superior to the middle ear, known as the attic. The long process of the incus attaches to the head of the stapes. The stapes occupies the oval window and is surrounded by the annular ligament, which attaches to its bony margin. The middle ear is mostly lined by a simple cuboidal epithelium, but there are tracts of mucus-secreting cells within it. The middle-ear space is connected to the nasopharynx by the Eustachian tube, which is responsible for maintaining the middle ear at atmospheric pressure.

Inner ear

The inner ear consists of a series of spaces – the membranous labyrinth – surrounded by a bony shell, the otic capsule. The interior of the membranous labyrinth is filled by a fluid called endolymph; the bony labyrinth is filled with perilymph. The cochlea is a coiled tube with the oval window at one end and the round window at the other. The vestibular portion of the inner ear consists of three semicircular canals and the saccule and utricle. The acoustic nerve and the three vestibular nerves combine in the internal auditory meatus and pass medially to the brain stem. The facial nerve enters the temporal bone by the internal auditory meatus and passes laterally to the geniculate ganglion. It passes through the middle space superior to the oval window and turns inferiorly to exit at the stylomastoid foramen.

Physiology

The pinna collects sound and funnels it into the ear canal. The tympanic membrane and ossicular chain combine to act as an impedance-matching transformer, so that vibrations in air are transferred to the cochlear fluids without excessive loss of energy. The cochlea converts vibrations in endolymph into electrical impulses in the auditory nerve. This is achieved by stimulation of hair cells in the organ of Corti. The maximum response to high frequencies occurs in the basal turn of the cochlea, whereas low frequencies produce maximal stimulation at its apex. Auditory neurons connect via the brain stem to the auditory cortex. Different groups of cells within the cortex are stimulated by nerve impulses coded for different frequencies. The semicircular canals have ampullae which contain hair cells, and which are stimulated by angular acceleration. The saccule and utricle are stimulated by linear acceleration. Information from the labyrinths, eyes and limbs is combined within the brain stem. Connections from the vestibular nuclei pass to the cortex and the cerebellum (Fig. 32.3).

Assessment

Symptoms

Conductive deafness is due to disorders of the external or middle ear and results from impairment of the transmission of sound to the inner ear. Sensorineural deafness results from lesions of the cochlea or acoustic nerve. Deafness is often associated with a noise in the ear (tinnitus). Ear pain (otalgia) may be due to ear disease, but may also be referred from other sites (Table 32.1). Ear-related disorders of balance usually cause a sensation of movement, usually rotation (vertigo). Some patients describe unsteadiness, but this symptom usually has a non-otological cause. Patients with ear disease do not fall to the ground or lose consciousness.

Examination

Inspection of the ear canal and tympanic membrane is carried out using an otoscope. A rigid telescope can also be used and is particularly useful for photography. A more detailed examination of the ear can be made using a binocular microscope. This method is also useful when there is a need

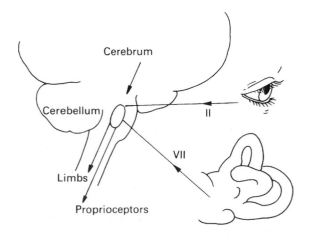

Fig. 32.3 The vestibular system.

Table 32.1	Causes of referred otalgia
Throat	Tonsillitis
	Tonsillectomy
	Tumours
Mouth	Dental disease
	Tumour
Temporomandibular (TMJ) joint	TMJ dysfunction
	Arthritis
Neck	Cervical spondylosis
	Tumour
Paranasal sinuses	Maxillary sinusitis

to remove wax or discharge from the ear. Tuning fork tests can be used to differentiate between conductive and sensorineural hearing loss. In normal individuals, and in sensorineural deafness, a tuning fork is heard better via the ear canal (air conduction) than via the mastoid process (bone conduction). When there is a conductive hearing loss, the tuning fork is heard better by bone conduction (Rinne's test). When there is symmetrical sensorineural hearing loss, or normal hearing in both ears, a tuning fork placed on the forehead is heard equally well on both sides (Weber's test). If a conductive hearing loss is present in one ear, the tuning fork is heard better in the deaf ear. If there is a unilateral sensorineural deafness it is heard better in the good ear.

Audiometry

Hearing can be assessed by pure tone audiometry, in which sounds of known pitch and loudness are presented to the patient via headphones. Bone conduction can also be tested via a bone conductor applied to the mastoid process. The patient's ability to hear speech can be tested by presenting lists or words of known loudness via the headphones. The percentage correctly identified at different levels of amplification allows a speech reception threshold and a speech discrimination score to be determined. Middle-ear function can be assessed by tympanometry. The amount of sound reflected back from the tympanic membrane is measured while the pressure in the ear canal is varied. This allows drum compliance to be determined. Compliance is maximal when the pressure in the ear canal is the same as that in the middle ear. Tympanometry is particularly useful for confirming the presence of fluid in the middle ear.

Imaging

In patients with unilateral sensorineural hearing loss, MRI scans are of value in confirming the presence of acoustic neuromas. At present the value of CT and MRI in the diagnosis of other diseases is limited, but it is likely that the role of MRI will increase as the technology improves.

Diseases of the pinna

Bat ears

A developmental abnormality results in the absence of the antihelical fold (Fig. 32.1). This produces prominent ears that cause embarrassment. The abnormality can be corrected surgically.

Trauma

Trauma may result in a haematoma that strips the perichondrium off the underlying cartilage. Secondary infection may lead to loss of cartilage, resulting in a 'cauliflower ear'. To avoid this, haematomas should be drained.

Tumours

Basal cell and squamous carcinomas may occur on the pinna and require excision.

Diseases of the external auditory meatus

Wax

Wax (cerumen) is found normally in the ear canal. The ear canal has a migratory epithelium that carries wax to the opening of the external auditory meatus. Wax seldom causes complete deafness, but does impair hearing if it becomes packed against the eardrum.

Otitis externa

This is an inflammatory condition of the ear canal skin. Secondary infection with bacteria or, less frequently, fungi may occur. It is managed by cleaning the ear followed by local treatment with ear drops, sprays or ointment containing a steroid with or without antibiotics. Uncommonly, chronic otitis externa causes stenosis of the ear canal.

Tumours

Squamous carcinoma of the ear canal is uncommon and is treated by a combination of surgery and radiotherapy.

Otitis media

Acute otitis media is a bacterial infection of the middle-ear space, usually caused by *Streptococcus pneumoniae* or *Haemophilus influenzae* and occurring most commonly in young children (3 years and under). The child presents with a combination of ear pain (otalgia), fever and malaise. On examination, dilated blood vessels are seen on the drum surface in the early stages. The drum then becomes red and begins to bulge. Perforation with discharge frequently occurs. Most of these perforations heal spontaneously. Antibiotic therapy shortens the episodes and provides protection against the development of complications. In the preantibiotic era infection commonly spread to the mastoid process, causing bone destruction and the development of a subperiosteal abscess (mastoiditis). This is now seen only infrequently. Occasionally facial palsy or meningitis may complicate middle-ear infection.

Otitis media with effusion (OME), or 'glue ear', is a condition in which fluid accumulates in the middle-ear space. It is much more common in children than in

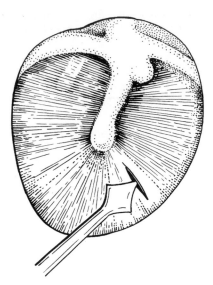

A

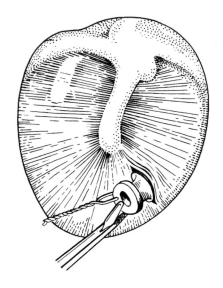

B

Fig. 32.4   Myringotomy and grommet insertion.

adults. Most cases are idiopathic, but a minority are caused by nasopharyngeal tumours and systemic disease. Childhood OME causes hearing loss and may interfere with the acquisition of language and performance at school. Virtually all cases resolve spontaneously, but can take as long as 10 years. Initial management involves documentation of the presence of an effusion and the degree of hearing loss during a period of 'watchful waiting'. If the effusion persists, hearing may be improved by drainage and insertion of a ventilation tube (Fig. 32.4). In children, removal of the adenoids leads to resolution in a proportion of cases. Spontaneous resolution may also occur in adults,

but effusions often persist. Ventilation tubes can also be of value, but some cases are better managed with a hearing aid.

Chronic suppurative otitis media (CSOM) causes aural discharge and deafness. Tubotympanic or mucosal disease is characterized by the presence of a perforation of the tympanic membrane. Discharge is common, but not universal. Swimming and other activities that involve water entering the ear may precipitate discharge. Greater degrees of hearing loss occur when there is erosion of the ossicular chain, most commonly the long process of the incus. Discharge can be controlled by cleaning the ear and introducing ear drops. Recently, there has been concern about the possible ototoxic effects of aminoglycoside drops used in this way. Surgery is indicated to prevent discharge, improve hearing and allow the patient to swim. An operation designed to repair a perforation is called a myringoplasty. Defects of the ossicular chain can be repaired by removing the incus and repositioning it to bridge the gap between the malleus and stapes, or by the use of a prosthesis (ossiculoplasty).

Atticoantral or squamous disease is associated with the development of cholesteatoma. This consists of a retracted area of the drum in which keratin accumulates. The drum tissue around the periphery of the cholesteatoma is known as matrix. It produces a number of chemical mediators that stimulate osteoclast activity. This means that cholesteatoma is capable of eroding the surrounding bone, and can be associated with complications such as facial palsy and intracranial sepsis. Surgical treatment is mandatory in all but the elderly and those who are medically unfit. The operation employed to eradicate cholesteatoma is called a mastoidectomy. Erosion of the ossicular chain is more likely to occur in association with cholesteatoma. However, the priority of surgery is to eliminate the disease rather than to improve hearing.

Otosclerosis

This is a condition in which the stapes becomes fixed by new bone formation. It is more common in females and sometimes runs in families. It can be treated by an operation called stapedectomy, in which the stapes is replaced by a piston attached to the incus. This produces excellent hearing improvement in the majority of patients, but in a minority the hearing is made worse by inner ear damage. The hearing loss can also be managed with a hearing aid.

Diseases of the inner ear
Deafness

Deafness is most commonly due to changes in the cochlea. Ageing produces a gradual deterioration in hearing acuity hydrops) produce a combination of fluctuating deafness, tinnitus and vertigo known as Ménière's disease. Initially, this is treated medically, but in some cases an operation to facilitate the drainage of endolymph (endolymphatic sac decompression) may be required. If this fails, destruction of the labyrinth, either surgically or by using an vestibulo-toxic drug such as gentamicin, or sectioning the vestibular nerve, can produce symptomatic improvement.

Benign positional vertigo is a condition in which debris floating in the posterior semicircular canal stimulates the hair cells in its ampulla. This happens when the affected ear is downmost and the episodes typically occur when the patient turns over in bed. Debris can be displaced by positioning the head so that it floats out of the canal (Epley's manoeuvre). If this fails, division of the ampullary (singular) nerve or occlusion of the posterior semicircular canal are beneficial.

Vestibular neuronitis is a condition that causes severe vertigo for up to several weeks. The hearing remains normal. It is due to severe temporary reduction of vestibular function in the affected ear. Patients are managed by bed rest and vestibular sedatives, such as prochlorperazine.

Disorders of the facial nerve

Facial palsy may result from temporal bone fractures or surgical trauma. When the nerve is divided it may be repaired by end-to-end anastomosis or a cable graft derived from a sensory nerve of the right size, such as the sural nerve. Bell's palsy is an idiopathic facial palsy that usually improves spontaneously. Steroid therapy given soon after the onset may be beneficial. Herpes zoster infection of the geniculate ganglion causes facial palsy, often associated with deafness and vertigo (Ramsay Hunt syndrome). Vesicles may be seen on the palate and on the tympanic membrane. Antiviral treatment appears to influence the course in a favourable manner. Intracranial tumours and malignant tumours in the neck can also cause facial palsy.

NOSE

Anatomy

The nasal skeleton consists of two nasal bones superiorly and two paired cartilages inferiorly (Fig. 32.5). The nasal septum, which comprises cartilage anteriorly and bone posteriorly, divides the nasal cavity in two. Three turbinate bones protrude from the lateral wall of the nose (Fig. 32.6). Between the inferior and middle turbinates is the middle meatus of the nose. Most of the paranasal sinuses open into this area under cover of a soft tissue flap known as the uncinate process. Obstruction of the sinus ostia in this area can cause sinus pain and lead to sinus infection. Superior to

known as presbycusis. The cochlea may be damaged by chronic noise exposure, blast injuries and temporal bone fractures. Significant noise exposure may occur in heavy industry, agriculture, from shooting and from playing in rock bands. Deafness may also be inherited or be a manifestation of systemic disease. Some drugs, for example aminoglycosides and cytotoxic agents such as cisplatinum, can damage the cochlea. Viral infections such as mumps and rubella can also cause sensorineural deafness. Unilateral hearing loss occurs in acoustic neuroma. Most cases of inner-ear deafness are managed with a hearing aid, but in cases of profound deafness hearing may be restored by a cochlear implant. This consists of a series of electrodes that are introduced into the cochlea surgically. A speech processor converts sound into electrical energy that stimulates the cochlear nerve.

Vertigo

In some cases balance disorders are due to abnormalities of the vestibular portion of the inner ear. Abnormal fluctuations of fluid pressure within the inner ear (endolymphatic

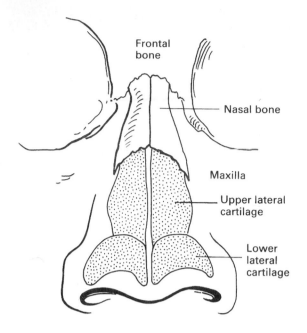

Fig. 32.5 Anatomy of the nasal skeleton.

the superior turbinate is an area of olfactory epithelium from which arise the nerve fibres of the olfactory nerve. The anterior portion of the nasal septum is called Little's area.

Physiology

The functions of the nose are to filter, warm and moisten inspired air. Olfaction is important in its own right and as an adjunct to taste.

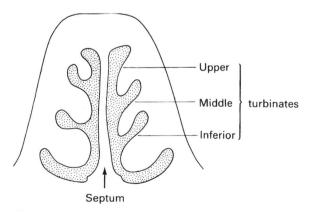

Fig. 32.6 Anatomy of the nasal cavity.

Assessment

Symptoms

Nasal obstruction is a common symptom with a number of causes. Sneezing and rhinorrhoea are generally due to chronic rhinitis. Purulent nasal discharge and facial pain occur in sinusitis. Loss of smell may be due to nasal blockage that prevents odours from reaching the olfactory epithelium. It may also be due to dysfunction of the olfactory epithelium or damage to the olfactory nerves. Smell is an important part of taste and reduced taste sensation is usually also reported.

Examination

The nasal cavity can be inspected using a nasal speculum or an otoscope. More detailed examination, particularly of the posterior part of the nose, can be carried out with a rigid telescope.

Imaging

Plain films can be used to assess disease in the maxillary and frontal sinuses but do not show the ethmoid labyrinth well. CT scans show all the paranasal sinuses well and also give information about the middle meatus of the nose, where the sinus ostia are sited, and variations in the anatomical relationships between the sinuses and the orbit and skull base.

Diseases of the nose

Trauma

This may result in fracture and displacement of the nasal bones. Such fractures should be reduced within 14 days, as after this it becomes difficult to mobilize the bones. There may also be displacement and fracture of the septal cartilage and bone, leading to a deviated nasal septum. Treatment consists of resection (submucous resection, SMR) or repositioning (septoplasty) of cartilage, and should be carried out at a later date when the results of trauma to the soft tissues have settled. Bleeding into the septum causes a septal haematoma, resulting in severe nasal obstruction. This should be drained under aseptic conditions as infection may cause loss of cartilage and collapse of the nasal bridge.

Chronic rhinitis

In some cases this condition is a manifestation of sensitivity to inhaled allergens such as pollen or dust. In others no allergies can be demonstrated, and it appears to be a reaction to environmental conditions such as temperature and humidity. It may be seasonal (usually summer) or perennial. Patients complain of nasal blockage that often switches from side to side, sneezing and rhinorrhoea. Most cases are best managed medically with a steroid nasal spray. In severe cases with nasal obstruction, reduction of the inferior or middle turbinates may provide relief.

Nasal polyps

Oedematous paranasal sinus mucosa extrudes through sinus ostia to produce nasal polyps. When they arise from the ethmoid labyrinth the polyps are multiple, but when the origin is the maxillary antrum a large single polyp protruding posteriorly into the nasopharynx is produced (antrochoanal polyp). The extent of sinus involvement is best determined by CT scanning (Fig. 32.7). Temporary improvement in the resulting nasal obstruction can be produced by topical or systemic steroids, but definitive treatment consists of surgical excision, with or without clearance of the sinus(es) of origin. Nowadays this is usually carried out endoscopically, sometimes with the assistance of a device called a microdebrider. Recurrence is common.

Epistaxis

Nose bleeds may be associated with a number of disease processes (Table 32.2). They are common in healthy children and young adults. Bleeding usually arises from Little's area and can be controlled by squeezing the nose (Fig. 32.8). In the elderly, more severe bleeding from further back in the nose may occur. In these cases a nasal pack may be required to arrest the bleeding (Fig. 32.9). In this group bleeding may be associated with the use of non-steroidal anti-inflammatory drugs.

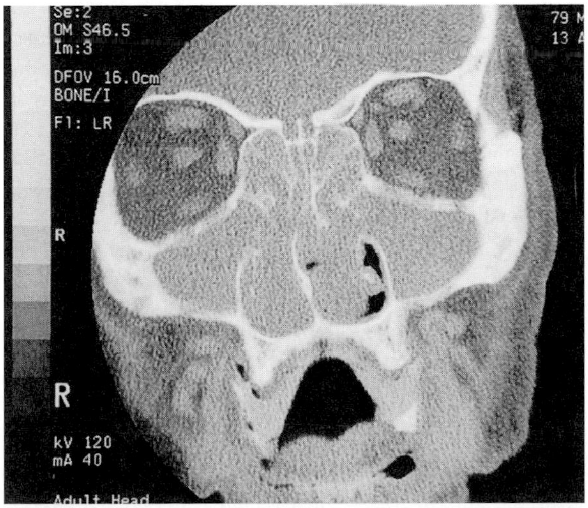

Table 32.2 Diseases associated with epistaxis	
Bleeding disorders	Haemophilia Thrombocytopenia Von Willebrand's disease Excessive anticoagulation (warfarin)
Systemic disease	Liver disease Renal disease Hypertension Hereditary telangiectasia

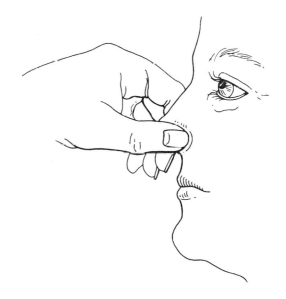

Fig. 32.8 Stopping epistaxis by squeezing the nose.

Fig. 32.7 CT scan showing gross nasal polyposis.

PARANASAL SINUSES

Anatomy

The paranasal sinuses are air-filled cavities that open into the nasal cavity, mostly into the middle meatus of the nose (Fig. 32.10). The maxillary sinuses occupy the cheeks and have ostia that are situated closer to the roof of the sinus than to the floor. The ethmoid labyrinth consists of a number of air cells lying between the orbit and the lateral wall of the nose. The frontal sinus is an ethmoid air cell which has migrated into the frontal bone and is connected to the nose via the frontonasal duct, which passes down to the middle meatus. The sphenoid sinus is posterior to the ethmoid labyrinth, inferior to the pituitary fossa.

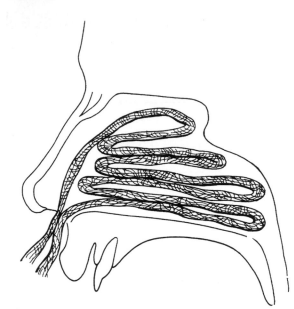

Fig. 32.9   Nasal packing.

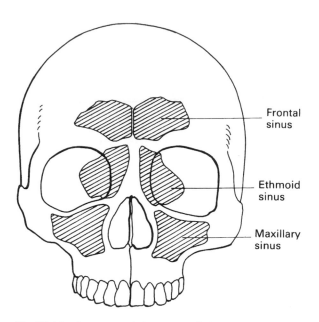

Fig. 32.10   Anatomy of the paransal sinuses.

Diseases of the sinuses

Sinusitis

The site of the pain caused by sinusitis depends on which is affected: the most commonly involved is the maxillary sinus. Pain arising from the maxillary sinus is felt in the cheek; from the ethmoid labyrinth over the nasal bridge; from the frontal sinus in the forehead; and from the sphenoid sinus over the occipital region. Acute sinusitis is most commonly caused by *Streptococcus pneumoniae* or *Haemophilus influenzae*, and typically follows an upper respiratory infection. When the origin of the infection is a dental abscess, Gram-negative organisms may be isolated. Uncommonly, fungal infection may occur. Acute sinusitis is usually managed medically. Chronic sinusitis may result from failure of resolution of acute infection, or may arise insidiously. Surgical treatment is frequently required and consists of enlargement of the natural ostium of the maxillary sinus. Chronic infection of other paranasal sinuses also usually calls for surgical intervention. Infection may spread from the sinuses, usually the ethmoid or the frontal, to involve other areas such as the cranial cavity or orbit.

> **SUMMARY BOX**
>
> *Epistaxis*
>
> - Epistaxis in young patients usually arises from a small blood vessel in Little's area; in older individuals it arises from an arteriosclerotic vessel located more posteriorly.
> - Pressure on Little's area by compressing the anterior septum usually stops the bleeding, and topical applications of 1 in 1000 adrenaline may be helpful.
> - Bleeding arising more posteriorly may require balloon compression or packing.
> - Coagulation defects should always be excluded in patients with troublesome bleeding. In a proportion of patients these can be caused by alcohol or non-steroidal analgesics.
> - In persistent epistaxis it may be necessary to ligate one of the arteries supplying the nose, e.g. the maxillary artery.

Tumours

The most common neoplasm found in the paranasal sinuses is squamous carcinoma, but adenocarcinomas are seen in workers in the furniture industry. The most common sites of origin are the maxillary and ethmoid sinuses. Spread outside the primary site is usually evident at presentation (Fig. 32.11). These relatively uncommon tumours are managed by a combination of surgery and radiotherapy, or local surgery combined with topical chemotherapy.

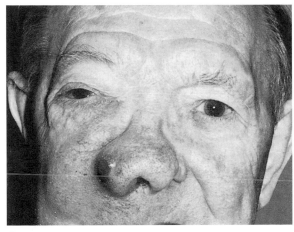

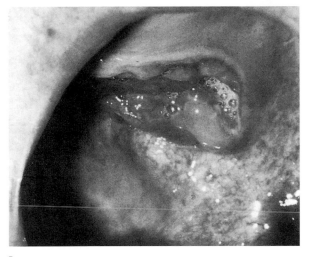

A   B

Fig. 32.11 Spread of sinus cancer. **A** There is evidence of spread into the cheek and orbit, with displacement of the eye. **B** There is ulceration of the hard palate, indicating spread into the mouth.

NASOPHARYNX

Anatomy

The nasopharynx lies posterior to the nasal cavity and superior to the oropharynx. Superiorly is the skull base; the Eustachian tubes open into its lateral walls.

Diseases of the nasopharynx

Adenoids

The adenoids consist of lymphoid tissue and in young children they occupy a significant proportion of the space within the nasopharynx. They increase in size until the age of 4 and then become progressively smaller, disappearing altogether by the time the individual is an adult. In some children adenoid hypertrophy causes nasal obstruction. They also have a role in the pathogenesis of childhood otitis media with effusion (OME) and sleep apnoea syndrome. Surgical removal may be indicated in these circumstances.

Tumours

Carcinoma of the nasopharynx is common among the inhabitants of southern China. The Epstein–Barr virus has been implicated in its pathogenesis. It may present with middle ear effusion or cervical adenopathy, as well as local symptoms such as nasal obstruction or epistaxis. Treatment is by radiotherapy. Young boys may develop a benign but locally invasive tumour called an angiofibroma. This presents with nasal obstruction and epistaxis, and is treated by surgical excision.

MOUTH

Anatomy

The floor of the mouth is occupied mainly by the tongue. The ducts of the submandibular salivary glands open anterolateral to it. The roof is formed by the hard and soft palates. Its lateral walls are the medial aspects of the cheeks. The parotid ducts open just above the second upper molar teeth.

Diseases of the mouth

Stomatitis and gingivitis

Inflammation of the oral mucosa and gums is often associated with poor oral hygiene. It may also be a manifestation of a systemic disorder, such as anaemia (e.g. Patterson–Brown–Kelly syndrome). *Candida* is an opportunist infection that may affect the oral cavity. It is characterized by white spots on the mucous membrane. Removal of the white material causes bleeding. Infection in the floor of the mouth may occur secondary to dental sepsis (Ludwig's angina). Pain, dysphagia, trismus and even airway infection may occur.

Mouth ulcers

Aphthous ulcers are the most common type. They have a punched-out appearance and are painful. They are thought to be due to a local failure of the mechanisms that protect the oral mucosa from damage. They resolve spontaneously, but this process can be speeded by the use of local treatment with steroid pellets. Oral ulceration is also seen in systemic disorders such as pemphigus and mucous membrane pemphigoid. Rarely, oral ulceration may be due to TB or syphilis.

Retention cysts

Mucous retention cysts may occur anywhere in the oral cavity. Those inferior to the tongue are called ranulas. They result from blockage of the openings into mucus and minor salivary glands. This may clear spontaneously, but otherwise excision may be required.

Leukoplakia

Leukoplakia (white patches) may develop on the oral mucosa as a result of chronic irritation, for example by tobacco and alcohol, causing hyperkeratosis. Leukoplakia is a premalignant condition. Removal of the patches together with avoidance of the causative factors can prevent progression.

Tumours

Squamous carcinoma of the tongue is the commonest neoplasm seen in the oral cavity. Lesions cause induration of the tongue, usually with ulceration. Lymphatic spread occurs to the submental nodes and thence to other deep cervical nodes. Smoking and heavy spirit drinking are predisposing factors. Small lesions can be treated by local excision or radioactive implants (iridium wires), but more extensive tumours require excision with a margin of normal tissue. This often includes excision of part of the mandible.

OROPHARYNX

Anatomy

The oropharynx lies posterior to the oral cavity, between the nasopharynx superiorly and the hypopharynx and larynx inferiorly. At the junction of the mouth and oropharynx are the tonsils, which consist of lymphoid tissue. Together with the adenoids (see above) and the lingual tonsil in the base of the tongue, they form a lymphoid system known as Waldayer's ring. This system is important in the development of immunity during early infancy, but subsequently can be removed without ill effect. The pharynx itself is surrounded by three constrictor muscles arranged one inside the other like a stack of bottomless beakers.

Diseases of the oropharynx

Pharyngitis

Viral infection of the pharynx is common and is often associated with coryza. Symptomatic relief can be obtained from analgesics. A sore throat with exudate over the tonsils is a common manifestation of infectious mononucleosis (glandular fever). This disease is caused by the Epstein–Barr virus, which also causes cervical adenopathy and hepatosplenomegaly. Irritation of the pharynx may be due to tobacco smoke and acid reflux.

Tonsillitis

Bacterial infection of the tonsils, usually with *Streptococcus pyogenes*, causes tonsillitis. Patients present with episodic sore throat associated with fever and malaise. Tonsillitis must be differentiated from viral sore throats, which are not usually associated with pyrexia and often form part of a more generalized upper respiratory tract infection. Infectious mononucleosis (glandular fever) can easily be confused with tonsillitis. Tonsillitis may be complicated by the development of a peritonsillar abscess (quinsy), which may require incision and drainage. Recurrent tonsillitis can be successfully treated by tonsillectomy.

Snoring and sleep apnoea

Snoring arises because of obstruction within the pharynx during sleep, or from vibration of the soft palate. In some cases it is associated with apnoeic episodes. These individuals tend to sleep poorly, wake unrefreshed and become drowsy during the day. If significant apnoea is confirmed by overnight monitoring, the use of nasal continuous positive airway pressure (CPAP) may be indicated. Simple snoring can be improved by weight loss and reduc-

---

SUMMARY BOX

Tonsils and adenoids

- Adenoids are large in small children, but become smaller with age.

- They may cause nasal obstruction and be involved in the pathogenesis of otitis media with effusion and sleep apnoea in children.

- Tonsils may require removal because of recurrent tonsillitis or peritonsillar abscess in adults and children. Children with sleep apnoea may also benefit from tonsillectomy.

- Unilateral tonsillar enlargement may be due to squamous carcinoma or lymphoma.

tion of nocturnal alcohol intake. Sleep apnoea syndrome can also occur in children, in whom it is usually cured by adenotonsillectomy.

Tumours

Lymphomas occur in the younger age group and cause enlargement of the affected tonsil, producing a smooth swelling. Squamous carcinoma occurs in older patients and usually presents with ulceration of the tonsil. Treatment is by radiotherapy or surgery. Kaposi's sarcoma occurs in patients with AIDS.

HYPOPHARYNX

Anatomy

Below the oropharynx the aerodigestive tract divides into an air passage (larynx/trachea) and a digestive passage (oesophagus). The entrance to the air passage is protected by the epiglottis, a mobile cartilaginous structure, and by the ability of the vocal cords to close together. The entry of material into the oesophagus is controlled by a ring of muscle, the cricopharyngeus. Lateral to the larynx, the pharynx continues inferiorly on both sides into a blind-ended pit known as the pyriform fossa.

Physiology of swallowing

Swallowing is achieved by the coordinated contraction and relaxation of muscles. It is initiated by the tongue, which pushes the bolus to the back of the mouth. The pharyngeal constrictor muscles propel it towards the oesophagus and the cricopharyngeus relaxes to receive it. A peristaltic wave then carries it on down the oesophagus to the stomach.

Assessment

Symptoms

Obstruction of the oesophagus, and disorders that interfere with the muscle activity involved in swallowing, cause dysphagia. Physical obstruction causes dysphagia worse for solids, whereas neurological disorders cause more difficulty with liquids. Pain may be felt locally in the throat, in the retrosternal area, or may be referred to the ear (Table 32.1).

Examination

The pharynx can be assessed in the clinic using a mirror, rigid telescope or flexible fibreoptic rhinolaryngoscope. Under anaesthesia the pharynx and oesophagus can be directly inspected using rigid endoscopes. A fibreoptic oesophagoscope can be used to examine the oesophagus with local anaesthetic and sedation.

Imaging

A barium swallow will show structural abnormalities within the pharynx and oesophagus, and also gives some information about the dynamics of swallowing. Video recording can be used to increase the yield of information concerning swallowing. CT scanning can be used to identify the spread of oesophageal lesions into surrounding areas and to image external lesions causing oesophageal compression.

Diseases of the hypopharynx

Pharyngeal pouch

This is formed by mucosal herniation through the weakest part of the pharyngeal musculature, Killian's dehiscence (Fig. 32.12). It develops when pharyngeal muscle contraction is not associated with adequate relaxation of the cricopharyngeus. It causes dysphagia for solids and regurgitation of food, sometimes several days after it was swallowed. The diagnosis can be confirmed by a barium swallow. In most cases it is possible to divide the wall between the pouch and the oesophagus and staple the edges together with a specialized instrument, introduced via an endoscope. This creates a segment of oesophagus that is

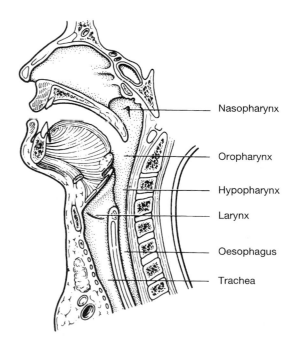

Nasopharynx

Oropharynx

Hypopharynx

Larynx

Oesophagus

Trachea

Fig. 32.12 Anatomy of the pharynx and larynx.

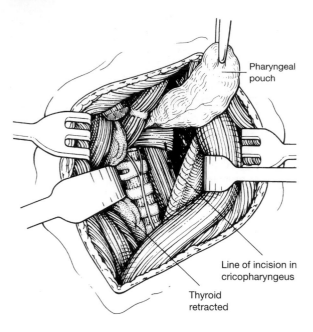

Fig. 32.13 External excision of pharyngeal pouch.

wider than the rest. If this is not possible the pouch can be excised via a neck incision (Fig. 32.13).

Tumours

Squamous carcinoma may arise from the pharyngeal walls, the epiglottis, the pyriform fossa or the upper oesophagus (postcricoid region). Postcricoid carcinoma is sometimes preceded by the development of a thin membrane in the upper oesophagus, a postcricoid web. This is associated with iron deficiency anaemia, glossitis and stomatitis (Patterson–Brown–Kelly syndrome, also known as Plummer–Vinson syndrome). The web itself causes some dysphagia, and treatment of the anaemia can prevent progression to tumour. Other pharyngeal tumours are associated with smoking. Hypopharyngeal tumours are treated by radiotherapy or surgery.

LARYNX

Anatomy

The larynx has a cartilaginous framework. Superiorly it is supported and protected anteriorly by the thyroid cartilage. Inferiorly lies the cricoid cartilage, which connects to the trachea (Fig. 32.12). Within the laryngeal lumen two soft tissue folds pass from anterior to posterior. The superior

limits of these are the ventricular bands or 'false cords'. Inferiorly lie the (true) vocal cords, which are responsible for phonation. These consist of a vocal ligament covered with mucosa. The free edge of the mucosa is important in achieving glottic closure and determines voice quality.

Physiology of voice

Voice production requires an air supply from the lungs, the presence of normally functioning vocal cords to create vibrations, and the tongue and mouth to articulate the vibrating air source into speech.

Assessment

Symptoms

Hoarseness of the voice is the cardinal symptom of laryngeal dysfunction. Patients may also complain of pain locally or referred to the ear (Table 32.1). The voice is weak and breathy in unilateral vocal cord palsy, but rough and husky in severe chronic laryngitis and laryngeal cancer. Patients with psychogenic dysphonia often have a squeaky voice quality.

Examination

The larynx can be inspected in the clinic using a mirror, rigid telescope or flexible fibreoptic rhinolaryngoscope. Under anaesthesia a better view can be obtained using a rigid endoscope and operating microscope.

Imaging

CT can be used to assess the spread of laryngeal lesions into surrounding areas.

Diseases of the larynx

Congenital disorders

A number of congenital abnormalities of the larynx may occur, but most are rare. The most common is laryngomalacia, a condition in which the laryngeal cartilages are not stiff enough to prevent collapse of the larynx during inspiration. This causes inspiratory stridor and dyspnoea, which becomes worse during upper respiratory infections. Most children grow out of the problem by the age of 2 and do not require active intervention. In severe cases surgical division of the ventricular bands can produce improvement.

Laryngitis

Inflammation of the vocal cords is the most common cause of hoarseness. Acute laryngitis frequently follows an upper respiratory tract infection. Antibiotics are of no value, but steam inhalations may be helpful. The common predisposing factors for chronic laryngitis are smoking, acid reflux and excessive voice use. During the acute phase the vocal cords appear red or pink. In chronic laryngitis they may be markedly swollen (Reinke's oedema). This pattern occurs in smokers who talk a lot. In these cases surgical drainage of the submucosal space produces improvement. In other cases thickened, red cords or keratotic plaques (leukoplakia) may be seen.

Individuals who abuse their voices may develop vocal nodules, situated at the junction of the anterior third and the posterior two-thirds of the vocal cords. These can be removed, but may recur if voice abuse is not modified. In many patients the vocal cords appear normal and the problem is functional rather than structural. Speech therapy is often helpful in these cases.

Vocal cord palsy

Unilateral cord palsy is the most commonly seen variant. Left vocal cord palsy may be caused by invasion of the recurrent laryngeal nerve by a bronchial carcinoma. The right recurrent nerve is not at risk because it does not enter the chest. Damage to the recurrent laryngeal nerves in the neck may occur as a result of surgery, trauma or neoplastic invasion. The voice may be improved by the injection of Teflon or fat lateral to the vocal ligament. Bilateral cord palsies cause airway obstruction rather than dysphonia.

Tumours

Carcinoma of the larynx is the commonest form of head and neck cancer and is almost always squamous. The most important aetiological factor is smoking, but a few cases are seen in non-smokers. Patients complain of a hoarse voice. Uncommonly, they present with airway obstruction or haemoptysis. Tumours may arise from any of the three regions of the larynx – glottis, supraglottis or subglottis (Fig. 32.14). The most common site is the vocal cord. As this area has no lymphatics these tumours only metastasize to lymph nodes when they spread into an adjacent area. Tumours arising from the other regions do not cause hoarseness at first and therefore tend to present later. Most laryngeal tumours are treated by radiotherapy. In T1 lesions of the vocal cord this modality produces cure in up to 90% of cases. The outlook is less favourable in more advanced tumours and there may be a case for primary surgery. Surgery also has a role in cases where radiotherapy fails to control the tumour. Operative treatment usually involves total removal of the larynx. In these circumstances the trachea is brought out on to the surface of the neck as an end tracheostome. Patients can regain speech by swallowing air and using a segment of the pharynx to make it

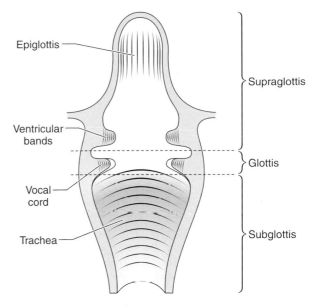

Fig. 32.14   Regions of the larynx.

vibrate when it is expelled. Alternatively a device with a one-way value can be inserted between the pharynx and the trachea, allowing air from the trachea to be diverted into the pharynx.

SUMMARY BOX

Carcinoma of the larynx

- Persistent hoarseness in smokers should be assumed to be carcinoma of the larynx until proved otherwise.

- T1 glottic tumours can be cured by radiotherapy in up to 90% of cases.

- More extensive tumours and those not cured by radiotherapy may require removal of the larynx.

- Following laryngectomy the trachea is brought out on to the surface of the neck. Speech may be regained by using swallowed air or by creating a fistula containing a one-way valve between the trachea and the pharynx.

Tracheostomy

Tracheostomy may be required to relieve acute upper airway obstruction (Table 32.3). It is carried out by creating a window in the anterior tracheal wall at the level of the second and third tracheal rings and introducing a suitable tube. When short-term airway support and the causative

Table 32.3	Causes of upper airway obstruction
Children	Inhaled foreign body
	Acute epiglottitis
	Laryngotracheobronchitis
Adults	Inhaled foreign body
	Acute epiglottitis
	Tumour
	Laryngeal trauma
	Bilateral vocal cord palsy

pathology allows, the situation is better managed by passing an endotracheal tube. Cricothyrotomy (Fig. 32.15) provides a rapid short-term solution to airway obstruction and can be carried out with makeshift equipment. Foreign bodies in the upper airway can be displaced by turning a small child upside down. In a larger individual a 'bear hug' around the chest and abdomen may expel the item (Heimlich's manoeuvre). Tracheostomy may also be of value to reduce the dead space in patients with respiratory disease and to facilitate artificial ventilation.

NECK

Anatomy

A knowledge of the anatomy of the neck is essential if the likely origin of neck masses is to be determined

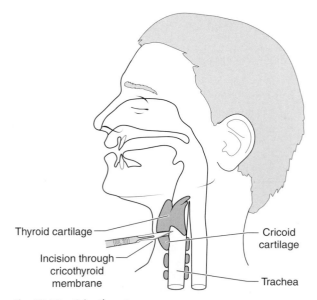

Fig. 32.15   Cricothyrotomy.

Thyroid cartilage

Incision through cricothyroid membrane

Cricoid cartilage

Trachea

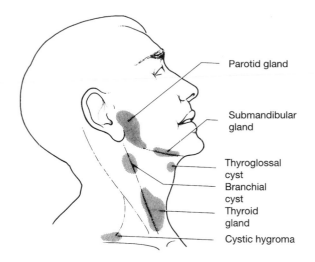

Fig. 32.16   Locations of swellings in the head and neck.

Parotid gland

Submandibular gland

Thyroglossal cyst
Branchial cyst
Thyroid gland

Cystic hygroma

(Fig. 32.16). In the midline lie the pharynx, larynx and trachea anteriorly. The oesophagus is deep to the trachea. The thyroid gland lies anterior and lateral to the trachea in the lower neck. Laterally, the sternomastoid muscles run from the sternum and clavicles inferiorly to the mastoid process superiorly. Between them and the midline structures is a space containing the carotid arteries and jugular veins. The vagus nerve is closely related to the great vessels. Along the course of the jugular vein lies a chain of lymph nodes. There are also lymph nodes in other regions of the head and neck (Fig. 32.17). In the submental region lie the submandibular salivary glands; these have ducts that run in the floor of the mouth to open anterior to the tongue. The parotid salivary glands lie posterior to the angle of the mandible and anterior to the external auditory meatus (Fig. 32.18). The parotid duct opens into the mouth in the cheek, close to the second upper molar tooth. The facial nerve runs through the parotid gland and emerges as a number of branches. The sublingual salivary gland lies in the floor of the mouth anteriorly (Fig. 32.19). The mucosa of the mouth contains numerous small accessory salivary glands.

Assessment

Symptoms

Most neck masses are painless, but infection and malignant disease may cause pain. Rapid enlargement of a mass makes malignant disease more likely. Salivary gland swellings due to duct obstruction enlarge when the patient eats; there may also be a bad taste in the mouth.

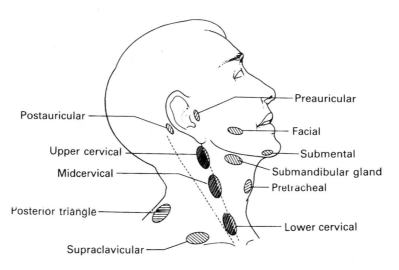

Fig. 32.17 Lymph node groups in the head and neck.

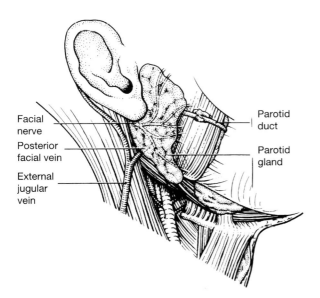

Fig. 32.18 Anatomy of the parotid gland.

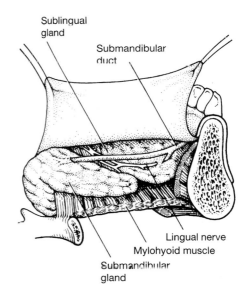

Fig. 32.19 Anatomy of the submandibular salivary gland.

Examination

Palpation of the neck should generally be carried out from behind. It is important to establish the size, shape, site and consistency of the swelling. Fixation to the skin or underlying structures should be established.

Imaging

CT can be used to assess many forms of neck mass and will sometimes reveal the presence of lymph node swellings that have not been detected clinically. Both CT and MRI are of value in evaluating salivary gland swellings. The introduction of contrast into the duct of a salivary gland (sialogram) can be used to confirm the presence of stones and demonstrate inflammatory changes. Cystic swellings can be differentiated from solid ones by using ultrasound.

Diseases of the neck

Skin and subcutaneous swellings

Sebaceous cysts occur commonly in the head and neck region and may require removal. They are characterized by the presence of a punctum. Furuncles or boils arise as a result of infection in hair follicles. Drainage may be required. When infection spreads to involve the dermis and subcutaneous tissue, a carbuncle is produced. These may have multiple discharging sinuses. In some cases wide excision may be required. The possibility of underlying diabetes mellitus should be considered. Kaposi's sarcoma occurs in patients with AIDS.

Thyroglossal cyst

This is a midline swelling usually situated just above the upper border of the thyroid cartilage (see Ch. 26). It moves on swallowing or tongue protrusion. Thyroglossal cysts can become infected, and must therefore be differentiated from thyroid tissue by carrying out an isotope or ultrasound scan. Treatment is by surgical excision. The centre of the hyoid bone and the persistent thyroglossal duct up to the base of the tongue should be excised with the cyst to ensure complete removal.

Branchial cyst and fistula

Swellings lying laterally in the upper neck may be branchial cysts. They are thought to be remnants of the second and third branchial arches, but this is not certain. They more often present in adult life, which calls into question their status as congenital abnormalities. The cysts contain opaque fluid containing cholesterol crystals. Lymphoid tissue is found in the wall. They may become infected and usually require excision. Branchial fistulae may occur between the skin surface low in the neck and the tonsil. Infection often occurs and excision is usually required.

Other cystic swellings

Cystic hygroma is a rare benign lymphangioma of the neck that usually presents in early life. Complete excision is difficult, leading to frequent recurrence. Dermoid cysts may be found in the upper neck. They occur as a result of sequestration of squamous cells during development. Laryngoceles occur as a result of herniation of laryngeal mucosa laterally into the neck. They distend with air during the Valsalva manoeuvre, and may become infected. Excision is usually required.

Lymphadenopathy

Lymph nodes in any of the groups present in the head and neck may become enlarged in response to infection in their area of drainage. Primary neoplasms (lymphomas) and secondary deposits, usually from squamous carcinomas of the head and neck region, should always be considered as a possible cause (Table 32.4).

Table 32.4	Causes of lymphadenopathy
Infective	Bacterial (pyogenic infection in drainage area e.g. streptococcal tonsillitis) Tuberculosis Brucellosis Viral Infectious mononucleosis Cytomegalovirus HIV Protozoal Toxoplasmosis
Neoplasm	Lymphoma Metastatic squamous carcinoma Other metastatic tumours
Systemic disease	Collagen diseases Sarcoidosis Amyloidosis

When cervical adenopathy is noted the upper aerodigestive tract must be carefully examined to exclude a tumour. This usually involves direct examination of the mouth, pharynx, nasopharynx, larynx and oesophagus. When inspection of these areas does not reveal an abnormality, palpation of the tonsils and tongue may reveal an occult tumour. Random biopsies from the nasopharynx may also reveal an unsuspected tumour. If no tumour can be found there may be a need to excise the swelling for histological examination. However, small mobile lymph node swellings can be observed and only removed if they enlarge.

Salivary gland disease

Swellings of the submandibular salivary gland are more likely to be due to obstruction of the submandibular duct by a stone or chronic inflammation. In contrast, swellings of the parotid gland are usually benign tumours.

Calculi cause salivary gland swelling by blocking the duct. Some, but not all, are radio-opaque (Fig. 32.20). Calculi may pass spontaneously, but are more likely to remain in situ. Provided they are in the main duct it is possible to remove them by opening the duct. If they are within the substance of the gland they are usually not accessible, in which case removal of the gland may be required. In other cases, although there are no calculi, inflammatory changes can be demonstrated within the duct system of the gland. Chronic sialadenitis may also be an indication for removal of the submandibular gland. Removal of the parotid gland should be avoided if possible because of the risk of damage to the facial nerve.

SUMMARY BOX

Lymphadenopathy

- Nodes become palpable when their diameter exceeds 1 cm, but impalpable nodes may contain tumour.

- Tender nodes are usually inflammatory, whereas non-tender nodes may be malignant.

- The head and neck, and in particular the oral cavity, nose, pharynx and larynx, must be examined to detect a primary cause for lymphadenopathy.

- Fine-needle aspiration cytology can be diagnostic for secondary head and neck tumours or lymphoma.

- CT scanning helps to find the extent of the lymphadenopathy.

- Painless neck nodes in patients over 45 are often due to metastases from carcinoma. In most cases the primary is within the head and neck. Such nodes must not be biopsied in the first instance; a thorough search for a primary lesion is the key to diagnosis.

- In lymphoma:
  - the nodes are often bilaterally enlarged, rubbery, firm and discrete
  - there is underlying immunosuppression in some cases
  - extranodal disease is commoner in non-Hodgkin's lymphoma
  - excision biopsy is diagnostic
  - bone marrow examination and CT scanning are used in staging.

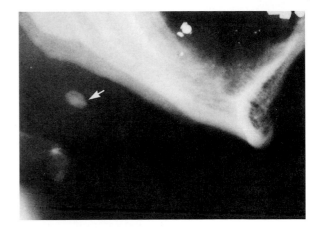

Fig. 32.20 X-ray showing submandibular salivary calculus.

Table 32.5	Parotid neoplasms
Benign	Pleomorphic adenoma Adenolymphoma
Intermediate	Oncocytoma Mucoepidermoid tumour
Malignant	Squamous carcinoma Adenoid cystic carcinoma Adenocarcinoma Lymphoma

Salivary gland tumours

A large number of different tumour types are found in the salivary glands (Fig. 32.18). The most common are the pleomorphic adenoma (mixed salivary tumour) and the adenolymphoma (Warthin's tumour). These tumours are benign, but malignant tumours and others of variable behaviour also occur (Table 32.5). Benign parotid tumours are treated by excision with a cuff of normal tissue (superficial parotidectomy). Care must be taken to avoid damage to the facial nerve, which runs through the gland between the deep and superficial lobes. Submandibular gland tumours are treated by excision of the gland. Malignant tumours are treated by more radical surgery with or without radiotherapy. The typical radiological appearance of a parotid tumour is shown in Figure 32.21.

SUMMARY BOX

Salivary gland swellings

- Swellings in the submandibular gland are more often due to calculi, but those in the parotid gland are commonly benign neoplasms.

- The most common salivary gland tumours are pleomorphic adenomas and adenolymphomas (Warthin's tumour).

- Parotid swellings generally require removal with a cuff of normal salivary tissue (superficial parotidectomy).

- The facial nerve runs through the parotid gland as a series of branches and is at risk during parotid surgery.

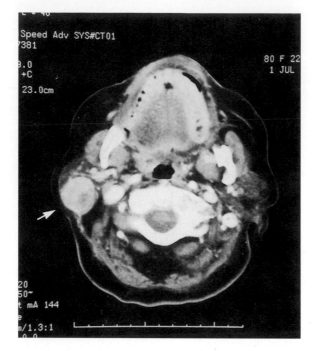

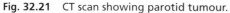

Fig. 32.21 CT scan showing parotid tumour.

Carotid body tumours

Chemodectomas of the carotid body are rare tumours arising from chemoreceptor tissue in the carotid body. They present as pulsatile swellings in the upper neck at the level of the carotid bifurcation. The diagnosis is best confirmed by duplex ultrasound. Biopsy is hazardous because of the risk of bleeding. Surgical excision is recommended.

Index